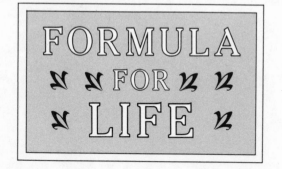

FORMULA
FOR
LIFE

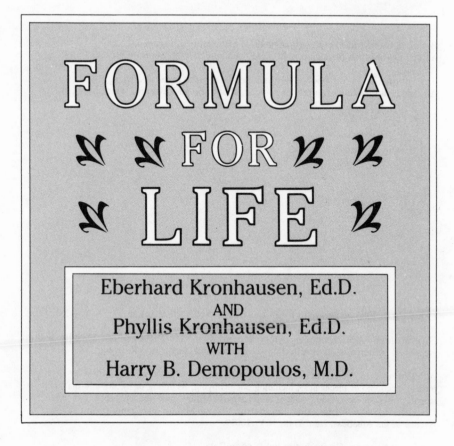

FORMULA FOR LIFE

Eberhard Kronhausen, Ed.D.
AND
Phyllis Kronhausen, Ed.D.
WITH
Harry B. Demopoulos, M.D.

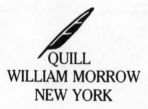

QUILL
WILLIAM MORROW
NEW YORK

Before beginning this or any other medical or nutritional regimen, consult a nutrition-oriented physician to be sure it is medically appropriate for you.

The information in this book is not intended to replace medical advice. Any medical questions, general or specific, should be addressed to your physician.

Library of Congress Cataloging-in-Publication Data

Kronhausen, Eberhard, 1915–
Formula for life / Eberhard and Phyllis Kronhausen with Harry B. Demopoulos.
p.   cm.
ISBN 0-688-09426-0
1. Longevity. 2. Anti-oxidants—Health aspects. 3. Nutrition.   4. Vitamins. 5. Active oxygen—Health aspects. I. Kronhausen,
Phyllis, 1929–   . II. Demopoulos, Harry B. III. Title.
RA776.75.K76   1989
613—dc 19   88-38660
                                                                          CIP

Printed in the United States of America

     3 4 5 6 7 8 9 10

BOOK DESIGN BY JAYE ZIMET

For

LINDA,

the best German shepherd

ever,

whom we lost because we

were away so long,

working on this book

PREFACE

*D*rs. Eberhard and Phyllis Kronhausen have written a comprehensive treatise on practical health matters that touch virtually everyone. They have combined their own in-depth, professional experiences, their personal experimentation, and knowledge from an impressively wide spectrum of disciplines to produce a scholarly work that anyone can understand.

This is their book. They did the work. They thought, interviewed, wrote, rewrote, revised, haunted the libraries, stuck microphones into people's faces to get their ideas recorded, and put it all together to benefit mankind.

As a medical science consultant, I have attempted to provide some guidance in several areas.

The recommendations made by the Kronhausens are responsible and are generally accompanied by words of caution. In particular, we all agree that before any of the recommendations are followed, the reader consult with a physician who has an interest in such matters and seek advice.

Some areas, which just a few years ago were avant garde, have been entering the mainstream of medicine. This includes dietary restrictions of fat, sensible fiber intake, high consumption of fruits and vegetables, moderate exercise, abstinence from dangerous habits and addictions, and even the use of high doses of safe, broad-spectrum anti-oxidants to that fight off the incessant, insidious free-radical attacks that cause so much infirmity and disease.

The Kronhausens bring to the reader the background knowledge, the rationale, and the practical approaches that they have dubbed "Formula for Life." It is a valid, scholarly work that can reshape your life.

—HARRY B. DEMOPOULOS, M.D.

ACKNOWLEDGMENTS

If there are angels, many must be in human form, if our own experience is any guide. Without several of these human angels, this book would never have come into being. First of all, there was Shirley MacLaine, who early on put confidence in Dr. Demopoulos's "formula for life"—his spectrum of anti-oxidants and vitamin co-factors. She graciously provided shelter for us in the Big Apple during the initial research for this project, otherwise it might have never gotten off the ground.

Our next angel was the writer Erica Jong, who also believed in Dr. Demopoulos's science and in us as long-standing friends and interpreters of that science. She and her motherly housekeeper, Margaret Kiley—together with Katya Spiegelman, Erica's brilliant research assistant, her precocious, upcoming actress daughter, Molly, and a clownish Bichon named Poochini—put up with us for one whole year. If it hadn't been for Erica making us part of "her extended family," as she liked to call this ménage, we would never have been able to continue our research in New York City.

The third angel was our friend Steve Katz, who literally turned over his spacious loft (and his two cats) to us for several months during the final work on this book. As it turned out, we needed the kind of space only a New York loft can provide to spread out a huge amount of scientific research papers (and we needed Susie and Sally, Steve's two mischievous cats to keep us grounded).

To these four principal angels—Shirley, Erica, Margaret, and Steve—goes our deepest gratitude. Each one in turn not only saved this book, but possibly a lot more.

Lynn Nesbit, another early believer in Dr. Demopoulos's science, and former president of International Creative Management, a prestigious New York talent agency, provided a fifth angel in the person of Bob Tabian, member of ICM and one of the best literary agents in the country. It was he who convinced Jim Landis, publisher and editor-in-chief of William Morrow and Company, that our half-finished manuscript would be an important state-of-the-art compendium on the role of anti-oxidants in preventive health care and life extension. And thanks to Jim Landis for having the good judgment to see that Bob was right.

There were a number of other "minor" angels, who were essential for bringing this book project to fruition, among them Joel Ross, technical director, and Dr. Myron Seligman, vice-president, Research and Development, at Health Maintenance Programs. They gave us many helpful suggestions for the improvement of the manuscript, which underwent various transformations in the course of the two and a half years from its inception to its completion.

We would like to thank Steve Blechman, vice-president, Research and Development, Twinlab, Inc., for providing valuable information from his company's research files and his vast personal experience in the manufacture of high-quality micronutrients.

Nor do we want to forget the initial help rendered to us by our friends Durk Pearson and Sandy Shaw, authors of *Life Extension,* the encyclopedic and much contested "primer" on the use of micronutrients in the service of life extension. They were good teachers and patient friends in helping us over the first hurdles in doing research for this book.

Much thanks is also due our several editors. First of all, we want to thank Renni Browne, head of a private editorial service, The Editorial Department, as well as her colleague, actress and novelist Judith Searle, an old friend of ours. Mary Haran, another member of the Editorial Department family, made several chapters containing complicated technical detail more readable.

Thanks, too, to senior editor Randy Ladenheim-Gil and copyeditor Sonia Greenbaum at our publishers, William Morrow and Company.

For critically stepping on our toes, where necessary, and for his many helpful suggestions, additional scientific information on the medicinal properties of many vegetables, herbs, and spices, and for much appreciated permissions, we have to thank Dr. James A. Duke, chief, Germplasm Resources Laboratory, U.S. Department of Agriculture. His professional input on the medicinal, health-promoting properties of natural foods made for a better balance between the protective properties and the various toxicities of some of these and other plant foods, as pointed out by Dr. Bruce Ames, chief of biochemistry, University of California at Berkeley—who also graciously answered some of our questions.

We would also like to extend our appreciation to Dr. Bela Toth of the University of Nebraska for his personal communications regarding the real and much underrated toxicities in the most commonly eaten mushrooms. Another famous researcher at the University of Nebraska and a specialist in free radicals and aging, Dr. Denham Harman, deserves our sincere thanks for allowing us to consult him by phone about his personal conviction that supplemental anti-oxidants are indeed "good health insurance" and may extend our life span. We would like to express our thanks to California pneumologist Dr. Irwin Ziment for granting us a phone interview on the role of anti-oxidants in certain spices and their use in the treament of upper respiratory infections. Thanks also to Dr. Daniel Kesden of Fort Lauderdale, Florida, for important pointers on the anti-oxidant crocetin in saffron. And special thanks to Dr. Ann Kennedy of the University of Pennsylvania for clearing up some questions we had about certain plant compounds called *protease inhibitors*—and their potential for protecting our health.

Many thanks, too, to Dr. Rita Demopoulos for her emotional support of this project, and Nellie Zigurides, her and Dr. Harry Demopoulos's assistant.

Our sincere appreciation must be extended to our friends radiologist Dr. Milos Sovac of Rancho Santa Fe, California, biologist-turned-businessman "Daugh" Daughenbaugh of Boston, author Kathleen Tynan, and John Czapek of La Paz, Bolivia, our nephew-in-law, for their critical reading of parts of the manuscript, leading to important improvements in it.

Finally, our immense gratitude to faithful Miguel Canales and his good wife, Maria, who kept the plants growing on our farm in Costa Rica and took such good and loving care of our German shepherd family—Pancho, Amy, Kron, Della, and Arthur—during our long absences.

—DRS. EBERHARD AND PHYLLIS KRONHAUSEN

CONTENTS

13

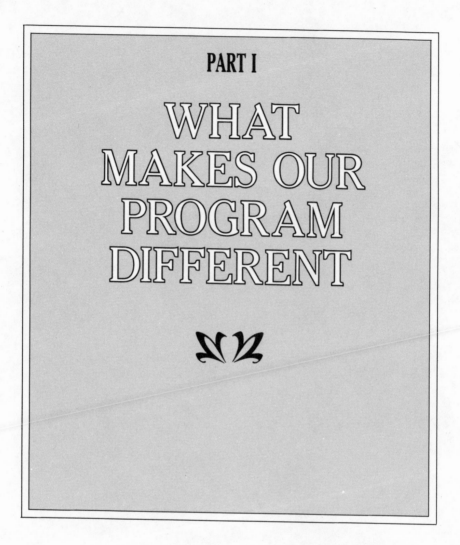

PART I

WHAT MAKES OUR PROGRAM DIFFERENT

CHAPTER 1

WHY THIS BOOK?

*W*e decided to write this book because we had news too good to keep to ourselves. And we came to it *after* reaching and passing the age when most people resign themselves to a progressive decline in their abilities and capacity for enjoyment. Remember the mythical Fountain of Youth? People entered on one side bent over, decrepit, full of aches and pains; they came out the other side standing tall, happy, healthy, and smiling. Well, we don't expect you to believe us right away, but the fact is that what we've discovered over the past few years has come very close to producing exactly these effects in us.

It wasn't that way ten years ago. At that time, we were no better off physically and mentally than most people our age. Eberhard, fourteen years older than Phyllis, logically showed more signs of aging, but Phyllis was far from content with her own physical state.

There were two circumstances that probably prevented matters from being worse than they were. One was that a few years earlier we had stopped eating meat, not so much for health as for philosophical reasons. (We were, however, still eating high-fat cheeses, butter, sugar, and salt, and drinking wine with most of our meals.)

The other thing was that although Eberhard had now reached retirement age, we had no pension to retire on. This meant we had to keep busy making a living—a circumstance we now feel amounted to a blessing in disguise. We had seen too many friends in our same age bracket retire and promptly start deteriorating.

Having decided that a total change in life-style might be an adventure to keep us young at least in spirit, we recklessly bought some land in Costa Rica—a place most people go to for retirement, not for a new career—and proceeded to build up a little tropical farm.

Whatever else it did for us, this new venture certainly provided a lot more adventure than we had bargained for. Much of it came in the form of manual labor, an automatic exercise workout that lasted from dawn to dusk.

Things weren't exactly easy for us those first years as we tried to build a new life in such a different environment. But there was one redeeming feature that made things more tolerable than they might have been otherwise: Despite a lifetime of not precisely health-conscious living, neither of us was plagued by any of the major degenerative diseases that make their appearance after the age of fifty or so. We were and are profoundly grateful for that. On the other hand, we were not spared the usual minor symptoms of advancing age—our bodies tired far more quickly than they used to and, much worse, our minds weren't firing on all cylinders. Eberhard especially was becoming progressively forgetful. And the process of learning anything new— such as a foreign language (Spanish), not to mention tropical agriculture—turned out to be much slower and more difficult than we had anticipated.

Most dispiriting of all was the prevailing, undermining assumption that all of this was "only to be expected" at our age. In the past we had been able to cope much more easily with whatever problems had come our way, even the most serious ones. Now, however, even relatively minor problems often seemed beyond our ability to cope. And all we could see ahead at the end of this tunnel was another tunnel, and another, and another.

Without any exaggeration, we say that we had definitely arrived at the most serious crisis point in our lives. We had already done what we could to improve our outward circumstances, which remained difficult, to say the least. Now we were telling ourselves: *If* only we were twenty years younger; *if* only we were physically stronger; *if* only we could still depend on our good minds; *if* only we had more energy; *if* only we were up at least as much as down, and so on. If piled upon if, while our spirits sank even lower.

As mental health professionals we were of course perfectly aware that this sort of outlook wasn't going to solve anything or get us anywhere. We had to try to find out what, if anything, might be done about the decline we were experiencing so painfully.

The message of traditional medicine—like that of conventional wisdom—was loud and clear: Stop kidding yourselves; there is no Fountain of Youth; you've reached the age when your body's deterioration accelerates, and your mind simply isn't going to work anymore the way it used to. That's life, like it or not.

We heard the message, all right. But neither of us was inclined to take such a hopeless verdict lying down. Instead, we agreed to leave no avenue unexplored that offered—even theoretically—any possibility of our keeping the faculties we still had and perhaps getting back some of the ones we had lost.

We were perfectly aware that the mainstream medical community regards such a goal as neither realistic nor legitimate. That realization only encouraged us to start looking outside mainstream medicine for the answer—if, indeed, there *was* an answer.

We knew of the "live cell therapy" practiced by some European clinics, and of Dr. Ana Aslan's procaine treatment to restore youth. But we had neither the kind of money these "therapies" take nor much faith in them, since some of our more affluent friends had embraced them with less than impressive results.

We kept improving our diet, bit by bit. While far from ideal, it was nonetheless a lot better than it had been before. Basically it was a semivegetarian diet that contained abundant fresh vegetables and fruits from our own farm. And we had virtually stopped drinking wine.

As our diet improved, so did we. We also kept up the search for a program that would offer more than a little slowing down of the process of deterioration. So we turned briefly to some of the "naturopathic" approaches to health and longevity.

At first this avenue seemed promising. These offbeat "therapies" were at least addressing the issues that most concerned us, such as preventing disease, slowing down the aging process, and in general keeping the human body and mind functioning to the fullest capacity possible. They held out hope to us—as they do to millions of others whose deep-seated yearnings for a better, healthier, fuller, and longer life are ignored or ridiculed by mainstream medicine, mainstream nutrition, mainstream psychiatry, even mainstream religion.

Hope wasn't all the health cults had to offer. Their advocates encouraged people to stop smoking and drinking, to cut down on or cut out red meat, and add fresh fruits and vegetables to their diet, to get exercise—all commendable practices, to be sure. Unfortunately, the health cults abounded with fanatics and self-appointed diet gurus. No sooner were you nodding agreement over the benefits of getting closer to nature, raising your consciousness, and rejecting the junk-food culture, than you found yourself stopped cold by unscientific theories that flew in the face of all logic, or by bizarre dietary practices and irrational "detoxification" rituals that could not but offend your common sense.

Though disappointed with our explorations into the uncharted and treacherous waters of health cultism, we were not willing to give up the search for realistic suggestions to improve health and general functioning. Maybe, around the next corner, we would find new research, new theories that *would* stand up under close scrutiny.

It was at this point that, almost accidentally, we turned just such a corner. We began to tap into the life-extension movement that had first quietly and then noisily sprung up in America while we were tending our crops in Costa Rica.

We knew from the beginning that we were dealing not with another fad or cult but with a legitimate new branch of the natural sciences. Its gurus were not starry-eyed health faddists, but serious people from medical, biochemical, and other scientific fields.

In a way these scientists almost seemed to be modern counterparts of the alchemists of old—for they, too, were in a sense looking for a kind of Fountain of Youth. Only they were using not wands but state-of-the-art scientific apparatus, such as scanning electron microscopes and electron paramagnetic resonance spectrometry, to discover what might enable people to live longer and better.

We met these scientists, listened, asked questions—and, during visits to the States, immersed ourselves in the scientific literature that had already developed around their work. We soon began to catch the life-extension fever: Not only was their research solid, but it did not involve costly, questionable "miracle drugs" or rejuvenation treatments.

The implications were exciting indeed: If we combined the high-complex-carbohydrate, low-fat (about 20 percent of total calories), high-fiber diet we had adopted by then with the anti-oxidants and vitamin co-factors these scientists had been experimenting with for a number of years, we'd have a winning combination. It definitely had the potential to maximize the benefits of sound nutrition, while adding the protective and therapeutic effects of the anti-oxidants and vitamin co-factors.

Anti-oxidants are natural or man-made substances that prevent oxidation; vitamin co-factors are vitamins that help the anti-oxidants (most of which are technically also vitamins) do their job better and perform specific therapeutic functions, all of which we shall discuss in this book.

Why do we need anti-oxidants, since oxygen is absolutely essential to life? Because oxygen is also a highly toxic gas whose destructive effects can most easily be seen in the corrosion of metals—iron, copper, and many other substances can be totally destroyed by "rusting," the popular term for oxidation. And so all living organisms—plants and animals and human beings—need natural anti-oxidants so as to be able to live in the oxygen-rich atmosphere of our planet.

It is with great difficulty that the body controls such a highly reactive substance. For instance, after playing its necessary role in important metabolic processes, oxygen may keep on burning, oxidizing, and breaking down our cell membranes and the molecular structure of all our vital organs.

Oxygen causes this damage by generating still more destructive and reactive compounds called *free radicals,* about which we will have a great deal to say later on. For now, let it suffice to emphasize that our system has a critical need for anti-oxidants to prevent destructive oxidation.

While tremendously excited by what we learned about anti-oxidants, nonetheless we saw that some life-extension researchers seemed to underestimate the importance of the diet we ourselves had belatedly come to appreciate. And some of the man-made and possibly life-extending substances being experimented with seemed, on closer look, not yet proven safe or effective enough to be advisable in the long run.

We also found a great deal of confusion among the experts as to the recommended dosages and right combinations of anti-oxidants and vitamin co-factors to be taken. Only Dr. Harry B. Demopoulos—a distinguished professor of pathology at New York University, who was to become our chief medical consultant—had researched extensively enough to determine the right combinations and dosages of anti-oxidants and vitamin co-factors for a safe and effective life-extension program.

More conservative in his approach than most others working in this field, Dr. Demopoulos had ruled out all substances—however promising—that could possibly cause trouble. The leading researcher, then and now, in what is known as "free-radical pathology," Dr. Demopoulos set out to put his twenty years of research to work. Having discovered a method of combining a number of anti-oxidants and vitamin co-factors in a single capsule—without the use of common manufacturing additives, which can be allergenic and harmful—he eventually established a distribution company* to ensure a readily available source of the right combinations and dosages for each of the essential metabolic micronutrients required for any serious life-extension program.

However, our information on how you can implement Dr. Demopoulos's anti-oxidant program will not be limited to his recommendations or those of anyone else. More about that presently.

For the moment, let us return to what adding anti-oxidants and vitamin co-factors to our basic diet and physically active life-style has meant to us personally. To begin with, they have had a dramatic energizing, stabilizing, antidepressant, and positively mood-enhancing effect on both of us. Now, when problems come our way that are anything but funny, we tend to see the funny side of them. Friends tell us that our dispositions, especially Eberhard's, are sunnier than during any period they've known us. This is of particular interest, for mood stabilization and improvement are not fringe benefits of the program—they're critical to the majority of older people who experience depression and mood swings with aging.

---

* Health Maintenance Programs (HMP). See Appendix A, "List of Suppliers," for details.

The changes in our mental functioning have been quite wonderful. By any criteria, our mental faculties have greatly improved—we figure, conservatively, by at least 50 percent. Short-term memory has greatly improved for both of us. We have been carefully noting, first, the number of times during the day when we fail to remember something; then we note the number of times we make mistakes because of lapses of memory, lack of concentration, or confusion. The German language has a perfect if untranslatable term, *Fehlleistungen,* for the kind of misdirected, off-target acts of daily living we are talking about, such as turning off an appliance when you've just turned it on.

Our physical health has improved so dramatically over the past two or three years that our friends can hardly believe we are the same people. Unbelievable as it sometimes seems even to us, we have considerably more energy than many of our much younger friends and colleagues. Though Phyllis is pushing sixty and Eberhard is well past the biblical threescore and ten, we regularly work a fourteen-hour day without feeling the need for a siesta. This represents quite a change for Eberhard, who says:

It's true. I no longer embarrass myself and Phyllis by dozing off in front of company at nine-thirty in the evening. But as much as I welcome the renewed energy, my physical improvement is more dramatic and more specific.

First, I had been suffering from the kind of chronic prostate infection and enlargement typical in older men. Not wanting to undergo one of those disagreeable prostate operations so thoroughly publicized thanks to President Reagan, I had been taking one kind of antibiotic or another for several years. Of course, you can't stay on antibiotics indefinitely; besides, the bacteria kept adapting to them, just as flu germs adapt to the latest virus. So every time I discontinued an antibiotic to give my system a respite, the infection would come right back. Not only was my urologist running out of antibiotics to prescribe, but I was spending more time on them than off.

I'm sure male readers past middle age will find this syndrome all too familiar. Well, the unfamiliar, almost unbelievable news after I'd spent some months on the anti-oxidant program is this: I realized that for the first time in several years, I wasn't on antibiotics. To this day, my prostate is behaving itself—or rather it's behaving like the prostate of a much younger man.

I've had improvement that's almost as dramatic in another chronic condition. I was one of those millions who suffer from recurrent lower-back pain. At times the pain was mild, at times so excruciating that I could barely make it to the chiropractor for an adjustment. The visit usually helped, but the next week the pain might be back and I might need one or more further adjustments. Sometimes I'd then be free of pain for weeks or even months. Then I'd make a wrong move, literally, and there came the pain, back again. Phyllis was sympathetic, for she had her own lower-back problems. Her attacks were less severe than mine, but the pain *was* getting worse each year.

So, what happened?
We are not about to tell you that taking anti-oxidants puts bones or spinal disks back where they belong. But they are known to help with

arthritis, rheumatism, and other inflammatory diseases, and much of what goes under the catchall term "lower-back pain" is really just another manifestation of these problems.

Another most welcome benefit has been in our improved immune systems. Neither of us has had a severe cold or flu for the last two years, even when everybody around us is sick; and Eberhard used to be capable of catching a cold just by *thinking* about bad weather.

Certain improvements are cosmetic: We know we look better because our friends tell us and because we can see it in each other. The basic reason, of course, is that a better general state of health is reflected in our appearance. But more specifically, some of the anti-oxidants we are taking have marvelous effects on our skin, notably vitamin B_5 (calcium pantothenate) and pure liquid vitamin E (not to be confused with capsules containing vitamin E, suspended in vegetable or mineral oil; see our discussion on pages 45–47). After being on the program for only a few weeks, we both noticed that our hair, especially Phyllis's, was noticeably shinier and silkier. Chronic dandruff, for which we had used special shampoos, had simply disappeared.

This last change did not surprise us, since it is known that certain peroxidation (rancidification) processes in the sebaceous glands of the scalp play a large role in this annoying affliction, for which a low-fat diet and anti-oxidants are the only logical therapies.

We very much enjoyed throwing out the dandruff shampoos—which use external anti-oxidants such as pyrithione zinc to control the problem externally, but fail to touch its cause, as is the case with so many other symptomatic treatments. (It is, for instance, eminently so with most popular over-the-counter remedies for common gastrointestinal ailments like hemorrhoids, heartburn, and constipation; see Part IX, pages 265–290.)

One final comment on hair: Phyllis's has definitely returned to the light-blond color it had begun to lose, and Eberhard's graying process seems to have slowed down, and has begun to get back some of its original brown hue.

We had never heard of this happening as a result of anti-oxidants alone—without the vitamin and cell-membrane stabilizer PABA (para-aminobenzoic acid), which is said to restore color to graying hair in about 10 percent of cases. But though Eberhard had also been using a little PABA, Phyllis never did and seemed to have gotten the same results.

Even more important, Phyllis had been losing hair, by the brushful, ever since menopause:

I was put on an estrogen-replacement regimen, which certainly helped, but I was still losing far too much hair. This was particularly upsetting to me because, frankly, I've always had pretty hair. My excessive hair loss stopped within three weeks of my going on the anti-oxidant program. Dr. Demopoulos explained it this way: Once the anti-oxidants began to get more nutrients to my scalp—including more of the estrogens—less and less hair fell out. Today the amount of hair I find on my brush is within perfectly normal limits.

This, then, is our story. We got older; we didn't like the effects. We combined a healthy diet with the right spectrum of anti-oxidants and vitamin co-factors—and we stopped most of the distressing ill effects of aging. We don't speculate about what our lives might have been like had we known years earlier what we know now about anti-oxidants, nutrition, and life-style. Ten or twenty years ago, even Dr. Demopoulos—like any of the other scientists working on age retardation and life extension today—wouldn't have had much more to offer than some interesting theories—certainly he would have had no practical suggestions. What's more, it's doubtful that we would have been receptive to such information, even had it been possible to know exactly what to do to avoid the physical and mental problems we would soon develop. There is, after all, an element of readiness involved in getting on the right track with anything—certainly in seriously taking care of yourself. The sad truth is that many people find it hard to get interested in these matters until they themselves start to experience a loss of faculties or develop a serious disease.

These days we counsel a great many people about nutrition and anti-oxidants and life-style. Despite some initial skepticism, they usually write or telephone to let us know that "the diet and the anti-oxidants, vitamins, whatever, really work!"

We *know* they work. We ourselves have never been better off physically and emotionally then we are right now. This highly personal assessment is corroborated by the regular laboratory tests and medical checkups we undergo for research purposes. Our blood pressure is perfect, our cholesterol levels are around 130, and neither of us is overweight.

For people of our age, this is a remarkable state of affairs—certainly it's beyond anything one could reasonably expect from any health-enhancing regimen.

We believe that whatever irrevocable damage to our system occurred, it has now been "frozen." No health problem seems to be getting worse for either of us, and in many respects the damage has been rolled back to put us in a state of health comparable to the one we enjoyed many years ago.

This happy outcome, we are convinced, is the result of having combined a scientifically worked-out spectrum of anti-oxidants and vitamin co-factors with sound nutrition, gentle but effective exercise, and a generally health-conscious life-style. How to do this with minimal effort—but to maximum effect—is the message of this book.

PREVENTION

Twas a dangerous cliff, as they freely confessed,
  Though to walk near its crest was so pleasant;
But over its terrible edge there had slipped
  A duke and full many a peasant.
So the people said something would have to be done
  But their projects did not all tally.
Some said, "Put a fence round the edge of the cliff."
  Some, "An ambulance down in the valley."

But the cry for the ambulance carried the day,
  And it spread through the neighboring city;
A fence may be useful or not, it is true,
  But each heart became brim full of pity
For those who slipped over the dangerous cliff,
  And dwellers in highway and alley
Gave pounds or gave pence, not to put up a fence,
  But an ambulance down in the valley.

Then an old sage remarked, "It's a marvel to me
  That people give far more attention
To repairing results than to stopping the cause,
  When they'd all better aim at prevention."
"Let us stop at its source all this mischief ," cried he.
  "Come neighbors and friends; let us rally.
If the cliff we will fence we might almost dispense
  With the ambulance down in the valley."

"Oh, he's a fanatic," the other rejoined;
  "Dispense with the ambulance? Never!
He'd dispense with all charities, too, if he could.
  No, no, we'll support them forever!
Aren't we picking up folks just as fast as they fall?
  And shall this man dictate to us? Shall he?
Why should people of sense stop to put up a fence
  While the ambulance works in the valley?"

But a sensible few, who are practical too,
  Will not bear with such nonsense much longer;
They believe that prevention is better than cure,
  And their party will soon be the stronger.

Encourage them, then, with your purse, voice and pen
  And while other philanthropists dally
They will scorn all pretense and put up a stout fence
  On the cliff that hangs over the valley.

—Joseph Melvin*

* G. S. Goldstein, "Institutional barriers to alcohol and drug abuse prevention," *Int. J. Addictions,* 1985; 20:1:217–231.

CHAPTER 2

WHY DON'T WE TAKE BETTER CARE OF OURSELVES?

We are taking good care of ourselves.

That's what we would have said ten years ago. And, in a sense, we would have been right. We were eating "good" food. We weren't smoking tobacco, or anything else, for that matter. Yes, we were drinking wine rather freely, but then we were living in Paris at the time and the wine was practically free. Besides, half a bottle of wine with lunch and dinner, in France, put us in the light-drinker category.

We were eating extremely well by most standards. Food prices were so low in Europe that we could buy the best meats, cheeses, seafood, vegetables, and fruits from our neighborhood markets on the Left Bank.

It's true that the wonderful cheeses, the meats, the cream sauces, the rich pastries, had pushed our cholesterol right into the critical zone for stroke and heart attack. And it's also true that today—older and wiser and much healthier—there are times when we still miss the terrines and pâtés, and especially the soft, scented cheeses that went so well with a nice red wine. All this means is that while we still love wonderful-tasting food, we are not willing to die for it. Especially since we now know there is wonderful-tasting food that *doesn't* kill you.

Of course, if we failed to take better care of ourselves a decade ago

One in 5 American adults suffers from some type of disability.

Difficulty in walking is the most common disability. Over 19 million people can walk as little as ¼ mile only with some difficulty; 7.9 million cannot make such a walk at all.

Eighteen million people say they cannot even climb 1 flight of stairs without stopping to rest; 5 million report they cannot make such a climb at all.—*The New York Times*, December 23, 1986

in France and earlier in America, it wasn't a matter of willful neglect. Nor is it with most people we counsel. Most of them are more confused than unwilling: who would suspect that fine foods that have been enjoyed for hundreds of years are bad for you? And which advice about diet should one take seriously?

Another basic factor is the extent to which food choices are tied up with activities other than eating: recreation, work, social life, even sex. In warm weather, American family life and social life often revolve around the outdoor barbecue. Barbecued ribs are black soul food. And what's a Fourth of July picnic without hot dogs and roasted marshmallows? Or a birthday or wedding without the obligatory cream-filled layer cake?

It's hard to imagine an American child without cookies and soda, a Frenchman without cheeses and wine, Germans without sausage and beer. Given such deeply ingrained eating and drinking habits, one doesn't win popularity contests by informing people that their traditional ways of eating are loading their arteries with atherosclerotic plaque or will give them cancer. People are likely to think they are taking pretty good care of themselves, and are more than likely to resent being told otherwise. They perceive health activists like us as overly interested in their private affairs and overeager to impose their own values on the rest of the world. We find this attitude quite understandable—since ten years ago we felt the same way.

Understandable or not, the effect of this attitude on the individual is always negative. Denial of the obvious can go to unbelievable lengths. For instance, we had a friend who suffered from such severe emphysema that he had to spend most of his time in an oxygen tent. What did he do during his brief intervals out of it? You guessed it—he lit up a cigarette!

We are also reminded of the published case of a seventy-four-year-old gentleman, a heavy smoker and drinker who developed cancer of the throat. This type of cancer has a mortality rate of 10 percent, but he turned out to be one of the lucky 90 percent. He was successfully operated on, the cancer was removed, and even his swallowing mechanism and speech were restored.

With such a close call, anyone would quit smoking—right? Wrong. Ten years later, and now eighty-four years old, the patient was back in the hospital with a new smoking-induced cancer, this time on his tongue. Again, the doctors were able to remove the cancer and, after further reconstructive surgery, restored his swallowing mechanism and ability to talk for the second time—although, for a while following the latter operation, he had to communicate with pencil and paper. When a friend came to visit him at the hospital and asked whether he was still smoking, the man wrote out his answer on a notepad: "Yes, I still drink and smoke. At eighty-four, I can't last that long."

HEALTH-PROMOTING ATTITUDES

1. Healthy people feel that they are in control of their own lives, rather than victims of circumstances beyond their control.
2. Healthy people do not underestimate or overestimate their capacities. They are aware of their physical and mental limitations and accept them, but continually strive to improve themselves to realize their potential.
3. Healthy people make personal decisions on the basis of rational rather than emotional considerations.
4. Healthy people are not prejudiced, but are open to rational argument.
5. Healthy people are not stubborn or willful, but proceed in the light of the most logical course of action.
6. Healthy people are not overly flattered by praise and recognition, nor unduly influenced by lack of recognition and criticism.
7. Healthy people have a strong, personal value system and are therefore immune to corrupting influences and greed.
8. Healthy people have a realistic appraisal of human frailties and shortcomings. Such realization does not prevent them from readily entering into trusting and meaningful relationships with others.
9. Healthy people have interests and concerns beyond their own personal welfare and happiness, or that of their immediate family and circle of friends. They see themselves as members of the larger world community and accept the responsibilities this entails.
10. Healthy people conduct themselves in full knowledge of their ultimate mortality and have come to grips with it emotionally. These people do not harbor a morbid fear of death or dying, but are sustained by a strong sense of the underlying continuity in the perpetual changes and transformations observable in nature.

Such a remark is not surprising. We're too used to hearing people say things like, "Well, we all have to die sometime, so what's the use in worrying?" But the question, surely, is not *whether* one has to die but *how soon* and under what circumstances.

Of course, there are many of us who have had one or more friends or relatives who ate fatty foods, smoked cigarettes, and drank alcohol all their adult lives and lived into their eighties or even nineties. Never mind that most of them lived in nursing homes and could no longer do as much as tie their own shoelaces. Somehow they still made it into the longevity decades—even if in a wheelchair. The few exceptions to this usual state of affairs only confirm the rule.

"A diplomat's life is made up of three ingredients: protocol, Geritol, and alcohol."—Adlai E. Stevenson, *The New York Times*, November 5, 1986

Sometimes, the "don't tell me" argument is used in reverse. When we warned a friend of ours in a letter about his cigar smoking and his diet, he replied by return mail: "You should remember that Mr. Pritikin is dead, as are four of George Burns's doctors who advised him to give up smoking cigars." We refrained from pointing out that Nathan Pritikin might have suffered a recurrence of his leukemia years sooner if it hadn't been for his strict diet.

Denial of the facts of aging and the ill effects of certain life-styles on health are especially prevalent among younger people. During the first two decades or so of life, there's a near-universal tendency to deny our very mortality—along with an inability to believe that any really life-threatening illness could befall us personally.

Nor is this tendency necessarily outgrown. A case in point: A California woman who has undergone three skin cancer operations notes that her son seems to be developing a lesion but refuses to have it checked—while her daughter continues exposing herself as much as ever to the sun, totally disregarding her mother's sad experience. "They think they'll live forever," the woman says with a sigh.[1]

This reluctance to apply unpalatable truths to themselves is one of the biggest obstacles in motivating people to modify their life-styles. As Dr. Lawrence W. Green, director of the Center for Health Promotion Research and Development at the University of Texas Health Sciences Center in Dallas, put it in an interview with *New York Times* health columnist Jane Brody: "The person has to get beyond anonymous statistics to realize that this could happen *to him*."[2]

Dr. Green is right, of course. We have to apply health information to ourselves before we can reap any benefit from it whatsoever. While this is true, there is a reverse side to it: *Not* applying the statistics to themselves may not only be killing many people, but keeping others alive.

How does this reverse psychology work? Well, as cancer surgeon Dr. Bernie Siegel explains in *Love, Medicine, and Miracles,* many cancer patients beat the mortality statistics of their supposedly "terminal" disease by firmly believing that the statistics do *not* apply to them. Instead of sitting around and waiting to die, some of them just go on with their lives in a "business as usual" manner. Others go even further, acting as if they had already been given a new lease on life by believing the doctor when he tells them that they are *not* statistics, and that there's always a chance of beating the odds. They are, in short, Dr. Siegel's "exceptional patients."

We have observed the same principle working with some of our friends and clients: They are doing literally everything to make themselves sick and shorten their life span. They eat high-fat foods, smoke like chimneys, and drink like fish. Yet, although they may not really thrive on such reckless life-styles, they are surviving—often into their late seventies and eighties, occasionally even beyond.

When we talk to these people about the serious health hazards they are courting, they usually cut us short—often rather aggressively—insisting that there is no real scientific proof that smoking and drinking "moderate" amounts of alcohol, or eating high-fat foods is so bad for them. But more important, they point out that even if they aren't eating right, or are smoking and drinking too much, they somehow feel "special" or "different" from others. They have "good genes," they usually tell us, or anyway nothing bad is going to happen to them, regardless . . .

Of course, their optimism is totally irrational and their supreme confidence is based on what psychologists call the "mechanism of denial."* But there they are, doing all the wrong things from a more health-conscious point of view, and apparently getting away with it. If they are our friends, we worry about them, knowing that sooner or later they will have to pay the price. On the other hand, it seems that by their mental high-wire act they are able to postpone that day of reckoning by years—sometimes decades. So we have come to accept—if ever so reluctantly—that these extraordinary "deniers" are better left alone and spared our well-meaning health-educational attentions. Chances are, the truth might shatter their fragile illusions and take away the magic protection on which they are surviving.

* In another context, we shall refer to studies showing that seriously ill patients who are "not facing reality," as far as their illnesses are concerned, often fare better than those who do (see pages 204–205).

Dr. Green and his colleagues at the Health Sciences Center in Dallas have found what is necessary for most people to become motivated to take better care of themselves is for them to appreciate the severity of the problem—to see that it really is worth their concern.

Finally, a person must come to believe that he or she is not just a helpless victim of circumstances, but can actually do something about the situation. This is especially true in cases of substance dependency (tobacco, liquor, drugs).

But even without substance dependency, why change your diet, engage in more physical exercise, and take anti-oxidants if you aren't convinced that these changes will result in a healthier, happier, and longer life? Such a belief or conviction doesn't come easy living, as we do, in a culture that is by and large not even aware of the health hazards we are talking about.

> Even in the armed forces, where the means of indoctrinating troops with preventive nutrition is theoretically at hand, more attention is paid to food lobbyists, worried mothers, congressional complaints and the unthinking cravings of youth than to presently known knowledge on disease prevention by nutritional means.
>
> [This includes] the National Aeronautics and Space Agency where hardware considerations and astronaut whims ... have received higher priority. Other agencies are no less remiss.—Robert S. Good-hart and Maurice E. Shils, eds. *Modern Nutrition in Health and Disease: Dietotherapy* (Philadelphia: Lea & Febiger, 1973)

Of course, there is some awareness in society at large that smoking is bad for you, that cholesterol levels should be brought down a bit, that drinking too much isn't a good idea, and that, *theoretically* speaking, you should take more exercise. But that's about as far as it goes. People might even accept eating more fresh fruits and vegetables. However, the idea that you don't necessarily have to get old and decrepit, that serious illness is largely avoidable, and that you might be able to dramatically extend your life span, are not a part of public consciousness—to say nothing of taking anti-oxidants to help achieve these goals.

On the other hand, sometimes it's easier to convince people to take anti-oxidants or vitamins than to make dietary and life-style changes or alter their attitudes. Of course, the fact that the anti-oxidants on our program allow for a somewhat more relaxed diet than would be necessary without them is often a big inducement. In these cases, we try to make sure that dietary leeway doesn't develop into dietary irresponsibility. Swallowing numerous capsules filled with anti-oxidants and other nutrients—no matter how potent and effective—does *not* cancel the necessity for making drastic changes in our food habits.

Getting onto a life-extension program such as ours also requires reshuffling our financial priorities. Both extra savings and extra expense are involved. A shift from steak and chocolate cake to an emphasis on vegetables, fruits, and grains saves money, as does cutting out cigarettes and booze.

Better health means lower medical bills and less time lost because of illness. Implementing our anti-oxidant program does cost money, even if you make your own powder mix (see pages 63–64 and 593–595), and the regular medical checkups and laboratory tests every life-extender accepts as essential can be quite expensive, especially in America.

For most of us, a one-, two-, or three-week residential health and weight-control program like those at the Canyon Ranch in Tucson, Arizona, or the Pritikin Longevity Center in Santa Monica, California, to mention just two of the most famous, are well beyond our means. This is unfortunate because these programs offer an excellent practical education on how to take better care of oneself. Such programs are a godsend, especially to people with heart disease, diabetes, or any other physical condition known to respond well to nutritional treatment—a category that includes many more diseases than you might think. In such cases, even a price tag of several thousand dollars for a two- or three-week program can actually be a bargain. In any event, it is often a viable alternative to undergoing bypass operations or other invasive and costly medical procedures.

Our own comprehensive, nonresidential regimen of diet, exercise, and anti-oxidants offers an option that is far from second-best, even for those who do have a serious health or weight-control problem. This is not to say that you shouldn't enroll at least once in such a residential course, if you can afford it. It would give you a fine head start on our program, especially if you have, or suspect that you have, cardiovascular or diabetic problems.

We think there's another, quite basic reason why many of us find it so hard to consistently take better care of ourselves when it comes to food choices. We have all been conditioned to salivate at certain cues—not at a ringing bell, like Pavlov's dogs, but at the sight or smell of certain kinds of foods.

The foods that evoke a positive conditioned response often trigger childhood associations with parental love and affection. What, for instance, does the average parent offer a young child as a sign of approval? The reward isn't likely to be an apple or a dish of strawberries. Rather, it's apt to be an ice cream cone, a chocolate candy bar, a piece of cake, or some cookies. And the richer the sweet treat, the more loving the sentiment behind it—at least, that's the way the subconscious soundtrack goes.

Meat, butter, milk, and cheese are other foods of dubious nutritional value that we've all been conditioned to appreciate from early childhood. In the past, what parents who could afford meat and butter would have had second thoughts about letting their children have them? Even today, most parents cannot imagine (nor will they be informed by pediatricians) that meat should be eaten only sparingly because of its high fat and cholesterol content. In fact, many parents still believe that growing children need plenty of meat for their protein requirements.

Parents are even less likely to suspect milk and cheese. Aren't they rich sources of protein children need for growth, and of calcium for proper bone development?[3] Yes, but cow's milk happens to have the wrong kind of protein, namely *casein,* which promotes atherosclerosis in everybody, including children. Cow's milk is also a highly allergenic food that many people—in fact, whole populations, including most blacks and Asians—cannot tolerate because their bodies lack the necessary enzyme to digest it. Whole milk is high in fat, and most cheeses even higher. That's another atherogenic (contributing to atherosclerosis) factor—for children too!

Item: The National Health Council's breakfast fare is reputed to be of dubious nutritional quality. If so, it's not the kitchen's fault. When the breakfast menu offered high-fiber cereals, only two or three of the 200 assembled medical and health experts chose them. The rest went for the "customary broad array of calories, cholesterol, and nitrites: eggs, sausage, fried potatoes and pastries."—*The New York Times,* "Washington Talk," December 1986

One doesn't have to look far to find the reason why teenagers don't take better care of themselves: It has been calculated that the average American sixteen-year-old has already seen about 360,000 TV food commercials, plus countless newspaper and magazine ads—all pushing what we call "unfriendly," that is, fatty, sugary, or salty, foods.

In addition, there is tremendous peer-group pressure. The group standards for teens extend as much to what is eaten as to what kind of clothes are worn or music is listened to. For a teenager to eat differently, or to dare to be different in other respects such as turning down an afternoon spent suntanning, or an alcoholic drink, or a cigarette or joint—requires a strength of character not often found in people so young.

Not that adults are exempt from peer-group pressure when it comes to eating, especially when they dine out with friends who do not share their views. Here the issue is not so much the need to conform as it is the unwillingness to upset a well-meaning hostess who has served us something she "knows" we can eat—fish, for example, but deep-fried or smothered in butter.

And of course teenagers and adults alike are subjected to constant bombardment with advertising and television commercials proclaiming the delights of all the worst kinds of food. How can we reasonably expect teenagers to listen to somebody who says all these products are eventually going to clog up their arteries or give them cancer?

Item: Senator Edward M. Kennedy is a devoted cigar smoker. Usually he heeds his staff's advice to refrain from smoking when before television cameras because . . . it does not present a good role model.

"But last week the Massachusetts Democrat threw caution to the winds as he lit up and puffed away while the cameras rolled at a committee hearing. He was delighted at improved prospects for a favored piece of legislation—a comprehensive health-care package."—Wayne King and Robin Toner, *The New York Times*, January 20, 1987

Nor do members of the medical profession have many opportunities to offer much help in educating their patients toward healthier eating habits and life-styles. If your doctor doesn't have the time or doesn't seem concerned about what you eat, or whether you smoke, why should you? In some countries, the medical profession sets an even worse example than here in America. For instance, in Spain, the prevalence of smoking is higher among doctors than in the general population (*BMJ*, 1988; 297: 441).

In schools, colleges, and universities, health education that seriously covers sound nutrition is all but unheard of, while greasy hamburgers are served in the school cafeteria. Then there's hospital food, not to mention what the doctors and nurses eat in the hospital cafeteria. In the armed forces, we find a ray of hope: Experimental alternative, healthier diet programs have been surprisingly successful and could become more widely available. Meanwhile, the typical high-fat, high-protein, low-complex-carbohydrate, low-fiber army chow reigns supreme in the mess hall. And hamburgers and french fries are served almost on demand in the armed forces.

One could obviously make a very long list of examples and reasons why most of us are not taking better care of ourselves. Basically, as we have tried to show, it all comes down to a single fundamental principle: *conditioning*. This forming of dietary habits and the adoption of certain life-styles begin very early in life. In America they are perhaps more pronounced and accelerated because of the intensive advertising of food, alcoholic drinks, cigarettes, and over-the-counter drugs. This kind of bombardment with commercial propaganda makes eating the wrong kind of foods, then taking nonprescription drugs for heartburn, upset stomach, diarrhea, or constipation, seem the most natural thing in the world. At the same time, it glamorizes and trivializes unhealthful life-styles that involve smoking and drinking.

The problem, of course, is not specifically American but worldwide. Even without commercial advertising of consumer products and the profit motive, the wrong kind of habit forming and conditioning goes on even in the Soviet Union. In a recent discussion via satellite hookup between leading American and Soviet heart specialists, the Russian physicians expressed comparable concerns about these matters.

Item: Representative Charles P. Rangel, a Democrat from the Harlem district of New York City, is a believer in the Pritikin diet. You can count on him to get behind health bills in the U.S. Congress. He recently sponsored a bill, introduced by Senator Howard P. Metzenbaum, requiring disclosure of the cholesterol content of foods.

But don't look at his formidable size or take a peek at what he has on his plate if you happen to run into him lunching in the congressional restaurant—you might have a heart attack just watching him eat!

Focusing on prevention rather than surgical techniques, the American and Russian cardiologists agreed that they were facing very similar public health problems. Dr. Raphael Organov, director of the Institute for Preventive Cardiology of the Soviet Cardiology Center, saw the problem specifically as that of "getting people to change long-standing habits so they can reduce their risk of suffering or dying from heart disease."

The Soviet scientists went on to say that they believe it is important to teach children in their preteen years about low-fat diets and other ways of staying healthy. "We feel it is at this stage," Dr. Organov said, "that life-long habits are formed,"[4] echoing the view expressed by many American doctors that children as young as two could benefit from low-fat diets.

Besides early conditioning, there is only one other reason why people who are genuinely concerned about their health may find it hard to get off traditional foods and onto a healthier diet: It is not easy to find or prepare a variety of healthful foods that really satisfy them the way cheese and chocolate and hamburgers or steaks "satisfy."

It is true that in adopting a health-conscious diet, we discover new and exciting foods. But it requires a different way of shopping; much more thought in planning meals, and it may involve unaccustomed ways of food preparation. For instance, finding substitutes for ingredients in recipes takes quite a bit of rethinking in the kitchen.

Item: Mayor Michael Boyle of Omaha, Nebraska, has had to face a recall petition because of an alleged drinking problem. He's tried several times to change his life-style, but not successfully.

Said Mayor Boyle, as he was making another attempt at personal reform: "I think I needed, and still need, to take better care of myself. . . . So I intend this Monday . . . there's always another Monday—to begin a program of exercise and to begin to take better care of myself as to my diet and my drinking habits."—*The New York Times,* December 9, 1986

We shall discuss all of this in some detail in later sections dealing with diet and nutrition; here we only want to acknowledge the deliberate effort and enormous mental energy it takes to go against the culture and overcome long-established dietary patterns. True, there also is a sense of adventure and excitement in learning how to shop differently, cook differently, and generally adopt a brand-new life-style. But at times not eating the way one has been used to for many years can get pretty frustrating, and there is always the temptation to revert to the old, bad but familiar ways of feeding oneself and the family—even in the full knowledge that they are dead wrong!

For all these reasons, we entertain no illusion that any more than perhaps one in a thousand people reading this book will actually follow our recommendations all the way. We'll be happy if 10 percent of our readers go only part of the way with us on diet but faithfully take the anti-oxidants, adhere to a minimal exercise program, and dedicate themselves to cultivating positive mental attitudes.

Our hope is that more and more people—however unthinking they may have been in the past—will never have to say, "I wish I'd taken better care of myself."

SOURCES

1. *Newsweek,* June 9, 1986.
2. Brody, Jane E. "Why Many Efforts Fail to Change Unhealthy Habits." *The New York Times,* April 29, 1987.
3. Schuette, S., and H. Linksweiler, in their review of calcium in: *Present Knowledge in Nutrition,* 4th ed. Washington, D.C.: The Nutrition Foundation, 1985, pp. 405–406.
4. "Satellite Conference Links Heart Specialists." UPI report in *The New York Times,* December 17, 1985.

CHAPTER 3

WHY PEOPLE GIVE UP ON VITAMINS

In this health-conscious age, half the people you know may be trying to take better care of themselves—and perhaps you are among them. These people may have modified their diet or taken up exercise; they're almost certain to have tried taking some vitamins. "Tried" is the operative word: The most common object in the American household may be the half-empty bottle of multivitamins in the medicine cabinet. "And you're trying to get people to take more?" a friend of ours, himself a health professional, asked. "Lots of luck!"

"Not vitamins," we were quick to answer. "At least, not in the usual sense of the term. We try to get people to take *anti-oxidants* and *co-factors,* many of which also happen to be vitamins."

We went on to explain that we were not talking about "multivitamins" taken as food supplements, in dosages adequate to prevent deficiencies. We use vitamins in much larger but safe dosages to scavenge and quench the dangerous oxygen-derived free radicals in our bodies, stop their potentially lethal chain reactions, and prevent the rancidification of our body fats. The vitamins have to be absolutely pure and taken in the right combination and strength to do the job.

All of that takes a lot of explaining. Many of you—maybe even most of you—are disenchanted with vitamins, and for good reason. Some people who take them have reported side effects ranging from upset stomachs, headaches, and diarrhea to skin rashes and other allergic reactions. Some have complained to us about vitamin preparations that have an unpleasant odor. Just sniff a bottle of some multivitamin tablets and you'll see what they mean. And *most* have discontinued taking vitamins for the same compelling reason: They produced no discernible benefits.

41

When you add to these problems the controversy among various authorities over the value of vitamins in the first place and the correct dosages in the second, many people simply throw up their hands and walk away.

Yet, there is a "gut feeling" among many that vitamins should be taken nonetheless—and they're right. Take, for instance, Marjorie Holmes, author of *God and Vitamins,* * who describes getting violently ill from food poisoning one night while on a book promotion tour. The first thing she did was pray for her recovery. Very soon, she writes, she felt certain that the worst was over. Then, in her own words: "I crept back to the bathroom and washed my face. Then something told me to take the vitamins I'd brought along, to replenish my strength." It worked. "God and vitamins," as she put it, had pulled her through. She was able to continue her book tour without interruption.

She went on to become an enthusiastic spokesperson for vitamin therapy. "I pray for strength," she says, "and I fortify myself with extra vitamins and minerals." She also became an outspoken critic of the U.S. Food and Drug Administration (FDA), calling the Washington health bureaucrats on many false and misleading statements about vitamins.†

The *current* FDA administrators seem to be far more enlightened. The policies on manufacturers' informing consumers about fiber and anti-oxidants in cancer prevention is quite heartening. While direct claims still require definitive clinical testing, the indirect statements in current advertising of fiber and anti-oxidants are apparently not running afoul of the FDA today.

Another example of this gut feeling about vitamins that made a deep impression on us is related in *Life and Death in Shanghai,* Nien Cheng's immensely touching account of China's Cultural Revolution during the 1960s and her harrowing experiences as one of its millions of victims.‡ In frail health and knowing that she faced years of incarceration, Madame Cheng was convinced that she would never survive without some vitamin supplements. Her gums had already started bleeding—the first sign of scurvy—because of a lack of vitamin C.

Fortunately, she had, by sheer accident, been carrying a small sum of money when she was arrested. The prison authorities agreed to keep it for her "on deposit" for possible later use following a lengthy period of

---

* Now reissued by Doubleday under the title *Secrets of Health, Energy, and Staying Young.* This book makes interesting reading, even if we cannot follow her all the way on her dietary recommendations. Nor are "bonemeal" and "desiccated liver" our idea of gourmet nutrient supplements. In fact, there are good scientific reasons why they can be more harmful than helpful. Having said this, we would like to add that Marjorie Holmes's whole attitude toward life is so positive that her book is worth reading for that alone.
† For an excellent but disturbing discussion of the role and attitudes of the FDA in the matter of vitamins and a possible conflict of interests because of the agency's intimate ties with the food industry, see the chapter entitled "Vitamins and the FDA" in Marjorie Holmes's *Secrets of Health, Energy, and Staying Young* (New York: Doubleday, 1987).
‡ Nien Cheng, *Life and Death in Shanghai* (New York: Grove Press, 1987), p. 245.

good behavior, Maoist ethics evidently forbidding its outright confis-
cation.

As Nien Cheng's health kept deteriorating under the conditions of
incarceration, the brutal interrogations, and the prison food that was
barely keeping the inmates alive, she had to be transferred to the prison
hospital. While there, she was lucky to find a young doctor who, unlike
the prison doctor, agreed that some vitamins should be purchased for
her from the money kept for her on deposit.

Unfortunately, there was no vitamin C to be had in all of Shanghai, so
she eventually lost all her teeth. (Apparently there was just enough
vitamin C in the rice and the small amount of cabbage she was
receiving to prevent full-blown scurvy from developing.) But the guards
did buy her some cod liver oil capsules and vitamin B-complex tablets,
which she credits with helping her survive the six years of her ordeal.

In this country where, it is hoped, such extremes do not exist even in
the worst of prisons, a large segment of the public nevertheless
senses—despite all the adverse publicity surrounding vitamins—that
we do need some micronutrient supplements in our diet. Nor is the lay
public alone in hedging its bets for health maintenance with vitamins.
Many members of the medical profession and other scientists, whose
official line may be "You don't need vitamin supplements," pop a few
vitamins themselves, "just in case." (If you thought this kind of
hypocrisy was limited to politicians, we suggest that you read the
July 1986 *Medical Tribune* report on an American Cancer Society
conference entitled "What the Experts Do—Unofficially—to Dodge
Cancer."

The vitamin critics in the official medical and nutritionist camps are
talking about the haphazard taking of low-dosage—and probably
impure—vitamins, while we are talking about taking a carefully formulated broad spectrum of *anti-oxidants,* with *co-factors* to help the
anti-oxidants work to best advantage. Never mind that many of them
are also chemically known as vitamins. In the new way the micronutrients are used in our program, they become something quite different.
They do *not* serve as food supplements to ensure getting enough
nutrients to prevent deficiencies. We absolutely agree with those who
say this purpose is admirably served by a health-promoting diet. But
our program's aims are quite different: taking anti-oxidants and vitamin
co-factors to counteract free-radical activity—in other words, for
optimum health maintenance. This means strengthening our immune
system, getting some cancer protection, and postponing, if not altogether preventing, other degenerative diseases such as heart attack,
stroke, and general senescence.

That's a tall order, and we're not so naïve as to suggest that
anti-oxidants, with or without co-factors like the B vitamins, are any
cure-all in and of themselves. We feel strongly that the vital issues of

health and longevity can only be approached from a comprehensive—what some people term a "holistic"—point of view.

In counseling our clients we always take the whole human being into account—body, mind, and life-style. Our recommendations are based not only on a person's physical problems and emotional state, but also on such factors as relationships, home environment, diet, recreation, sex life, degree of physical activity and exercise, even moral values and philosophy of life. It is only in this wider context that a health-maintenance and life-extension program based on anti-oxidants and vitamin co-factors can realize its full potential. It is no different from what a good doctor does—treat the whole person.

This is perhaps an idealistic point of view. Certainly it is an all-encompassing approach not everyone is ready to take. The last thing we want to do is assume a die-hard, all-or-nothing stance that would discourage large numbers of people from taking at least partial measures to safeguard their health. We have, however, established certain priorities in our program: (1) to minimize those life-style factors that are the most damaging, primarily drugs, alcohol, dietary fats, and smoking; (2) to guide you to optimally healthful nutrition according to the most recent knowledge; and (3) to encourage at least a minimum amount of daily exercise. It is in the context of these objectives that we urge you to take anti-oxidants and vitamin co-factors.

THE PROBLEM OF IMPURITIES

The major drawback with many mass-market or off-brand vitamins that sometimes find their way even onto the shelves of respectable health-food stores and drugstores is the amount of potentially harmful substances they contain. Many of these cheaper vitamins are made from raw materials that are only *food grade* rather than USP *pharmaceutical grade*. The problem is that manufacturers are not required to declare on the label what type of raw materials they use. Even if they did, it probably wouldn't help matters: People understandably assume that anything labeled FOOD GRADE is pure enough for human consumption. In the case of vitamins, however, we cannot make such assumptions. For example, some of the food-grade vitamins, inspected chromatographically under ultraviolet light, show forty or more "spots," each signaling some kind of contaminant.

Why do some vitamin manufacturers use questionable raw materials? The answer, of course, is cost. Pharmaceutical-grade vitamin materials are ten times more expensive than food-grade materials.

Unfortunately, the bad news about some of these cheaper, off-brand vitamins does not end with inferior raw materials. The process of forming vitamins into tablets or capsules can add a sinister host of additional contaminants to the end product. Tree saps and gums may be added to hold the tablets together; shellac to coat the pills; talc and sand for stretchers or fillers. Worst of all, soaps and detergents such as magnesium stearate are often added as lubricants to help move the powders through the encapsulating and tableting machines in the factory.

Manufacturers are not required by law to list all these added substances by name. If they are shown at all on the label (most of the time they don't), it is in such innocent-sounding terms as "inert substances" or "excipients." The trouble is that these additives are often neither innocent nor inert. They may, in fact, be highly active and reactive, capable of causing allergic reactions and stomach upsets.

Not surprisingly, when some people take these twice-contaminated vitamins, they get sick. When this happens, they generally blame the vitamins. Or they may conclude that they are "allergic" to vitamins, not realizing that the problem lies not with the vitamins but with the contaminants.

This situation is not helped by the manufacturers' eagerness to tell you what is *not* in their product while neglecting to mention everything that *is*. How many labels have you read that say: NO CORNSTARCH OR SOYA PRODUCTS, NO SALT OR SUGAR, NO ARTIFICIAL COLOR OR FLAVOR, NO PRESERVATIVES? And have you ever read a label that mentioned talc, sand, tree sap, shellac, or soap—all common ingredients in many commercial vitamins?

Another deceptive marketing practice is the touting of products as "all natural" or "pure." The sand found in many of these preparations is certainly natural and pure, but that doesn't mean it's good for you. Chances are, if the sand is listed on the label at all, it will be termed "silica," or "silicon dioxide," which does not sound quite as bad as "sand."

Other potentially harmful substances like tree sap and shellac can also be described as "natural." Manufacturers of vitamins that contain soap, usually listed as "magnesium stearate," will tell you it breaks up harmlessly in the stomach into magnesium and stearic acid—which, they claim, is "a fat that will simply be digested."

Unfortunately, this is not true. Magnesium stearate does *not* break down in the tissues, but instead is absorbed and circulated through the body as an intact soap molecule, acting as a detergent that destroys cell membranes.

The polyunsaturated vegetable oils in vitamin E capsules are another "natural" substance that may have unhealthy effects. Manufacturers suspend vitamin E in oil to give an impression of greater quantity, so consumers seem to be getting their money's worth. Certainly the amount of actual vitamin E in each capsule would be unimpressively small if left by itself.

We might allow this deceptive practice to pass were it not for the fact that polyunsaturated vegetable oils readily become rancid (peroxidize). When the capsules are filled, oxygen dissolves in the oil and enters the capsules right along with it. The only way to avoid this would be to fill the capsules under nitrogen, something no manufacturer does because it would escalate the production costs.

Moreover, the liquid vitamin E that has to be mixed in with the vegetable oil is a viscous substance of the consistency of, say, a heavy syrup or honey. For it to go through the filling machinery at a rapid flow, it must be heated up. Under higher temperatures, the oxygenated vegetable oil, mixed with the heated vitamin E, produces peroxides—that is, the oil becomes thoroughly oxidized (rancid) all the faster. And these oxidation processes involve free-radical activity, which will continue even inside the hermetically closed capsules.*

We take our vitamin E as pure, unadulterated, liquid dl-alpha tocopheryl acetate. In dry-based preparations about half of the vitamin E has undergone degradation during the drying process, and unfortunately it is used as a powder added to many multivitamin preparations.

To confuse the issue further about the relative merits of vitamin E in various forms, a large segment of the public has been sold on "natural" vitamin E. The origin of this hot topic was the development some years ago of a process that extracts vitamin E from by-products of flour milling, a complicated and costly procedure requiring no less than twenty-seven different chemical steps.

Whether it is proper and logical to call a product at the end of such a tortuous chemical route "natural" seems questionable. A more precise label might be DERIVED FROM NATURAL SOURCES. But the important question is, does this "natural" (or rather natural-*source*) vitamin E have properties that make it in any way superior to synthetic vitamin E, as the companies promoting it claim?

Well, you have to use 5 percent more synthetic vitamin E per dose than of "natural" vitamin E. But in terms of International Units (I.U.), a much more realistic yardstick, 1,000 I.U. of "natural" vitamin E are absolutely identical to 1,000 I.U. of synthetic vitamin E. So why spend more money on it?

The question of cost is also relevant to those "natural" vitamin E products "made from cold-pressed wheat germ." Not only is this the most expensive form of vitamin E you can buy, it is ironically also the most hazardous. Containing a high percentage of polyunsaturated oils, the preparation is rich in estrogens. While these female sex hormones are useful to women who need estrogen-replacement therapy after

---

* Unesterified, mixed tocopherol in soft-gel capsules are potent *in vitro* anti-oxidants. Consequently, vitamin E products like Twinlab's Super-E Complex, which contains Vitamin E from unesterified, mixed tocopherol, are highly resistant to peroxidation (rancidity), along with Health Maintenance Program's Pure Liquid Alpha Tocopheryl Acetate.

menopause, they are highly unsuitable for the general population. If vitamin E extracted from wheat-germ oil is taken in high enough doses, the estrogens can cause testicular degeneration and loss of sex drive in men, and may incidentally accelerate the growth of unrecognized cervical and uterine cancer in women.

Among the preparations of vitamin E made from wheat-germ oil, there is one vacuum-distilled version made from natural plant sources that is pure and free of estrogens. However, it is very expensive and offers no serious advantages over either the liquid or dry-base synthetic vitamin E.

Before we leave the subject, we must note one problem common to many commercial vitamin E preparations. As we said, vitamin E must be chemically stabilized while outside the body, a process best accomplished by adding acetate to a specific oxygen-hydrogen group of the vitamin. In our digestive system, the protective acetate is chemically split off by enzymes and thus liberates the active vitamin E.

THE DEGRADATION PROCESS IN VITAMINS

Various vitamin C preparations on the market generally pose no similar problems as for vitamin E. Most people take their vitamin C either in tablet form, to be chewed or swallowed, or in an effervescent form, which dissolves in water. Both forms are effective, and the effervescent variety is especially good if you have a sore throat.

The only caution we would make about the effervescent vitamin C is this: Do not drop a tablet into a glass of water and drink only half of it, planning to finish it later. Once dissolved in water, vitamin C is no longer as stable as in the dry state. Even within an hour or two, part of it will already have started to turn into its degradation product, dehydroascorbic acid—which is the opposite of vitamin C (ascorbic acid). (Thanks to stomach acids, this does *not* happen in your digestive system.)

As for the degradation of vitamin preparations in general, we suggest you take care, once a bottle is open, that the vitamins do not absorb moisture from the air and oxidize. Vitamin C is relatively stable if kept in a tightly closed container, but some of the B vitamins (our co-factors) spoil rapidly if exposed to air or humidity, and especially to light. The same is true for the triple amino acid glutathione in our anti-oxidant Menu (see pages 59 and 118–121), which is especially light-sensitive and vulnerable to oxidation.

Unfortunately, the difficulties with degraded vitamins don't begin with preparations that have been sitting for years in your medicine cabinet. We know of people who have bought already degraded vitamin

B_{12}, oxidized vitamin A, and peroxidized beta-carotene. We ourselves once got severe bellyaches from trying just one oxidized "high-potency" B-complex capsule of the off-brand type, distributed by a cut-rate outlet chain.

At this point, you may be wondering how vitamins that have already started to degrade can be sold in America. Doesn't the Food and Drug Administration (FDA) serve as a watchdog over this kind of thing? The unfortunate truth is that when it comes to degraded vitamins, you are really on your own. All the FDA is able to do presently is determine whether the strength per tablet listed on the label is still valid after a couple of years of storage.

To comply with this basic requirement, manufacturers market their product with what is known as "overage." Certain pharmaceutical calculations can predict how much of a certain substance will degrade over a particular period, and that amount is simply factored into the product. This ensures that at the end of two years the declared amount of the active ingredient will still be there and the labeling will be perfectly accurate—as far as it goes. It neglects to mention that 25 to 30 percent of the ingredients may have degraded into unknown or potentially toxic substances.

Since the directions on the labels clearly state that you are supposed to take only one to two tablets a day, the manufacturers are not particularly concerned about these toxic by-products. In the small recommended dosages, the impurities and degradation products are unlikely to cause much harm. The reasoning seems to be that if the consumer takes more than directed on the label and suffers from side effects, he has no one but himself to blame.

The trouble is, people who take only the suggested mini-doses of vitamins probably won't get much benefit from them and will soon stop taking them. And those who take higher doses than the manufacturer recommends—enough to make them work as anti-oxidants—may get sick from the impurities in the raw materials or from additives, or degradation products. Either way, vitamins get a bad name and consumers are deprived of the benefits of pure vitamins.

By now we hope to have given you some motivation to throw away those half-empty bottles of spoiled vitamins. It will free up some shelf space in your cabinet—and can free *you* to start our program of pure anti-oxidants and vitamin co-factors, explained in the chapters that follow.

CHAPTER 4

HOW ANTI-OXIDANTS CAN SUPPLEMENT GOOD DIET AND EXERCISE

A "prudent diet" like the one promoted by the American Heart Association—based on a modest cutback to 30 percent of calories from fat (far too modest, from our point of view) and encouraging greater consumption of complex carbohydrates, with less emphasis on meat—is certainly a step in the right direction.

The same is true for similar diets advocating greater consumption of fresh vegetables, fruits, and grains while drastically cutting back on fats. The most severe of these remedial diets is the one originated by the late Nathan Pritikin, a brilliant electronics engineer and inventor who devised it primarily to save his own life when he had advanced coronary heart disease.

The Pritikin diet is basically a high-complex-carbohydrate, low-fat, high-fiber diet in which fats (of *all* kinds) make up no more than 5 to 10 percent of total caloric intake. Over time, as Pritikin and more people like him benefited from it in dramatic ways, the Pritikin diet was publicized in book form and institutionalized as "The Pritikin Program for Diet and Exercise."*

* See Nathan Pritikin's book by the same title, first published in 1979 by Grosset and Dunlap and in a Bantam paperback 1980 edition. See also: *The Pritikin Promise—28 Days to a Longer, Healthier Life,* first published in 1983, then in a paperback edition by Pocket Books in 1985.

Pritikin believed vitamin supplements to be unnecessary for anyone on his type of diet. From his point of view, this belief was partly justified: If you eat plenty of fresh fruits and vegetables—especially raw—along with unprocessed grains, you're probably fairly safe without extra vitamins. You'll certainly be taking the ultraconservative minimum amounts of the Recommended Daily Allowances (RDAs) for vitamins. And since a person who is on the Pritikin diet gets hardly any oils and fats that could oxidize either outside or inside the body, there is perhaps not as much need for fat-soluble anti-oxidants like vitamin E or beta-carotene (pro-vitamin A) to counteract oxidation—although we would not want to bet our health on it.

We take a dim view of not taking supplemental vitamins and anti-oxidants even under the most "ideal" dietary conditions (this is not to say that we consider the Pritikin diet is "ideal" for *everybody,* even though it might well be just that for serious heart conditions or advanced diabetes). One must keep in mind that when Nathan Pritikin was saying that there was no need for adding vitamins to those already present in the foods in his diet, he was thinking of vitamins not as anti-oxidants and co-factors or co-antioxidants, but strictly as *food supplements.* He wasn't and isn't alone in this respect. Most physicians and nutritionists—unless they believe, like Dr. Demopoulos and ourselves—in the concept of oxidative damage to the molecular structure of our bodies—think of vitamins and other micronutrients only as food supplements and nothing else.

From this semantic confusion arises a host of other misunderstandings. Again and again, in our discussions with other health professionals who do not think of micronutrients in terms of potential anti-oxidants and free-radical quenchers, we find we are literally "talking by each other."

While traditional nutritionists see little need for supplemental vitamins and other micronutrients, given what they call a "well-balanced diet" (more about that later), we see many good reasons for such supplementation. Just to start with, there is our contaminated environment. From that there is no escape, either for the big-city dweller pounding the asphalt, or for the farmer walking on his own land. The EPA and the Public Health Service have just informed the American public that radon gas is so ubiquitous, and in such high concentrations, that it plays a major role in causing approximately twenty thousand lung cancers each year. We need not tell you about the polluted air most of us have to breathe, or about the many noxious substances in our water supply and our food. But we can tell you with a high degree of confidence that the supplemental anti-oxidants and vitamin co-antioxidants we recommend can be good insurance against all these environmental contaminants; at least, they have been so proven in many animal experiments. And even though there is as yet no absolute

ENVIRONMENTAL DETERMINANTS OF CANCER
Predominant Sets of Factors in Developing Cancer

Estimated Relative Percentage	Approximate Number of Such Cancer Deaths
35% of cancer deaths are predominantly due to smoking high-tar cigarettes and consuming excess amount of distilled liquor (this includes 90% of the cancers of the lungs, mouth, larynx, esophagus and liver, plus 40% of cancers of the urinary bladder).	350 cancer deaths/day
45% are predominantly caused by disordered nutrition, with the following subcategories: a) excess calories; b) excess fat ingestion, including saturated and unsaturated fats, as well as cholesterol; c) obesity, of a magnitude of 40 pounds or more overweight, for the average individual; d) nutritional deficiencies, especially dietary fiber and retinoids (the latter includes vitamin A deficiency; however, only the recommended daily allowance is needed; excesses are extremely dangerous).	
(The cancers that relate to disordered nutrition are mostly cancers of the colon, rectum, stomach, breast, and many of the cancers of the ovaries and endometrium.)	450 cancer deaths/day
5% or less of the present deaths are due predominantly to occupational exposures that occurred in the past when the dangers were not known (the cancers that are generally included represent a small proportion of the malignancies of the urinary bladder, lung, nasopharynx, stomach, hemolymphatic system, liver, bones and skin).	50 cancer deaths/day
3% are predominantly due to ionizing radiation; about ⅔ of these are due to "background" or naturally occurring radiation, and ⅓ to radical radiation.	30 cancer deaths/day
2% are due predominantly to pre-existing, benign medical disorders such as chronic fibrocystic disease of the breast, ulcerative colitis, regional enteritis, and chronic atrophic gastritis.	20 cancer deaths/day
1% are due predominantly to the administration of prescribed pharmaceutical agents such as cancer chemotherapeutics, excess estrogens in miscalculated estrogen-replacement therapy, and possibly some antihypertensive drugs.	10 cancer deaths/day

scientific proof that they work equally well with humans, we prefer to play it safe and take our chances *with* them rather than do without them. Medical researchers like Dr. Demopoulos of New York University, Dr. Denham Harman of the University of Nebraska, and others have for years been demonstrating the life-extending and protective effects of anti-oxidants against free-radical damage in countless animal experiments. Admittedly, that's still no absolute proof that it works the same way in humans. But one cannot very well expose humans to the same risks, just to satisfy all the Doubting Thomases.

Let's not delude ourselves: Even the vegetables, fruits, and grains on the best of diets are not free of residues from pesticides and chemical fertilizers, or possible contamination by the radiation treatment used to keep produce fresh longer. In addition, plants generate their own chemical defenses against insects and fungi, some of which can be very toxic even to humans (see the section "Toxicities in Natural Foods").

Meats, poultry, and seafood have of course their own toxicity problems: The growth-stimulating hormones given to cattle, the antibiotics in both cattle and poultry feed, the pollutants such as lead and mercury found in lakes, rivers, oceans—and fish. Here again there is good reason to believe that anti-oxidants provide at least some measure of protection from these chemical assaults.

There is legitimate hope too that anti-oxidants and their vitamin co-factors are able to blunt the destructive impact of the kinds of toxins most of us are voluntarily inviting into our systems. We need only mention the combustion products of tobacco and the metabolic products of alcohol—to say nothing of even more destructive substances.

Last but not least, there are the equally inescapable stresses and strains associated with living in a highly competitive, high-tech, high-pressure society. They also call for supplemental anti-oxidants and vitamins in very specific ways that should be understood in order to appreciate fully how they can help us deal with all kinds of physical and psychosocial stress.

Any kind of stress causes the massive release in our brain of a group of chemicals called *catecholamines.* One of them, adrenaline, is pumped into the bloodstream when we get angry or frightened and triggers the "fight-or-flight" mechanism. Mind-driven chemical secretions, such as adrenaline, are essential for survival in critical situations, but once the crisis is resolved they must be removed from our system as soon as possible. If they are not, the consequences are usually serious and sometimes fatal.

The dynamic involved in this destructive process is, once again, the production of free radicals: Each molecule of adrenaline produces two oxygen radicals as it metabolizes in the body. While nature has equipped us to handle the occasional release of small amounts of catecholamines and the free radicals generated thereby, too much is too much, and some damage to nerve cells and other tissue will result. Hence again the need for anti-oxidants to neutralize the free radicals released by the stress-induced production of adrenaline.

Society allows for only so much adrenaline-driven aggression: It's not advisable to beat up your boss or the cop at the corner! In fact, it may be that the high physical-assault rates among some socioeconomic groups are not only due to frustrations, economic problems, and other sociological factors but may also have to do with a deficiency of vitamin C in the diet. Vitamin C is known not only to have an energizing, but also a decidedly calming effect.

Another result of mental or physical stress is the release of an additional group of brain chemicals called *endorphins.* Endorphins function as tranquilizers, helping us to cope with stress. They are incidentally also responsible for the pleasant high that sometimes follows aerobic exercise. In more critical situations, endorphins can take the edge off intense physical pain—they are, after all, the body's chemical equivalent to morphine.

Again, too much of a good thing can be disastrous. With prolonged stress, our body tends to overproduce endorphins. The excessive supply causes these normally helpful brain chemicals to become potentially *neurosuppressive*—that is, they may prevent millions of nerve cells in our brain, heart, and the whole central nervous system from firing properly.

What's worse, the excess endorphins also become *immunosuppressive:* They weaken our resistance to disease by destroying the T4 (helper) cells, NK (natural killer) cells, and macrophages that make up the core of our immune system and protect us from invading bacteria, viruses, toxins, and cancer cells. The tragic consequences of destroying the immune system are all too visible in the disease of AIDS.

Still another result of the overproduction of endorphins and similar substances under stress is *hormonal suppression.* Our endocrine system is incredibly complex, consisting of delicate checks and balances among the various hormones. Upsetting this balance can have serious physical and mental consequences, including emotional disturbances, as well as sexual dysfunction and even cancer. All this is well known and amply documented in the scientific literature.

Taking all these factors together, their most outstanding and most visible effect is on mental health. If we need any further evidence of this, we have only to look at Valium sales in the United States. Over the past two decades billions of dollars' worth of this popular tranquilizer have been sold, making it the single biggest moneymaker on the ethical-drug market. Clearly, we are buying this drug because we need it to cope with the stresses in our lives. And so it goes with the rest of the tranquilizers, sleeping pills, and antidepressants that make fortunes for their manufacturers.

Even more money is being made on the *illicit* drug market—for the same reason. Street peddlers push uppers and downers. Mood improvers, from marijuana and hashish to crack and heroin, are readily available. Not that a drug like heroin makes people all that happy. But it does desensitize them neurologically to the point where no pain or stress can get through. The drug haze enfolds body and mind like a cocoon, which is one good reason drugs are so addictive.

Though the situation may not be quite so dramatic in the average middle-class household, it is frequently just as dangerous. Even in an environment free of illegal drugs, people come home from work mentally and physically depleted. Having to live day after day with such common stresses as time pressure, competition, job insecurity, and uncertainty about the future cannot help taking its toll on emotional equilibrium. Resulting tensions in relationships provoke further stress.

To feel better, or to help us cope, many of us might—quite understandably—have a couple of drinks, or cigarettes, or both. We might also try to console ourselves with favorite foods associated with good feelings, indulge our sweet tooth with candy, cakes, and ice cream. Again, it's only human . . . all too human! But the trouble is that most "solace foods" happen to be bad for us, just as we're not doing ourselves any favors by smoking and drinking to "relax" or "forget."

In all situations of emotional stress and mental fatigue for which people take legal and illegal drugs—and which frequently have far-reaching, devastating personal and social consequences—does it not seem reasonable to give anti-oxidants and vitamin co-factors a chance to prove *their* mood-enhancing and revitalizing capacities?

As if all this were not reason enough for taking anti-oxidants, medical experts estimate that 85 percent of all human cancers are in effect self-inflicted. Of the 1,000 cancer deaths that occur every day just in the United States, 350 are the direct result of tobacco and alcohol use or abuse. (Tobacco- and alcohol-related cancers include those of the mouth, esophagus, larynx, and, of course, the lungs.) But these substances also have an indirect effect on a number of other cancers.

Another 450 cancer deaths are caused by disordered nutrition. By that we mean the average American-European diet with its emphasis on meat, highly processed foods, excess fats, and cooking methods like deep-frying, barbecueing, and grilling, and its shortfalls of complex carbohydrates (vegetables, grains, and fruit), with a consequent lack of fiber. (Nor do the figures take into consideration other diet-related causes of death such as heart attack and stroke.)

Another 3 percent of cancers are caused by natural background radiation and from X rays, nuclear power plant accidents, and atmospheric tests of nuclear weapons. In addition, one thousand skin cancers are produced every day by ultraviolet irradiation, mostly a result of sunbathing. Fortunately, most of these skin cancers are of the relatively harmless basal-cell or squamous-cell types. Only about 4 percent are deadly melanomas, but that's 4 percent too many! (See our chapter "Sun Exposure: 'Deadly Pleasure #4.' ")

The important thing to note is that all these cancers are promoted or indirectly affected by free-radical activity—and that an unknown but presumably considerable percentage of them could undoubtedly be prevented by providing better anti-oxidant protection for ourselves. Ideally, the needed anti-oxidants and vitamin co-factors should come from both natural food sources and—because it is difficult if not impossible to get a sufficient degree of protection from food sources alone—from anti-oxidant supplements as well.

This is especially true for those of us who are interested not just in remaining in reasonably good health and not dying off prematurely, but also in peak performance and the prospect of extending our lives—in good health and for many, many years beyond the norm. Even to approach the present average life spans in good health, we are absolutely convinced that what is called for is not only stricter adherence to dietary ideals and physical fitness, but also anti-oxidants and vitamin co-factors.

In the chapters that follow, we will be telling you which anti-oxidants and co-factors we recommend for our daily anti-oxidant Menu, in what dosages they could be taken, the different safe ways in which you can put such a micronutrient Menu together, and the reasons why each anti-oxidant and co-factor is included.

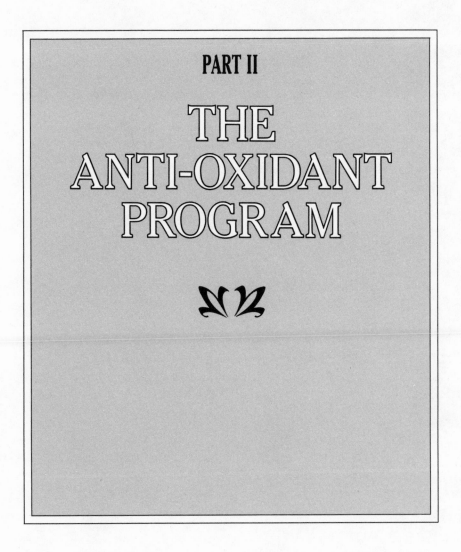

PART II

THE ANTI-OXIDANT PROGRAM

THE FULL MICRONUTRIENT MENU*

ANTI-OXIDANTS	PER SERVING
Ascorbic acid (vitamin C)	2,000 mg
D1-alpha tocopheryl acetate (vitamin E)	100 I.U.
Glutathione (a triple amino acid)	50–100 mg
Beta-carotene	15 mg†

ANTI-OXIDANT CO-FACTORS (B VITAMINS)

Thiamine (B_1)	80 mg
Riboflavin (B_2)	8 mg
Niacinamide	30 mg ⎧or 40 mg straight
Niacin (B_3)	10 mg ⎩niacin if preferred
Calcium pantothenate (B_5)	240 mg
Pyridoxine hydrochloride (B_6)	80 mg
Cyanocobalamin (B_{12})	400 mcg (micrograms)
Ergocalciferol (D_3)	125 I.U.

MINERALS

Calcium (as calcium carbonate)	250 mg

* We are following the spectrum of dosages of anti-oxidants and vitamin co-factors proposed by Harry B. Demopoulos, M.D. (*See* H. B. Demopoulos et al., "Free Radical Pathology: Rationale and Toxicology of Antioxidants and Other Supplements in Sports Medicine and Exercise Science." In: *Sport, Health, and Nutrition, The 1984 Olympic Scientific Congress Proceedings,* Vol. 2, F. I. Katch, ed. (Champaign, Ill.: Human Kinetics Publishers, Inc.).

† 15 mg of beta-carotene are potentially equivalent to 25,000 I.U. pro-vitamin A, if needed. Excess vitamin A, however, will not be formed. For best therapeutic effects, we recommend three full nutrient servings per day taken with your main meals (maximum, five per day).

The spectrum of anti-oxidants and vitamin co-factors on this program has been carefully worked out and tested over the years for safety and maximum effect by our medical consultant, Dr. Demopoulos. Every single micronutrient is included because it fulfills a specific role, either in quenching and scavenging free radicals, or in helping them to carry out these anti-oxidant functions.

However, only those substances have been included that also occur in many forms of nature, and to which the body is therefore already accustomed. True, this ultracautious attitude does, for the present, rule out some very promising and tempting substances which may someday turn out to be both life-extending and safe. But at our current state of knowledge, it seems more prudent not to include them in the program, and we advise you to do likewise.

Rest assured our program does include all the essential metabolic vitamins and other anti-oxidants you need to achieve your goals for optimum health protection, disease prevention, peak performance, and life extension. If, as we sincerely hope, anything new should be discovered in the future that can safely be added to the program, we fully intend to let you know about it in future updates of this book.

HOW TO IMPLEMENT THE ANTI-OXIDANT PROGRAM

Okay, you might say, I'd like to see what your anti-oxidant program can do for me, but how can I get on it?

Perhaps the best way of explaining how to get on our program would be to tell you how *not* to do it. Let's say for starters that the worst possible way would be simply to go to a health-food store or pharmacy and start taking bottles of vitamins and micronutrients off the shelves.

For one thing, micronutrients are commonly offered in various combinations—such as multivitamins, B-complex preparations, and so on—which usually provide too much of some substances and too little of others, making it practically impossible to get the right dosages. Micronutrient combinations of this kind may also include substances which—for good reasons—are *not* included on our program.

Individual vitamins and other micronutrients like glutathione and beta-carotene are of course also available. However, the prudent shopper would be well advised to stick wherever possible with the suppliers listed in Appendix C. Where that is not possible (for instance, in some areas outside the United States), great care should be taken to choose only top name brands, even if these products are considerably more expensive than others.

In other words, shopping for micronutrients to put yourself on an effective anti-oxidant program requires some planning and care. But we shall try to show that it's not all that difficult.

In the United States, there are basically three options of getting on the anti-oxidant program: Option 1 is to take the Performance Packs, formulated by Dr. Demopoulos,* which correspond exactly to the spectrum and dosages of micronutrients in the table on page 59.† Option 2 puts the same combination together with individual, ready-made micronutrients from various recommended suppliers. Option 3 shows you how to make your own anti-oxidant mix from micronutrient raw materials readily available in the USA. This latter option is obviously the most economical one, but it requires that you spend more time and effort than in using ready-made products, as in options 1 and 2.

OPTION 1

With this option you would simply use HMP's Performance Packs or Twinlab's new MaxiLIFE. The recommended dosages of these two products give you what we call "The Full Micronutrient Menu"—or the "Full Menu" for short—as in the table. The core of HMP's Performance Packs (each of which contains four capsules) are two large yellow capsules containing the vitamin C and all the B vitamins. Since HMP also offers these separately as Ascorbic-B capsules, which can be used instead of or to supplement the Performance Packs in order to achieve economies. For this reason, we actually use them twice a day between meals instead of the packs, as we shall explain more fully later on.

As far as Dr. Demopoulos's Performance Packs and Ascorbic-B capsules are concerned, we would only add that the technology of combining all those vitamin B co-factors with vitamin C in a single capsule, without their degrading each other, is not easy. Vitamin C, for instance, must be prevented from coming into direct contact with vitamin B_{12} lest it deactivate and spoil it. Obviously, you want to take as few capsules as possible, so this patented process has its advantages. However, we shall be telling you how to keep the number of capsules to a minimum, even if you are using other products (as in option 2).

In addition to the Ascorbic-B capsules, the Performance Packs also

* The Performance Packs are manufactured by Health Maintenance Programs Inc. (HMP), of Elmsford, New York.
† The new MaxiLIFE capsules by Twin Laboratories, Inc., Ronkonkoma, New York, also correspond roughly to the spectrum and dosages of anti-oxidants and vitamin co-factors shown in the table on page 59, only they also contain a number of optional but very well balanced minerals and trace elements, as well as a few other substances that are not included in our basic Demopoulos spectrum.

contain a capsule with the triple amino acid glutathione. Since glutathione is a very delicate and highly oxidizable substance, in this capsule it is put up with four times the amount of vitamin C to keep it in its "reduced," active state. (Do the same if you make your own mix!) It is not that oxidized (degraded) glutathione or, for that matter, degraded B_{12}, is known to do any outright harm, but if half the amount in the capsule has already been deactivated, it can't do you any good either.

Aside from the two Ascorbic-B capsules and the capsule with glutathione, including the additional vitamin C used as a preservative, each pack also contains a tiny soft-gel capsule, or "pearl," containing beta-carotene. The beta-carotene is put up with a small amount of liquid vitamin E acetate, which keeps the beta-carotene in its fresh, "reduced" state due to the lipoidal nature of the E acetate.

Included also is enough calcium (as calcium carbonate), together with just the right amount of vitamin D for better absorption.

So, if you take one of these Performance Packs at least three times a day, or the equivalent number of MaxiLIFE capsules, you are actually already on the program and don't need to take anything else. To our mind, that's quite frankly the "ideal" way of doing it, provided you live in the United States or, as of recently, in Europe.* It is, however, not necessarily the cheapest or by any means the only way of getting onto the program, as we shall explain under options 2 and 3.

OPTION 2

This option consists of implementing the program with ready-made, individual micronutrients obtained from high-quality suppliers (see Appendix C). There are both advantages and disadvantages in using option 2. It may not necessarily result in any savings, since here we are dealing again with ready-made products. However, it provides a feasible alternative. Also, it makes for greater flexibility in the program. It gives you the option of choosing between several excellent calcium products; or taking an only recently available type of beta-carotene, developed from clear-water algae; or using a sublingual micropill of vitamin B_{12} with excellent absorption qualities.

Obviously, taking option 2 involves more studying and shopping around to get everything in dosages that are as close as possible to those in the table on page 59. But doing so is important in order to be

* A Dutch firm, HB Healthy Body Products, Prinsclauslaan 4, 1171 LD Badhoevedort, Holland, is currently importing the Performance Packs and other Health Maintenance Programs products. From Holland, the products can be shipped duty-free within the entire Common Market area.

sure that you are getting a sufficient supply of every anti-oxidant and vitamin co-factor, while not taking too much of anything and maybe overdosing. (You will find detailed instructions on how to go about this in Appendix A.)

It should be fairly easy to use this option outside the United States, at least in Europe and in Japan. In both of these areas, high-quality micronutrients are available; in fact, practically all of the glutathione used in the United States is imported from Japan.

In many other areas—for instance, Central and South America—it might be impossible to put our program together with only locally available products. You will have to get supplies somehow from the United States, although, we know, since we live part of the year in Costa Rica, this can take some doing. But we still consider it a small price to pay to stay healthy and maybe enjoy life on the planet a few more years.

One more thing: Wherever you happen to be living, whether in the United States or abroad, please make sure to use only the very highest-quality micronutrients available. If you don't, you will run the risk of being subject to all kinds of allergic reactions from manufacturing contaminants we mentioned earlier.

This is not such a serious problem if you take vitamins the way people usually do, namely in only very small quantities, say, one to two tablets or capsules a day. But when you are taking them in higher dosages to function as anti-oxidants and co-factors, the common contaminants in inferior products can give you stomach pains, headaches, and other flulike symptoms.

OPTION 3

With this option, you can make your own micronutrient mix from commercially available powders based on the same spectrum and dosages as in the table. Although there are a number of suppliers of the necessary raw materials, we favor Vitamin Research Products of Mountain View, California, which seems to have the most complete list of pure USP pharmaceutical grade micronutrients in powder form. You can buy the powders in bulk instead of in capsules or tablets. Also—important for the beginner—the company's product catalog provides detailed instructions on the technicalities of mixing bulk vitamins and other substances in various proportions. They even offer several very useful and inexpensive gadgets like calibrated measuring spoons and simple chemical scales to make the job easier for you.

If you are on a very limited budget but are serious about getting on an effective anti-oxidant program, this is the way to go about it. The only drawback is of course that it takes more time. On the other hand, we know some people for whom making their own micronutrient mix has become an enjoyable activity that they look forward to on weekends. (See Appendix B for more information on this option.)

Just a word of caution before closing: If you use options 2 or 3, you will be dealing with suppliers who—although they utilize the highest-grade raw materials—also offer other products that we cannot recommend. Some of them produce broad-spectrum micronutrient preparations that contain all of the anti-oxidants and vitamin co-factors on our program. However, they may also contain substances that we and our medical consultants consider unwise to take at this point of our knowledge.

MORE IDEAS ON HOW TO ECONOMIZE

One way to economize on the program, if you use either option 2 or option 3, is to cut out the glutathione, which is the most expensive part of it. It would, however, really be a pity if you had to do this because glutathione is an important anti-oxidant and detoxifier.

On the other hand, if a cutback has to be made, this is the place to do it, no matter how regretfully. In our own case, we have opted for a compromise by taking the Full Menu three times a day, including the glutathione; but two additional times only we take what we call the "Short Order," namely vitamin C with all the B-vitamin co-factors. Another way to do it would be to make your own anti-oxidant mix (option 3), in which case you save so much, compared with using any ready-made products, that you'll probably find you can afford to include the glutathione.

On the other hand, if, like us, you are either too busy or don't want to make your own anti-oxidant mix, just take the vitamin C with all the B-vitamin co-factors in either option 1 or option 2, plus the vitamin E, beta-carotene, and one or the other recommended forms of calcium. We strongly feel that it would be a pity to have to strike any one of these vital anti-oxidants and co-factors from your list for economic reasons.

If there is absolutely no other choice, do take at least three to five times a day all the vitamin C and vitamin B co-factors, either as the rather inexpensive Ascorbic-B capsules (from HMP), or by combining the spectrum from individual, ready-made micronutrients (option 2). It would be even better, finances allowing, if you could add vitamin E to this combination, because it synergizes so well with vitamin C and will protect the fat molecules in your cell membranes from free-radical damage, something vitamin C cannot do.

If your finances improve—people who have changed to a healthier life-style often find their earning power increases dramatically—we would add the beta-carotene. This is especially important if you're past forty, because from then on, you can use all the anticancer protection you can get. Only after that—if a choice has to be made—would we add the glutathione. Not because we consider it only the "frosting on the cake"—it's far too important for that—but because it is more expensive than vitamin E and beta-carotene put together.

Let's hope you'll never have to compromise on your anti-oxidant program at all and can take the Full Menu all the way. However, many of us can have ups and downs in our financial fortunes, and sometimes we simply do have to cut corners. It is for that reason alone that we have added these words of counsel, giving you the same advice we would give ourselves.

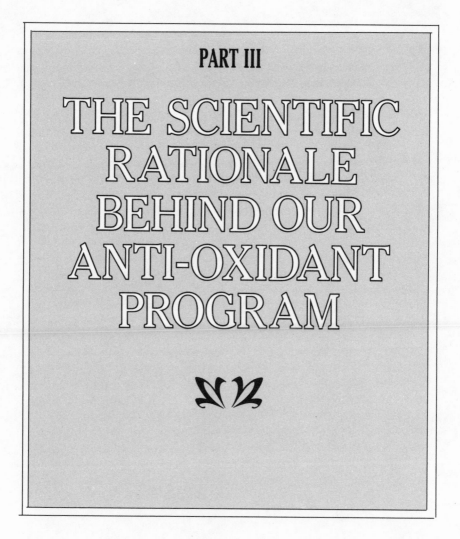

PART III

THE SCIENTIFIC RATIONALE BEHIND OUR ANTI-OXIDANT PROGRAM

CHAPTER 5

WHAT ARE FREE RADICALS AND ANTI-OXIDANTS?

2 In searching for a simple way to explain free radicals and anti-oxidants, we thought of the little boy who returned a book on penguins to his local library and said to the librarian, "It told me more about penguins than I really wanted to know."

Some of our readers are likely to be as fascinated as we are by the scientific nuts and bolts of biochemical processes, and for them we offer Chapter 6: a fairly detailed account of free-radical theory and the ways in which anti-oxidants work to protect our bodies against destructive free-radical processes. In this chapter, you will find some of the same information but in sharply abridged form.

Let's start by spelling out what is meant by "anti-oxidant." Simply put, an anti-oxidant is any substance that prevents another substance from getting oxidized.* In the food industry, for instance, anti-oxidants are used to prevent the oxidation, or spoiling, of foods. Manufacturers frequently add such man-made anti-oxidants as BHT (butylated hydroxytoluene) or BHA (butylated hydroxyanisole)—harmless in the small amounts in which they are used—to cooking oils, canned meats, and sausages to prevent the oxidation of the fats these products

---

* Oxidation is the combination of a substance with molecular oxygen (O_2), or a loss of hydrogen, or a loss of electrons.

contain, a process called *peroxidation.* * Vitamins like ascorbyl palmitate, the fat-soluble form of vitamin C, and the active (de-esterified)
form of vitamin E (alpha tocopherol) are also often used for that
purpose.

While these commercial applications of anti-oxidants are well known
and widely practiced, their use for preventive health care or in the
treatment of diseases is a truly novel and revolutionary concept based
on the free-radical theory. So exactly what, then, is a free radical?

Well, we all know that matter is made up of tiny particles, atoms, that
combine in any number of different ways to form molecules. Atoms
themselves consist of still tinier particles, one of which is the electron.
Electrons carry a negative electrical charge and revolve around a
positively charged nucleus.

The organs and tissues of our bodies are composed of stable
molecules and atoms, meaning that the electrons spinning around the
nucleus come in pairs and cancel out each other's electrical charge. A
stable molecule carries neither a positive nor a negative charge: It is
electrochemically neutral.

Some atoms and molecules, however, have only an odd or a single
electron in their outer circumference, or orbital. These are called *free
radicals.* They are electrochemically unbalanced and incomplete,
therefore highly unstable. Free radicals are also highly reactive: They
seek to combine with neighboring atoms or molecules to complete
their own configurations. The problem is that the single electrons of the
free radicals are highly "promiscuous," as scientists like to say. They
just love to break up the happy marriages of paired electrons in
neighboring molecules and steal an electron partner, thereby creating
hosts of other free radicals and setting up a vicious circle. That's the
bad news about free radicals on the loose.

The good news is that when free-radical reactions occur normally
and under the full control of our physiological mechanisms, they fulfill
a number of very useful functions. They are, for instance, responsible
for generating energy in our cells and in the production of melanin
pigment. The latter is crucial to human vision, for when a photon of
light impinges on the retina, melanin is needed for the conversion of
certain molecules without which we would not be able to form images
of what we see.

Also, there are free-radical reactions in nature without which life on
this planet would be unthinkable. For example, free radicals are
involved when light, working on the chlorophyll of plants, results in the
exchange of oxygen and carbon dioxide that produces the earth's
atmosphere. Similar free-radical reactions occur when UV (ultraviolet)

---

* Fats are oxidized by the effect of highly oxidized compounds (called peroxides), like
hydrogen peroxide (HO_2), which form during contact with oxygen.

light interacts with oxygen molecules (O_2) in the topmost layers of the stratosphere, producing ozone (O_3). The ozone in turn absorbs 98 percent of the sun's UV rays, thereby preventing the destruction of life on earth. We are all acutely aware of the vital importance of these matters as industrial pollution with chlorofluorocarbons is suspected of depleting the protective ozone shield above our planet.

But there is a very destructive side to free-radical activity and, hence, a need for anti-oxidant protection. Without such protection, free radicals can form branching chain reactions that are capable of doing enormous damage to the molecular structure of our cells. What's more, all this mischief is done within microseconds of time.

Given the need for anti-oxidants in the face of such real and ever present danger, where are they to come from?

One anti-oxidant is vitamin C. Scientists think that as "recently" as 250,000 years ago the human body was able to synthesize its own vitamin C. Somewhere along the line of evolution we lost that ability, so today we have to get our vitamin C from food sources and from vitamin supplements. Vitamin E, beta-carotene, and glutathione are also important dietary anti-oxidants. So are several other natural plant substances to be discussed later on. As for the B vitamins, they are, however, not so much true anti-oxidants in their own right as they are co-factors or co-antioxidants. That is, they assist the anti-oxidants proper to do their job better and for much longer periods of time than would be true without them.

We do, however, have three built-in enzyme systems (about which more later) that produce chemical substances (enzymes) that are highly effective in neutralizing oxygen-derived free radicals. It is safe to say that without them we wouldn't be able to survive.

These self-manufactured and food-derived anti-oxidants are usually sufficient until we reach our forties, although just *how* sufficient depends on such factors as stress, smoking, and drinking—not to mention what kind of food we're eating. But even under the most benign circumstances, by middle age, the store of anti-oxidants in our bodies begins to decline and the amount we obtain from our food can't take up the slack. It is then that the onset of the killer diseases usually occurs: cancer, heart attack, stroke, and so on. Prudence and common sense therefore suggest that people in their forties take serious measures to resupply their systems with anti-oxidants.

Better yet would be to begin doing so in childhood, gradually increasing anti-oxidant supplementation in adolescence and young adulthood to build a strong immune system and prevent later depletion of our anti-oxidant stores. We realize that this goal, however ideal, is not realistic. We'd be happy just to see our adult readers from as early on as possible pay increasing attention to their nutrition, make sure they get the right amount of exercise, and take our spectrum of anti-oxidants and vitamin co-factors. That way they would at least be spared most of the health problems of advancing age.

Still, it's unfortunate that more young people cannot be persuaded to take better care of themselves earlier in life. Ideally, this would include taking a broad spectrum of anti-oxidants, since even young and healthy bodies are subject to more free-radical activity than even the best nutrition and their own anti-oxidant enzyme systems can fully handle.

To repeat: Young and old, we are all under more stress than we ought to be. We breathe polluted air, we may be drinking polluted water, and we take in all sorts of toxins along with the food we eat. And many of us drink alcohol or smoke cigarettes. In short, nearly everyone—regardless of age or life-style—can benefit from an anti-oxidant program in addition to sound diet and regular exercise.

Before going on to all the practical applications of our anti-oxidant program, we would like to encourage you to read Chapter 6. In this chapter we explain precisely how free radicals affect our lives, the role of oxygen in free-radical activity, and how anti-oxidants protect us from life-threatening environmental hazards.

CHAPTER 6

THE FREE-RADICAL THEORY OF DISEASE AND AGING

The study of free radicals and the damage that their uncontrolled activity can do to all the organs of the body has led, for the first time in medical history, to a unified theory of disease and aging. Free-radical pathology (the study of disease processes associated with free-radical activity) has given us a better understanding not only of such degenerative diseases as atherosclerosis and cancer, but also of the aging process—the shrinking of the internal organs and the mental deterioration (senile dementia) that often accompanies it. Further, free-radical pathology plays a part in immune-system suppression and the body's resulting susceptibility to infectious diseases.

You will recall that any atom or molecule with a single or unpaired electron in its outer orbital is, by definition, a free radical. As the single electron spins around the atom's nucleus, it creates a weak but detectable magnetic field, measurable by electron paramagnetic resonance (EPR) spectrometry, also known as electron spin resonance (ESR) spectrometry.

We mentioned earlier that it is the extreme excitability of free radicals that makes them so dangerous to living organisms. Uncontrolled free-radical activity can tear apart cell membranes—and, in so doing, destroy many different types of molecules (proteins, carbohydrates, fatty acids, and phospholipids) in the various layers of the membranes and cell interiors. If we think of the molecules that make up cell membranes as their skeletal framework, the attack of free radicals on these critical components of our anatomical infrastructure literally breaks their bones.

By puncturing the cell membranes, free radicals cause cell fluids to leak out and, at the same time, prevent the intake of vital cell nutrients, literally starving the cells. Free radicals even attack the nucleic acids in the very heart of our cells—DNA and RNA—producing mutations in the chromosomes that carry the genetic blueprint. Mutant cells behave strangely, take on abnormal forms and shapes, and suddenly start reproducing wildly. In short, they cause cancer.

Free radicals also cause an uncontrolled fusion of large cell molecules, called *cross-linking*. This process is responsible, among other things, for hardening of artery walls, a factor in atherosclerosis and hypertension. Cross-linking is also responsible for removing the elastic "give" from lung tissue, causing the disease known as emphysema, a very serious condition usually associated with smoking. Cross-linking is involved in a process responsible for the wrinkling of skin and the loss of flexibility with age—just as it also takes part in rigor mortis, when there is no more anti-oxidant activity to counteract the rapid stiffening of body tissues.

Since most free radicals—superoxide, singlet oxygen, and the hydroxyls—are oxygen dependent, it's important to understand the critical role of this element in our body.

If molecules had faces, oxygen would be Janus-faced, one side smiling, one side scowling—or, perhaps, like the Hindu goddess Kali, bestowing life with one hand and snatching it away with the other. The destructive effects of oxygen are visible all around us. Witness rusty nails and screws, ugly brown spots on our car bumpers, corrosion on copper pipes, tarnish on silverware. Sliced apples turn brown, meat turns gray, fats and oils go rancid (peroxidize), all because of oxygen.

The production of ozone is typical of oxygen's two-faced nature. The same ozone that protects our atmosphere is a highly oxidized form of oxygen and a highly excitable gas that is inherently dangerous to humans. If we breathe it in by sitting under sunlamps, which generate oxygen through ultraviolet radiation, or by working for long periods of time with ozone-producing machines, ozone can become a threat to our health.

Oddly enough, the earth's atmosphere was originally devoid of molecular oxygen. Only with the development of the first life forms (similar to blue-green algae) was oxygen first released into the atmosphere as a by-product of photosynthesis. These primitive life forms utilized light energy to synthesize glucose via fermentation, without the need for oxygen. In so doing they generated oxygen as a by-product.

For the first time in evolutionary process, all living organisms had to contend with the accumulation of oxygen, both inside their cells and in the outside environment. This development forced plants and animals at this early stage to develop protective mechanisms for detoxification in order to defend themselves against the ravages of oxidation. Thus all botanic and zoologic life, while living off oxygen, developed endogenous (body-produced) anti-oxidants, without which the evolution of the human race would have been stopped dead in its tracks.

The reaction of anaerobic bacteria to oxygen dramatically illustrates this point. These organisms, having never developed anti-oxidant defenses, die instantly upon exposure to atmospheric oxygen. For example, when a patient is suffering from an anaerobic infection such as tetanus or gas gangrene, one good form of treatment is to get oxygen under high pressure (hyperbaric oxygen) into the infected area.

Unlike anaerobic bacteria, we humans, like all other living organisms, not only survive in the presence of oxygen but have in many ways prevailed over it. The human body has learned to use this highly toxic gas to its own advantage—we breathe in oxygen and metabolize it into the primary source of energy for our cells. But this delicate conversion process depends on the built-in anti-oxidant defenses nature has provided for us: first, our three free-radical–neutralizing enzyme systems; second, whatever anti-oxidants we can get from food sources.

As it happens, the various physiological mechanisms that utilize free radicals for our benefit are such marvels of efficiency that most of them are detoxified in the same process. However, a small percentage of highly reactive species of free radicals frequently escapes. We might visualize it as sparks escaping from a fireplace despite a protective screen.

One of the characteristics of this type of free radical is a tendency to generate chain reactions that rapidly branch right out of control. And it is precisely this uncontrolled free-radical activity that wreaks havoc with so many different systems in the human organism. Take, for example, the nervous system. Uncontrolled free-radical activity can upset the critical and delicate interrelationships of nerve chemicals upon which all our higher functions depend. Nerve cells "talk" to one another by making contact with each other's neural fibers (dendrites and axons) at synapses (points of junction). At these points, minute molecular droplets of chemicals, called *neurotransmitters,* are released. They are passed along certain routes in the brain or spinal cord to the target point and then removed or destroyed so that a particular transmission ends.

Dr. Demopoulos and his co-workers have demonstrated that if free-radical activity interferes with these exquisitely delicate neurological processes, the result will be distorted transmission or no transmission at all; the particular circuit involved, though anatomically still intact, will simply stop functioning. Such free-radical interferences in the central nervous system can have devastating effects on reflexes, organ regulation, muscle contractions, and control of blood flow, as well as on memory and learning ability. That's why ascorbic acid (vitamin C) is actually concentrated fifty to seventy times more in the brain and spinal cord than in other tissues, a protective mechanism that ensures that our vital central nervous system will always have the highest possible levels of this food-derived anti-oxidant.

Uncontrolled free-radical activity represents such a serious threat to cell integrity that it has to be promptly deactivated. This necessitates ample supplies of chain-breaking anti-oxidants that can readily donate hydrogen and then form stable molecules themselves to *stop* these runaway reactions. That's exactly what makes ascorbic acid (vitamin C) and alpha tocopherol (vitamin E) such good anti-oxidants.*

On the other hand, free-radical activity under proper control by the body can serve many useful, even essential functions. For example, the immune system can use potentially dangerous free radicals for our own protection.

Here's how it works: Two different types of white blood cells form an important part of the immune system. Some of these defender cells are called *PMNLs* (polymorpho-nuclear leukocytes); the others are very large cells, histiocyte macrophages, which circulate in our bloodstream and tissues. Both of these types of cells are usually inactive but can become highly aggressive when stimulated into action by some alarm system going off in the body (say, an inflammation) in which case they start gobbling up, PacMan-like, anything in the bloodstream or tissues—for instance, such "garbage" as rancid cholesterol, bacteria, viruses, even cancer cells. The most astonishing thing in all this is that to kill invading organisms, these cells actually generate superoxide and other free radicals that do the job.

Obviously, these toxic free radicals are able to kill not only the invading parasites but the leukocytes and macrophages as well. It's as if the "garbage collectors" were being killed while carrying out the garbage. But that doesn't need to happen—and, in fact, does *not* happen—if we provide additional anti-oxidant protection for our valiant defenders. To use another image: It's like putting firefighters into asbestos suits so they can go into the fire without getting burned up themselves.

Similarly, without certain controlled free-radical reactions, there would be no synthesis of the hormone-like prostaglandins and related

---

* These two vitamins are both members of the hydroxyl groups (-OH) of compounds that, after having donated hydrogen, become stable quinoid groups (= O). Likewise, glutathione, a member of the thiol (-SH-) group, can give up hydrogen, with the resulting sulfur free radical (S·), joining another sulfur radical (S·) to form a stable disulfide (-S-S).

compounds that regulate many of our physiological functions. Dr. Demopoulos and fellow researchers have speculated that the inability of many aged people to respond to infections with the normal inflammatory reaction or fever might be due to diminished prostaglandin production, in turn resulting from a disturbance of necessary, controlled free-radical reactions. The reasoning is that prostaglandins and related compounds, such as leucotrienes, act as agents in attracting helper leukocytes to zones of inflammation—in the same way that heat-sensitive missiles are guided to their targets.

Free radicals even play a role in the synthesis of major biomolecules (proteins, carbohydrates, lipids, and nucleic acids) and the detoxification of chemicals inside ultramicroscopic organelles (called *peroxisomes*) in the interior of cells. Also, normally occurring free-radical reactions play a part in generating cellular energy in the power-generating units of our cells called *mitochondria.*

These are the primary useful functions of controlled free-radical activity in the normal physiological processes on the molecular level. However, given the threat to the integrity of our cells from the uncontrolled activity of highly reactive species of free radicals, it is critical that we supply a steady and ample number of anti-oxidants to neutralize them. We have already touched briefly on the different mechanisms by which nature has provided a certain amount of anti-oxidant "insulation" for us. Most of the food-derived anti-oxidants and vitamin co-factors are substances that react one-on-one with free radicals. One molecule of beta-carotene, for instance, can react with and deactivate only one single oxygen radical and get used up in the process. Vitamin C, however, is twice as effective in that it can catch two free radicals and deactivate them, since it has two hydroxyl (–OH) groups.

More effective still are the three previously mentioned enzyme systems: superoxide dismutase (SOD), catalase, and glutathione peroxidase. In each system a single enzyme molecule can handle *several thousand* free radicals before the enzyme's protein structure breaks up. These enzymes also have the advantage of already being in place when a free-radical challenge occurs. It's similar to the fire department being already at the site of a fire before it starts. This is crucial because free-radical fires (chain reactions) can develop too rapidly for other anti-oxidants (such as those from food sources or supplements) to get to the right place soon enough to prevent damage.

The functioning of the three enzyme systems is interconnected, each system serving to reinforce the action of the others. For instance, in the process of deactivating superoxide, the enzyme superoxide dismutase (SOD) will throw off other free radicals, which then also have to be promptly deactivated. This is accomplished with equal efficiency by the enzyme catalase, which specifically decomposes hydrogen peroxide, one of the most dangerous by-products of the free-radical process.

Similarly, other challenges by free radicals are met by the third enzyme system of the human organism, glutathione peroxidase, which uses available selenium, an essential mineral nutrient, to fight them off. But this enzyme, too, can finally become depleted and need outside anti-oxidant reinforcements.

We can get the most abundant micronutrients with anti-oxidant properties from common food sources. The anti-oxidants include vitamin C from citrus fruits; beta-carotene and related carotenoids from carrots, squash, yams, sweet potatoes, green, leafy vegetables, and oranges; and alpha tocopherol (vitamin E) from grains. A large variety of food sources also provide us with the B-vitamin co-factors, which at times take on even more direct anti-oxidant functions.

Despite all these endogenous (body-made) and exogenous (food-derived) anti-oxidants, not all of the uncontrolled free-radical activity can always be neutralized. This means there's a cumulative effect of free-radical assaults over the years, against which we are about as defenseless as against the actions of terrorists.

How, for example, are we to protect ourselves adequately against environmental pollutants? Nor is the pollution all external: Most of us lay ourselves wide open to serious free-radical damage by eating peroxidized fats in aged cheeses and meats, or smoked and barbecued foods (full of highly dangerous hydrocarbons), to mention just a few of the worst offenders. In addition, some of us smoke tobacco, drink alcohol, or expose ourselves to free-radical attack through overexercising and overworking—in short, burning the candle at both ends.

Even nonsmokers who are very careful about what they eat and drink are not totally protected. Who, in our society, with all the cards stacked against sound nutrition and sane living, can follow an ideal diet *all* the time and avoid *all* the many traditional but ultimately unhealthy customs that we simply take for granted?

Not even the strictest vegetarian whose produce is organically grown is exempt. In the unlikely event that no chemical fertilizer or pesticide has come near a vegetable or piece of fruit, it will still not be completely toxin-free. Why? Because plants develop their own "pesticides"—self-protective substances concentrated mostly in the skin or seed shell—to discourage insects and other small predators.

Although these poisons usually are not in high enough concentrations to do any serious harm to large predators like ourselves, they nonetheless have to be deactivated and bound to some other substance in the body in order to be finally eliminated. In these chemical processes, too, free radicals are generated and anti-oxidants are needed.

The good news is that now, for the first time, there is something we can actually do to counteract and offset much of this free-radical damage, voluntary or not. We can eat plenty of vegetables and fruits high in anti-oxidants *and* supplement them with effective man-made anti-oxidants to quench and neutralize free radicals—even cut into their chain reactions.

Obviously, it is not just the older generation that is in dire need of anti-oxidants to maintain health, supply extra energy, and slow down the aging process. Younger people, too, are exposed to external and internal pollutants and typically experience intense school, career, marriage, or family stresses. Young or old, the way in which we live unavoidably suppresses the immune system and invites free-radical attack. That's why everybody needs protection to a greater or lesser extent. That protection calls for a steady supply of anti-oxidants. In fact, if our ultimate goals are not just survival in reasonably good health but peak performance, maximum immune protection, and age retardation, we need greater anti-oxidant supplies than can be gotten from even the most "ideal" diet. In the next chapter, we shall go into many other reasons why we feel so strongly that anti-oxidant supplementation is the most logical route to take.

ADDITIONAL BACKGROUND READING

Arfors, K. E., Chairman, Pharmacia Symposium No. 1. "Free radicals in medicine and biology." *Acta Physiol. Scand.* (Supplement 492), 1980; 492:1–153.

Bendich, A., P. Diapolito, E. Gabriel, and L. J. Machlin. "Interaction of dietary vitamin C and vitamin E in guinea pig immune responses to mitogens." *J. Nutr.,* 1984; 114:1588–1593.

Bendich, A., L. J. Machlin, O. Scandurra, G. W. Burton, and D. M. Wayner. "The antioxidant role of vitamin C." *Adv. Free Radical Biol. Med.,* 1986; 2:419–444.

Beutler, E., O. Duron, and B. M. Kelly. "Improved method for the determination of blood glutathione." *J. Lab. Clin. Med.,* 1963; 61:882–890.

Bielski, B. H. "Chemistry of ascorbic acid radicals. Ascorbic acid: chemistry, metabolism, and uses." *Adv. Chem. Ser.,* 1982; 200:81–100.

Bodannes, R. S. and P. C. Chan. "Ascorbic acid as a scavenger of singlet oxygen." *FEBS Lett.,* 1979; 105:195–196.

Bulkley, G. B. "The role of oxygen free radicals in human disease processes." *Surgery,* 1983; 94(3):407–411.

Burton, G. W., D. O. Foster, B. Perly, T. F. Slater, I.C.P. Smith, and K. U. Ingold. "Biological antioxidants." *Philos. Trans. R. Soc. Lond. B. Biol. Sci.,* 1985; 311:565–578.

Burton, G. W. and K. W. Ingold. "Beta carotene: an unusual type of lipid antioxidant." *Science,* 1984; 224:569–573.

Casaril, M., G. B. Gabrielli, S. Dusi, N. Nicoli, G. Bellisola, and R. Corrocher. "Decreased activity of liver glutathione peroxidase in human hepatocellular carcinoma." *Eur. J. Cancer Clin. Oncol.,* 1985; 21:941–944.

Cerutti, P. A. "Prooxidant states and tumor promotion." *Science,* 1985; 227:375–381.

Chow, C. K., R. R. Thacker, C. Changchit, R. B. Bridges, S. R. Rehm, J. Humble, and J. Turbeck. "Low levels of vitamin C and carotenes in plasma of cigarette smokers." *J. Am. Coll. Nutr.,* 1986; 5:305–312.

Cohen, G. "Oxidative Stress in the Nervous System." In: *Oxidative Stress.* H. Sies, ed. New York: Academic Press, 1985, pp. 383–403.

Combs, J. F., Jr. "Protective roles of minerals against free radical tissue damage." *Nutrition.* Bethesda, Md.: American Institute of Nutrition, 1987.

Corrocher, R., M. Casaril, G. Bellisola, G. B. Gabrielli, N. Nicoli, G. C. Guidi, and G. De Sandre. "Severe impairment of antioxidant system in human hepatoma." *Cancer,* 1986; 58:1658–1662.

Corrocher, R., M. Casaril, G. C. Guidi, G. B. Gabrielli, O. Miatto, and G. De Sandre. "Glutathione peroxidase and glutathione reductase activities of normal and pathologic human liver: Relationship with age." *Scand. J. Gastroenterol.,* 1980; 15:781–786.

Crump, B. J., et al. "Free radicals and alcoholism" (letter). *Lancet,* October 26, 1985; 955–956.

Cutler, R. G. "Aging and Oxygen Radicals." In: A. E. Taylor, *Physiology of Oxygen Radicals,* S. Matalon and P. A. Ward, eds. Bethesda, Md.: American Physiological Society, 1986, pp. 251–285.

Demopoulos, H. B., W. B. Jones, B. Lavietes, M. L. Seligman, P. Coleman, and R. Poser. "Manipulation of Free Radicals in Pigmented Melanomas: Effects on Metabolism and Growth." In: *Pigment Cell Biology,* Vol. 2. Basel: Karger, 1976, pp. 347–364.

Demopoulos, H. B., E. S. Flamm, M. L. Seligman, J. A. Mitamura, and J. Ransohoff. "Membrane perturbations in CNS injury: Theoretical basis for free radical damage and a review of the experimental data." In: *Neural Trauma, Seminars in Neurological Surgery,* Vol. IV, A. J. Popp, R. S. Burke, L. R. Nelson, and H. K. Kimelberg, eds. New York: Raven Press, 1979, pp. 63–68.

Demopoulos, H. B., D. D. Pietronigro, E. S. Flamm, and M. L. Seligman. "The possible role of free radical reactions in carcinogenesis." *J. Env. Path. and Toxicol.,* 1980; 3(4):273–303.

Demopoulos, H. B., E. S. Flamm, D. D. Pietronigro, and M. L. Seligman. "Free radical pathology and the microcirculation in the major central nervous system disorders." *Acta Physiol. Scand.* (Supplement 492), 1980; 91–120.

Demopoulos, H. B., E. S. Flamm, M. L. Seligman, and D. D. Pietronigro. "Oxygen Free Radicals in Central Nervous System Ischemia and Trauma." In: *Pathology of Oxygen.* A. Autor, ed. New York: Raven Press, 1980, pp. 127–155.

Demopoulos, H. B., et al. *The Possible Role of Free Radical Reactions, Cancer and the Environment.* Illinois: Pathotox Publishers, Inc., 1980, pp. 273–303.

Demopoulos, H. B., E. S. Flamm, M. L. Seligman, and D. D. Pietronigro, op. cit., 1982, pp. 127–155.

Demopoulos, H. B., E. S. Flamm, M. L. Seligman, D. D. Pietronigro, J. Tomasula, and V. DeCrescito. "Further studies on free radical pathology in the major central nervous system disorders: effect of very high doses of methylprednisolone on the functional outcome, morphology, and chemistry of experimental spinal cord impact injury." *Can. J. Physiol. Pharmacol.,* 1982; 60:1415–1424.

Demopoulos, H. B., D. D. Pietronigro, and M. L. Seligman. "The development of secondary pathology with free radical reactions as a threshold mechanism." *J. Am. Col. Toxicol,* 1983; 2(3): 173–184.

Demopoulos, H. B., E. S. Flamm, D. D. Pietronigro, and M. L. Seligman. "Free Radical Pathology and Antioxidants in Regional Cerebral Ischemia and Central Nervous System Trauma." In: *Anesthesia and Neurosurgery*, 2nd ed.,

James E. Cotrell and Herman Turndorf, eds. St. Louis, Mo.: C. V. Mosby Company, 1986, pp. 246–279.

Demopoulos, H. B., J. P. Santomier, M. L. Seligman, and D. D. Pietronigro. "Free Radical Pathology: Rationale and Toxicology of Antioxidants and Other Supplements in Sports Medicine and Exercise Science." In: *Sport, Health and Nutrition,* the 1984 Olympic Scientific Congress Proceedings, Vol. 2. Frank I. Katch, ed. Champaign, Ill.: Human Kinetics Publishers, Inc., 1986, pp. 139–189.

Demopoulos, H. B., M. L. Seligman, and E. S. Flamm. "The Role of Free Radical Pathology in Cerebral Ischemia and the Resulting Dementia." In: *Senile Dementia: Early Detection.* London, England: John Libbey and Company, Ltd., 1986, pp. 281–292.

Demopoulos, H. B. "Control of free radicals in the biologic systems." *Fed. Proc.,* 32:1903–1908, 1973a.

Demopoulos, H. B. "The basis of free radical pathology." Ibid., 1859–1861, 1973b.

Demopoulos, H. B., E. S. Flamm, M. L. Seligman, E. Jorgensen, and J. Ransohoff. "Antioxidant effects of barbiturates in model membranes undergoing free radical damage." *Acta Neurol. Scand.* (Supplement 64), 1977; 56:152.

Dormandy, T. C. "Free radicals and alcoholism" (letter). *Lancet,* October 26, 1985; 956.

Dormandy, T. L. "Free-radical oxidation and antioxidants." *Lancet,* March 25, 1978; 647–650.

Dormandy, T. L. "An approach to free radicals." *Lancet,* October 29, 1984; 1010–1014.

Fahrenholtz, S. R., F. H. Doleiden, A. M. Trozzolo, and A. A. Lamola. "On the quenching of singlet oxygen by alpha-tocopherol." *Photochem. Photobiol.,* 1974; 20: 505–509.

Fantone, J. C., and P. A. Ward. "Role of oxygen-derived free radicals and metabolites in leucocyte-dependent inflammatory reactions." *Am. J. Pathol.,* 1982; 107(3):397–418.

Fiala, S., A. Mohindru, W. G. Kettering, A. E. Fiala, and H. P. Morris. "Glutathione and gamma glutamyl transpeptidase in rat liver during chemical carcinogenesis." *J. Natl. Cancer Inst.,* 1976; 57:591–598.

Fink, R., et al. "Increased free radical activity in alcoholics." *Lancet,* August 10, 1985; 291–294.

Flamm, E. S., H. B. Demopoulos, M. L. Seligman, J. Tomasula, V. DeCrescito, and J. Ransohoff. "Ethanol potentiation of central nervous system trauma." *J. Neurosurgery,* 1977; 46:328–335.

Flamm, E. S., H. B. Demopoulos, M. L. Seligman, R. G. Poser, and J. Ransohoff. "Free radicals in cerebral ischemia." *Stroke,* 1978; 9:445–447.

Flamm, E. S., H. B. Demopoulos, M. L. Seligman, J. A. Mitamura, and J. Ransohoff. "Barbiturates and Free Radicals." In: *Neural Trauma,* pp. 289–296.

Flohe, L., R. Beckmann, H. Giertz, and G. Loschen. "Oxygen-centered free radicals as mediators of inflammation." In: *Oxidative Stress,* H. Sies, ed. New York: Academic Press, 1985, 405–437.

Freeman, B. A., and J. D. Crapo. "Biology of disease: free radicals and tissue injury." *Lab. Invest.,* 1982; 47:412–426.

Fridovich, I., and B. Freeman. "Antioxidant defenses in the lung." *Ann. Rev. Physiol.,* 1986; 48:693–792.

Fukuzawa, K., and J. M. Gebicki. "Oxidation of alpha tocopherol in micelles and liposomes by the hydroxyl, perhydroxyl, and superoxide free radicals." *Arch. Biochem. Biophys.,* 1983; 226:242–251.

Ganther, H. E., D. G. Hafeman, R. W. Lawrence, R. E. Serfass, and W. G.

Hockstra. "Selenium and Glutathione Peroxidase in Health and Disease. A Review." In: *Trace Elements in Human Health and Disease,* Vol. 2, Prascil, A., S. Prasad and D. Oberleas, eds. New York: Academic Press, 1976, pp. 165–235.

Garcia-Buñuel, Luis (letter). "Oxygen radicals and cell damage." *Lancet,* September 8, 1984, p. 577.

Gey, F. "On the antioxidation hypothesis with regard to atherosclerosis." *Bibl. Nutr. Dieta.,* 1986; 37:53–91.

Gey, L. F., G. B. Brubacher, and H. B. Stahelin. "Plasma levels of antioxidant vitamins in relation to ischaemic heart disease and cancer." *Am. J. Clin. Nutr.,* 1987; 45:1368–1377.

Girotti, A. W., et al. "Xanthine oxidase-catalyzed crosslinking of cell membrane proteins." *Arch. Biochem. Biophys.,* 1986; 251(2):639–653.

Halliwell, B., and J.M.C. Gutteridge. "Lipid peroxidation, oxygen radicals, cell damage, and antioxidant therapy." *Lancet,* June 23, 1984; 1:1396–1397.

Halliwell, B., and J.M.C. Gutteridge. *Free Radicals in Biology and Medicine.* Oxford, England: Clarendon, 1985.

Hemila, H., et al. "Activated polymorphonuclear leucocytes consume vitamin C." *FEBS Lett.,* 1985; 178:25–30.

Hirschelmann, R., and H. Bekemeier. "Effects of catalase, peroxidase, superoxide dismutase and 10 scavengers of oxygen radicals on carrageenin edema and adjuvant arthritis of rats." *Experientia* (Basel), 1981; 37:1313–1314.

Horvath, P. M., and C. Ip. "Synergistic effect of vitamin E and selenium on the chemo prevention of mammary carcinogenesis in rats." *Cancer Res.,* 1983; 43:5335–5341.

Jamieson, D., et al. "The relation of free radical production to hyperoxia." *Ann. Rev. Physiol.,* 1986; 48:703–719.

Johnson, J. E., Jr., R. Walford, D. Harman, and J. Miquel, eds. *Free Radicals, Aging, and Degenerative Diseases,* Vol. 8. New York: Alan R. Liss, Inc., 1986.

Kunert, K. J., and A. L. Tappel. "The effects of vitamin C on in vivo lipid peroxidation in guinea pigs as measured by pentane and ethane production." *Lipids,* 1983; 18:271–274.

Levin, S. A., with P. M. Kidd. *Antioxidant Adaptation. Its Role in Free Radical Pathology.* San Leandro, Calif.: Biocurrents Division, Allergy Research Group, 1985.

Littarru, G. P., S. Lippa, P. De Sole, A. Oradei, F. Dalla Torre, and M. Macri. "Quenching of singlet oxygen by d-alpha-tocopherol in human granulocytes." *Biochem. Biophys. Res. Commun.,* 1984; 119:1056–1061.

Machlin, L. J. *Vitamin E: A Comprehensive Treatise.* New York: Dekker, 1980.

Machlin, L. J., and A. Bendich. "Free radical tissue damage: protective role of antioxidant nutrients." *FASEB J.,* 1987; 1:441–445.

McCay, P. B. "Vitamin E: interactions with free radicals and ascorbate." *Ann. Rev. Nutr.,* 1985; 5:323–340.

McCord, J. M. "Oxygen-derived free radicals in postischemic tissue injury." *N. Eng. J. Med.,* 1985; 312:159.

Marx, J. L. "Oxygen free radicals linked to many diseases." *Research News,* January 30, 1987; *Science,* 235:249–531.

Mathews-Roth, M. M. "Beta carotene therapy for erythropoietic protoporphyria and other photosensitivity diseases." *Biochemie,* 1986; 68:875–884.

Mayne, S. T., and R. S. Parker. "Subcellular distribution of dietary beta carotene in chick liver." *Lipids,* 1986; 21:164–169.

Menkes, M. S., G. W. Comstock, J. P. Vuilleumier, J. P., K. J. Helsing, A. A. Rider, and R. Brookmeyer. "Serum beta carotene, vitamins A and E, selenium and the risk of lung cancer." *N. Eng. J. Med.,* 1986; 315:1250–1254.

"Metal chelation therapy, oxygen radicals, and human disease" (editorial). *Lancet,* January 19, 1985; 1:143.

Nishikimi, M. "Oxidation of ascorbic acid with superoxide anion generated by the xanthine-xanthine oxidase system." *Biochem. Biophys. Res. Commun.,* 1975; 63:463–468.

Novi, A. M. "Regression of aflatoxin B1-induced hepatocellular carcinomas by reduced glutathione." *Science,* 1981; 212:541–542.

Novi, A. M., R. Flörke, and M. Stukenkemper. "Glutathione and aflatoxin-B1-induced liver tumors: Requirement for an intact glutathione molecule for regression of malignancy in neoplastic tissue." *Ann. N.Y. Acad. Sci.,* 1982; 397:62–71.

"Oxygen radicals and cell damage" (letter). *Lancet,* 1984; 2:1095.

Ozawa, T., A. Hanaki, and M. Matsuo. "Reactions of superoxide ion with tocopherol and model compounds: correlation between the physiological activities of tocopherols and the concentration of chromanoxyl-radicals." *Biochem. Int.,* 1983; 6:685–692.

Peskin, A. V., Y. M. Koen, and I. B. Zbazky. "Superoxide dismutase and glutathione peroxidase activities in tumors." *FEBS Lett.,* 1978; 1:41–45.

Pietronigro, D. D., H. B. Demopoulos, M. Hovsepian, and E. S. Flamm. "Brain ascorbic acid depletion during cerebral ischemia." *Stroke,* 1982; 13:117.

Player, T. J., P. L. Mills, and A. A. Horton. "Age-dependent changes in rat liver microsomal and mitochondrial NADPH-dependent lipid peroxidation." *Biochem. Biophys. Res. Commun.,* 1977; 78:397–402.

Proc. Nutr. Soc., 1987; 46:1–156. Symposium on "Nutritional Aspects of Free Radicals."

Rose, P., et al. "Dietary antioxidants and chronic pancreatitis." *Human Nutrition: Clinical Nutrition,* 1986; 40C: 151–164.

Salonen, J. T., R. Salonen, R. Lappetelainen, P. Maenpaa, G. Alfthan, and P. Puska. "Risk of cancer in relation to serum concentrations of selenium and vitamins A and E: matched case-control analysis of prospective data." *Brit. Med. J.,* 1985; 290:417–420.

Seligman, M. L., E. S. Flamm, B. D. Goldstein, R. G. Poser, H. B. Demopoulos, and J. Ransohoff. "Spectrofluorescent detection of malonaldehyde as a measure of lipid free radical damage in response to ethanol potentiation of spinal cord trauma." *Lipids,* 1977; 12:945–950.

Sies, H. "Oxidative Stress: Introductory Remarks." In: *Oxidative Stress,* H. Sies, ed. New York: Academic Press, 1985, pp. 1–8.

Simmons, K. "Defense against free radicals has therapeutic implications" (Medical News). *JAMA,* 1984; 251(17):2187–2192.

Singh, T. S. "Oxygen radicals and cell damage" (letter). *Lancet,* September 8, 1984; 577.

Slater, T. F., et al. "Free radical mechanisms in relation to tissue injury." *Proc. Nutr. Soc.,* 1987; 46:1–12.

Slater, T. F. *Free Radical Mechanisms in Tissue Injury.* London: Pion, 1972.

Smith, M. T., and S. Thompson. "Free radicals and alcoholics" (letter). *Lancet,* October 5, 1985; 774–775.

Stähelin, H. B., F. Rösel, E. Buess, and G. Brubacher. "Cancer, vitamins, and plasma lipids: prospective Bosel study." *J. Natl. Cancer Inst.,* 1984; 73:1463–1468.

Taj, M., et al. "Free radicals and alcoholism" (letter). *Lancet,* October 26, 1985; p. 957.

Tate, R. M., and J. E. Repine. "Phagocytes, Oxygen Radicals and Lung Injury." In: *Free Radicals in Biology,* Vol. 6, W. A. Pryor, ed. New York: Academic Press, 1984, pp. 199–212.

Taylor, A. E., S. Matalon, and P. A. Ward, eds. *Physiology of oxygen radicals.* Bethesda, Md.: American Physiological Society, 1986.

Urbach, C., K. Hickman, and P. L. Harris. "Effect of individual vitamins A, C, E and carotene administered at high levels and their concentration in the blood." *Exp. Med. Surg.,* 1951; 10:7–20.

Vernie, L. N. "Selenium in carcinogenesis." *Biochem. Biophys. Acta,* 1984; 738:203–217.

Wirth, P. J., and S. S. Thorgeirsson. "Glutathione synthesis and degradation in fetal and adult rat liver and Novikoff hepatoma." *Cancer Res.,* 1978; 38:2861–2865.

CHAPTER 7

THE TROUBLE WITH THE "RECOMMENDED DAILY ALLOWANCES" (RDAS)

12 The careful reader will have noticed that the amounts of micro-nutrients (anti-oxidants and vitamin co-factors) shown on our peak-performance and life-extension Menu are often far in excess of the U.S. "Recommended Daily Allowances" (RDAs). This is worrisome to some people, since almost everyone has read somewhere that taking more of any micronutrient than the RDA might do more harm than good.

Statements of this type have been made by members of the medical profession, nutritionists, dietitians, and even consumer groups. Usually, the not-so-veiled implication is that the whole vitamin industry is ripping us off. The effect of the antivitamin propaganda is to scare the public away from micronutrient supplements altogether, which are characterized as useless at best, outright dangerous at worst.

In Chapter 3, "Why People Give Up on Vitamins," we went into some justifiable grounds for not using the cheaper, mass-market–type vitamins. They can indeed be useless and even harmful if taken in the higher dosages necessary for them to work effectively as anti-oxidants and co-factors. This is why we recommend only the highest-quality micronutrients.

As for the RDAs themselves, they do not relate to the concept of vitamins and other micronutrients used as anti-oxidants and co-antioxidants. They apply only to vitamins as constituents of foods or as food supplements.

The historical background of the RDAs lies in the not-so-distant past, when vitamin-deficiency diseases were rampant. During long voyages, more sailors died from scurvy—a disease caused by lack of vitamin C—than from shipwrecks or pirates. Back on shore, matters were not much better. Until the early 1900s, it was common for the rural poor of the American South to develop an odd disease, pellagra, whose symptoms mimicked those of schizophrenia and which was nicknamed "the 3 Ds," for dermatitis, diarrhea, and dementia, its symptoms.

Physicians of the day believed pellagra to be an infectious disease, a result of the poor sanitation in rural areas. However, it turned out that pellagra was actually caused by a vitamin deficiency—lack of niacin (vitamin B_3)—resulting from a diet based mainly on corn.

Pellagra, rarely seen in the United States today except in serious cases of chronic alcohol abuse or malnutrition, is still a very real problem among the Bantus of South Africa, in certain rural areas of Egypt, and among the maize (corn)-eating population of the Deccan Plateau in India. In the city of Hyderabad, pellagra still accounts for 8 to 10 percent of admissions to mental institutions.

At the same time that pellagra was rampant in the American South, the islands of Indonesia were the scene of another unusual medical drama. No sooner had the Dutch installed themselves on the island of Java than many of the natives fell ill with a mysterious disease that caused severe weakness, irritability, depression, and mental confusion. Nobody knew just what was wrong. The finger seemed to point at the Dutch—but why then were none of the Dutch getting sick?

It so happened that the Dutch, soon after their arrival, had installed rice mills on Java because it was much cheaper to process the rice on the spot rather than in Holland. They bought up practically all the rice from the villages, processed it into white rice, shipped most of it to Holland, and used the rest as wages for the Indonesians.

The Indonesians were pleased with this arrangement—white rice was the white man's food (surely superior to their own brown rice) and could be cooked much faster than brown rice (thus saving on firewood and on the time needed to prepare the family meal, which consisted of rice and little else).

No connection was made between the change in the traditional Indonesian diet and the onset of the new disease until a Dutch scientist on Java started feeding his chickens the white rice. They promptly got sick, whereupon his Indonesian housekeeper—thinking it a terrible waste to feed "good" white rice to sick chickens—obtained a sack of rice husks from the mill and fed that to the chickens instead. Within days the whole flock was well. And once the Dutch scientist convinced the authorities to give the Indonesians brown rice, the natives stopped getting sick as well.

This series of events led to the discovery of the thiamine deficiency called *beriberi*—the Indonesian term for "cannot do," expressive of the physical weakness that is one of the earliest and most characteristic symptoms of this disease. Most of the thiamine in rice is in the outer shell, which is removed in the milling process. The reason the Dutch on Java or in Holland didn't get sick was because, being more affluent than the native Indonesians, they ate a much more varied diet and thus obtained thiamine from other sources.

It is against this kind of background that one must view the U.S. Food and Drug Administration's noble resolve, some thirty years ago, to ensure that vitamin-deficiency diseases like scurvy, pellagra, and beriberi would remain forever diseases of the past. Working with the Food and Nutrition Board of the National Academy of Sciences, the FDA came up with a Recommended Daily Allowance (RDA) for the vitamins and minerals that, in the agency's own words, "people need each day to stay healthy."

What these scientists did, Dr. Roy Walford, a physician and life-extension researcher, has pointed out,[1] was to ask themselves, "How much vitamin C do you need to avoid scurvy? Well, it's not much. How much niacin to keep from getting pellagra? Again, not much," and so on down the line. Deficiency prevention was, then, the whole point—not *optimum* health or peak performance, and certainly not life extension. Further, the RDAs are based on the amounts of various nutrients present in the "typical American diet," no provision being made for sizable groups of people whose living conditions demand special nutritional attention. In fact, so large are these subgroups taken together that their numbers begin to look more like averages.

Take, for instance, the vitamin needs of all those who, like us (when not on our farm in Costa Rica), have to live and work in heavily polluted city environments, or have to work with toxic materials, as in many industrial plants, or have almost daily contact with dangerous pesticides, as in agriculture.

What about making allowance for the extra vitamin (read antioxidant) needs of heavy smokers? Or the millions of "social drinkers" who, though not qualifying as bona fide alcoholics, are under constant free-radical assault from the toxic metabolites of alcohol? And what about the special vitamin needs of women on oral contraceptives?

A particularly persuasive case can be made for the special micronutrient needs of pregnant and lactating women. Many a mother thinks that she can meet these special nutritional needs for herself and her baby by eating larger portions of food, especially meat for extra protein and dairy products for calcium. The trouble is that the extra protein will put more acid particles into the mother's bloodstream and leach out more calcium than all those glasses of milk and slices of cheese can supply.

The real problem is that a fetus needs extra amounts of micronutrients throughout the entire twenty-four hours of every day. The reason? During the first hours of the day and at night, the nutrient supply from the mother's regular diet is very low. The fetus, however, does not stop growing and needs the nutrients around the clock. Consequently, the most logical way for mothers to supply those needs is to take some specially formulated micronutrient supplements in the early morning and at bedtime.*

A similarly strong argument for micronutrient supplements can be made for the elderly. The diets of older people are notoriously deficient in vital nutrients. Yet few doctors will prescribe—or nursing homes provide—vitamins for them.

But to come back to the RDAs: It's interesting to note, as Durk Pearson and Sandy Shaw point out in *Life Extension,* that the National Research Council, on whose estimates the RDAs are based, has published much more generous nutrient requirements for laboratory animals than for humans. Monkeys and apes, for instance, have a recommended 100 milligrams of vitamin C per kilogram of food, *double* the RDA for human beings. And guinea pigs—which, like humans and the primates, are the only mammals that cannot make their own vitamin C—are allotted 200 milligrams per kilogram of food by the guidelines of the National Research Council,[2] or four times the amount recommended for human beings.

Food scientists at the Ralston Purina Company, which produces commercial feed for laboratory animals, apparently consider even these more generous allotments for animals to be insufficient. Ralston Purina Monkey Chow, a product widely used by zoos and laboratories, contains not 100 milligrams but 750 milligrams of vitamin C per kilogram of food, or thirteen times the RDA for humans!

There are such glaring discrepancies and contradictions in all these dietary recommendations that one does not know what to make of them all. We are not the first to suggest that the National Research Council take another look at the whole issue of micronutrients.

To arrive at an intelligent and informed decision on whether to take vitamins and other substances as anti-oxidants and co-factors in much higher dosages, we have to rely on specialists like Dr. Demopoulos, Dr. Linus Pauling, Dr. Denham Harman, and others who have given these matters considerable, informed thought. As Dr. Linus Pauling, winner of two Nobel Prizes but much criticized for his view that much larger

---

* Health Maintenance Programs (HMP) and two or three other manufacturers (e.g., Twinlab) market special micronutrient formulas for pregnant and lactating women. This, in fact, is one of the very few cases in which doctors are inclined to set aside their prejudices against vitamins and recommend supplements.

amounts of vitamins—especially of vitamin C—are needed than the RDAs provide, has stated: "They say the RDA is the amount needed to keep the average person in ordinary good health. I say it keeps them in ordinary bad health."[3]

SOURCES

1. Walford, R. *Maximum Life Span.* New York: Avon Books, 1984, pp. 136–137.
2. *Nutrient Requirements for Laboratory Animals,* No. 10, National Research Council, 1978, and *Nutrient Requirements for Nonhuman Primates,* No. 14, 1978.
3. Pauling, Linus. *How to Live Longer and Feel Better.* New York: W. H. Freeman & Company, 1986. See especially: Chapter 27, "The Low Toxicity of Vitamins," pp. 240–256; Pearson, Durk, and Sandy Shaw. *Life Extension.* New York: Warner Books, 1982. See especially: Part IV, Chapter 5, "FDA's Recommended Daily Allowances," pp. 392–407; Hendler, Sheldon S. *The Complete Guide to Anti-Aging Nutrients.* New York: Simon & Schuster, 1984, pp. 79–80; Berger, Stuart M. *How to Be Your Own Nutritionist.* New York: William Morrow, 1987, pp. 44–46; Johnson, J. E., Jr., R. Walford, D. Harman, and J. Miquel, eds. *Free Radicals, Aging, and Degenerative Diseases.* New York: Alan R. Liss, Inc., 1986.

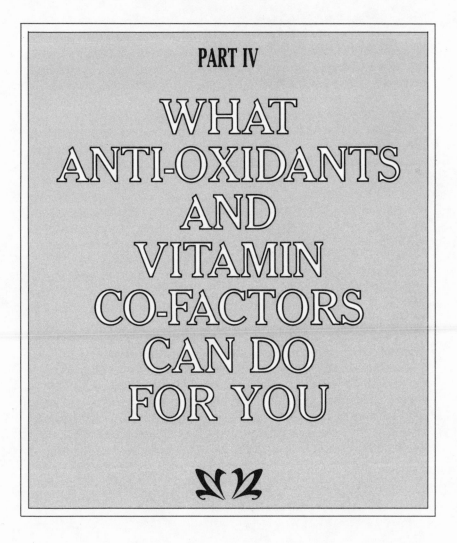

PART IV

WHAT ANTI-OXIDANTS AND VITAMIN CO-FACTORS CAN DO FOR YOU

Rule No. 1: Take only pure pharmaceutical (USP)-grade anti-oxidants and vitamin co-factors with no contaminants or additives.

Rule No. 2: Take these micronutrients in the recommended doses only—high enough to prevent free-radical damage, but not so high as to cause toxicities.

Rule No. 3: Take them only in a broad combination or spectrum, so that they can work together and recycle each other for maximum effectiveness.

I n observing these three basic rules, you are releasing the anti-oxidant power of each micronutrient, magnified by the power of all the other anti-oxidants and vitamin co-factors on our program. Technically this is called *synergism:* The interaction of the various nutrients with one another produces a total effect that is much greater than the sum of its parts.

But a great deal more is happening when you stop taking vitamins and other micronutrients haphazardly: One anti-oxidant, for instance, vitamin C, can help another one—say, vitamin E—stay active for much longer periods of time than if each were taken alone. Likewise, most of the B vitamins on the program not only provide specific benefits in their own right, but they also work as co-antioxidants to allow all the primary anti-oxidants—like vitamin C, vitamin E, beta-carotene, and glutathione—to keep on scavenging and quenching dangerous free radicals in your body much longer than would otherwise be possible.

Without this mutual protection that different micronutrients provide for each other when present in a sensible combination and dosage, some of the anti-oxidants themselves may actually become oxidized in the course of duty. When that happens, they can turn into other compounds that may be detrimental to your health.

For example, vitamin C could turn into its own toxic degradation product, dehydroascorbic acid (DHA). Other anti-oxidants, like glutathione and beta-carotene (pro-vitamin A), can oxidize into their own degradation products as well. Vitamin E (alpha tocopherol) can turn into tocopherol quinone, a very nasty substance indeed. Vitamin B_{12} also tends to degrade very quickly. All too often, these anti-oxidants have already started to go bad in the bottle—which they most certainly will if not properly preserved.* What's more, they can even become oxidized *after* you have taken them. In either case, they obviously

* That's why we are so fussy about recommending only micronutrients that we feel absolutely sure about and why we have added a list of trustworthy suppliers in Appendix C.

cannot do their job under these conditions. Having become free radicals themselves, they might be harmful to your health.

Again, the right way to take anti-oxidants and their vitamin co-factors is as part of a spectrum of mutually complementary micronutrients. Even Dr. Linus Pauling, a longtime advocate of high doses of vitamin C, recommends that it be taken along with other vitamins for best effect.

Which brings us to our fundamental rule:

> If you take vitamin C, you must also take vitamin E. If you take vitamin E, it's best also to take beta-carotene and glutathione. And if you take any of these anti-oxidants, you must take high doses of the B vitamins to provide a steady stream of electrons and hydrogen to reconstitute the anti-oxidants that would otherwise be sacrificed as they do their job of quenching free radicals.

CHAPTER 8

VITAMIN C

THE ANTI-OXIDANT THAT PREVENTS US FROM "RUSTING"

Let us start with the key anti-oxidant on our program—vitamin C, known chemically as ascorbic acid. In the first place, it is a first-class free-radical quencher. That's very important in itself, though there are other micronutrients—for instance, vitamin E, glutathione, and beta-carotene—that are also expert at rounding up dangerous free radicals.

What makes vitamin C so crucial for optimum heath is its ability to saturate every cell of the body, reaching not only very high blood serum levels, but impressively high tissue levels as well. It is the combination of these various properties of vitamin C that makes it the universal remedy for so many human ills, for which it has in recent times become increasingly and justifiably popular.

As already mentioned, most animals are able to produce vitamin C in their own bodies, while we humans cannot, though some scientists believe that a quarter-million years ago we probably could. The animals who *can* produce vitamin C must convert glucose in their livers, and glucose is the chief source of energy for living organisms. The amount of glucose in the body could become critical in a life-or-death fight where every last bit of energy counts. Therefore, humans probably have a survival advantage over other animals in not having to divert precious glucose to make vitamin C.

Some of the higher apes cannot make vitamin C either. The only other creatures sharing in this characteristic are the guinea pig, a rare

Indian fruit-eating bat, and a few equally rare Indian birds. The guinea pig also shares with us a susceptibility to a number of diseases, including diphtheria, pulmonary tuberculosis, and a type of viral leukemia that is indistinguishable from its human counterpart. None of the vitamin-C–synthesizing animals are subject to these human diseases.

If guinea pigs don't get enough vitamin C in their food, they develop a tendency toward a disease one would not expect these little animals to suffer from: atherosclerosis, the number-one vascular affliction of humans. Guinea pigs develop the same arterial lesions and high serum cholesterol levels as do we on the wrong kind of diet. But if they are given supplemental vitamin C, it inhibits the development of atherosclerosis.

Humans, of course, can also benefit from the atherosclerosis-inhibiting effect of vitamin C. Fifteen years ago, a carefully conducted study led by the same investigator (E. Ginter) who did the guinea pig study[1] showed that the cholesterol levels of people taking 500 milligrams of vitamin C three times a day were reduced by significant percentages. The vitamin C caused this reduction by encouraging the conversion of cholesterol into bile acids, which are eliminated in the feces.[2] But more important than vitamin C's cholesterol-lowering effect—vitamin B_3 (niacin) actually does an even better job of that—may be its ability, together with other anti-oxidants, like vitamin E, to prevent the oxidation of cholesterol and the other lipids in our arteries that form the dangerous atherosclerotic plaque.

Since humans can no longer synthesize vitamin C, can we get enough from food sources alone, as some claim? Are we really any better off in that respect than the guinea pig?

An animal weighing as much as an average human male, around 150 pounds, will make 10 grams of vitamin C per day, and several times more that amount when under stress. That's how cows, sheep, and large dogs get their vitamin C. But according to Linus Pauling, the most vitamin C humans can get from plant sources on an average 2,500-calorie diet would be 2.3 grams. His calculations also show that humans would need to drink more than 100 large glasses of orange juice daily to get 10 grams (10,000 milligrams) of vitamin C. The standard dosage on our program is 6 to 10 grams.

Why do we take so much? For one thing, vitamin C is absolutely vital to the human immune system. It leads to the production of more antibodies to fight infections. It also stimulates the activitiy of neutrophils and phagocytes, those white cells that identify, kill, and eat invading bacteria, viruses, arterial plaque, and even cancer cells. Vitamin C also enhances production of interferon, a protein with antiviral and anticancer properties that encourages antibody production.

VITAMIN C

(Ascorbic Acid)

Ascorbic acid

- is a key anti-oxidant (free-radical fighter).
- helps (with vitamin B_3) to control cholesterol.
- strengthens and protects the immune system (helps produce more antibodies, more leukocyte and phagocyte activity, more interferon).
- blunts the harmful effects of excessive endogenous opoids (endorphins) that are overproduced with stress (physical or psychological).
- helps to convert the amino acid tyrosine into adrenaline and other related neurotransmitters.
- fights cancer cells.
- is a helpful adjunct in radiation therapy.
- helps alleviate pain and fight inflammation (can be used instead of, or together with, aspirin, Tylenol, etc.).
- helps with allergies (makes antihistamines and asthma medication work better). Useful with insect bites; even makes snakebite serum work better.
- is good for wound healing, burns, etc.
- aids in recovery from heart attack.
- helps (with vitamin E) in preventing blood clots (thrombosis and embolism).
- is important in preparation for and after surgery, to prevent infections, speed healing, prevent deep vein clots.
- is useful in cases of male infertility.

A number of researchers have demonstrated for years that megadoses of vitamin C can either prevent the common cold or at least greatly reduce its debilitating effects and shorten the time it takes to get rid of it. We're convinced from our own experience that those for whom vitamin C doesn't work have simply not been taking enough of it. A realistic amount for someone suffering from a cold and not on a steady anti-oxidant program (people on our program rarely get colds or the flu) would be about 15 grams (15,000 milligrams) in divided doses throughout the day.

Of course, it is a serious mistake to start taking anti-oxidants only *after* getting sick. *Preventing* illness will become more important when you realize that every time you get sick, even with only a cold, you may suffer some residual damage that can shorten your life. On the other hand, every time you prevent an illness, you slow down the aging process and stand to live that much longer.

We were incredulous ourselves, at first, when we came across a reference by Dr. Robert Cathcart III, a physician specializing in vitamin C therapy, to "a 50-gram cold or a 100-gram cold." Surely 50,000 to 100,000 milligrams (12 to 25 teaspoons) was a fantastic amount of vitamin C to take in a twenty-four-hour period to fight a cold!* But when we both picked up a potent virus—the only one either of us has had since going on the anti-oxidant program—we discovered that Dr. Cathcart was possibly right. Instead of our being terribly ill for two weeks or more, the symptoms passed within a few days.

Dr. Cathcart advises to take ½ to 1 teaspoon of this vitamin C mixture every one to two hours, until you reach your bowel tolerance level— that is, until you develop diarrhea. Having reached that level, stay a little below that, but not too much. As you get better, you'll need less and will tolerate less vitamin C powder, so start gradually cutting down on the doses.

> To get rid of nasal congestion use sodium ascorbate, a form of vitamin C that is available in a health-food store or from one of the suppliers listed in Appendix C.
>
> Make a solution of 3 grams (about ½ teaspoon) of this powder in 100 milliliters (about ¼ cup) of water, and put 10 to 20 drops into each nostril with an eyedropper. It is at least as effective as any commercial decongestant advertised on TV, and much safer, not to mention cheaper.

You'll notice that if you have a cold, this therapy will dry up your sinuses. It will even dry up the mucous membranes of your mouth, so drink plenty of water!

We have more good news about this vitamin C therapy for upper respiratory infections: It actually prevents the lingering cough that usually hangs on, even after all other symptoms have long since disappeared. You do, however, have to keep on taking sufficient vitamin C and brave out some of the unavoidable discomfort (increased intestinal gas and more frequent bowel movements) to make this regimen really work for you.

---

* A very good way of taking such high doses of vitamin C is to use a highly buffered form. We like Twinlab's Ascorbate-C powder, or capsules, made from fully reacted calcium and magnesium ascorbates. For taking very large amounts of vitamin C, the powder is, of course, the only practical form.

A suggestion: Why not keep a supply of vitamin C powder mix on hand for emergency use? That way you won't have to scurry around shopping for it when the need arises. Besides, you'll get a jump on any incipient infection by having the perfect home remedy right at hand.

VITAMIN C COLD-FLU FORMULA*

Mix together 25 percent calcium ascorbate (a buffered form of vitamin C) and 75 percent crystalline ascorbic acid (pure vitamin C). Use powders only, not capsules or tablets, because of the large quantities involved. (Many health-food stores and pharmacies carry such powders; check Appendix C for mail-order suppliers.) In a pinch you can also use crystalline ascorbic-acid powder, which is sometimes more readily available than calcium ascorbate. In that case, take ¼ to ½ a Tums tablet every time you take the ascorbic acid.

Depending on the severity of your symptoms, take ½ to 1 level teaspon of ascorbic-acid powder or powder mix every hour during the day and as many times as you wake up during the night. (One teaspoon equals approximately 6,000 milligrams, i.e., 6 grams.) Wash the powder down with water; the taste is acidy but not disagreeable.

* Based on R. F. Cathcart, "The method of determining proper doses of vitamin C for the treatment of disease by titrating to bowel tolerance," *J. Orthomol. Psychiatry,* 1981; 10:125–132.

Dr. Cathcart has demonstrated that vitamin C in greater dosages than for the cold-flu formula can be effective against many other infectious diseases, including mononucleosis, viral hepatitis, viral pneumonia, tuberculosis, septicemia (blood poisoning), polio, encephalitis, measles, and herpes zoster. We're *not* suggesting that you should not take antibiotics or any other therapy your physician prescribes. We *are* saying that if you take lots of vitamin C too, you'll recover that much faster.

Dr. Cathcart has found that the sicker a patient is, the more vitamin C he or she needs and can tolerate before diarrhea results. When not sick or injured, most people cannot take more than 10 to 15 grams (10,000 to 15,000 milligrams) of the vitamin per day. Dr. Cathcart's "miraculous" finding is that when we become ill, or cut or burn ourselves, we can suddenly tolerate much more vitamin C than usual. The new tolerance level depends entirely on the severity of the illness or the seriousness of the injury.

We know we're sticking our necks out, but, yes, there's considerable evidence that vitamin C may help prevent and fight cancer. There are some suggestions, but no scientific proof that it might contribute to stopping abnormal cell development (mutation) through its anti-oxidant function, before the mutation becomes malignant. It works even better when given together with the two lipid (fat)-soluble anti-oxidants, vitamin E and beta-carotene, and better still if a third powerful anti-oxidant, glutathione, is added along with all the vitamin B co-factors, as in our program.[3]

One way in which vitamin C alone (and even more so in conjunction with vitamin E and vitamin B_5) helps prevent cancer of the colon is by not only scavenging free radicals in the area but also by speeding up the "transfer time" of foods passing through. The bacteria in the colon don't have much of a chance to produce mutagenic, cancer-causing toxins. If these toxins do develop, they won't stay in harmful contact with the intestinal mucous membranes for as long as usual, since they will be expelled by the increased peristaltic action encouraged by the vitamin C.

Dr. Pauling and his fellow researchers have found in studies of cancer patients that there is a very low concentration of vitamin C in these patients' blood plasma and in their leukocytes (the white cells of the blood whose chief function is to destroy invading bacteria, viruses, and cancer cells). If there isn't enough of the anti-oxidant vitamin C, the white cells can't do their job. Quite logically, Dr. Pauling and Dr. Cathcart suggest that cancer patients be given megadoses of vitamin C orally and intravenously in order to keep their bodily defenses as effective as possible. We would like to add that they should also be given other known cancer-fighting anti-oxidants such as vitamin E, beta-carotene, and glutathione.

Studies show that the characteristically low level of vitamin C in the urine of smokers is positively correlated to a higher incidence of bladder tumors.[4] When laboratory animals are given a dose of vitamin C corresponding to a human dosage of 1.5 grams per day, the vitamin appears to help prevent these tumors.[5]

It has been found that a toxic pellet implanted in the bladders of experimental mice produces tumors in the mice on a normal lab diet— and that no tumors develop if the animals are given extra vitamin C.[6]

Researchers have also found vitamin C to be helpful as an adjunct to radiation therapy for cancer patients. The vitamin seems to protect healthy tissue while increasing the response of the tumor to the radiation.[7] The researchers have thus far offered no apparent explanation for this phenomenon; but from the perspective of free-radical pathology, such findings are only to be expected. Radiation generates free radicals, and the introduction of an effective free-radical fighter such as vitamin C limits the damage. Since free radicals also play a direct role in the genesis of cancers, anti-oxidants add to the cancer-inhibiting effect of the radiation therapy while at the same time strengthening the patient's immune system.

High doses of anti-oxidants, of the type and dosages we are discussing, will not cancel out the antitumor effects of radiation or chemotherapy. While radiation and some cancer chemotherapeutic drugs work against tumors by causing free-radical reactions within the tumor cells, our anti-oxidant recommendations are not powerful enough to cancel out the antitumor effects that are concentrated in the tumors.

> We recommend high intake of a complete spectrum of anti-oxidants—with special emphasis, apart from vitamin C, on the proven anticancer nutrients alpha tocopherol (vitamin E), beta-carotene, and glutathione. Such a program is more important still for any cancer patient undergoing radiation or chemotherapy. (In this case, extra supplementation over and above our regular program is indicated for beta-carotene and glutathione.)

Even skeptics have come to admit that vitamin C—as well as vitamin E—has been shown effective against cancers of the upper respiratory organs. In one study, focusing specifically on cancer of the larynx, the effectiveness of vitamins C and E remained constant, even after adjusting for such factors as smoking and alcohol consumption.[8] These findings were confirmed by a 1986 Harvard University study on the protective effects of beta-carotene with regard to lung cancer and smoking.[9]

Vitamin C has recently been found remarkably effective against an abnormality in the cellular structure of the cervix that is known to be a forerunner of cervical cancer.[10]

Finally, there are the famous Pauling-Cameron (Vale of Leven) study, as well as a similar one conducted at the Fukuoka Hospital in Japan, involving vitamin C and terminal cancer patients. Both studies were conducted during the late 1970s, independently of each other, and both seemed to show definite positive gains from vitamin C therapy.[11] The patients treated with vitamin C lived on an average three hundred days longer than those without the benefit of extra vitamin C. A few of them actually continued to survive and remained symptom-free on continued megadoses of vitamin C, although detractors of Dr. Pauling are quick to point out that there are always some cases of spontaneous remission, regardless of the therapy used or if no therapy at all is administered.

The Mayo Clinic subsequently repeated theses studies without finding demonstrable benefits to the patients. The Mayo Clinic study was given wide publicity in this country by the media and used to refute, even ridicule, any anticancer claims for vitamin C. Dr. Pauling points out that "the Mayo Clinic doctors did not follow the protocols of those [Pauling/Cameron/Campbell] studies" and that their work therefore has "only small relevance to the question of how great the value of vitamin C is for cancer patients."[12] The Mayo Clinic gave the vitamin C in one dose, rather than in divided doses throughout the day, as in the Pauling/Cameron/Campbell protocols. Vitamin C is largely eliminated after four to six hours, so it is necessary to give divided doses for efficacy.

Without wishing to contribute further to this controversy, we might point out, however, that as a consequence of all the negative publicity surrounding Dr. Pauling's work, many cancer patients who had been taking vitamin C stopped taking it. To our minds, this is all the more regrettable, since—taking even the most conservative and skeptical position—vitamin C therapy would certainly have improved these patients' general health and strengthened their immune system, and at the very minimum, have had a beneficial effect on their illness.

Vitamin C's ability to help with pain and inflammation has been well documented.[13] According to Dr. Pauling, there is sufficient research indicating that vitamin C acts similarly to aspirin in inhibiting the synthesis of certain prostaglandins—(PGE_2 and PGF_2-alpha)— hormone-like secretions that play a part in inflammation, fever, and pain. However, in contrast to aspirin, vitamin C stimulates the production of another prostaglandin, PGE_1, needed for the production of lymphocytes (defender cells), which are such an important part of our immune system. Consequently, in the face of minor pain or discomfort, increasing your intake of vitamin C instead of reaching for the aspirin bottle might be a good idea. This is all the more advisable since aspirin is—contrary to popular opinion—a rather dangerous drug that can produce serious side effects (i.e., hemorrhaging in the brain; it is best to restrict aspirin to ½ tablet, twice a week, as a mild antiplatelet regimen, unless otherwise prescribed). On the other hand, if you find that vitamin C alone is not sufficient to kill enough of the pain or reduce the inflammation (for the latter you have to give the vitamin more time), take a little Tylenol or Advil/Nuprin along with the extra vitamin C. We have found that you don't need nearly as much other medication when you take it with plenty of vitamin C.

Vitamin C can greatly alleviate allergy problems associated with insect bites, asthma, and hay fever. Very high dosages can even slow down the massive histamine release that results from the painful and sometimes life-threatening effects of multiple bee stings, spider bites, or scorpion stings. Very high dosages can also boost the efficacy of conventional medical first-aid treatment for snakebite and for shock caused by a hypersensitivity toward certain drugs like penicillin.

Those of you on our anti-oxidant program already have partial protection from allergic reactions, including hay fever and asthma. We suggest that if you are prone to hay-fever attacks you should always carry some extra vitamin C to take with your prescribed medication.

If you are going into areas where there's a risk of poisonous insect or snakebites, you might have your doctor make up a kit containing snakebite serum, epinephrine, and antihistamine, together with instructions for using them in emergencies. Needless to say, you should add a small jar of crystalline vitamin C to the kit.

Vitamin C is needed for the production of collagen and elastin, proteins that hold the warp and woof of our tissues together. (Without them we would literally fall apart.) Norman Cousins, who gives much credit for his recovery from a most serious collagen disease to his large intake of vitamin C, has the following to say: "Additional supporting data on the improvement in my condition after taking ascorbic acid came from the Lederle Laboratories. Drs. Arnold Oronsky and Suresh Kewar reported on research in their laboratories showing that ascorbic acid is essential for the proper functioning of prolylhydroxylase, which in turn is essential for the synthesis of collagen. The significance of ascorbate in the treatment of collagen diseases such as arthritis, therefore, seems compelling."*

Vitamin C is an important factor in wound healing and repair of bone fractures. When the body is wounded or burned, it diverts as much vitamin C as it can spare (and often more!) to the site of the injury. Because the vitamin, while promoting healing, turns into its metabolite (dehydroascorbic acid), there has to be a constant new supply of it to make up for that lost during the healing.

We also highly recommend additional amounts of glutathione in injury and burn cases, even for people already on our basic program.

Vitamin C and other anti-oxidants encourage faster recovery from heart attacks. Cardiologists are learning this very well and are using them in some sophisticated heart centers. It is also interesting to note that white blood cells rush vitamin C to the heart from other organs after a heart attack, even at the risk of dangerous deficiencies in the donor organs.[14] Vitamin C and other anti-oxidants protect the oxygen-deprived (ischemic) area of the heart from further free-radical damage. Here, clearly, is another situation calling for emergency megadoses of vitamin C and certain companion anti-oxidants.

A combination of vitamins C and E is also effective in helping to prevent blood clots. This can be life-saving for patients in danger of developing deep vein clots, or at high risk for stroke. There are even

* Norman Cousins, *Anatomy of an Illness as Perceived by the Patient* (New York: W. W. Norton, 1979), p. 140.

studies that substantiate the role of vitamin C alone as an anticoagulant, a fact previously known only from clinical experience.[15]

Another reliable study shows that even a single intravenous administration of 2 grams of vitamin C can prevent the clumping of blood platelets. Platelets, irregularly shaped disks, can combine with cholesterol and other rancid fats in our arteries and veins to cause the *embolisms* that so often lead to stroke, heart attack, and other complications like varicose veins, ulcers, and thrombophlebitis.[16]

Those of us who are on an effective vitamin/anti-oxidant program that includes at least 6,000 milligrams of vitamin C need not worry too much about this problem. Experience has demonstrated that doses of 6,000 to 10,000 milligrams of vitamin C—especially in conjunction with 300 to 500 I.U. of pure liquid vitamin E—seem sufficient to prevent platelet aggregation and dangerous blood clotting.

Recent evidence suggests that vitamin C can help in cases of male infertility due to agglutination, the clumping together of sperm cells. In this condition, the motility of the sperm is inhibited and few if any sperm ever make it near the egg. Studies showed that when young, infertile men were given vitamin C supplements of 1 gram per day, even for just a few days, sperm motility reached normal levels. A high proportion of the young men involved were almost immediately able to impregnate their partners.[17]

In our bodies vitamin C acts like a major detoxification system. It does so by means of its ability to stop the superoxide radicals $\cdot\,O_2^-$ in their tracks before they get out of line and exceed their normal functions (just as other "radicals" are known to do!). You must understand that these superoxide radicals are perfectly normal byproducts of the body's metabolism. They are formed by respiration and a number of enzymes. However, there may get to be more of them than our built-in anti-oxidant systems can handle—for example, if we have to breathe polluted air from car exhaust, tobacco smoke, or anything else burning—not to mention city air, which all too often contains dangerous levels of ozone from industrial pollution.

Fortunately, there is plenty of evidence that ascorbic acid can protect our lungs against the destructive action of free radicals. We know this by the fact that ascorbic acid is found in lung fluid. The ability of vitamin C to protect us against chemical pollutants is also demonstrated by ascorbic acid having been shown to lower the mortality of laboratory rats exposed to cancer-causing carbon tetrachloride (that chemical we smell in dry-cleaning fluid). There are studies showing that vitamin C may even be important in preventing free-radical damage in the central nervous system.

In the Demopoulos spectrum of anti-oxidants, vitamin C also serves to "sacrificially stabilize" the vitamin E. Sometimes the chemical reaction also proceeds in the opposite direction, with vitamin E protecting the vitamin C. Basically, however, it is the B-vitamin co-factors that provide, as pointed out earlier, the steady stream of hydrogen and electrons to regenerate the spent vitamin C.

A WORD OF CAUTION

You may have heard or read about the danger of oxalate kidney stones forming as a result of taking vitamin C. The fact is that the percentage of people who develop kidney stones is exactly the same for those who take vitamin C supplements as for those in the general population.

One type of kidney stone—about 50 percent of all such stones—is typical for alkaline urine. In those cases, vitamin C actually helps to acidify the urine and prevent these stones from developing.

Another type of stone is produced by the opposite condition: If the urine is very acidic, it can lead to the formation of stones made up of calcium oxalate, uric acid crystals, or cystine. Dr. Pauling suggests taking vitamin C as sodium ascorbate or to take baking soda or some other type of alkalizer along with the regular ascorbic acid. Be certain to discuss this course of action with your doctor, because you don't want to increase your sodium intake if you suffer from hypertension or coronary heart disease.*

Dr. Demopoulos agrees with Dr. Pauling that there may be some people who have an abnormal tendency to form oxalate kidney stones. Vitamin C could possibly increase that tendency. If you have a history of forming oxalate kidney stones—you should probably refrain from taking supplemental vitamin C despite all its therapeutic benefits. By the same token, you should also avoid eating rhubarb and spinach as well as other plants containing larger amounts of oxalic acid. Above all, CONSULT A DOCTOR WHO IS KNOWLEDGEABLE ABOUT NUTRITION.

BIOFLAVONOIDS: THE OTHER HALF OF THE VITAMIN C EQUATION?

In 1928 a famous European scientist, Dr. Szent-Gyorgyi, discovered ascorbic acid. Shortly afterward, a friend of his developed bleeding gums. Dr. Szent-Gyorgyi thought that since this type of capillary

---

* New research seems to indicate that only sodium chloride (table salt), but no other sodium combination, causes hypertension.

breakdown was also one of the well-known symptoms of scurvy—long recognized as being caused by a deficiency in the substance he had just discovered—having his friend take some of it might help. All he had at the time was some raw vitamin C that still contained natural "contaminants," compounds of the citrus fruits from which he had derived the vitamin. On the theory that raw or unrefined vitamin C was better than no vitamin C, he let his friend try some of it.

The man's gums soon stopped bleeding and healed up very nicely. But since he ate very few vegetables and fruits, a year later he was back again with bleeding gums. This time Dr. Szent-Gyorgyi did not hesitate. Having now succeeded in purifying his ascorbic acid, he proudly gave his friend some of the "new, improved" vitamin C. This time, the magic did not work. When the man's gums refused to stop bleeding, Dr. Szent-Gyorgyi considered the possibility that the natural "contaminants" in the earlier raw vitamin C, rather than the vitamin itself, might have produced the healing effect. He decided to try treating the man with the "contaminants" alone—and, sure enough, they did the trick. We now know why: bioflavonoids are able to stabilize the membranes of our capillaries.

From then on, Dr. Szent-Gyorgyi was convinced that bioflavonoids—certain substances in the white skin and pith of citrus fruit, but present also in apricots, blackberries, and cherries—*alone* could heal scurvy and quite a few other diseases.

And so for a while thousands of European and many American physicians happily prescribed bioflavonoids, either alone or as part of the treatment, for numerous afflictions. Then in 1968, a Massachusetts physician, Edme Regnier, reported having treated groups of patients with colds in three different ways: (1) with ascorbic acid (vitamin C) alone; (2) with ascorbic acid plus bioflavonoids; (3) with bioflavonoids alone. A fourth, control, group was given a placebo. The result? Dr. Regnier had about the same success with the ascorbic-acid-plus-bioflavonoid treatment as with ascorbic acid alone. But giving people bioflavonoids alone helped no more than did giving them a placebo.[18]

That same year, 1968, the FDA decided to come out strongly against bioflavonoids on the grounds that they were allegedly "ineffective" in humans, though no claim was made that they were harmful. American physicians stopped prescribing them, but people did not stop buying bioflavonoids in health-food stores and taking them along with vitamin C—the popular notion being that we need them to make proper or optimal use of vitamin C. In all this controversy, the original, scientifically more valid reason for taking bioflavonoids—to help protect our *capillaries*—had somehow gotten lost.

Doctors are, however, again starting to prescribe bioflavonoids—albeit more selectively and not as a panacea—for specific capillary problems. It's reasonable to assume that people suffering from herpes lesions, for instance, may derive significant benefits from taking additional bioflavonoids. Otherwise we see no good reason for taking bioflavonoids in the form of supplements so long as we are eating whole citrus fruits rather than drinking just the juice.

SOURCES

1. Ginter, E., et al. "The influence of chronic vitamin C deficiency on fatty acid composition of blood serum liver triglycerides and cholesterol esters in guinea pigs." *J. Nutr.,* 1969; 99:261–266.
2. Ginter, E. "Cholesterol: Vitamin C controls its transformation to bile acids." *Science,* 1973; 179:702–704.
3. Hendler, Sheldon S. *The Complete Guide to Anti-Aging Nutrients.* New York: Simon and Schuster, A Fireside Book, 1984. See especially: pp. 61–63, "Why Supplements Should Help Antioxidant Impact on Cancer and Other Age-Related Diseases." Also: Pauling, Linus. *How to Live Longer and Feel Better.* New York: W. H. Freeman & Company, 1986.
4. Schlegel, J. U., et al. "Urine composition in the etiology of bladder tumor formation." *J. Urol.,* 1967; 97:479–481.
5. Schlegel, J. U., et al. "The role of ascorbic acid in the prevention of bladder tumor formation." *J. Urol.,* 1970; 103:155–159.
6. Schlegel, J. U., et al. "Studies in the etiology and prevention of bladder carcinoma." *J. Urol.,* 1980; 101:317–324.
7. Cheraskin, E., et al. "Effect of diet upon radiation response in cervical carcinoma of the uterus: A preliminary report." *Acta Cytologica,* 1968; 12:433–438.
8. Graham, S., et al. "Dietary factors in the epidemiology of cancer of the larynx." *Am. J. Epidem.,* 1981; 113(6):675–677.
9. Menkes, Marilyn S., G. W. Comstock, et al. "Serum beta carotene, vitamins A and E, selenium, and the risk of lung cancer." *N. Engl. J. Med.,* 1986; 315(20):1250–1289.
10. Wassertheil-Smoller, S., et al. "Dietary vitamin C and uterine cancer." *Am. J. Epidem.,* 1981; 114:714–724. Also: *Internal Medicine News,* 1983; 16(10):49.
11. Pauling, L., *op. cit.,* pp. 173–179.
12. Ibid.
13. Cameron, E., and A. Campbell. "The orthomolecular treatment of cancer. II. Clinical trial of high-dose ascorbic supplements in advanced human cancer." *Chem. Biol. Interacts,* 1974; 9:285–315.
14. Hume, R., et al. "Leucocyte ascorbic acid levels after acute myocardial infarction." *Brit. Heart J.,* 1972; 34:238–243.
15. See two editorials in *Lancet,* 1973; 2:199–201. Also: Sarji, et al. *Thrombosis Research,* 1979; 15:639–644, and *Atherosclerosis,* 1980; 35:181.
16. Cardova, C., et al. "Influence of ascorbic acid on platelet aggregation in vitro and in vivo." *Atherosclerosis,* 1982; 41:15–19.
17. Gonzalez, Elizabeth R. "Sperm swim singly after vitamin C therapy." *JAMA,* 1983; 249:2747–2751.
18. Regnier, E. "The administration of large doses of ascorbic acid in the prevention and treatment of the common cold, Parts I and II." *Review of Allergy,* 1968; 22:835–846, and 948–956.

CHAPTER 9

VITAMIN E

THE ANTI-"RANCIDITY" VITAMIN

M "Man is rusting and going rancid simultaneously," as Dr. Sigmund A. Weitzman, a noted medical scientist at Northwestern Medical University, once remarked at a conference dedicated to discussing the damage that free radicals can do to the molecular structure of our cells.

"Rusting" and "rotting" (going rancid) are both caused by oxidation, albeit by different types, and oxygen-derived free radicals are always involved. However, the "rusting" is more like the oxidation reactions in our connective tissues (skin, ligaments) that render us progressively less flexible (cross-linking). That's why we sometimes talk of "creaky" bones and joints. In that respect, we are very much like any piece of machinery that has been left unprotected from the elements and whose moving parts can no longer move freely because they have accumulated rust.

The other type of oxidation—which can be likened to "rotting"— happens when the fat molecules in our cell membranes spontaneously oxidize under free-radical attacks from the oxidative compounds in smog, cigarette smoke, or the toxic metabolites of alcohol. This rancidification of fats in our tissues is what causes the gradual dropping out—literally the rotting—of millions and trillions of cells over the years, leading to the progressive shrinkage of all our internal organs with age (see page 223).

To prevent or undo the rusting type of oxidative damage, vitamin C is the anti-oxidant of choice. But vitamin C is water soluble and therefore cannot work in fatty tissue. For that reason, it cannot work against the

VITAMIN E

(Dl-Alpha Tocopheryl Acetate)

Vitamin E
- protects cell membranes against free-radical attack.
- prevents rancidification of body fats (e.g., cholesterol).
- helps prevent blood clots (thrombosis).
- encourages production of the Teflon-like coating (prostacyclin, or PGI_2) for the inside lining of the arteries, thereby providing protection against atherosclerosis and heart attack.
- is good for prevention and treatment of nonmalignant breast tumors (fibrocystic breast disease).
- is helpful in prevention and treatment of breast cancer.
- is the only known remedy for painful cramping in legs and arms (intermittent claudication).
- protects against many environmental pollutants (especially in the lung cells).
- is good for hair and skin.
- improves the quality of sleep.

rotting, or rancidification, of fat molecules in our cell membranes and other tissues. That's where lipid-soluble vitamin E comes in handy because it can go to work in all those places vitamin C cannot enter, including the fat-containing tissues of the heart, the brain, the spinal cord, and the liver.

Since lipids are highly susceptible to oxidation, inside as well as outside the body, a fat-soluble anti-oxidant like vitamin E is sorely needed. Cell membranes are basically made up of lecithin-like fat molecules and can be seriously damaged through the free-radical–generating process called *peroxidation*. This process happens continuously in our bodies. Cell contents may leak out or entire complex enzyme systems inside the cells may be damaged and unable to carry on the complicated exchange of secretions that depends on an intact cellular surface.

The good news is that vitamin E, acting as a membrane stabilizer, can effectively protect against damage to the cell membranes. In fact, free-radical researchers have pointed out that one molecule of vitamin E can protect up to 1,000 membrane lipid molecules from peroxidation. This protection becomes even greater when ample vitamin C is present, as in our program.

An example of this kind of damage is hemolysis, the rupture of red blood cells associated with free-radical damage to blood cell membranes. Actually, the usual way to test serum vitamin E level is to see how much of a beating the blood in a test tube can take before the blood cell membranes rupture. The more vitamin E, the harder it is to crack the cell membranes.

Vitamin E also helps prevent blood clots especially if taken with vitamin C. After surgery, when the danger of blood clots forming is at its greatest, vitamins E and C might mean the difference between life and death. The common medical belief is that vitamin E encourages bleeding, prevents normal coagulation, and interferes with the synthesis of collagen for wound healing—all clinical evidence to the contrary.

Vitamin E has been shown over and over again to interfere not with normal coagulation but only with the *abnormal* formation of blood clots. Patients undergoing surgery who have very high serum vitamin E levels do not have unusual bleeding problems. In fact, their wound-healing and recuperation time is generally shorter than that of patients with low E levels. We think that vitamin E may protect the production of prostacyclin (PGI_2), a hormone that puts the Teflon-like coating on the inside of our veins and arteries. This coating facilitates blood flow and prevents the accumulation of cholesterol (plaque) and other debris that can form clots. This would explain why vitamin E can prevent abnormal blood clots without interfering with normal coagulation and wound healing.

We would like to mention, in this connection, that vitamin E is not an "antiplatelet" chemical, the way aspirin and indomethacin are. The two latter drugs actually poison an important enzyme in platelets and render them useless. This is why you tend to get bleeding reactions with aspirin. Vitamin E, however, does not inactivate platelets or their enzymes. It merely prevents excessive lipid peroxidation that makes platelets excessively "sticky." It is important to realize this distinction between the effects of antiplatelet drugs like aspirin and the "normalizing effects" of anti-oxidants in protecting against occlusions of blood vessels.

Vitamin E in doses of 800 I.U. can help prevent deep vein clots from forming, even in postoperative patients who have to remain immobile for long periods of time, a situation in which the mortality rate is extremely high. In addition, the patient taking vitamin E might avoid the often nasty side effects of conventional anticoagulant medication.[1,2]

Since vitamin E is such a helpful anticoagulant agent, it is not surprising to learn that it has proven extraordinarily helpful in several serious circulatory conditions, including heart disease.*

Among some of the other known protective effects of vitamin E we must mention a condition called *fibrocystic breast disease,* which

---

* We urge the interested reader to consult the following books: Wilfred E. Shute and Harold J. Taub, *Vitamin E for Ailing and Healthy Hearts* (New York: Pyramid House, 1969) and Evan Shute, *The Heart and Vitamin E* (London, Canada: The Shute Foundation for Medical Research, 1969).

The positive effects of vitamin E in cardiovascular disorders are certainly consistent with its proven ability to prevent the peroxidation of fats inside and outside the body, especially polyunsaturated vegetable oils, which are more prone to direct attack by molecular oxygen than are saturated animal fats, including butter. Vitamin E is also known to offer protection against rancid (peroxidized) cholesterol, which builds up dangerous arterial plaque.

affects 20 percent of American women. Vitamin E provides protection for these women*—as opposed to surgery, which often has to be repeated as new cysts make their appearance. Fibrocystic breast disease is frequently the forerunner of breast cancer, and breast cancer is related to high fat consumption.† This brings us right back to the problem of peroxidized fats with their cancer-causing free radicals, and to vitamin E's role in preventing the peroxidation of fats. It is also a prime example of how a combination of diet and anti-oxidant therapy is the most effective means of preventing and controlling a wide range of diseases—including most cancers and precancerous conditions like fibrocystic breast disease.

Another condition for which vitamin E is an effective treatment is a circulatory disorder called *intermittent claudication,* which produces painful cramping in legs and arms. One carefully conducted medical study in Sweden concluded that "exercise and alpha-tocopherol [are] the best therapy" for this disease.[3]

It has long been known that vitamin E can prevent the damage to our lungs caused by air pollution—especially from the ozone in smog—by keeping the pollution from peroxidizing the fat molecules in the lungs' cell membranes. The same kind of protection, though by no means complete, works against the internal "pollution" caused by smoking. Most smokers don't realize that smoking generates large quantities of toxic phenoxy free radicals and carbon monoxide, the deadly gas found in automobile exhaust that inhibits the hemoglobin in red blood corpuscles from transporting oxygen to the brain and other organs. Anti-oxidants like vitamin E reduce this damage through their free-radical–scavenging activity. The same applies to the cross-linking effect of hydrocarbons in tobacco smoke that render lung tissue of

* For a discussion of vitamin E and fibrocystic breast disease with references to several scientific papers, see Sheldon S. Hendler, *The Complete Guide to Anti-Aging Nutrients* (New York: Simon & Schuster, 1981), p. 123.

† For an excellent discussion of breast disease and breast cancer by a nutrition-oriented doctor, see John A. McDougall, *A Challenging Second Opinion* (Piscataway, N.J.: New Century Publishers, Inc., 1985) pp. 19–51.

smokers more and more rigid. When that happens, the lungs can no longer expand and contract freely (*emphysema*).

In addition to these major and well-established benefits of vitamin E, there are several minor ones too. For instance, we noticed that after having taken ½ to 1 teaspoon of liquid vitamin E at bedtime to improve the quality of our sleep, there was a marked improvement in our hair. Vitamin E was definitely giving it a more silky feel and appearance.

You will remember reading in Chapter 1, "Why This Book?," that going on an anti-oxidant program solved a long-standing dandruff problem. The anti-oxidants—particularly the lipid-soluble vitamin E—prevent peroxidation of the oils from the sebaceous glands of the scalp, a major cause of dandruff.

We even put a teaspoon of liquid vitamin E into the food for each of our three German shepherds. Result: It has made their fur "shine like mink," as one friend remarked—not to mention that it has nearly eliminated their "doggie" smell (the characteristic unpleasant odor of cat and dog fur is basically due to peroxidized fats).

LIQUID VITAMIN E

Practical Applications

Useful on minor cuts and abrasions, and for eczema, dry, scaly skin, etc. In winter put vitamin E on a Q-tip and swab the inside of nostrils dried out from cold or central heating. Helps prevent nose bleeding. Also, cold and flu viruses are less likely to get an entry via the nasal passages if the mucous membranes are intact. Useful as well for herpes lesions on lips and nostrils.

Extremely helpful inside the mouth—inflamed gums, periodontal disease, and gingival (gum) dentistry will be helped by holding some liquid vitamin E in the mouth and swishing it around. Let the vitamin E remain in the mouth, in contact with such sore, inflamed areas, as long as practical. Do this every time you have your teeth cleaned!

WARNING   We do have a warning about vitamin E. It may cause a small, *temporary* rise in blood pressure. People with high blood pressure, and heart patients in general, should therefore start with a small amount, about 100 I.U. per day, and work up slowly to a larger dose. We think the risk in that respect is very small and definitely outweighed by the potential gains of vitamin E therapy, especially for heart patients. However, you should consult your physician before taking vitamin E, and make sure it is free of other oils.

Even though vitamin E has not been found to interfere with blood coagulation in *normal* people, a warning is indicated for people with vitamin K deficiencies who are on anticoagulant medication. Dr. Demopoulos, admittedly biased in favor of vitamin and anti-oxidant therapy, favors the replacement of more toxic anticoagulant medications with the much less hazardous vitamin E and a diet that is high in fresh, cold-water fish. But this should be decided individually in consultation with your physician.

Despite these warnings, we would like to point out that vitamin E, even though it is fat soluble, can be taken safely within the general limits of the program (300 to 800 I.U. per day). It is not cumulative in the body, as some people still think. The only difference between vitamin E and the water-soluble vitamins is that while water-soluble vitamins take only three to six hours to be metabolized and completely eliminated, vitamin E takes twenty-four hours.

SOURCES

1. Ochsner, A., M. E. DeBakey, and P. T. DeCamp, "Venous thrombosis." *JAMA,* 1950; 144:831–834.
2. Ochsner, A. "Thromboembolism." *N. Eng. J. Med.,* 1964; 271:211.
3. Haeger, K. "Walking distance and arterial flow during longterm treatment of intermittent claudication with d-alpha-tocopherol." *Vasa,* 1973; 2(3):280–287.

CHAPTER 10

BETA-CAROTENE

THE ANTICANCER NUTRIENT

Beta-carotene is a forerunner (technically a "precursor") of vitamin A and is therefore also called *pro-vitamin A*. In our opinion, beta-carotene is without question the most underrated micronutrient, even among life-extenders. We say this because of its proven anticancer properties—which make it the top point in what we think of as the anticancer triangle, with vitamins C and E at the two corners of the triangle's base line.

Furthermore, even though some beta-carotene stays in our fatty tissues, it is perfectly *safe* to take even in high doses. Its worst side effect is the slight orange-yellow cast it gives to your skin, imparting a perpetual light suntan without exposure to ultraviolet radiation. In other words, beta-carotene provides an effective internal kind of biochemical "sunscreen." This doesn't mean you shouldn't use a sunscreen too, but the beta-carotene does add extra protection from the sun's UV rays.

Just to give you an idea of how safe beta-carotene is: There is a strange, and fortunately rare, disease (erythropoietic protoporphyria) that makes the skin of some children hypersensitive to even the slightest bit of sunlight. Protoporphyrin, a substance in their bloodstream, enters the skin tissues and, when light hits it, produces a lot of free radicals. Children with this congenital blood abnormality used to be routinely thrown into insane asylums because whenever they went into the sunshine to play, they would run back in screaming and hide under the bed or in a closet (back then, an obvious sign of insanity).

BETA-CAROTENE

(Pro-vitamin A)

Beta-carotene

- enables the body to produce its own vitamin A according to needs.
- has proven anticancer properties.
- traps singlet-oxygen radicals and destroys perhydroxy radicals.
- helps to protect against the effects of atherosclerotic arteries that have become seriously narrowed.
- helps to decrease acute and chronic inflammation.
- is impossible to overdose on (therefore is preferable to taking vitamin A).
- provides radiation protection (acts as an internal kind of "sunscreen").
- renders radiation therapy more effective by protecting the normal tissues near the radiated site.
- synergizes with vitamin E, thus enhancing effectiveness of both anti-oxidants as anticancer nutrients.
- is present in many forms of nature (plumage of birds, coloration of fish, plants, flowers).

When doctors eventually studied the urine of these children, they found massive amounts of protoporphyrin were being excreted. Next it was discovered that the disease was treatable with dosages of beta-carotene high enough to turn the children's skin completely orange. Long-term studies now show that people can take these megadoses of beta-carotene for many years without developing any serious problems.[1]

Our astounding tolerance for beta-carotene becomes less surprising when you consider that it is present in substantial amounts in many life forms. You have no doubt often unknowingly admired its effects in the pink plumage of the flamingo, the rainbow hues of tropical fish, the pale rose or deep purple of flowers and plants. As with vitamin C, if there was ever a natural substance that is present in almost everything, it would be beta-carotene.

In America and Europe, the principal dietary sources of beta-carotene are, as the name implies, carrots. But it is present also in yellow squash, sweet potatoes, oranges, cantaloupes, papayas, and other yellow vegetables and fruit, as well as in green, leafy vegetables.

Our small intestine manufactures from beta-carotene just the amount of vitamin A our bodies need, but no more. The fraction that is converted to vitamin A actually decreases as the amount of beta-carotene we take in with our food or in the form of supplements increases. This means that we can never overdose on vitamin A if we take it as beta-carotene rather than directly as vitamin A.

In fact, it seems to be not so much the vitamin A the body produces from beta-carotene—though vitamin A also has such properties[2-5]—as the portion of beta-carotene that is absorbed unchanged from the intestine and circulated in the body that is responsible for most of its cancer protection. Free-radical pathology offers a logical explanation: As one researcher put it, beta-carotene is "the most efficient quencher of singlet oxygen thus far discovered."[6] Beta-carotene's effectiveness as one of nature's primary anticancer substances is further strengthened by its ability to trap certain other cancer-initiating or cancer-promoting free-radical species.

By the same token, beta-carotene provides protection against the dangers of radiation—and hence against radiation-induced cancer—for animals and humans, just as it does for plants. In plants beta-carotene's chief function is to neutralize the singlet-oxygen free radicals produced by photosynthesis (the process by which plants use sunlight and their chlorophyll to produce nutrients from carbon dioxide and water).

In 1986 Dr. Eli Seifter of the Albert Einstein College of Medicine in New York reported to the Federation of American Societies for Experimental Biology that when mice with cancer were given both radiation therapy and beta-carotene, their tumors disappeared.[7]

Also in 1986, researchers at the Johns Hopkins School of Hygiene and Public Health in Baltimore reported that people with low levels of beta-carotene in their bloodstream were about four times more likely to develop a common form of lung cancer called *squamous-cell carcinoma.* They concluded "that beta-carotene might protect against cancer is biologically plausible, since it is known to deactivate free radicals and excited oxygen, both of which have been implicated in carcinogenesis."[8] These scientists also found a similar increase in lung cancer risk for those with low levels of vitamin E.

There is also a strong possibility that in addition to being protective against cancer, beta-carotene may actually retard the aging process itself. The scientific rationale for this possibility lies in the observation that aging and cancer have a number of characteristics in common. This has led one noted researcher, Dr. Richard G. Cutler of the Gerontology Research Center, National Institute on Aging in Baltimore, to the interesting hypothesis that the life span of animal species "may be governed in part by the same mechanisms as those processes governing species' differences in their age-dependent probability of developing cancer."[9] In other words, beta-carotene may not only protect against cancer, but also plays a key role in determining how long an animal or a person is going to live.

Dr. Cutler thinks that carotenoids like beta-carotene may not only function in a living organism as anti-oxidants but also, by other unknown mechanisms, to "stabilize the differential state of cells." The shorter-lived animal species generally have less concentrations of carotenoids in their blood serum and brain, although there are some surprising exceptions. Dr. Cutler takes these findings to mean that the role of carotenoids in determining the life span of animals "may have evolved only in the longer-lived species, reaching a peak expression in human."

Be that as it may, obviously anything that is as clearly protective against cancer as has been proven for beta-carotene must at minimum have a profound effect on individual life span. Here again a good case can be made for synergism: Vitamin C, which also appears to protect against cancer, is water soluble. Beta-carotene and vitamin A, in contrast, are lipid (fat)-soluble, which means they can get into all the body tissues, like the lipid-containing cell membranes, that vitamin C and the water-soluble B vitamins cannot penetrate. Furthermore, beta-carotene functions particularly well as an anti-oxidant at the low oxygen pressures that prevail in most mammalian tissues, including our own.

SOURCES

1. Mathews-Ross, M., et al. "Beta carotene therapy for erythropoietic protoporphyria and other photosensitive disease." *Arch. Dermatol.*, 1977; 113:1229–1232.
2. Wylie-Rosett, J., et al. "Influence of vitamin A on cervical hysplasia and carcinoma in-situ." *Nutrition and Cancer,* 1984; 6:49–57.
3. Palgi, A. "Vitamin A and lung cancer." *Nutrition and Cancer,* 1984; 6:105–119. Also: Shekelle, R. B., et al. "'Dietary vitamin A and risk of cancer in the Western Electric study." *Lancet,* 1981; 2:1185–1190.
4. Kummet, T., et al. "Vitamin A. Evidence for its preventive role in human cancer." *Nutrition and Cancer,* 1983, 5:96–106.
5. Menkes, M. S., and G. W. Comstock. "Vitamin A and E and lung cancer." *Am. J. Epidem.,* 1984; 120:491 (Abstract).
6. Peto, R., et al. "Can dietary beta carotene materially reduce human cancer rates?" *Nature,* March 19, 1981; 290:201–207.
7. Hendler, op. cit., p. 88. Also: Harris, R.W.C. "Cancer of the cervix, uteri, and vitamin A." *Brit. J. Cancer,* 1986; 53:653–659; Shekelle, R. B., M. Lepper, S. Liu, et al. "Dietary vitamin A and risk of cancer in the Western Electric Study." *Lancet,* 1981; 2:1185–1190.
8. Menkes, M. S., G. W. Comstock, et al. "Serum beta carotene, vitamins A and E, selenium, and the risk of lung cancer." *N. Eng. J. Med.*, 1986; 315(20):1250–1289.
9. Cutler, Richard G. "Carotenoids and retinol: their possible importance in determining longevity of primate species." *Proc. Natl. Acad. Sci. USA,* 1984; 81:7629–7631.

CHAPTER 11

GLUTATHIONE

THE LONGEVITY "GOLD DUST"
FROM JAPAN

12 The single amino acid cysteine is the central molecule among the three making up glutathione—which, using its thiol group (-SH) to quench free radicals, works as an anti-oxidant in its own right. Cysteine can, for instance, help reduce acetaldehyde damage from cigarette smoke, smog, alcohol, and atherosclerosis. It has cancer-prevention properties. It helps slow down cross-linking. It strengthens the immune system. It helps prevent damage from peroxidized fats in our diet.

With such an impressive list of benefits, we faithfully took cysteine along with our other anti-oxidants every day—until we found that as a free-radical scavenger, cysteine can turn into its own degradation product, cystine. Cystine is not easily soluble and may precipitate kidney stones. For this reason we switched to the cysteine-containing triple amino acid glutathione. Unlike cysteine, glutathione is *not* degraded in our bodies into anything that can do us harm. It is absorbed totally from the intestinal tract and cannot crystallize in the kidneys. Equally important, glutathione can be recycled in the body by certain enzymes and thus work more efficiently.

The only requirement for this elegant system to function is the presence of plenty of hydrogen. Fortunately, glutathione is able to take hydrogen from the naturally occurring coenzyme NADPH and from other electron donors such as vitamin C and the B vitamins. And not only can glutathione be recycled by enzymatic activity, as described,

GLUTATHIONE

Glutathione's main functions include amino acid transport and synthesis of prostaglandins and leukotrienes. Glutathione

- contains the amino acid cysteine and has similar effects, e.g., protection from acetaldehyde damage due to smoking, alcohol, or air pollution.
- is more effective and safer than cysteine (cysteine's metabolite, cystine, can cause kidney stones).
- is important in keeping our own glutathione-peroxidase enzyme system working to quench free radicals.
- can recycle spent (oxidized) vitamins C and E.
- works as an effective detoxifying agent, e.g., binds to organic toxins, like DDT, and to heavy metals, like mercury, lead, and cadmium, and carries them out of the body via the urinary system.
- seems to have anti-aging effects (older cells contain 20 to 30 percent less glutathione than younger ones).
- helps PacMan-like defender cells of the immune system protect us against bacteria, viruses, and cancer cells.
- helps repair liver damage (e.g., in alcoholic cirrhosis).
- offers cancer protection, similar to beta-carotene.
- protects against radiation damage.
- protects against the harmful effects of excessive endogenous opioids (endorphins) produced as a result of physical or psychological stress.
- useful in eye surgery.
- the optic lens of the eye has the very highest levels of glutathione; cataracts develop in the lens when this and other anti-oxidants are "overworked."
- has no known toxicity level, when pure and in chemically "reduced" form.

but it can return the favor and recycle degraded (oxidized) vitamin C (dehydroascorbic acid) back into reduced, fresh vitamin C (ascorbic acid). Fresh (reduced) glutathione can do the same for spent (oxidized) vitamin E (tocopherol) that has turned into toxic tocopheryl quinone.

Our bodies contain large amounts of a very important enzyme, glutathione peroxidase. This selenium-containing and selenium-dependent enzyme directly deactivates free radicals, especially those of the dangerous lipid-peroxide type (like rancid cholesterol) in our arteries. Reduced glutathione (GSH) feeds right into this crucial anti-oxidant system. In that respect it works like a second defensive line for vitamin E, which fights a constant, running battle on the molecular level against free-radical attacks on cell-membrane lipids in every part of our bodies.

Now, we must keep in mind that glutathione peroxidase functions only in the presence of glutathione. While our bodies do make some glutathione, the supply is not nearly enough to prevent fat molecules in cell membranes, serum cholesterol, and ingested dietary fats from peroxidizing. Moreover, our own glutathione production is insufficient to keep detoxifying our system from environmental pollutants and self-inflicted free-radical assaults from smoking, alcohol, and certain foods.

In its internal clean-up process, glutathione works as a detoxifying agent by attaching itself to toxic substances such as epoxides (a kind of sticky resin, like epoxy glue), halides (compounds that include the toxins chlorine, iodine, bromine, and fluorine), and heavy metals such as lead, cadmium, and mercury. Having joined itself to these substances, glutathione carries them out of the body via the urinary system.

In addition, glutathione itself may actually slow down the aging process. Animal studies have disclosed that older cells contain 20 to 30 percent less glutathione than do younger cells. The lower concentrations of glutathione in aged cells may be due to an accumulation of toxic substances with aging, making increasing demands on glutathione peroxidase and transferase activities, resulting in a progressive depletion of the intracellular pool of reduced glutathione (GSH). Researchers are currently trying to determine whether the same applies to humans. The Japanese, who consume tons of glutathione a year in the form of supplements, are already convinced that it does.

Even plants are smart enough to use glutathione to their advantage. When injured, the plants rush extra glutathione to the damaged tissue. Unfortunately, insects are even smarter and come to feed on these injured plants to obtain the extra glutathione, which makes them stronger, bigger, and more destructive than ever. Fortunately for us humans, glutathione is highly beneficial to damaged human tissue.

Glutathione, for instance, is protective of the liver, and it is therapeutic in liver damage caused by alcohol or hepatitis, and probably also liver cancer. Dr. Roberto Corrocher of the Policlinico di Borgo in Rome, Italy, and colleagues discovered that the glutathione content was extremely low in tumors and even in tumor-free tissue of patients with liver cancer.

In view of all these well-established benefits of glutathione, it's not hard to understand why more and more medical scientists are studying it. For example, in eye surgery, glutathione is sometimes given intraocularly. They bathe the *inside* of the eye (both the anterior and posterior chambers) with high concentrations of glutathione rather than with the traditional saline solution.

In other types of surgery in which ischemia (lack of blood in the affected tissue, caused by some obstruction) is an important factor, free-radical researchers believe that glutathione may prove to be equally beneficial. Heart surgery would be a case in point, as well as plastic (reconstructive) surgery, where fast healing and avoidance of skin discoloration is of special concern.

We can close our discussion of this important anti-oxidant on the happy note that, as in the case of beta-carotene, there appears to be no toxicity associated with glutathione, even at rather high dosages.* Dr. Demopoulos has monitored patients with liver damage who were taking 1 gram (1,000 milligrams) of glutathione per day, without finding any problems. In fact, your wallet may be the only realistic limit as far as this expensive nutrient is concerned: 2.2 pounds of glutathione is worth an ounce of pure gold!

SOURCES

1. Hazelton, G. A., and C. A. Lang. "Glutathione contents of tissue in the aging mouse." *Biochem. J.*, 1980; 188:25–30.
2. Corrocher, R., et al. "Severe impairment of antioxidant system in human hepatoma." *Cancer,* 1986; 58:1658–1662.

VITAMIN CO-FACTORS

The B vitamins in our program are called co-factors or co-antioxidants because they step up the activity of one of the body's natural anti-oxidant systems involving two coenzymes, NADH and NADPH,[†] and serve as hydrogen carriers able to recycle oxidized anti-oxidants.

The B vitamins have many other protective and healing qualities you should know about. In the chapters that follow we will be giving you evaluations of each of these important micronutrients. We shall be focusing only on those aspects that have been sufficiently verified by scientific research to justify their inclusion here. So, if there is no discussion of a claim you have heard for one or more of these vitamins, you can rest assured that such omissions simply indicate the lack of sufficient evidence.

---

* Health Maintenance Programs (HMP) now offers an extra-strength glutathione capsule (glutathione forté) containing 250 milligrams of glutathione, plus 750 milligrams of ascorbic acid (vitamin C).
† NADH and NADPH (abbreviations for complex molecules made out of niacin) are used within the "furnaces" of the cells (the mitochondria) to carry hydrogen atoms along a system that eventually leads to the production of energy, a lot of which is stored as chemical energy. ATP is the abbreviation of the specific molecule that stores chemical energy, which can then be used, like "money in the bank," when you need it. A "thinking" bunch of brain cells needs a lot of ATP, for example.

CHAPTER 12

VITAMIN B₁₂

BLOOD BUILDER AND BRAIN FOOD

12 Among the B vitamins, B_{12} is the only one that has nothing to do with generating hydrogen or electrons to recycle anti-oxidants. It does, however, have a great deal to do with other vital processes. B_{12} is critical for blood synthesis, and a deficiency of it will cause anemia and serious nervous system problems.

The principal food sources of B_{12} are organ meats, egg yolks, some fermented cheeses, and bivalves such as clams and oysters. None of these foods is on the menu for strict vegetarians, who sometimes develop severe vitamin B_{12} deficiences.

The principal reason this does not happen more often is that even though vegetarians consume no animal products, some of the bacteria that produce B_{12} are ingested inadvertently. Also, only very small amounts of this vitamin are needed to avoid gross, noticeable deficiencies. But the fact that they do occasionally occur ought to be sufficient reason for strict vegetarians to supplement their diet with B_{12}.

Vitamin B_{12} is absent in fruits, vegetables, grains, and grain products because the plants themselves cannot synthesize this vitamin. Its production in nature depends entirely on the work of microorganisms, which means the only possible vegetable source of B_{12} is from seaweeds which contain this vitamin because microorganisms inside this special group of aquatic plants synthesize it. (Unfortunately, the much touted spirulina does not qualify in this or any other respect.)[1]

On the other hand, large amounts of B_{12} are produced by the microorganisms in the human colon. One would therefore assume that

VITAMIN B$_{12}$

(Cobalamin)

Vitamin B$_{12}$

- is crucial for proper transmission of nerve impulses in the brain and the rest of central nervous system (including operation of nerve cells in heart and skeletal muscles).
- deficiency is slow in onset, but can cause pernicious anemia with mental deterioration, as production of important molecules slows down.
- should be taken supplementally by strict vegetarians because there are no supplies of this vitamin in vegetables, fruits, and grains.
- absorption problems can be overcome by taking sufficient amounts (mass action), as on our program. (Exceptions: people with pancreatic disease, or who have had part of the stomach or small intestine removed. In these cases, B$_{12}$ is better supplied by a nasal spray or injection.)
- claims that vitamin C destroys B$_{12}$ are unfounded. When inside the body, carelessly manufactured supplements that freely admix vitamin C and B$_{12}$, without manufacturing precautions, may contain B$_{12}$ that has been destroyed or degraded by vitamin C, with the result that a toxic form of B$_{12}$ is produced.

even the strictest vegetarian ought to get sufficient B$_{12}$ from this self-manufactured source alone. The problem is that we cannot absorb vitamin B$_{12}$ from the colon, no matter how much is produced there, because it is simply excreted in the feces. Meat and meat products contain vitamin B$_{12}$ because the animals have ingested microorganisms that contain it. Also, animals can absorb the vitamin B$_{12}$ produced by microorganisms higher up in their alimentary tract, which differs greatly from ours. They are therefore able to store food-derived B$_{12}$ in their tissues so that it can, in turn, be ingested by meat-eating and dairy-product–consuming humans.

A second problem is that dairy products—including even low-fat and no-fat milk, as well as egg yolks—should be unacceptable food sources for all health-conscious dieters, whether they are vegetarians or not. (See Chapter 41 for our discussion of this point.) Fortunately, some seafood, for instance, clams, oysters, crab, rockfish, salmon, and sardines, also contains at least moderate amounts of B$_{12}$. Smaller but still significant amounts are present in lobster, scallops, flounder, haddock, swordfish, and tuna. Occasional consumption of these foods is undoubtedly sufficient to prevent vitamin B$_{12}$ deficiencies.

The inclusion of vitamin B_{12} in our micronutrient program, in addition to preventing deficiency, serves very different purposes. Vitamin B_{12} is absolutely critical to the integrity of cell membranes, especially those in the central nervous system. Picture the surfaces of nerve cells as resembling carefully laid-down paving stones in a road. Only, instead of car traffic, nerve impulses in the brain, the spinal cord, the heart, and the skeletal nerve cells that control motion and coordination are constantly traveling back and forth across these surfaces. The "pavements" must therefore be kept nice and smooth, with no "stones" (molecules) sticking up or lying crooked. If there are any "potholes" or "kinks" in the surface, transmission stops as abruptly as when you click off your TV set. Advanced pernicious anemia, a vitamin B_{12} deficiency disease, is a very serious case in point. Here we see both the anemia itself and the terrible symptom of central nervous system malfunction—mental deterioration.

Even without B_{12} deficiency, none of us always fires mentally on all cylinders. The wear and tear of modern living is enough in itself to put some nasty kinks and potholes into our delicate brain-cell surfaces. One of the main reasons we need sleep is to give our bodies time to repair this daily damage. You might think of sleep as a night crew filling in the potholes while the city slumbers: There's little traffic (few nerve impulses), so nerve transmissions can proceed along a smooth surface the next day.

Unfortunately, our bodies are not always able to repair overnight a day's worth of cumulative damage—which is why sometimes we cannot cope even with the kind of routine mental tasks we normally handle with ease. What do most of us do when we're mentally sluggish? Have a strong cup of coffee, which will give us a lift but won't repair a single nerve-cell membrane. So the day goes: a little boost from coffee or cigarettes, followed by a letdown, followed by a need for more caffeine and nicotine, followed by more of the same. Sound familiar?

Every cup of coffee, every cigarette only causes more damage. Not only are we putting still more potholes and kinks into our brain cells, we're also damaging nerve cells in our heart muscle and even our skeletal muscle cells.* Nor can those of us who avoid coffee and cigarettes prevent other types of assaults on the central nervous system. It's no wonder that we often don't think as clearly, don't remember as easily, and aren't as well coordinated as we'd like to be.

Obviously, we need strong vitamin B_{12} support to repair nerve-cell membranes as rapidly as possible. But that is easier said than done, because the way most people take vitamin B_{12} does them no good. To be effective, B_{12} has to be absorbed in the small intestine. This absorption, however, depends on a sufficient amount of *intrinsic factor,*

---

* Smoking actually destroys vitamin B_{12}, as does alcohol.

a substance secreted by the stomach. Most of us don't produce very much intrinsic factor and therefore don't absorb vitamin B$_{12}$ well, whether it comes from a food source or from vitamin supplements. For this reason, physicians usually suggest that vitamin B$_{12}$ be given by injection.

Fortunately, Dr. Demopoulos and his fellow researchers have discovered another way to get the B$_{12}$ absorbed: by *mass action*, that is, when enough of the pure vitamin is taken by mouth. (See our anti-oxidant Menu, page 59, for the correct dosage.) The mass-action method may not work if you have pancreatic disease or have had part of your stomach or small intestine removed, in which case your physician should monitor your vitamin B$_{12}$ absorption and use injections or nasal sprays if necessary.

For most people, however, the oral absorption of very large amounts of B$_{12}$ by Dr. Demopoulos's mass-action technique has proved to be suitable. This is important for still another reason: There has been some controversy in the scientific community over the past ten years as to whether or not vitamin C can destroy B$_{12}$. Some scientists say it can, others say that it does not, and still others say that the effect, if any, is so minimal as to be negligible.* In any case, our program provides stable forms of B$_{12}$, so there's nothing to worry about.

SOURCE

1. Herbert, V., and G. Drivas. "Spirulina and vitamin B$_{12}$." *JAMA,* 1982; 248:3096–3097.

---

* For an excellent review of the controversy about vitamin C in relation to vitamin B$_{12}$, see Dr. Linus Pauling, *How to Live Longer and Feel Better* (New York: W. H. Freeman & Company, 1986), pp. 262–263.

CHAPTER 13

VITAMIN B₆

FRIEND OF WOMEN AND
ARTHRITIS SUFFERERS

We all need plenty of vitamin B_6 to ensure the proper functioning of several vital enzyme systems. Without these enzymes, the conversion of amino acids into certain hormone-like secretions called *neurotransmitters* would not be possible. These chemical substances, in turn, are necessary for smooth communication between nerve cells. In that respect, vitamin B_6 complements the function of vitamin B_{12}, providing yet another example of the need for full-spectrum vitamin/ anti-oxidant supplementation.

Vitamin B_6 is essential to children, whose adequate growth and mental development depend on it.

Since arthritis and rheumatism are degenerative diseases initiated and promoted by free-radical activity, vitamins like B_6—together with anti-oxidants like C and E—are of great therapeutic value.

The joints in our bodies are lined with tough coatings (synovial membranes) that act like the surface bearings in a piece of machinery. By generating their own lubricating fluid, the surfaces are actually self-lubricating—no small engineering feat of nature! If oxidized, rancid fats get into our joints, these marvelous mechanisms become clogged up. Free-radical attacks on the synovial membrane linings make them enlarged and swollen. The joints no longer move freely, and the pressure on nerve endings produces the painful symptoms of arthritis and rheumatism.

Vitamin B_6 takes a leading role, together with vitamins A and C, in

126

VITAMIN B$_6$

(Pyridoxine)

Vitamin B$_6$

- is vital for proper growth and mental development of children.
- is best known for its ability to reduce the distressing symptoms of premenstrual tension.
- is necessary for production of important neurotransmitters (communication between nerve cells).
- helps prevent and control arthritis and rheumatism.
- protects myelin insulation around nerves.
- reduces pain and inflammation of wrists in a chronic condition called *carpal tunnel syndrome.*
- fights atherosclerosis.
- is possible to overdose on. Dosages on our program are well within wide safety margin, but should not be exceeded.

shrinking swollen joint membranes and dissolving rancid fat deposits. Pain is reduced and the sufferer regains some of the lost mobility in the joints.

Vitamin B$_6$ also protects the insulating myelin sheath around nerves, without which the raw nerves would be exposed—another instance of this vitamin's ability to control pain in arthritic and rheumatoid conditions.

It also offers protection in an excruciatingly painful inflammatory condition of the wrists called *carpal tunnel syndrome.* Doctors sometimes treat this ailment by surgically blocking the nerves. Surgery will stop the pain, but it does not stop the underlying inflammation in the swollen synovial membranes—nor does it clear up the debris from rancid fatty acids. In fact, mobility of the wrists is restored only partially, and that's only because the patient no longer feels the pain and therefore moves the wrists more freely.

An important source of help for this condition seems to be vitamin B$_6$. In one double-blind study, patients with carpal tunnel syndrome who were given therapeutic doses of B$_6$ (approximately 500 milligrams per day in divided doses) showed marked improvement, while those given placebos showed none.[1] This study is a rather dramatic illustration of a single vitamin's working not only as a co-factor but as an anti-oxidant in its own right to relieve an otherwise "incurable" condition. That is remarkable enough. We can only guess at how much more effective a complete spectrum of anti-oxidants and vitamin co-factors could have been for such patients!

Vitamin B_6 has been shown to help break down atherosclerotic plaque. First, we know from earlier findings (1945) that vitamin B_6 deficiency causes atherosclerosis in baboons.[2] Twenty-four years later, in 1969, it was discovered that children suffering from a metabolic disorder (homocystinuria) that produces all the symptoms of advanced atherosclerosis had the same enzyme defect as the atherosclerotic baboons; again, the cause was a vitamin B_6 deficiency. In fact, for those children whose atherosclerosis was a secondary effect of their primary metabolic disorder, vitamin B_6 supplementation actually improved their atherosclerotic symptoms.[3]

Vitamin B_6 is perhaps best known for its ability to relieve the symptoms of premenstrual syndrome (PMS) so troublesome to many women: breast tenderness, weight gain due to water retention, head-aches, nervous tension, and irritability. These symptoms can be alleviated by supplementation with 500 milligrams of vitamin B_6 per day, in divided doses, 100 milligrams per day above the upper limit on our program, but well below the possibly hazardous threshold (a problem to which we shall return presently).

However, we have found that, once again, broad-spectrum supple-mentation is far more effective in even severe cases of PMS than just B_6 therapy alone. We counsel women suffering from PMS gradually to start increasing their anti-oxidant/vitamin intake about a week before the expected onset of the syndrome. By the time PMS would normally hit, they should already be up to the maximum anti-oxidant intake. In addition, a PMS sufferer should be taking a magnesium supplement (200 to 400 milligrams per day), which is most effective if combined with potassium.*

At the same time, women in the throes of full-blown PMS should be extra careful with their diet. This is no time to indulge in sweets, "unfriendly" fatty foods, coffee, alcohol, and nicotine. Not that you can't have a glass of wine or a cup of coffee and a couple of cookies, but you know what we mean by "indulge"! Also, a woman suffering from PMS should definitely practice some kind of relaxation technique, be it meditative yoga, Dr. Herbert Benson's relaxation response, or whatever is most congenial to your personality and life-style. If these basic principles are adhered to, we have yet to see a case of PMS that didn't soon become a barely remembered thing of the past.

* We can recommend Twinlab's liquid magnesium-potassium "cocktail" called Liqui-K Plus (1 teaspoon provides 100 milligrams of magnesium aspartate and 99 milligrams of potassium aspartate and citrate). It isn't the greatest-tasting stuff, but that way you can avoid taking more tablets or capsules, and it's very well absorbed in this form. Best taken during a meal so the awful taste is erased with the next bite of something good; that's what we do. We do so because even a health-conscious, low-sodium diet such as ours provides more sodium than potassium.

Vitamin B$_6$ deficiencies are common in women who are on birth control pills,[4] a depletion that is greatly increased if the woman drinks any alcohol. Also, during pregnancy, women frequently develop vitamin B$_6$ deficiencies for similar hormonal reasons. Fortunately, in either case, such deficiencies are easily corrected by preventive supplementation.[5,6]

In the light of all the well-documented potential benefits of this important vitamin co-factor (and sometime anti-oxidant), we must say a few words about the alleged dangers of overdosing on B$_6$. This apprehension is essentially based on a single, much-publicized study published a few years ago and calling for, in not-so-veiled language, federal intervention in the availability of vitamin B$_6$ in health-food stores and pharmacies.[7]

The study in question is based on the case histories of just seven people (five women and two men) who had been grossly and bizarrely overdosing on B$_6$ for many months. The women had been taking B$_6$ to relieve premenstrual syndrome, two of them on the advice of their gynecologist. One of the men had been taking it on the advice of his psychiatrist. All of them, however, had kept increasing the dosage more and more on their own.

Now, it's perfectly true that you *can* overdose on B$_6$, but not without working hard at it. You would have to take 200,000 percent (yes, *two hundred thousand percent*) of the RDA (Recommended Daily Allowance) for B$_6$ to reach the danger level. And you would have to continue overdosing even after the initial symptoms of toxicity (tingling and numbness in your fingertips and toes) told you that something was wrong.

As it turned out, no permanent damage was done to the seven overdosers. Once they were taken off the B$_6$, their peripheral nervous system symptoms gradually receded, and within a few months they returned to normal.

Since the B$_6$ dosage on our own program—like all dosages—is based on Dr. Demopoulos's long-term research, no one who follows our guidelines can possibly overdose. In fact, you would have to exceed the recommended intake by ten to twenty times in order to reach toxic levels. In seven years of experience with thousands of clients, we have yet to see this happen. And we are confident that our readers, like our clients, will understand perfectly that more is *not* always better.

VITAMIN B$_6$ UPDATE

We have always been sensitive to MSG (monosodium glutamate), so every time we got a dose of it in Chinese food we would get an upset stomach and headache (Chinese restaurant syndrome). Over the past few years, however, we haven't been affected by MSG anymore. Since we frequently eat Chinese food when we are in the United States, we thought this welcome relief was due to our bodies' finally having become inured to it.

Then we came upon a study[8] showing that vitamin B$_6$ has a strong protective action against the effects of MSG in susceptible individuals. In double-blind trials, in which neither the human test subjects nor the researchers knew who was and who wasn't getting vitamin B$_6$ along with MSG, it transpired that those who had been given the vitamin did not get the Chinese restaurant syndrome, although they had all been prone to it previously. It was only then that we realized our immunity to MSG was owed to the B$_6$ on the Demopoulos spectrum, which includes 240 to 400 milligrams.

SOURCES

1. Ellis, J. M., et al. "Response of vitamin B$_6$ deficiency and the carpal tunnel syndrome to pyridoxine." *Proc. Nat. Acad. Sci. USA,* 1982; 79:7494–7498.
2. Rinehart, J. F., and L. D. Greenberg. "Arteriosclerotic lesions in pyridoxine-deficient monkeys." *Am. J. Pathol.,* 1969; 25:481–486.
3. Barber, G. W., and G. L. Spaeth. "The successful treatment of homocystinuria with pyridoxine." *J. Pediatr.,* 1969; 75:463–478.
4. Brown, R. R., et al. "The effect of vitamin supplementation on the urinary excretion of tryptophan metabolites by pregnant women." *J. Clin. Invest.,* 1961; 40:617–623. Also: *Lancet,* April 10, 1976, pp. 788–789.
5. Adams, P. W., et al. *Contraception,* 1972; 6:265–271; and "Influence of oral contraceptives, pyridoxine (vitamin B$_6$), and tryptophan on carbohydrate metabolism." *Lancet,* April 10, 1976, pp. 759–764.
6. Brown, op. cit.
7. Schaumburg, H., et al. "Sensory neuropathy from pyridoxine abuse." *N. Eng. J. Med.,* 1983; 309:445–448.
8. Folkers, K., et al. "The biochemistry of vitamin B$_6$ is basic to the cause of the Chinese Restaurant Syndrome." Hoppe-Seyler, *Zeitschrift für physiologische Chemie,* 1984; 365:405–414.

CHAPTER 14

VITAMIN B₃

THE CHOLESTEROL FIGHTER

Vitamin B$_3$ is highly important to one of the body's natural anti-oxidant and hydrogen transfer systems, NADH and NADPH,* as well as to about two hundred other enzyme systems.

Aside from this, vitamin B$_3$ has a pivotal position in our program because of its demonstrated ability to lower serum cholesterol levels. In one study—involving only a small number of people but with very high cholesterol levels—the researchers succeeded in lowering serum cholesterol by an average of 25 percent and triglycerides by 30 percent.[1]

These results were obtained with 3,000 milligrams per day of niacin in divided doses, within an incredibly short time (two weeks). However, since in these types of experiments niacin is purposely not accompanied by any health-promoting dietary changes, niacin therapy had to be continued during an entire follow-up period of eight and a half years to maintain improvements.

Another long-term study, the Coronary Drug Project (1975), in which 3,000 milligrams of niacin also were given to chronic heart patients, produced an average cholesterol reduction of only 10 percent, but a 26 percent average reduction in triglyceride levels. Even more important was the finding that the niacin therapy resulted in a "statistically significant lower incidence of definite, nonfatal myocardial

---

* NADH and NADPH are abbreviations of chemicals that transport hydrogen in the mitochondria (the "furnaces" of the cells) and in other parts of the cells.

VITAMIN B$_3$

(Niacin)

Vitamin B$_3$

- is crucial to one of the body's important anti-oxidant systems (NADPH) and many other enzyme systems.
- lowers serum cholesterol and triglycerides.
- reduces risk of heart attack.
- is helpful with allergies (hay fever, asthma, etc.).
- can be used instead of tranquilizers because it binds to same brain-cell receptors as do Valium, Librium, Dalmane.

infarction"—in other words, a reduced rate of nonfatal heart attacks—better than 25 percent over the eight-and-a-half-year follow-up period.[2]

Unlike other studies involving the same relatively high but commonly prescribed doses of niacin in such cases, several undesirable side effects were reported, among them heartbeat irregularities and "acute gouty arthritis." These reactions are so unusual that we cannot help wondering whether they were not caused by contaminants in the niacin preparation used, or by some other unknown factor, rather than by the niacin itself.

This impression gains strength with the findings of a 1981 study on niacin treatment for dangerously elevated cholesterol levels, which involved doses of niacin identical to those in the earlier study. The researchers made a point of stating that there were "no significant side effects" in any of the twelve patients. There was a 22 percent average drop in their serum cholesterol over a period of five weeks. Even more impressive was a 52 percent drop in another type of fat/protein molecules called *VLDLs* (very low-density lipoproteins), from which our bodies manufacture the threatening LDLs (low-density lipoproteins) of cholesterol (see Chapter 34, "Cholesterol and Triglycerides," pages 231–233).

Summing up their findings, these investigators said: "To our knowledge, no other single agent has such potential for lowering both cholesterol and triglycerides." And this despite the absolutely atrocious diet the patients had been eating, including 40 percent of fat "mostly in the form of lard" [pork fat!].[3]

Niacin also favorably tilts the balance between the two types of fat/protein molecules (LDLs and HDLs) that make up cholesterol. The "good" HDLs (high-density lipoproteins) increase, and the "bad" LDLs decrease. However, we must not make so much of this single positive factor that we are lulled into false confidence. Substances like alcohol can also raise the level of HDL—but some researchers say it is an HDL of the wrong kind. A diet high in polyunsaturated oils can do the same thing. In fact, a favorable HDL:LDL ratio may merely be covering up unfavorable total cholesterol.

Many people make the mistake of taking B$_3$ only in its niacinamide form—some because they don't realize that there are two different types of vitamin B$_3$, others in order to avoid the "niacin flush" they get from taking B$_3$ on an empty stomach. This mild prickly heat on the face, and occasionally the neck and chest, is not unlike the "sex flush" that many women experience prior to orgasm, and it is just as harmless. Some people actually like it. What causes both the niacin flush and the sex flush is a sudden release of histamine. In the case of niacin, the release is accompanied by the dilation of the small blood vessels (capillaries) in the skin and elsewhere.

This dilation eases the flow of oxygen and nutrients to the skin surface as well as to the heart muscle and the tiny blood vessels of the brain. Smokers with chronic constriction of the fine blood vessels in the brain caused by nicotine sometimes experience a slight headache when starting to take niacin. But as these blood vessels open up and become more normal, this annoying initial side effect usually disappears. By the way, even if you don't experience the niacin flush, you're still benefitting from this important dilating effect, only the histamine release proceeds more slowly (either because you have food in your stomach, or for individual physiological reasons).

Niacinamide, another form of vitamin B$_3$, does not produce the flush, but neither does it lower your cholesterol. So, if you have to use additional niacin to bring high cholesterol under control—for which you need about 3,000 milligrams per day, you had better use a time-release form of it.

With much smaller doses of niacin, as on our regular program, the flush is experienced only if you take the full anti-oxidant Menu, which provides for 40 milligrams of niacin at one time (three to five times per day) on an empty stomach. If it's time to take your anti-oxidant spectrum, but it happens to be between meals, take only half of it then, and take the other half about fifteen minutes later. For us this eliminates the flush (which isn't really much of a problem with our program).

If niacin is taken on a regular, daily basis, it causes a constant small drain of histamines. This has a buffering effect on the distressing symptoms, caused by histamine release, that are characteristic of asthma, hay fever, and other types of allergic reactions. For this purpose, however, somewhat larger amounts of niacin than are called for on our program (in the range of 1,000 to 3,000 milligrams per day, depending on the individual case) will have to be taken to achieve more noticeable relief.

Vitamin B_3 can also help with sleep problems: This vitamin has the ability to bind to the same nerve-cell receptors in the brain as do tranquilizers like Valium, Librium, and Dalmane. If you have both a cholesterol and a sleep problem, we suggest taking some extra niacin (200 to 300 milligrams) at bedtime. (If you have no cholesterol problem, we recommend taking pure liquid vitamin E to improve the quality of sleep.) In either case, you're much better off taking either niacin or vitamin E instead of tranquilizers or sleeping pills. Nutrients are not addictive, nor do they have negative side effects, as is the case with most drugs.

SOURCES

1. Miettinen, T. A., et al. "Glucose tolerance and plasma insulin in man during acute and chronic administration of nicotinic acid." *Acta Med. Scand.,* 1969; 186:247–253. Also: Miettinen. "Effects of nicotinic acid on catabolism and synthesis of cholesterol in man." *Acta Clin. Chim.,* 1968; 20:43–51.
2. The Coronary Drug Project Research Group. "Clofibrate and niacin in coronary heart disease." *JAMA,* 1975; 231(4):360–381.
3. Grundy, Scott M., et al. "Influence of nicotinic acid on metabolism of cholesterol and triglycerides in man." *J. Lipid Res.,* 1981; 22:24–36.

CHAPTER 15

VITAMIN B$_1$

THE VITAMIN THAT DOES A LITTLE OF EVERYTHING

In our bodies, high concentrations of vitamin B$_1$ (thiamine) are found in the skeletal muscles, heart, liver, kidneys, and brain. In fact, about half of all the thiamine in our bodies is found in the muscles—a measure of how important it is to physical performance.

Vitamin B$_1$ covers many bases in its capacity as a co-antioxidant. Together with several other co-factors and anti-oxidants, it has a role in the production of energy inside our cells. Also, it joins forces with other vitamin co-factors and anti-oxidants, especially vitamins B$_6$ and E, in fighting atherosclerosis (hardening of the arteries) and arthritis.

Vitamin B$_1$ helps prevent cross-linking—the abnormal bonding and stiffening of collagen and elastin, the "protein glue" in the white fibers of our tendons, bones, cartilage, skin, and all other connective tissue. By counteracting this bonding of our tissues, vitamin B$_1$ aids in keeping us youthfully flexible, provided we start taking it early enough in life. But even after much damage has already been done, B$_1$ and the other micronutrients can at least prevent or slow down any further cross-linking of connective tissue. Judging by our own experience, they seem even to be able to undo a certain amount of established damage.

Along with several other anti-oxidants and vitamin co-factors on our Menu, B$_1$ is a strong immune system stimulant and anticancer factor. It helps to detoxify the cancer-causing chemicals in different kinds of

VITAMIN B$_1$

(Thiamine)

Vitamin B$_1$

- is important for generating cell energy.
- helps fight atherosclerosis and arthritis.
- keeps us flexible by counteracting cross-linking (hardening) of skin and connective tissue.
- is a good immune stimulant and anticancer factor.
- helps detoxify environmental pollutants.
- counteracts effects of smoking and alcohol.
- helps prevent stroke and heart attack.

smoke—from cigarettes, a smoldering pile of leaves in the yard, automobile exhaust, or the coals of your barbecue grill.

Together with several other nutrients, vitamin B$_1$ plays a role in stroke and heart attack prevention.

Vitamin B$_1$ has a very special function in counteracting the effects of alcohol by helping to protect the liver and the brain from alcohol's metabolite, acetaldehyde, and other toxic compounds. On the other hand, much of the body's B$_1$ (like vitamins C and B$_6$) is destroyed by alcohol and must be promptly replaced.

Vitamin B$_1$ also helps combat smoker's cough.

Vitamin B_5 (calcium pantothenate) is basically an energy and antistress vitamin. In one classic study done in 1953, the effect of vitamin B_5 on rats enduring artificial stress was tested. The rats were made to swim in cold water, and the time it took for them to reach the point of exhaustion with and without the benefit of vitamin B_5 was clocked. Those rats given no vitamin supplement could swim for an average of three minutes; those who received a small dosage of B_5 lasted four minutes; and those given a high supplement of B_5 were able to swim in the cold water for an average of twelve minutes, or four times as long as those who had not been given B_5.

In cold-water submersion tests with humans, these same researchers found that B_5 supplementation increased antibody production—that is, it increased these subjects' resistance to stress.[1]

In experiments with frogs, giving them vitamin B_5 increased their total muscular output but not their peak output. In humans vitamin B_5 may be able to increase stamina and endurance through its special role in the energy cycle of an enzyme conversion called the *Krebs Cycle* or *Citric Acid Cycle*. As of this writing, there is still no positive proof of this benefit—which, if confirmed, would have implications for athletes to whom endurance rather than peak output is of the essence.

Vitamin B_5 has also long been credited with having a beneficial effect on arthritic and rheumatoid conditions. Researchers in England discovered as early as 1963 that people with rheumatoid arthritis had

VITAMIN B$_5$

(Calcium Pantothenate)

Vitamin B$_5$

- improves endurance and stamina in animals and probably humans.
- may have benefits for endurance sports.
- helps with arthritis and rheumatism, morning stiffness, etc.
- is needed for production of neurotransmitters (similar to B$_6$).
- helps protect against air pollution (similar to E and B$_1$).
- has cosmetic effects: good for skin and hair; helps (with B$_3$) to remove "age spots" (lipofuscin).
- helps digestion; shortens food transport time.

lower blood levels of B$_5$ than others. Those with the *lowest* blood levels were, the investigators said, "in nearly every case badly crippled, and in two cases bedridden. Injections of B$_5$ [in some instances together with royal jelly, the food of queen bees] were able to provide at least temporary relief to these arthritis sufferers."*[2]

Similar results were obtained—this time with oral administration of vitamin B$_5$—in relieving the symptoms of osteoarthritis, first, in a study done the same year (1963, Annand), and later (1980), with patients suffering from rheumatoid arthritis. In the latter study, the patients were given increasing doses of B$_5$ until they could tolerate without stomach upset one 500-milligram tablet four times per day for a combined daily dose of 2,000 milligrams. The total treatment time, including the first week of gradually increasing dosages, was eight weeks.

Vitamin B$_5$ was very successful in alleviating the suffering of these arthritic patients for the duration of the treatment. As the researchers reported, "highly significant effects were recorded for calcium pantothenate [B$_5$] in reducing the duration of morning stiffness, degree of disability, and severity of pain." The patients in a control group who had received a placebo did not experience any such effects.[3]

In addition, vitamin B$_5$ has an essential place on the metabolic "assembly line" that produces the neurotransmitter acetylcholine— essential to good mental functioning. Our type of high-complex-carbohydrate diet gives us plenty of lecithin, which comes mostly from beans, peas, and other legumes. Lecithin contains choline, which is known to improve learning, memory, long-term planning ability, and

* See also our discussion of the anti-inflammatory effects of fish oils, page 452.

mental focus. But the body must first convert choline to acetylcholine in the intestines, which requires an adequate supply of B$_5$.

Vitamin B$_5$ helps to protect us from the toxic effects of all kinds of smoke, in an action similar to that of vitamin B$_1$. Here again is one of the many instances in which several different co-factors or co-antioxidants complement one another or syngergize with each other to produce greater benefits.

Vitamine B$_5$ shares with several other micronutrients—among them vitamins E, A, B$_3$, and, of course, vitamin C—certain cosmetic properties for the skin and, possibly, the hair. With regard to B$_5$'s cosmetic effect on the skin, it seems to play an important role (with B$_3$) in the gradual removal of lipofuscin, those unsightly brown "age spots" that are chemically rancid fats. (Our anti-oxidant Menu tends to make these spots disappear, although it may take two to three years.)

As for vitamin B$_5$'s reputed ability to prevent hair from graying, or even to restore it to its original color, the meager evidence for this is inconclusive. The same is true for PABA (para-aminobenzoic acid), another B vitamin for which similar claims are made. There is no solid evidence for any of these claims except that some animal studies suggest such an effect.[4] But we do know that the graying of human hair is, in part, free-radical–mediated, which is probably the reason why a full-spectrum vitamin/anti-oxidant program sometimes does indeed slow down the graying process. Sometimes there is even a dramatic return to the original color, as has to a large extent been true in Eberhard's case. (Most people simply assume that he's using an artificial hair-coloring rinse, as they cannot imagine anyone in his seventies not being totally gray.)

Finally, we should mention that vitamin B$_5$ gently stimulates peristalsis; that is, it encourages the contractions of the colon that propel its contents forward for excretion. Most people on our high-complex-carbohydrate, low-fat, low-protein, high-fiber diet have no problems with constipation, which means that the suggested amount of vitamin B$_5$ is just right for them. But if you want to speed up food transport time, by all means take a little extra B$_5$ (250 to 500 milligrams). Certainly B$_5$ is a better choice than commercial laxatives. (See also our discussion of constipation, pages 273–276.)

ROYAL JELLY: THE ELIXIR OF YOUTH?

In concluding our discussion of vitamin B$_5$, we want to mention in passing a controversial natural substance, royal jelly, of which vitamin B$_5$ is one of the main constituents. This thick, viscous, whitish substance, secreted by the salivary glands of worker bees, is indeed the food of queen bees—whose life span it dramatically extends. Instead of dying within a month, like normal bees, the jelly-fed queen lives for six to eight years—an absolutely astronomical (seventy to ninetyfold) extension of a bee's maximum life span!

If royal jelly could do only half as much for us humans as it does for bees, it would be the fabled Elixir of Youth its proponents claim it to be. Alas, a royal jelly for human beings has yet to be discovered; and if it is ever found, it will undoubtedly be some combination of anti-oxidants more powerful than any we know today.

Researchers in England did discover as early as 1959 that either royal jelly or a compound in it—10-hydroxydecenoic acid—seems to be able to inhibit completely the development of a common type of leukemia and another kind of cancer in mice. Their report "appears to be the first unequivocal demonstration of an anti-tumor activity in royal jelly."[5] But as of this writing, there has been no follow-up to these promising experiments.

In 1963 English scientists discovered that if they injected patients suffering from severe rheumatoid arthritis with a mixture of the same compound, 10-hydroxydecenoic acid, fortified by the same amount of vitamin B_5 (calcium pantothenate), the patients improved. For a group of vegetarian patients who had higher vitamin B_5 levels than non-vegetarian patients, this combination "produced rapid disappearance of symptoms in all cases [fourteen days]."[6] These rheumatoid arthritis sufferers experienced relief from their symptoms *only while continuing the treatment, but not much beyond*—a reminder that anti-oxidant treatment, whether preventive or therapeutic, must be continuous.

SOURCES

1. Rally, E. P., and M. Dumm. "Relation of pantothenic acid to adrenal cortical function." *Vitamins and Hormones,* 1953; 11:133–157.
2. Barton-Wright, E. C., and W. A. Elliot. "The pantothenic acid metabolism of rheumatoid arthritis." *Lancet,* October 26, 1963, pp. 862–863.
3. Report No. 199 of the General Practitioner Research Group (coordinator, Dr. David Wheatley, Twickenham). "Calcium pantothenate in arthritic conditions." *Practitioner,* February 1980; 224: 208–211.
4. Goodman, L. S., and A. G. Gilman. *The Pharmacological Basis of Therapeutics,* 6th ed. New York: Macmillan, 1985, p. 1572.
5. Townsend, G., et al. "Activity of 10-hydroxydecenoic acid from royal jelly against experimental leukemia and ascitic tumors." *Nature,* 1959; 183:1270–1271.
6. Barton-Wright and Elliott, op. cit.

CHAPTER 17

VITAMIN B$_2$

CO-FACTOR OF THE ANTI-OXIDANT GLUTATHIONE

$\mathcal{V}$ Vitamin B$_2$, riboflavin, is a water-soluble, yellow-colored vitamin. It causes the urine of supplement users to turn a bright lemon yellow as it is eliminated by the kidneys.

Vitamin B$_2$'s primary function on our program is to help the enzyme glutathione reductase—from which your body makes the powerful anti-oxidant glutathione. This vitamin helps recycle oxidized, degraded glutathione back to the reduced state in which the glutathione can work to your advantage.

B$_2$ supplements (much like vitamin B$_{12}$ supplements) are especially important for strict vegetarians and others who either do not eat any meat and dairy products—the major dietary sources for vitamins B$_2$ and B$_{12}$—or do so in too small quantities to provide enough to help recycle used-up glutathione and prevent possible deficiency symptoms (for example, cracks at the corners of the mouth, itching eyes, and sensitivity to light).

Among others who may run short of B$_2$ are, generally, elderly people on inadequate diets, and also another group, which one would not suspect of having any shortfalls—namely, those who do strenuous aerobic exercises.[1] Also, people on very calorie-restricted diets have all the more reason to be on a full-spectrum anti-oxidant/vitamin program, like ours, that includes vitamin B$_2$.[2] Actually, marginal B$_2$ deficiencies are not uncommon, since this vitamin is easily destroyed by exposure to light, cooking, and alcohol (the Demopoulos spectrum

VITAMIN B$_2$

(Riboflavin)

Vitamin B$_2$

- helps body recycle oxidized glutathione.
- strict vegetarians risk shortfalls because main sources for B$_2$ are meat and dairy products.
- those doing aerobic exercises, or on calorie-restricted diets, and the elderly may also need extra B$_2$.
- is easily destroyed by light, cooking, and alcohol.
- crucial in forming flavin-based molecules that are essential in the hydrogen-electron transport system of the mitochondria (the "furnaces" of cells).

provides a more than adequate amount to cover any of these contingencies).

SOURCES

1. Belko, A. Z., et al. "Effects of exercise on riboflavin requirements of young women." *Am. J. Clin. Nutr.,* 1983; 37:509.
2. Belko, A. Z., et al. "Effects of aerobic exercise and weight loss on riboflavin requirements of moderately obese, marginally deficient young women." *Am. J. Clin. Nutr.,* 1984; 40:553.

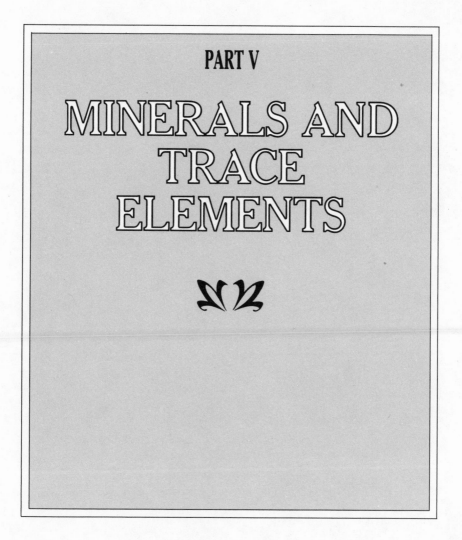

PART V

MINERALS AND TRACE ELEMENTS

CHAPTER 18

CALCIUM

THE MINERAL SUPPLEMENT WE NEED MOST

Although 99 percent of the body's calcium is stored in our bones and teeth, it is the 1 percent in solution that keeps us alive. The calcium in our blood serum and other fluids maintains normal heartbeat, keeps the nervous system functioning, makes muscle contraction possible, keeps complicated enzyme systems going, fosters proper hormone secretion, ensures that cells hang on to each other, and aids in the proper coagulation of blood. Calcium is now also recognized as an important secondary messenger for the neurons in our brain; it can facilitate the transmission of signals between neurons or cause more of a neurotransmitter to be released.

With all these vital roles for calcium in our system, and all the different demands made on it, it is amazing that the 1 percent that circulates in our bodies generally is enough to do the job. A calcium shortfall often does occur, oddly enough, with the 99 percent that is stored in our bones. And the moment there is a deficiency, our bodies start taking calcium from the storehouse of the bones. This insidious process culminates in the progressive condition called *osteoporosis,* (softening of the bones).[1]

In this country fully 200,000 people break their hips every year because they have become deficient in calcium over time. Add to broken hips the other types of fractures caused by weak bones that lack calcium, and you have a total 1.3 million fractures per year. The annual

CALCIUM

- only mineral supplement needed by most people.
- body takes calcium out of bones if it doesn't get enough from dietary sources.
- the average American diet provides for only about one half of the calcium required for good bone maintenance (vegetarians get even less).
- amount on our program makes up the difference.
- vitamin D (mostly produced by sunlight) is necessary for proper calcium absorption. Again, our spectrum of micronutrients provides the correct amount.
- calcium supplementation may lower blood pressure.
- helps prevent colon and rectal cancer.

cost of medical care for this easily preventable problem amounts to a staggering $3.8 billion.

The reason this problem is so widespread is because the average American diet—as well as our own personal, semivegetarian one, which excludes meat and dairy products (except low-fat yogurt)—provides only about one half (750 milligrams) of the 1,500 milligrams per day of calcium required to prevent osteoporosis. These numbers reflect the recent shift in American eating habits to greater health consciousness, away from calcium-rich but cholesterol- and casein-laden dairy products that promote atherosclerosis and can lead to serious allergic reactions, such as migraine headaches and chronic bronchitis (see our discussion of milk and dairy products in Chapter 49).

Our program provides for a daily supplement of 750 to 1,250 milligrams of calcium, depending on whether you take the micronutrient Menu three, four, or five times a day. Three capsules of 250 milligrams each per day suffices to supplement fully a totally dairy-product–free diet (as we advocate).

We start losing calcium much earlier in life than is generally believed. For white males and black females, the loss begins at about age thirty; for white women it begins at age eighteen. But black men are unaccountably exempt.

Most people are not aware of this loss until many years later when the all-too-visible sign appears, especially in older women: the dowager's hump, or curvature of the back. Once the damage is done, the condition can be slowed down by taking calcium supplements, but it can't be reversed.

Why is osteoporosis in our society especially prevalent among post-menopausal women? For one thing, the female hormones called *estrogens* play an important role in bone metabolism. Estrogens don't make new bone tissue, but they do slow down the rate of bone breakdown. That's why osteoporosis becomes much more acute in postmenopausal women, whose estrogen production is greatly reduced. This is also the case for women who have their ovaries removed.

In order to make up for the shortfall of estrogens in their postmenopausal or postoperative women patients, physicians usually prescribe estrogen-replacement therapy with calcium supplementation. Nowadays, physicians use both estrogens and progesterone for "estrogen-replacement therapy." Very often, this decision is the right one. But there is more to consider than just the prevention of bone softening and bone fractures. The advisability or inadvisability of estrogen-replacement therapy depends on several factors. If the woman is in sound health and has no history of any precancerous or cancerous condition, there's no reason for her not to take estrogens. But if she has undergone a hysterectomy—even for nonmalignant tumors—or has nonmalignant breast disease, not to mention breast cancer—the use of estrogen therapy must be seriously weighed in the light of possibly increased cancer risks.

Scientists have discovered a hormone that transfers calcium from the bones to the bloodstream—alas, sometimes overdoing it and thereby contributing to osteoporosis and possibly cancer. Such, at least, can be assumed from the fact that large amounts of this hormone—called *parathormone* because it's made by four small "buttons" of tissue behind the thyroid gland—have been found in the blood of patients with lung cancer, leukemias, and cancers of the female reproductive system.[2] Once researchers find out more about this complicated hormone (a protein made up of 141 amino acids!), we might be able to prevent osteoporosis not only with supplemental calcium—a rather crude, symptomatic therapy that doesn't address itself to the real causes of osteoporosis—and with estrogen-replacement therapy (which carries its own cancer risks), but also with a therapy that would inhibit the action of this hormone.

The fact that calcium absorption is largely dependent on vitamin D has been known for some time. Incidentally, it should perhaps be called a hormone rather than a vitamin because its molecular structure is similar to cortisone and estrogen. Incidentally, vitamin D not only aids in the absorption of calcium, but also in absorption of phosphorus, another element essential to bone structure.

The amount of vitamin D we get from food sources depends very much on diet. The fewer animal products eaten, the less vitamin D we get. For vegetarians or semi-vegetarians, we suggest taking some supplemental vitamin D for that reason alone. (Arguments by vegetarians that this is unnecessary are unconvincing.)

Now there are indications that there may also be a mind-body connection that influences calcium absorption. For instance, it was noted that young obese women on weight-reduction programs suddenly developed a negative calcium balance. This despite the fact that they were getting the same amounts of dietary calcium as they were before starting weight reduction. What made the difference? One explanation—and a very logical one—is that the emotional stress and frustration connected with the dieting might be responsible for this strange phenomenon.

The hunch was later confirmed by a study on ten young pregnant unmarried women, some of whom had serious emotional problems, while others appeared to be relatively free of disturbance. It transpired that calcium retention varied inversely to the amount of self-reported emotional stress.*

These findings were in turn confirmed by a study on adult male prisoners. Here again, calcium absorption was clearly influenced by the emotional state of the individual. As the emotional state of an inmate improved, so did his calcium utilization.[3]

Notwithstanding all the factors that influence calcium absorption, supplementation with vitamin D is still a good idea. This is true even considering that we actually get most of our vitamin D from the sun's action on certain cholesterol-like oils in the deeper layers of our skin. Since in the Northern Hemisphere we get virtually no vitamin D from the sun during the long winter months, we must rely more heavily on food sources (or supplements) during that period.

Older people, often already undersupplied with nutrients (including calcium) because of poor diet, also tend to spend less time outdoors and thus get less sun exposure. As a consequence, they are likely to be short on vitamin D. To make matters worse, older people are less able to synthesize the metabolically active form of vitamin D, calcitriol, which regulates the production of proteins required for intestinal calcium absorption,[1] which is all the more reason why calcium supplements should be balanced by vitamin D.†

Another problem that has only recently come to light is that many calcium supplements do not disintegrate fast enough in the stomach to do much good. Scientists at the University of Maryland School of Pharmacy tested thirty-five popular brand calcium supplements to find out how long they would take to dissolve in a solution similar to our gastric juices.[4,5] To their shocked surprise, almost one half of these

---

* We are convinced that if similar studies were done on the relationship between emotional states and the absorption of other nutrients, one might find that the same principle applies all across the board.

† Excellent calcium supplements with vitamin D are supplied by several companies, including Health Maintenance Programs, Twin Laboratories, and Vitamin Research Products.

products do not dissolve within half an hour, to the extent of 75 percent the USP standard. Most of the calcium in these products, it was found, actually passes through the alimentary canal without a chance of being absorbed. (The reason such a situation can exist is that the FDA currently requires only calcium-containing *drugs,* not supplements, to meet the USP guidelines.)*

In addition to all the previously mentioned benefits of calcium, there is evidence now that, in cases of mild to moderate hypertension, calcium supplements can actually lower blood pressure. In a 1985 study, hypertensive patients received 1,000 milligrams of oral calcium supplements for a period of eight weeks, while a control group received a placebo. Those on the calcium supplements showed a marked improvement in normalizing blood pressure; the control patients showed no improvement.[6]

This study, the first clinical trial of supplemental calcium on blood pressure in humans, represents an important breakthrough. Merely doubling the amount of calcium already on our Menu can be a valuable adjunct in the treatment and prevention of hypertenion.

Psychologists at Texas A & M University discovered in 1987 that moderate amounts of calcium seem to enhance mood, while large amounts have a depressive effect. As the researchers put it, ". . . smaller increases in calcium intake might enhance mood because they enhance the activity of certain neurons that are associated with mood and emotion, whereas larger increases might exacerbate mood because they suppress the activity of these sensory neurons.[7] There is little danger that most of us will take in too much calcium (over 3,000 milligrams per day); chances are, if you were tested for calcium level, you'd find yourself on the short end. So, by all means, take your calcium supplement, and keep the dose around 1,500 milligrams per day.

Furthermore, animal and human studies suggest that calcium supplementation may be one of several factors preventing a certain percentage of the rectal and colon cancers from which six million Americans alive today will eventually die. Most Europeans and Americans share the high-fat diets that encourage these cancers by producing up to ten times the normal level of bile acids, along with large quantities of anaerobic bacteria that appear to convert bile acids into carcinogens. Researchers at Sloan-Kettering Cancer Memorial Center in

* The calcium supplements we recommend have the extra advantage of being in capsule form rather than tablets, which must contain some kind of binder that would further inhibit disintegration in the stomach. Interesting, too, was the finding of the University of Maryland scientists that sometimes one calcium supplement made by a given company passed the disintegration test, while another manufactured by the same company failed it. For instance, AARP Pharmacy's Calcium 600-D (Formula 314) passed with flying colors, while its Oyster Shell Calcium with Vitamin D (Formula 310) flunked the test. Among other popular calcium supplements that did *not* pass were K Mart Extra strength O. S. Calcium, Pathmark Calcium 600-D, and Schiff Oyster Shell Calcium, 500 milligrams.

New York City have shown that calcium binds very strongly to bile acids and fatty acids, and in so doing short-circuits this cancer-causing process.[8]

The average American-European diet is not only notoriously rich in fats, but also much too rich in protein. While the fats promote cancers, atherosclerosis, and heart disease, excess protein causes too much calcium to be excreted and is hard on the kidneys.

Many people are now wisely cutting down on dairy products. Some of them do so mostly because of the high fat and cholesterol content of these foods. Others are concerned about casein, the milk protein, which is not only allergenic but also suspected of being a major contributor to atherosclerosis. Then there are the whey proteins, which are also highly allergenic and must be avoided by those with milk allergies. For all these reasons, many people's dietary sources of calcium have become rather limited, even more so for vegetarians, who must get all theirs from plant sources. The question then arises whether a vegetarian diet alone can supply sufficient calcium to prevent osteoporosis?

Some say it can, often citing in support of this view the example of the African Bantu, who live on a calcium-poor diet but do not develop osteoporosis. However, the Bantu engage in strenuous physical activity, at a level long known to protect against loss of calcium from the bones. Even a daily routine of jogging, yoga, or aerobic exercise is no comparison for the Bantu's energetic, day-in, day-out outdoor existence.

Being black offers a certain protection against osteoporosis. Black men have the biggest advantage in that respect. There are obvious implications here for manned space exploration: The weightlessness experienced in outer space takes calcium out of the bones at a fast clip. In longer space flights, white astronauts risk getting "jelly bones." Blacks could stay in outer space much longer and would therefore make ideal astronauts.

To recap quickly: Black men enjoy the most protection against osteoporosis; next in line for relative protection are white males; third in line are black women, and the most vulnerable to osteoporosis are white women. A white woman should therefore start taking calcium supplements long *before,* rather than after, menopause. By the end of her reproductive period, much irreversible bone loss has already occurred. A white female should ideally begin calcium supplementation not later than the beginning of her second decade. (White men should start in their early thirties.)

If you are on Dr. Demopoulos's spectrum of anti-oxidants and vitamin co-factors, you'll automatically be getting all the additional calcium you need. However, anyone else should do herself or himself the favor of preventing the unnecessary disfiguring and crippling fractures that will more than likely occur with advancing age by taking one of the excellent, inexpensive calcium supplements recommended here.*

SOURCES

1. Zaloga, G. P., and B. Chernow. "Endocrine Metabolic Problems in the Critically Ill Immunocompromised Patient." In: *The Critically Ill Immuno-suppressed Patient,* J. E. Parillo and H. Masur, eds. Rockville, Md.: Aspen Publications, Inc., 1987.
2. As reported in *The New York Times,* July 21, 1987.
3. Goodhart, R. S., and M. E. Shils, eds. *Modern Nutrition in Health and Disease, Dietotherapy,* 5th ed. Philadelphia: Lea & Fabiger, 1973, p. 88.
4. *American Pharmacy,* Vol. NS27, No. 2, February 1987, p. 56.
5. *Nutrition Action Health Letter,* June 1987, p. 9.
6. McCarron, D. A., and C. D. Morris. "Blood pressure response to oral calcium in persons with mild to moderate hypertension." *Ann. Int. Med.,* 1985; 103:6, Part I: 825–831.
7. As reported in *APA Monitor,* Vol. 18, No. 12, December 1987.
8. Lipkin, M., and H. Newmark. "Effect of added dietary calcium on colonic epithelial-cell proliferation in subjects at high risk for familial colonic cancer." *N. Eng. J. Med.,* November 28, 1985; 313(22):1381–1384.

* Recent research seems to indicate that the trace element boron is vitally important in preventing the demineralization of bones and for proper blood levels of certain hormones, including estrogens. A diet rich in fruits, especially pears, apples, and grains, provides ample quantities (about 4 to 5 milligrams per day). On the other hand, meat, fish, and dairy products are poor sources of boron.

CHAPTER 19

SELENIUM

GOOD INSURANCE, IF YOU LIVE IN A SELENIUM-POOR AREA

1 The one mineral (more accurately, trace element) we are most often asked about is selenium. Until a few years ago, medical opinion was dominated by fears about selenium's potential toxicity (liver damage) and the possibility of it being able to cause cancer. Although overdosing on it is certainly dangerous, it is now generally agreed that the toxic potential of selenium taken in recommended dosages has been greatly overestimated. As to fears that it may be carcinogenic, more recent studies suggest quite the opposite: Selenium appears to help prevent and inhibit rather than cause or promote cancers. According to the National Research Council of the National Academy of Sciences in 1982: "A large accumulation of evidence indicates that supplementation of the diet or drinking water with selenium protects against tumors induced by a variety of chemical carcinogens and at least one viral agent."[1]

In America researchers correlated the selenium content in the soils and drinking water of various states with the incidence of cancer. They found that people living in high-selenium areas had a lower cancer mortality rate than those living in low-selenium areas. Since South Dakota turned out to have the most selenium content and Ohio the least, it's not surprising that Rapid City, South Dakota, had the lowest cancer rates in the nation, or that Ohio's cancer rates were nearly twice as high.[2,3]

In a follow-up study, one group of investigators extended these geographic comparisons to twenty other countries.[4] The result was always the same: The less selenium in the soil and drinking water (hence in the diet), the higher the incidence of the most common cancers. Venezuela with its selenium-rich soil[5] had one quarter the mortality rate from cancer of the colon than the United States. And much lower rates of breast cancer were found among Japanese women living in Japan than among Japanese women living in the United States. Apparently, Japanese women in their homeland, eating a selenium-rich, fish-based diet,[6] enjoy a certain degree of protection from breast cancer, while their sisters in America, eating an essentially meat-based diet, have as high breast cancer rates as do American and European women.

However, is one justified in crediting only the selenium for this cancer protection? Probably not. A diet based on seafood instead of meat is essentially a low-fat diet. And we know that a high-fat diet promotes breast cancer. There is also some indication that the fish oils and seaweeds in the typical Japanese diet may have a protective effect with regard to certain cancers.*

As to the low colon cancer rate in Venezuela, selenium is an important dietary factor but surely not the only one. Rice and beans (*gallo pinto*) are commonly eaten at least once and often two or three times a day by the poorer classes throughout all of Latin America, as are other bean dishes, such as bean paste and bean soup (*sopa negra*). In addition, more fruit is eaten in these tropical countries than in many other parts of the world. Beans are high in guar gum, and fruit contains a lot of pectin—both the gum and pectin are water-soluble fibers with a known protective effect on colon cancer. They also contain other anticancer compounds (indoles, phenols, protease inhibitors, etc.), discussed in later chapters of this book. Selenium's credit for the low colon cancer rate in Venezuela should therefore probably be shared with several other protective factors in the national diet.

On the other hand, there can be little doubt from not only the above-mentioned population studies, but from animal studies as well that selenium has a protective effect against chemically induced cancers,[7,8] and that it is able to slow down or even totally prevent tumor growth.[9]

In keeping with these findings, other animal studies have shown that

* It is astonishing that the benefits of the lower fat content of the traditional Japanese diet override even the highly carcinogenic effect of the pyrilyzates (toxic compounds from scorched proteins) produced by broiling fish, a popular cooking method in Japan. Fortunately, the Japanese also eat fish prepared in other ways, for instance, as in *tempura* (deep-frying, but not as dangerous as broiling), or as raw *sushi* and *sashimi*. Moreover, breast cancer is much less affected by the carcinogens in broiled foods than are colorectal and stomach cancers (see also our discussion of the effects of different cooking methods on proteins in the chapters on barbecuing [page 353–354] and on proteins [pages 365–366]).

selenium can strengthen the immune system by stimulating lymphocytes to produce more antibodies. Selenium encourages the activity of phagocytes, PacMan-like cells that engulf and gobble up even cancer cells along with the usual bacteria and viruses.[10–12]

Studies on humans have consistently shown higher cancer rates—particularly cancer of the large intestine and pancreas—in people with low blood levels of selenium.[13,14] In fact, adults suffering from cystic fibrosis (a childhood disorder of certain duct glands also marked by chronic respiratory infections) are more likely to develop cancer when their blood selenium concentrations are low.[15] These findings are less surprising when you consider that people with cystic fibrosis are deficient in vitamins A and E and show signs of abnormal free-radical activity (for instance, badly cross-linked tissues). All three anti-oxidants—selenium, vitamin A, and vitamin E—are free-radical quenchers and have proven anticancer properties.

The close anticancer link between selenium, vitamin A, and vitamin E was dramatically illustrated by a four-year follow-up study involving 12,000 Finnish people[16] begun in 1977. It showed that patients who died of cancer had a much lower mean selenium level and much lower vitamin A and E levels than those who did not develop cancer. Not surprisingly, most of these differences are accounted for by the smokers in the study, who had the lowest serum levels of all three anti-oxidants (smoking destroys these substances.) Men who smoked (none of the women in the smaller cancer group were smokers) had 25 percent less vitamin A in their bloodstream, and those with the lowest serum selenium levels had almost nine times the risk of fatal cancer as did those with the highest selenium values. People with both low selenium and low vitamin E levels had an eleven times greater risk of dying from cancer compared with those with higher levels, which amounts to saying that those with higher anti-oxidant levels had by far the most anticancer protection.

All indications suggest that selenium also protects against stroke and heart attack. American regional studies on the incidence of cardiovascular disease and soil levels of selenium show a remarkably high incidence of stroke and heart attack where the soil is low in selenium.[17] That's why parts of Georgia and the Carolinas have been nicknamed the "stroke belt" of the United States.* And the previously mentioned Finnish study revealed that those who have low blood levels of selenium are three times more likely to die from heart attacks and twice as likely to suffer from nonfatal heart attacks as those with higher selenium levels.

---

* The New England states, western Oregon, and parts of the Midwest have selenium-poor soils. In contrast, Colorado, Kansas, Nebraska, North and South Dakota, and Wyoming are very high-selenium areas.

Interestingly enough, the people in this heart disease study who had low blood selenium levels were later found to have low levels of EPA, the fatty acids in fish oils that seem to protect against stroke and heart disease. Conversely, people who were free of these cardiovascular diseases had more EPA in their bloodstream. The Finnish researchers were thus inclined to blame the low EPA levels rather than the low selenium levels for the incidence of heart disease.[18]

Since the selenium content of soil and drinking water in Finland is low, we suspect that the people in the study who did not develop heart disease and had high selenium *and* high EPA blood levels probably ate more fish—the only source of EPA, and the only reliable source for selenium. This suggests that a more inclusive approach to these problems makes more sense than looking at only one factor at a time, be it selenium or EPA.

Experimental evidence[19,20] suggests that combined supplementation of selenium and vitamin E may help protect against tissue damage when there is insufficient blood flow and, hence, too little oxygen supply to an organ. Angina* sufferers who received 1 milligram (1,000 micrograms) of selenium and 200 I.U. of vitamin E per day experienced considerable relief from the excruciating chest pain that characterizes this heart condition. (Those in the study who received a placebo did not experience relief from pain.)

Pearson and Shaw[21] point out that free-radical damage to tissues (such as those of the heart) is usually more rapid and more severe when there is only a partial obstruction of blood flow, and hence only low or poor oxygen supply (hypoxia), rather than total shutoff of oxygen (anoxia). It is precisely this *partial* shutoff that causes most strokes. Cardiac arrest (heart attack), however, is most often caused by the rarer—but lethal—total shutoff of oxygen to the heart.

Most hypoxia is brought about by vasospasms (spasms of the smooth muscles surrounding our arteries). These spasms can be caused by many things, for example, alcohol. But platelet aggregation in the bloodstream, brought about by eating fatty foods or smoking tobacco is also quite sufficient to trigger a vasospasm. A good percentage of angina attacks as well as TIAs (transient ischemic attacks—really very mild strokes without permanent consequences) are undoubtedly due to spasms brought on by fatty foods or smoking, causing platelet aggregation. When platelet aggregation or anything else (like stress) brings on a vasospasm, the result is hypoxia and possibly an angina attack or a TIA. If the arteries are already partially obstructed because of atherosclerotic plaque, the vasospasm may cause a full-blown stroke

* Angina pectoris is a condition in which the individual suffers recurrent, extreme pain due to acute partial shutoff of blood and oxygen to the heart. These violent pains can be brought on by excitement, emotional stress, or overexertion, especially in the presence of atherosclerosis, the inevitable result of a high-fat diet.

or heart attack. We don't make the connection between events like these and our food habits because platelet aggregation peaks several hours after the ingestion of fatty foods. (That's why people usually don't suffer an angina attack or a TIA at the table, which might encourage a quick change of diet!)

In considering selenium's potential in helping prevent platelet aggregation and vasospasm, we must not overlook the effects of all the other anti-oxidants. Remember, for example, vitamin E's proven anticlotting effect and vitamin C's and niacin's well-established capacity to regress atherosclerotic plaque. Micronutrients, including selenium, are not comparable to, say, antibiotics, which work very well by themselves. Rather, they must be carefully "orchestrated" and used in a *complete system* if they are to work to our best advantage.

Selenium is credited by serious researchers[22] with being able to detoxify heavy metals such as mercury, lead, and cadmium, probably by forming harmless selenides with them. But we know that glutathione has the same ability to bind to these toxic metals and carry them out with the urine. And both glutathione and selenium play crucial roles in one of our primary anti-oxidant enzyme systems, glutathione peroxidase (each molecule of glutathione peroxidase has four atoms of selenium!).

For the same reasons, selenium detoxifies peroxidized fats and very possibly the toxic metabolites of alcohol and cigarette smoke. Selenium can also help detoxify various drugs, including a frequently used anticancer drug, Adriamycin, and *without* simultaneously neutralizing its tumor-inhibiting effect.[23]

THE BOTTOM LINE ON SELENIUM

Dietary selenium intake in the United States differs from state to state, depending on the selenium content of the soil and drinking water. Intake may be as low as 50 micrograms or as high as 150 micrograms a day, depending on where you live and on your food habits. (The best sources are seafood and meat; next, whole grains and cereals, and last, certain vegetables.)

There is no established RDA for selenium, but in 1980 a committee of the National Research Council proposed an "estimated safe and adequate daily intake" of 50 to 200 micrograms. There have been rumors that the National Cancer Institute is trying to have the council revise this estimate upward, and other scientists have shown that an upper dietary limit of 200 micrograms is too low.[24]

Dr. Sheldon Hendler suggests a daily supplement in the range of 100 to 200 micrograms of organic selenium, along with 100 to 400 I.U. of vitamin E, because of the known synergism between these two anti-oxidants. As for us, we're taking 250 micrograms of Twinlab's yeast-free sodium selenite at bedtime, together with ½ teaspoon of Health Maintenance Programs' liquid vitamin E. We think that that's the best way. Dr. Demopoulos still doesn't take selenium supplements because he calculates he gets most of his fruits and vegetables (which he consumes in prodigious quantities) from California, whose soil is generally selenium-rich. We can't always agree on everything.

SOURCES

1. *Diet, Nutrition, and Cancer.* Washington, D.C.: National Academy Press, 1982.
2. Shamberger, R. J., et al. "Antioxidants and cancer. Part VI. Selenium and age-adjusted human cancer mortality." *Arch. Environ. Health,* 1976; 31:231.
3. Schrauzer, G. N., et al. "Cancer mortality correlation studies. Part III. Statistical associations with dietary selenium intakes." *Bioinorg. Chem.,* 1977; 7:23.
4. Schrauzer, G. N., et al. "Selenium in human nutrition—dietary intakes and effects of supplementation." *Bioinorg. Chem.,* 1978; 8:303–318.
5. Mondragon, M. C., and W. G. Jaffe. "The ingestion of selenium in Caracas compared with some other cities of the world." *Arch. Latinoamer. Nutr.,* 1976; 26:341–352.
6. Sakurai, H., and K. Tsuchiya. "A tentative recommendation for the maximum daily intake of selenium." *Environ. Physiol. Biochem.,* 1975; 5:107–118.
7. Shamberger, R. J. "Relationship of selenium to cancer: I. Inhibitory effect of selenium on carcinogenesis." *J. Natl. Cancer Inst.,* 1970; 44:931.
8. Thompson, H. J., and P. J. Becci. "Selenium inhibition of N-methyl-N-nitrosourea-induced mammary carcinogenesis in the rat." *J. Natl. Cancer Inst.,* 1980; 65:1299.
9. Greeder, G. A., and J. A. Milner. "Factors influencing the inhibitory effect of selenium on mice inoculated with Ehrlich ascites tumor cells." *Science,* 1980; 209:825.
10. Spallholz, J. E., et al. "Anti-inflammatory, immunologic and carcinostatic attributes of selenium in experimental animals." Work reviewed in: *Advances in Experimental Medicines and Biology,* 1981; 135:43–62.
11. Desowitz, R. S., and J. W. Barnwell. "Effect of selenium and dimethyl dioctadecyl ammonium bromide on the vaccine-induced immunity of Swiss-Webster mice against malaria (plasmodium berghei)." *Infection and Immunity,* 1980; 27:87.
12. Ibid.
13. Spallholz et al., op. cit.
14. Desowitz, op. cit.
15. *Fed. Proc. Am. Soc. Exper. Biol.,* 1979; 38:2139.
16. Salonen, J. T., et al., "Risk of cancer in relation to serum concentrations of selenium and vitamins A and E: matched cse control analysis of prospective data." *Brit. Med. J.,* 1985; 290:417.
17. Ibid.

18. *Proceedings of the Symposium on Selenium-Telurium in the Environment,* Industrial Health Foundation, Pittsburgh, Pa., 1976, p. 253.
19. Miettinen, T. A., et al. "Serum selenium concentration related to myocardial infarction and fatty acid content of serum lipids." *Brit. Med. J.,* 1983; 287:517.
20. Van Vleet, J. F. "Effect of selenium-vitamin E on adriamycin-induced cardiomyopathy in rabbits." *Am. J. Veterin. Res.,* 1978; 39:997–1010.
21. Pearson, Durk, and Sandy Shaw. *Life Extension.* New York: Warner Books, 1982, p. 318.
22. Frost, D. V., and P. M. Lish. "Selenium in biology." *Ann. Pharmacol.,* 1975; 18:259.
23. Palmer, I. S., et al. "Selenium intake and urinary excretion in persons living near a high selenium area." *J. Am. Diet. Assoc.,* 1983; 82:511–515.
24. Meyer, E., et al. "Selenium Yeast Studies." In: *Selenium in Biology and Medicine,* J. E. Spallholz et al., eds. AVI, 1981.

CHAPTER 20

ZINC

VITAMIN E'S NEGLECTED TWIN BROTHER

12 Ironically, those who eat the right diet—rich in vegetables, high in fiber, and low in meats—are more likely to be short on zinc than those who do all the dietary "sinning." The reason is that plant foods have chemical substances called *phytates* and *oxalates* that bind to zinc and interfere with it absorption. Similarly, the high fiber content in vegetables, so good for us in most respects, works against us in this case by making it harder to benefit from whatever zinc the vegetables may contain. Most vegetables and grains don't have much zinc anyway—particularly when conventional chemical fertilizers have been used, which can cut in half the zinc available in the soil.[1] Unfortunately, while much of the zinc is taken out of grains in the milling process, cadmium—a very toxic metal often present from pollution or in the soil itself, and concentrated in the inner white part of the grain—will remain in the refined flour.

Cadmium is antagonistic to zinc, and as Dr. Sheldon Hendler points out, we already accumulate an average of 30 milligrams of cadmium, mainly in the kidneys.[2] We need to keep our zinc:cadmium ratio in favor of the zinc as much as possible, since zinc is protective and cadmium is anything but. (Cadmium can, for instance, produce sperm abnormalities and infertility.)* If we eat mostly bread, pasta, and

---

* In *A Complete Guide to Anti-Aging Nutrients*, Dr. Hendler writes that he had diagnosed his own fertility problem as being most likely due to his past smoking habit—cigarette paper contains cadmium, which is antagonistic to zinc and could therefore have produced a marginal zinc deficiency. His guess was obviously correct, for he was able to cure his infertility within a few weeks with nothing more than a daily supplement of 50 milligrams of zinc gluconate.

pastries made from refined white flour and ingest little or no meat, we run a risk of developing a zinc deficiency; in white flour the zinc: cadmium ratio is only 17:1, but it is 100:1 in whole-wheat flour.[3]

On the other hand, the bran in whole-wheat flour does, like all non-water–soluble fiber, interfere to some extent with zinc absorption. In India, where an unleavened type of bread called *chapati* is a dietary staple, special care is taken in milling the flour so that only the outer layer of bran (which contains most of the phytates) is removed while the other bran layers (containing most of the zinc and other minerals) remain in the flour.[4]

The antagonism between cadmium and zinc also figures in contradictory reports about the effects of zinc and selenium on cancer. If, as Dr. Hendler says, zinc antagonizes (neutralizes) the highly toxic cadmium, a protection against cancer may result. If, on the other hand, zinc antagonizes the cancer-protective selenium—a situation that might occur if a selenium deficiency already exists—there could be an *increased* risk of cancer.

Zinc is a biological catalyst in many enzyme systems, including those involved in the production of DNA and RNA. These systems are, among other things, necessary for cell growth, which is the reason why zinc deficiency can lead to dwarfism. But while the right amount of zinc furthers healthy, desirable, growth, too much zinc can promote atherosclerosis and malignant growth—a good reason not to go overboard with it and to balance supplementary zinc with selenium.

Zinc is important for keratin production, essential for healthy hair, skin, and nails. In fact, one of the telltale signs of marginal zinc deficiency can be nails that are speckled with many small white spots or that tend to buckle, curve, and show other abnormalities.

Another symptom of zinc deficiency is distortions of taste or smell. Certain foods or drinks may suddenly take on a disagreeable odor or taste. If you notice such changes, we suggest getting a blood test of your zinc level (a hair analysis is not at all reliable). If the blood test shows a level below 80 micrograms of zinc per 100 milliliters of blood serum, we recommend a zinc supplement (15 to 30 milligrams per day of zinc gluconate would be a reasonable amount in most cases). In any case, your doctor should regulate such treatment.

More than a hundred different enzyme systems depend on zinc for their proper functioning—among them, the pancreatic enzyme system, which is responsible for insulin production. In turn, the proper digestion of carbohydrates depends on insulin. This suggests that zinc deficiency might lead to glucose intolerance.

At least 25 percent of diabetics have abnormally low zinc levels and excrete excessive amounts of zinc in their urine.[5] Medical researchers therefore feel that diabetics probably have two simultaneous problems with zinc: (1) They don't seem to absorb it very well; and (2) they excrete too much of it in their urine (for some not fully understood reason). For these diabetics, some zinc supplementation seems logical.

Zinc supplementation might also help diabetics with two well-known chronic health problems: poor wound healing and proneness to infections. For wound healing, a combination of zinc and vitamin C is necessary to replace the collagen (the protein of the white fibers of skin, tendons, bones, and cartilage) and other proteins of connective tissues that were lost as a result of injury.

The medical literature contains proof of dramatic wound-healing acceleration with zinc supplementation. For instance, in 1967 in a clinical trial, a small group of patients were given 150 milligrams of zinc sulfate per day after major surgery; another group of patients were not given zinc. Those taking the zinc were completely healed in nearly one half the time it took the unsupplemented group to heal.[6] However, a similar experiment in 1970 did not confirm these findings,[7] which may indicate that improved wound healing occurs only in patients who have zinc deficiencies and not in others. At any rate, since zinc intake of 150 milligrams per day over several weeks' time is nontoxic, there seems to be nothing lost and possibly much to be gained by temporarily adding zinc to our basic anti-oxidant program when needed for wound healing. A doctor should supervise prolonged use of zinc at higher dosage regimens.

The wound-healing effect apparently extends to internal "wounds" such as gastric ulcers. In one study (1975), gastric ulcer patients who received 150 milligrams of elemental zinc per day had a three times better healing rate and experienced complete healing more often than patients given placebos.[8]

For ulcer patients a full spectrum of anti-oxidants and co-factors is preferable, assuming the patients can tolerate the increased acidity. Linus Pauling reports on the therapeutic effect of ascorbic acid (vitamin C), which is very acidic, even in patients suffering from gastritis and ulcers.[9] The Demopoulos spectrum uses straight, unbuffered ascorbic acid as well as niacin, another highly acidic micronutrient. And yet most ulcer patients seem able to tolerate this acidity surprisingly well, except for those with bleeding ulcers.

Anyway, people suffering from a serious ulcer problem should not go on our program or take any other micronutrients without their doctor's specific knowledge and consent. What such patients should do, however, besides taking appropriate medication, is go on our kind of diet, discussed in later chapters of this book, but leave out the "roughage," so the diet is soft. They also would be well advised to have a positive mental attitude and to practice some form of relaxation technique, also described further on. Once their ulcers are healed by use of a comprehensive therapy, chances are they will be able to tolerate and benefit from our anti-oxidant spectrum as much as anybody else.

As far as susceptibility to infections is concerned, zinc plays an important role by improving the functioning of the white blood cells (circulating T lymphocytes), which are among our main defenses against invading bacteria and viruses.[10] Zinc supplementation of 30 to 60 milligrams per day might therefore be a good idea for diabetics because they are so infection-prone. The same applies to postsurgical and injury patients. Of course, under any of these circumstances zinc supplements should be taken not in isolation, but, as always, within a broad-spectrum anti-oxidant program.

Other conditions for which zinc supplementation may be indicated are Crohn's disease and chronic kidney failure, when the patient is on dialysis. Zinc may also be helpful in cases of cystic fibrosis and Wilson's disease, another rare genetic disorder, in which copper accumulates in the liver and brain, threatening both these organs with severe damage. Since zinc is antagonistic to copper, using supplements seems logical in this case, provided it is done under a nutrition-oriented physician's supervision.

Zinc has also proven itself beneficial in anorexia nervosa, a partly psychological, partly physiological condition affecting mostly adolescent girls and young women, characterized by an inability or a refusal to eat, often resulting in life-threatening malnutrition. Although therapeutic success with zinc supplementation alone has been reported,[11,12] this is certainly one situation in which as broad a spectrum of anti-oxidants, vitamin co-factors, minerals, and trace elements as the patient can tolerate is indicated. (In fact, in extreme cases requiring intravenous feeding, all these micronutrients should be included in the IV solution.)

Finally, zinc supplementation may be useful in rheumatoid arthritis. Dr. Hendler reports that in a double-blind study conducted in England on a small group of patients who had not responded to other conventional treatments, considerable success was achieved with zinc. There was less morning stiffness, less joint swelling, improved walking ability, and improvement mentioned in the patients' subjective feelings about their condition.[13] Once again, the ideal supplementation is a broad spectrum of other anti-oxidants and vitamin co-factors, several of which seem to have a beneficial effect on rheumatoid arthritis (for example, vitamin B_5, especially if used with the active ingredient in royal jelly; see pages 139–140). Some researchers have speculated that it is also possible for zinc supplements to raise the zinc level within the joints themselves. If so, it may indeed have an anti-inflammatory effect at the very site of trouble, thereby directly causing reported pain relief.

A COUPLE OF MIRACLES ZINC CANNOT PERFORM

Having pointed out the various therapeutic possibilities of zinc, we must put in a strong disclaimer with regard to two frequently made claims. One alleges that zinc is beneficial in cases of prostate enlargement and infection. It's true that the prostate contains the greatest concentration of zinc in the body. But although zinc supplementation does seem to be helpful in cases of male infertility, no evidence for its alleged effectiveness with prostate problems has emerged. Nor is this a great loss: We know from Eberhard's own case, that an effective, broad-spectrum anti-oxidant program with plenty of vitamin C has a decidedly therapeutic effect on this common male affliction (see page 24).

The other disclaimer refers to the frequent misconception that supplemental zinc is helpful with hair loss and with skin problems such as acne. Zinc may have a beneficial effect on these conditions, but only where a severe deficiency existed before the supplementation began. *Topical* applications of creams containing zinc may, however, have a therapeutic effect on acne by being anti-inflammatory and by lowering the abnormal production of sebum (the oily secretion of the skin's sebaceous glands, composed of fat and skin debris), which may be clogging the pores.[14]

THE BOTTOM LINE

There is general agreement among experts that while serious zinc deficiencies are practically nonexistent in the developed world, marginal deficiencies are rather common. Dr. Rudolf Ballantine of the Himalayan International Institute in Honesdale, Pennsylvania, cites a study of college women who took in 12 milligrams of zinc per day but absorbed only 6.6 milligrams. The RDA for zinc is 15 milligrams, and these women, on an average American diet, were getting less than one half that amount.[15]

Nutritionist Dr. James Scala insists that only 2.5 to 4 milligrams of zinc per day are actually needed to avoid clinical zinc deficiency.[16] Again, this is a nutritional viewpoint that overlooks marginal deficiencies that might prevent optimal functioning and keep people from achieving their maximum life-span potential in good health and of a sound mind.

Dr. Jack Z. Yetiv—also not exactly a megasupplement advocate— cites[17] two important studies suggesting that "moderate zinc deficiency" can be expected in strict vegetarians because seafood, meat, and poultry are better sources of zinc than plant-derived foods. The elderly are also likely to suffer from subclinical zinc deficiencies—and not only the underprivileged but also the middle to upper-class elderly.[18,19] Such marginal shortfalls of zinc are especially detrimental in the elderly because their immune system is often already in decline and autoimmune diseases* more frequent. Therefore, if you are either a strict vegetarian or an elderly person, we suggest you take a preventive and yet conservative zinc supplement in the range of 15 to 30 milligrams per day. And if you suffer from any of the above-mentioned diseases involving abnormalities in zinc metabolism, do try a therapeutic zinc supplement in the recommended dosage ranges under the supervision of your doctor, who can monitor the serum zinc levels.

SOURCES

1. Sauchelli, V. *Trace Elements in Agriculture,* New York: Van Nostrand Reinhold, 1969, p. 120.
2. Hendler, Sheldon S. *The Complete Guide to Anti-Aging Nutrients.* New York: Simon & Schuster, A Fireside Book, 1986, p. 192.
3. Schroeder, H. *The Trace Elements and Man.* Old Greenwich, Conn.: Devin-Adair, 1973, p. 62.
4. Ballantine, R. *Diet and Nutrition: A Holistic Approach.* Honesdale, Pa.: The Himalayan International Institute, 1982, p. 251.
5. Kinlaw, W. B., et al. "Abnormal zinc metabolism in type II diabetes mellitus." *Am. J. Med.,* 1983; 75:273–277.
6. Pories, W. J., et al. "Acceleration of healing with zinc sulfate." *Ann. Surg.,* sulfate." 1967; 165:432–436.
7. Barcia, P. J. "Lack of acceleration of healing with zinc sulfate." *Ann. Surg.,* 1970; 172:1048–1050.
8. Frommer, D. J. "The Healing of Gastric ulcers by Zinc Sulphate." *Med. J. Australia,* 1975; 2:793–796.
9. Pauling, Linus. *How to Live Longer and Feel Better.* New York: W. H. Freeman & Company, 1986, p. 112.
10. Duchateau, J. "Beneficial effects of oral Zinc Supplementation on the immune response to old people." *Am. J. Med.,* 1981; 70:1001–1004.
11. Dinsmore, W. W., et al. "Zinc absorption in anorexia nervosa." *Lancet,* 1985; 1:1041.
12. Bryce-Smith, D., and R. I. D. Simpson. "Case of anorexia nervosa responding to zinc sulphate." *Lancet,* 1984; 2:350.
13. Hendler, op. cit., p. 194.
14. Schachner, L. *The Treatment of Acne: A Contemporary Review.* Pediatric Clinics of North America, 1983; 30(3):501–510.
15. Ballantine, R., op. cit., p. 250.

---

* In autoimmune diseases, antibodies or immune lymphoid cells are produced and directed against the body's own tissues.

16. Scala, J. *Making the Vitamin Connection.* New York: Harper & Row, 1985, p. 111.
17. Yetiv, Jack Z. *Popular Nutritional Practices.* Toledo, Ohio: Popular Medicine Press, 1986, p. 205.
18. Hendler, op. cit., p. 188.
19. Underwood, E. *Trace Elements in Human and Animal Nutrition,* 4th ed. New York: Academic Press, 1977, p. 229.

CHAPTER 21

MAGNESIUM

THE ENERGY MINERAL

21 A diet based on complex carbohydrates gives you a decided advantage because, unlike in the case of selenium and zinc, the grains and vegetables on this diet are rich in magnesium. The reason for this is that magnesium is the key element in the chlorophyll of plants, where it plays a role similar to that of iron in blood hemoglobin.

In animals, including humans, most of the magnesium—like calcium—is found in the bones. In fact, magnesium and calcium work very much in tandem in regulating many vital functions such as heartbeat, transmission of nerve impulses, and transformation of the interior of the cells into trillions of tiny generators of energy. However, if both minerals are not in perfect balance, these physiological processes will be seriously upset.

Considerations like these have led to an unfortunate misunderstanding among many health professionals who are in favor of vitamin and mineral supplementation: They believe that the ideal way of getting the right combination of calcium and magnesium is by taking bone meal. That way, their reasoning goes, a person will get not only the right amounts of calcium and magnesium in the most biologically compatible and easily absorbable form, but also fair amounts of phosphorus, which is stored in the bones.

The trouble is, bones accumulate highly toxic metals such as mercury and lead along with the useful minerals. When contaminated bone meal is ingested, the results can be disastrous. Dr. Rudolph

Ballantine[1] tells of some horrifying cases of lead poisoning from the same batch of bone meal: One woman became an invalid, another psychotic, and a third apparently died.*

Stories like these are fortunately rare, and of course not all bone meal is contaminated. But it is not comforting to realize that some commercial baby foods contain added bone meal (presumably to provide calcium!), or that the FDA has set no permissible limits for lead content in foodstuffs. Also, it is technologically next to impossible to extract all the fats from the complex grid structure of bones before they are ground into bone meal. Any fat residues are bound to be partly peroxidized before grinding, and will certainly be totally peroxidized in the fine bone meal when more surface is exposed to the air, just as happens with ground meat.

HOW CALCIUM AND MAGNESIUM WORK TOGETHER

Magnesium seems to be the gatekeeper of our cells, letting in the right amount of calcium to maintain heartbeat at a steady pace. But a magnesium deficiency that may have gone unnoticed can produce dangerous heartbeat abnormalities (cardiac dysrhythmia), and possibly even sudden death.[2,3]

Marginal magnesium deficiencies are very common but very hard to detect, not only because there may be no symptoms but also because routine blood tests may not pick them up. Since most doctors are not used to thinking about micronutrient deficiencies, they usually don't request information on mineral blood levels. The only way your doctor can be sure to catch a marginal magnesium deficiency is by having your blood level of magnesium and your *cellular* magnesium level checked by a first-class laboratory equipped to do that kind of analysis. ("Cellular" magnesium level means the concentration of this mineral in the white blood cells or lymphocytes, which are such an important part of our immune system.)

It is now known that high blood pressure (essential hypertension) is easier to control if magnesium supplements are taken.[4] This may be because people with high blood pressure are usually on diuretics, notorious for producing magnesium deficiencies.[5] The same applies to

---

* Such stories can give pause to dog lovers. (We have three German shepherds on our farm in Costa Rica.) Dogs need bones to clean their teeth, as well as to provide calcium and other minerals. But how can you tell whether the bones contain toxic metals, such as lead? It might be better to give your dog substitutes like Milk Bones instead of the real thing, or to limit your dog to a couple of bones a month.

medications containing digitalis, which are often prescribed to control heart dysrhythmias.*[6]

Women suffering from PMS (premenstrual syndrome) should know that some research suggests marginal deficiencies of magnesium—often accompanied by deficiencies of zinc and vitamins—may have a large role in PMS.[7] There are sufficient grounds to suspect that intake of too much refined sugar and too many dairy products exacerbates this condition because these foods are known to interfere with magnesium absorption, quite aside from their other physical and mental ill effects. This, in turn, might explain some of the psychological aspects of premenstrual tension (anxiety, irritability, mood swings). The reason may lie in the fact that adequate magnesium levels are needed for the proper synthesis of the brain neurotransmitter dopamine, upon which all the other brain chemicals depend. The good news is that broad-spectrum anti-oxidant supplementation, including magnesium, has brought clinically observed relief to women suffering from PMS.[8]

There is another large group of people who would be well advised to make sure their *cellular* magnesium levels are up to par: athletes, bodybuilders, runners, and anyone who performs strenuous exercise or physical work. As the title of this chapter indicates, magnesium is essential for cellular energy. In fact, magnesium is responsible (together with calcium) for the production of ATP (adenosine triphosphate), our most important high-energy phosphate compound. In addition, good magnesium levels are needed for optimal muscle contraction and to sustain the high oxygen consumption necessary for athletic performance. Research indicates that magnesium facilitates oxygen delivery to working muscle tissue,[9] all the more reason for physical high-performers to be sure they are not held back by marginal cellular magnesium deficiency.

THE BOTTOM LINE

Since marginal magnesium deficiencies are so common, you may want to take 200 to 300 milligrams of magnesium along with the calcium already provided on our program, if you feel that you may be a little short of it. Toxic accumulations of magnesium have thus far not been observed in those taking magnesium supplements, but that does not mean such a possibility doesn't exist (we suggest an upper dosage limit of 400 milligrams per day).

* Those of you who suffer from ventricular dysrhythmia will be interested to know that this condition has sometimes been controlled with magnesium supplements, even when conventional drug therapy has failed to do so. But a physician's supervision is crucial.

Others who might benefit from magnesium supplements are those who are now or until recently have been on a typical meat and dairy-products–based diet, that includes relatively few magnesium-rich whole grains and vegetables.

Magnesium has an important role in glucose metabolism, so diabetics probably should take magnesium—as should many people on diuretics or heart medications containing digitalis.

Pregnant women should take a little magnesium, provided their physician has no objections, and sports or exercise enthusiasts probably ought to supplement their basic anti-oxidant program with some magnesium as well. Finally, those who are on especially low-calorie diets should also be on a broad-spectrum anti-oxidant program, with added selenium, zinc, magnesium, and perhaps some copper (2 to 3 milligrams) just to counterbalance the zinc during the time they are on the diets. These mineral supplements should not be taken chronically, without some reason, and without supervision by a doctor who can monitor the serum or cellular levels.

Dr. Sheldon Hendler warns in his book, *Complete Guide to Anti-Aging Nutrients,* that people with serious kidney trouble and those with a certain heart condition,* should not take magnesium supplements. He sounds a warning to such patients to even be careful about using over-the-counter magnesium-containing antacids and laxatives (Milk Of Magnesia, etc.).

WHAT ABOUT IRON AND COPPER?

As far as iron is concerned, we can see the need for supplementation only in certain special cases, especially for pregnant women and maybe for poorly nourished children from disadvantaged environments. Apart from that, we can see no compelling reason, even for older but well-nourished people, to take iron supplements, unless a doctor prescribes it.

---

* The heart disease referred to is called atrioventricular or bifascicular block. In this condition, there is a defect in the functioning of the heart mechanism that receives blood from the pulmonary veins and delivers it to the ventricle of the same side. As Dr. Hendler points out, if magnesium slows down the heart rate and depresses neuromuscular function still further, it can result in blocking the atrioventricular mechanism to the point of complete failure. It can even result in venous blood backing up in the lungs, because the heart is not recycling it properly. Fortunately, worst-case scenarios like this would be extremely rare, but must be taken into consideration.

In the case of *any* heart condition, it is therefore imperative that you consult a nutrition-oriented medical specialist who can make the proper determination of whether it is safe for you to take magnesium supplements (If you are using a pacemaker, chances are that magnesium might actually do you a lot of good, because heart patients often have marginal magnesium deficiencies.)

American women, in particular, have been rather oversold on the alleged need for iron supplements during their reproductive years. However, the small loss of iron during menstruation is quickly made up by the body itself. There is therefore no realistic need for iron supplements unless the woman is already suffering from a degree of anemia.

With regard to copper, it is probably a good idea to take a small supplement, as already mentioned, if you are taking zinc, an antagonist of copper. There have also been reports of copper deficiencies developing with taking larger amounts of vitamin C, as on our program. However, Dr. Demopoulos has seen no evidence of this with thousands of cases over many years of careful clinical observation and monitoring of patients. Nor, for that matter, have Dr. Linus Pauling or Dr. Robert Cathcart III, the two most knowledgeable vitamin C experts.

Nevertheless, if you want a little copper along with your zinc, stay with the already indicated limit of 2 to 3 milligrams of copper to 15 to 30 milligrams of zinc per day. Copper may also provide some cancer protection and some benefits with regard to arthritis (probably by scavenging the toxic oxygen radicals that seem to play a crucial role in all inflammatory diseases like arthritis).

Having said all these positive things about iron and copper, we must now warn you about the possibility of their toxic accumulations in body tissue, especially the liver.[10] They must be chelated—that is, firmly bound to other substances—as is usual with mineral supplements, so that the metal ions cannot directly interact with other compounds in the body and cause damage on the molecular level of cells (for instance, by catalyzing the peroxidation of fats or the destruction of red blood cells).[11,12] We don't recommend cooking food in iron or copper utensils for that reason.

Also, if you live in an older metropolitan center, like New York, Pittsburgh, Philadelphia, Chicago, or Detroit, you may be getting a lot of copper in the drinking water. The reason is that many older buildings still have copper plumbing. Nor can one consider it accidental that the areas with high rates of coronary heart disease also have high concentrations of copper in the drinking water. In fact, Dr. Denhan Harman of the University of Nebraska, an eminent free-radical researcher and specialist on aging, suspects that the reasons for the common observation that the softer the drinking water in a given area, the higher the mortality rate from coronary heart disease, may in part be due to the higher copper content of soft water.[13]

So, those are the pros and cons about iron and copper supplementation. Personally, we'd like to confess that we do not take either iron or copper. Dr. Demopoulos's research shows that there is excellent iron and copper absorption from dietary sources with his spectrum of anti-oxidants and vitamin co-factors. There is also, frankly, a limit to how many capsules of anything even enthusiastic life-extenders like us are ready to swallow in any twenty-four-hour period.

However, we are looking forward to the discovery of new and even more potent anti-oxidants and maybe other life-extending substances that scientists will no doubt discover in the years ahead. If and when that happens, we shall happily add them to our arsenal of secret weapons against all those internal and external influences that would otherwise cut our creative life spans short. And we hope you'll do the same.

SOURCES

1. Ballantine, R. *Diet and Nutrition: A Holistic Approach.* Honesdale, Pa.: The Himalayan International Institute, 1982, p. 233. See also: Crosby, Wm., "Lead-contaminated health food." *JAMA,* 1977; 237:2627–2629.
2. Turlapaty, P. D., and B. M. Altura. "Magnesium deficiency produces spasms of coronary arteries: relationship to etiology of sudden death ischemic heart disease." *Science,* 1980; 208:198.
3. Iseri, L. T., et al. "Magnesium therapy for intractable ventricular tachyarrhythmias in noromagnesemic patients." *Western J. Med.,* 1983; 138:823.
4. Dyckner, T., and P. O. Wester. "Effect of magnesium on blood pressure." *Brit. Med. J.,* 1983; 286:1847.
5. Swales, J. D. "Magnesium deficiency and diuretics." *Brit. Med. J.,* 1982; 285:1377.
6. Cohen, L., and R. Kitzes. "Magnesium sulfate and digitalis-toxic arrhythmias." *JAMA,* 1983; 249:2808.
7. Abraham, G. E. "Nutritional factors in the etiology of the premenstrual tension syndromes." *J. Reprod. Med.,* 1983; 28:446–464.
8. Goei, G. S., and G. E. Abraham. "Effect of a nutritional supplement, Optivite, a symptom of premenstrual tension." *J. Reprod. Med.,* 1983; 28:527–531.
9. Lukaski, H. C., et al. "Maximal oxygen consumption as related to magnesium, copper, and zinc nutriture." *Am. J. Clin. Nutr.* 1983; 37:407.
10. Dianzani, M. U. "The role of free radicals in liver damage." *Proc. Nutr. Soc.,* 1987; 46:43–52.
11. Harman, D. "Free Radical Theory of Aging: Role of Free Radicals in the Origination and Evolution of Life, Aging, and Disease Processes." In: *Free Radicals, Aging, and Degenerative Diseases,* D. Harman et al., eds. New York: Alan R. Liss, Inc., 1986, pp. 3–49.
12. Ibid., p. 22.
13. Ibid.

CHAPTER 22

CHROMIUM

GLUCOSE TOLERANCE FACTOR

12 If you are eating the typical American diet with its highly processed foods, chances are that you may be low in the mineral chromium, because it is lost in the refining process. (This is true too for some of the other trace minerals, like selenium, zinc, magnesium, silicon, etc., but chromium is the most important with regard to sugar metabolism.)

The reason why it is so important, especially with regard to diabetes, is that without chromium, the body cannot produce an enzyme-like substance called *glucose tolerance factor* (GTF). We need this substance to potentiate the action of insulin so that it can work to best advantage in controlling our blood sugar.[1] This beneficial effect of chromium supplementation on carbohydrate (sugar) metabolism was noted not only on diabetics, but also on normal subjects.

Admittedly, there were some studies that seemed to cast doubt on the effectiveness of chromium supplementation. However, we suspect that it was again the small doses used in these trials, or some other flaw in their design, that accounted for these negative results.[2,3]

We are personally convinced from a thorough review of the scientific literature that chromium supplementation is effective in improving glucose tolerance if daily doses of 200 to 500 *micrograms* (*not* milligrams), are used.

In fact, when chromium-rich *brewers' yeast* is used instead of inorganic chromium, researchers found not only improved glucose tolerance, but also reductions in serum cholesterol and triglyceride

172

levels.[4-6] The beneficial effects on blood lipids (fats) was an unexpected bonus in these studies, and the scientists felt that they were probably due to other components of the yeast rather than the chromium.

To take advantage of this dual effect, we suggest you take chromium-rich yeast over inorganic chromium, unless you are allergic to it. You can find brewers' yeast in almost any health-food store or pharmacy. Twin Laboratories offers an organic, grain-grown type, as well as one called Nutritional Yeast, which is perhaps the best-tasting of them all. (To order this yeast direct, see Appendix C.)

Despite all the possible benefits of short-term chromium supplementation, we consider it no more than the proverbial "frosting on the cake," after correct diet, exercise, and our full anti-oxidant and vitamin co-factor spectrum. However, it could be a highly beneficial "frosting" on top of good medical management for diabetics.

SOURCES

1. Anderson, R. A., et al. "Chromium supplementation of human subjects: effects on glucose, insulin, and lipid variables." *Metabolism*, 1983; 32:894–899.
2. Glinsman, W. H., and W. Mertz. "Effect of trivalent chromium on glucose tolerance." *Metabolism*, 1966; 15:510–515.
3. Riales, R., and M. J. Albrink. "Effect of chromium chloride supplementation on glucose tolerance and serum lipids including high-density lipoprotein of adult men." *Am. J. Clin. Nutr.*, 1981; 34:2670–2678.
4. Doisy, R. J., et al. "Chromium metabolism in man and biochemical effects." In: *Trace Element Metabolism in Human Health and Disease,* A. S. Prasad, ed. New York: Academic Press, 1976, pp. 79–104.
5. Liu, V.J.K., and J. S. Morris. "Relative chromium response as an indicator of chromium status." *Am. J. Clin. Nutr.*, 1978; 31:972–976.
6. Offenbacher, E. G., and F. X. Pi-Sunyer. "Beneficial effect of chromium-rich yeast on glucose tolerance and blood lipids in elderly subjects." *Diabetes,* 1980; 29:919–925.

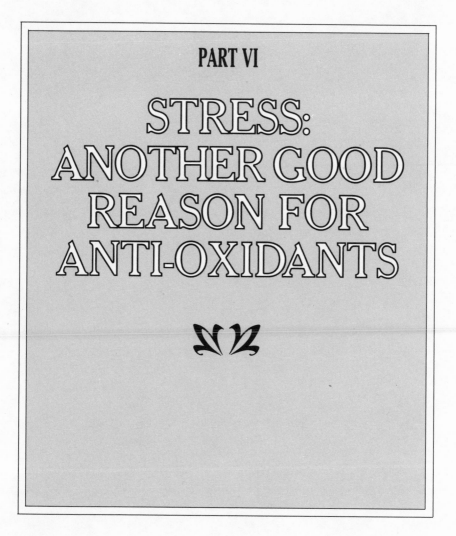

PART VI

STRESS: ANOTHER GOOD REASON FOR ANTI-OXIDANTS

CHAPTER 23

EMOTIONS THAT CAN KILL

12 In a provocative book,* Dr. Deepak Chopra, a Boston physician, tells the story of a fortyish patient with a mild heart condition who had worked himself into such an angry state over a slight delay in the waiting room that he collapsed and died there and then of a heart attack.

Chopra also tells of a young lawyer who had been brought to a hospital emergency room because of severe chest pains. The pains stopped, and initial tests did not seem to indicate a heart attack, so the man was sent home. His chest pains returned immediately, and he was brought back to the emergency room. This time Dr. Chopra was in charge. He decided to keep the patient overnight for observation, not so much because of his physical condition as because he was extremely anxious which, Dr. Chopra knew, put him at special risk.

Sure enough, further tests the next day revealed that the man had indeed suffered some damage to his heart the previous night. Enraged at this news, the man informed Dr. Chopra that he was going to sue the hospital and the other emergency room doctor who had first seen him for incompetency. Despite repeated admonitions to rest and relax, he began calling up lawyers immediately, right from his hospital bed. He did this for the next few hours, his blood pressure rising despite medications to control it, and an hour later suffered another—this time fatal—heart attack. The autopsy revealed that the weakened part of his muscle had literally been torn apart, undoubtedly by emotional tensions and self-generated agitation.

Hostility and anger are not, of course, the only emotions that can make us sick or even kill us. As Dr. Kenneth Pelletier puts it in his

* *Creating Health* (Boston: Houghton Mifflin Company, 1987).

177

definitive book *Holistic Medicine*:* "Throughout history there are reports of people dying suddenly while in the throes of great fear, rage, grief, humiliation, and even joy." He cites a researcher, George L. Engel, who collected newspaper clippings about incidents of sudden deaths and broke down the causes into four basic categories, beginning with the most common:

- traumatic events in a close human relationship
- situations of danger, struggle, or attack
- loss of status, humiliation, failure, or defeat
- moments of great personal triumph or joy

President Lyndon B. Johnson's fatal heart attack, mentioned in Dr. Pelletier's book, occurred the day after the newly elected Richard M. Nixon announced the total dismantling of Johnson's cherished Great Society programs. This might reasonably be classified as one of those sudden deaths that are due to a profound sense of failure and defeat.

The most common emotional factors in sudden death are traumatic events in close human relationships, such as the loss of a spouse, child, or other loved person vital to the emotional security and equilibrium of the individual. "Dying of a broken heart" is, in fact, not just an expression.

Bereaved persons suffer a general decline in health and become more susceptible to infectious diseases and malignancies. People who have suffered a loss tend to smoke more cigarettes, drink more alcohol, take more tranquilizers, and generally neglect themselves, which explains the frequency with which elderly spouses die within a very short time of one another.[1]

How often have you used the expression "I was worried to death"? Probably hundreds of times. What you didn't realize was how close you were to being literally right. The fact is that the all-too-common complex of anxious thoughts and imaginings called *worry* can, indeed, make us very sick.

Worry often begins with a vague, almost subconscious remembrance of past troubles, hurts, and problems. We then project this general uneasiness about what happened in the past onto the blank screen of the future, calling up all kinds of frightening and threatening images. Our minds are taking us back to unhappy past events and forward toward dreaded imaginary future troubles and dangers—which may never come to pass and are certainly not preventable by worrying about them in advance. Worry always keeps us from living fully in the

---

* *Holistic Medicine* (New York: Delacorte Press, 1979). We highly recommend this book to anyone seriously interested in a better understanding of a more comprehensive (holistic) view of human health.

present and—like hostility, anger, abiding resentment, overambition, power drive, greed, envy, jealousy, and similar negative emotions—is inarguably detrimental to good health and longevity.

Easily as destructive to one's health are intrapsychic (neurotic) conflicts and repressed wishes, thoughts, and fantasies, which can be erotic, hostile, dependent, or anything else we find unacceptable either socially or in terms of our "ideal" image of ourselves! Such repressed thoughts, feelings, or desires have a way of expressing themselves by physical symptoms—from peptic ulcers and irritable bowels to eczema, asthma, hypertension, heart disease, and, many experts suspect, even cancer. Often problems that are purely psychological are, as psychiatrist Leonard S. Zegan puts it, "transferred to a patient's body, where different organs or tissues enact a fantasied intra-psychic drama."[2] Or, as the nineteenth-century German physician and originator of the science of pathology Rudolf Virchow said, "Much illness is nothing but unhappiness sailing under a physiologic flag."

The term "psychosomatic medicine"—diagnosis and treatment of diseases that are partly mental (psycho-) and partly physical (somatic) in origin—was coined by psychoanalyst Dr. Franz Alexander,[3] who was the first to research systematically the transfer of emotional complexes and "unhappiness" to physical symptoms.

Some researchers still believe that certain characteristic neurotic complexes or types of neurotic family interactions produce certain kinds of physical symptoms or diseases. But today most medical scientists and psychologists (the authors of this book included) feel that one cannot be that specific. What we can say with a high degree of certainty is that almost *any* kind of intrapsychic conflict or neurotic family interaction is potentially able to express itself as physical ailment or type of disease. To oversimplify, neurosis may be dangerous, even fatal, to your health.

SOURCES

1. Helsing, K. J., and M. Szklo. "Mortality after bereavement." *Am. J. Epidem.,* 1981; 114:41–52.
2. Zegans, Leonard S. "The Embodied Self: Personal Integration in Health and Illness." In: *Advances.* Vol. 4, 1987, p. 40.
3. Alexander, F. *Psychosomatic Medicine: Its Principles and Applications.* New York: W. W. Norton, 1950.

CHAPTER 24

INTERNAL AND EXTERNAL STRESS

What are rage, unhappiness, and neurotic conflict if not forms of internal stress? Everything we said earlier about the ability of hostile, negative thoughts and unacceptable, repressed feelings and wishes to make us sick can be expressed in terms of stress and its effects on our bodies.

While not all stress is internal, we're all exposed to many sorts of external stress too, today more than ever. Much of what people assume to be inescapable external stress has a strong subjective aspect that renders it subject to some measure of control. But internal, self-generated stress is certainly the variety over which we have the *most* control.

Stress is as real as it is difficult to define. The young black carrying his oversized dual-speaker boom box on his shoulder on a walk through Central Park, his rap music blasting away, is putting other people—but not necessarily himself—under stress. His subjective experience is probably one of pleasure, while ours is one of stress or distress—both originating from the same source or stimulus.

In his series *Commentaries on Living*, J. Krishnamurti describes sitting on a park bench in India contemplating the beauty of the surrounding trees and flowers and the reflection of the sinking sun on a body of water. In the distance are the faint sounds of music from a transistor radio and traffic noise. Krishnamurti is aware of it all, but his focus is on the loveliness of the surroundings. Not so his neighbor, a middle-aged gentleman who seems to have focused on the intrusive music and traffic sounds. He complains that one can't go anywhere these days without being subjected to disagreeable noises. He is obviously right, but just as obviously, he is also missing the beauty that Krishnamurti is enjoying at the very same time.

The ramifications of the above encounter are interesting: One person is allowing an external stimulus (the intruding noises) to become a very real stressor that precludes his enjoyment of a beautiful sunset; the other is neither denying the existence of these disturbing noises nor permitting them to become stressors.

Is there, then, no objective definition of stress? Yes, there is. But it is crucial to make the distinction between stimuli that are potential stressors and our reaction to them—which may or may not result in the physiological syndrome called *stress.*

When a stressor such as the loss of a spouse, financial difficulty, or interpersonal conflict affects any of us, it sets into motion certain physiological reactions. These reactions rather than the stressor itself are what we experience as stress. Dr. Hans Selye, who coined the term "stress" in the 1930s, said that stress is the *"rate of wear and tear"* on the body, determined by our reactions to potential stressors regardless of origin—physical or psychological, internal or external.

For example, let's assume we are shipwrecked in a storm and suddenly find ourselves struggling to stay afloat in the pounding waves, a situation of very real *physical* stress (or, more precisely, physical *stressors*). If we know that the waters are shark-infested, we may also experience profound *psychological* stress in the form of fear. A person in this kind of situation is experiencing acute physical and mental stress at the same moment.

Although this example is extreme, from time to time we are all exposed to particularly stressful circumstances and confrontations that may make our blood freeze in fear or boil in rage. When that happens, our mind throws an automatic alarm switch that operates all the physiological survival mechanisms, often called the "fight-or-flight" response.

We don't normally associate the good things that happen to us with stress. And yet a promotion, with its increased responsibilities, somewhat different work environment, and new associates, may make heavy demands on the "lucky" person's entire intellectual and emotional household, to say nothing of the enormous strains that can ensue if the person is promoted way over his or her head.

Getting married is another example of a happy event, but it can be just as stressful as getting a divorce. So is becoming a parent, as most new parents will freely admit. You can undoubtedly think of other similar moments when something that was supposed to be a "lucky" event or a change for the better turned out to be hard to take.

Most external stress is, however, of the negative or distressing kind, and a lot of it is a by-product of the work environment. It is a known fact that stress has surpassed the common cold as the most prevalent health problem in America. Stress-related illness is costing the nation more than \$20 billion a year in lost industrial productivity.

Dr. Herbert Benson cites a recent Louis Harris poll that targets health problems associated with stress as the principal cause of absenteeism at work.* This fact is confirmed by findings of the national Centers for Disease Control (CDC) that show that stress in the work situation is causing "substantial health problems," including a variety of neuroses, depression, chronic anxiety, irritability, drug abuse, sleep problems, and a long list of psychosomatic conditions.

Interviews conducted by the CDC leave no doubt that most of these problems could be easily avoided if prevailing management attitudes in the workplace were different. Employees complain of feeling overloaded with work; of having little control over the way they do their jobs; of unsupportive bosses and co-workers, and of little or no opportunity for career advancement. And in the United States, the CDC concludes, matters seem to be getting worse rather than better.[1]

American sociologist Robert A. Karasek arrived at similar conclusions about the nature of work stress in Sweden, citing excessive workload (for example, at a rushed tempo) and low worker participation in decision making as the most damaging forms of work-related sress.[2] However, in Sweden, where public attitudes about work are more enlightened than in the United States, the outlook is considerably less gloomy.

Norway even went a big step further than its Scandinavian neighbor: In 1977 the Norwegian parliament enacted a work-environment law that actually makes it illegal for an employer to subject employees to "unnecessary stress," *including psychological stress!* [3,4] This law sets a precedent we hope other industrialized nations will follow in the future.

Meanwhile, we fear that millions of white-collar as well as blue-collar workers will continue to be exposed to chronic work stress. And it will continue to take its toll—in physical illness and premature death, in interpersonal conflict and emotional disturbance, and in lowered productivity and enormous public and private health costs. Apparently our society is still willing to pay that price, rather than try harder to eliminate unnecessary stress in the work environment.

SOURCES

1. Rosch, Paul J. "Stress and illness" (commentary). *JAMA,* August 3, 1979; 242:427.
2. Karasek, R. A., S. Russell, and T. Theorell. "Physiology of stress and regen-

* Herbert Benson, *Your Maximum Mind* (New York: Random House, Times Books, 1987).

eration in job-related cardiovascular illness." *J. Human Stress,* 1982; 8:29.
3. Theorell, T. "Research on stress and health in Sweden from 1950 to 1985." *Advances* (International Issue), Vol. 3, No. 4, 1986, p. 96.
4. Ursin, Holger. "Behavioral medicine in Norway." *Advances* (International Issue), Vol. 3, No. 4, Fall 1986, p. 107.

CHAPTER 25

THE PHYSIOLOGY OF STRESS

The better we understand just *how* stress undermines our health and can shorten our lives, the better equipped we will be to avoid it. What, then, actually happens to our bodies under stress? How exactly does the fight-or-flight response manifest itself?

We've all experienced it. Blood pressure and pulse rate shoot up; breathing is quick and shallow. The muscles tense, and blood is diverted to them from the skin and digestive organs and toward other areas vital to self-defense and survival, such as the heart, the lungs, and the brain. Under these circumstances it's not surprising if our hands and feet feel cold and clammy, cold chills run up and down our spine, and our throat feels as tight as a rope, or our stomach is tied up in knots. We may literally be trembling with fear or rage. If we could look at ourselves at such moments, all the color would seem to have gone out of our face and our pupils would be wide open.

There are many other manifestations of fight-or-flight that are impossible to observe. Clotting factors are released into the bloodstream to prevent excessive blood loss in case of injury. Powerful brain chemicals and hormones are also pumped into the bloodstream. One of these is adrenaline (epinephrine), the "fear hormone," from the adrenal glands of the kidneys. Another is noradrenaline (norepinephrine), the brain's own version of adrenaline, sometimes called the *anger hormone.* Both hormones are "revving up our engines," putting us at hair-trigger readiness either to lash out or run for our lives—even if the "crisis" is, say, nothing more than misplacing our housekeys or getting a flat tire.

The consequences of the system's getting revved up in such a manner can be serious, whether it is provoked by a true crisis or by an awkward social situation. We know that the morphine-like brain hormones called *endorphins* and *enkephalins* are released under stress—perhaps so they will already be in circulation should the need for a pain-killing substance arise. We also know that these only recently discovered peptide hormones have an uncanny capacity, when present in excess, to suppress the immune system.

In addition, other neurotransmitters and hormones suppress the immune system or contribute in other ways to a large variety of diseases. We have already mentioned the brain's nonadrenaline, as well as adrenaline, produced by the adrenal glands, as is cortisol. Adrenaline and cortisol are life-maintaining but can, when produced in excess during stressful situations, become life-threatening. Cortisol, for instance, can seriously weaken the body's immunity to disease by inhibiting the production of the antibodies and NK (natural killer) cells. All these substances seem to be governed by ACTH (adrenocorticotropic hormone), secreted by a master gland—the brain's anterior pituitary—which is exquisitely sensitive to any kind of emotional stress.

These are just a few of the physiological processes that affect the immune system and our entire physical and mental household under conditions of stress. It is only to be expected that all these biochemical upheavals in our bodies can literally make us ill, or even kill us outright.

CHAPTER 26

STRESS AND INFECTIOUS DISEASES

In In 1909 a brilliant physician, Sir William Osler, stated that "the care of tuberculosis depends more on what the patient has in his head than what he has in his chest." We can only imagine how this revolutionary statement must have been received by his colleagues at the turn of the century. Today, however, we have ample scientific proof that psychosocial factors indeed influence not only respiratory infections but also many other infectious and noninfectious diseases. Drs. Barbara Dorian and Paul E. Garfinkel of the Department of Psychiatry, Toronto General Hospital, Canada, have reviewed the scientific literature* addressing the way in which stress may "enhance vulnerability to certain diseases by exerting an immunosuppressive effect and especially to those diseases intimately connected with immunologic mechanisms such as infection, malignancy and auto-immune disease."[1]

Drs. Dorian and Garfinkel cite one study involving volunteers who were inoculated with one of the many strains of rhinoviruses that cause the common cold and other respiratory ailments. The results indicated that one could predict the severity of the infectious symptoms by evaluating a subject's recent life stress and degree of introversion (social isolation and consequent lack of emotional support).[2] Dr. S. Cohen-Cole and colleagues make a similar point, clearly establishing the connection between "negative life events over the preceding year" and the painful

---

* In this chapter, we shall base our discussion frequently on Drs. Dorian and Garfinkel's abstracts of the most recent studies in psychosomatic medicine, although our interpretations of the data may sometimes differ from theirs.

infection of the gums known as "trench mouth" (necrotizing ulcerative gingivitis).[3] These patients showed more anxiety and depression than normal when they first came for treatment, as measured by a psychological test, the MMPI (Minnesota Multiphasic Personality Inventory), long accepted as highly reliable. When given a general health questionnaire these subjects checked many items indicating distress from negative life events. At the same time, clinical tests confirmed that they were suffering from seriously impaired immunity.*

Tests have shown women under the stress of separation and divorce to be more susceptible to infection with the Epstein-Barr virus; having poor cellular immune system control over the latent virus, they consequently suffer more frequently from infectious mononucleosis than women not under similar stress.[4,5] Student nurses have a high incidence of cold sores, which are caused by the herpes simplex virus, during times of "unhappiness," as measured by the Clyde Mood Scale. A number of other factors, including colds, fevers, sunburns, and weakened immunity related to stress, can reactivate the herpes simplex virus too. There is even evidence that moderately severe emotional disturbance encourages the recurrence of genital herpes, which is caused by another form of the herpes simplex virus.[6] This confirms the common experience of genital herpes sufferers that emotional upset alone can provoke recurrences. (The same is true also for venereal warts [condylomata acuminata].)[7,8]

Examination anxiety can predispose students to a variety of infectious diseases. Researchers have studied a large group of West Point cadets over a four-year period with an eye to the relationship between academic stress and susceptibility to infectious mononucleosis. Of the new cadets, 20 percent became infected each year and 25 percent actually developed the disease. The researchers were even able to predict a cadet's susceptibility to mononucleosis by tracking his reactions to the high academic demands and his performance on quizzes and examinations.[9]

Dorian and Garfinkel list several studies, including one of their own, that show that the increase in such infections is in direct proportion to the degree of examination anxiety reported by the students.[10] These findings confirm similar studies on the link between academic stress and other infectious diseases. In one study, medical students were found to be most susceptible to three herpes viruses during periods of peak stress, especially those students who also reported feelings of acute loneliness.[11]

We have seen to what an extraordinary extent our emotions, and the resulting *stress,* predispose us to infectious diseases. We also know that this effect is achieved by stress suppressing the immune

---

* They exhibited depressed lymphoblast transformation and less polymorphonuclear leukotaxis and phagocytosis.

system. Even following a healthful diet, getting regular physical exercise, and taking anti-oxidants and vitamins are not sufficient to counteract the effects of stress. We must also keep destructive, immunosuppressive emotions like hatred, resentment, worry, and depression from getting the best of us.

It is wise to review our daily lives for factors that produce stress. Two scientists (Drs. Holmes and Rahe)[12] have devised a whole list of psychosocial stressors and have ranked them in order of importance: so many points for marital tensions, so many for being heavily in debt, so many for having lost a job, so many for having had recent surgery or a major illness, and so forth. There is not much we can do about many of these stressors, or so it would seem. But the truth is that to *some* extent we all write the scripts of our own lives. (German playwright Max Frisch has one of his characters say, "Do not call fate man's stupidity.") Whether it is because of "fate" or our own doing, some diseases are more likely triggered by distressing life events and negative attitudes than others: The infectious diseases we have just discussed are prime examples.

SOURCES

1. Dorian, B., and Paul E. Garfinkel. "Stress, immunity and illness—a review." *Psychol. Med.,* 1987; 17:393–407.
2. Totman. R., J. Kiff, S. E. Reed, and J. W. Craig. "Predicting experimental colds in volunteers from different measures of recent life stress." *J. Psychosom. Res.* 1980; 24:155–163.
3. Cohen-Cole, S., et al. "Psychosocial, endocrine, and immune factors in acute necrotizing ulcerative gingivitis ('trenchmouth')." *Psychosom. Med.,* 1981; 43:91–95.
4. Kiecolt-Glaser, J. K., et al. "Marital quality, martial disruption, and immune function." *Psychosom. Med.,* 1987 (in press).
5. Luborsky, L. "Herpes simplex virus and moods: a longitudinal study." *J. Psychosom. Res.,* 1976; 20:543–548.
6. Goldmeier, D., and D. Johnson. "Does psychiatric illness affect the recurrence rate of genital herpes?" *Brit. J. Venereal Dis.,* 1982; 58:40–43.
7. Ewin, D.M. "*Condyloma acuminatum:* successful treatment of four cases of hypnosis." *Am. J. Clin. Hypn.,* 1974; 17:73–83.
8. Goss, E. O. "Wart charming." *Radiography,* 1956; 22:75–77.
9. Kasl, S. V., et al. "Psychosocial risk factors in the development of infectious mononucleosis." *Psychosom. Med.,* 1979; 41:445–466.
10. Dorian, B. J., et al. "Stress, immunity and illness." *Psychosom. Med.,* 1986; 48:304.
11. Glaser, R., et al. "Stress, loneliness and changes in herpes virus latency." *J. Behav. Med.,* 1985; 8:249–260.
12. Petrich, J., and T. H. Holmes. "Life change and onset of illness." *Med. Clinics N. Am.,* 1977; 61:825–838. Also: Rahe, R. H., and T. H. Holmes. "Life crisis and disease onset; II—Qualitative and quantitative definition of the life crisis and its association with health change," and "Life crisis and disease onset; III—A prospective study of life crises and health changes" (unpublished manuscripts).

CHAPTER 27

SURVIVAL IN
THE AGE OF AIDS

12 If there is any prime example of an infectious disease in which life-style and every type of stress are the predisposing factors, it is AIDS. A recent *New York Times* article* calls AIDS a "product of high-risk behavior." According to the same article, the deadly disease is concentrated in the most economically depressed areas of New York City: the Lower East Side of Manhattan, the South Bronx, and the poorest sections of Brooklyn. What the article does not say is that these areas are precisely those that contain the highest degree of environmental and socioeconomic stress, areas where there is extreme density of population, terrible housing conditions, chronic unemployment, malnutrition, the highest rates of disease (hypertension, heart attack, stroke, cancer, infant mortality), pervasive crime, and so forth.

Not surprisingly, all these factors generate not only more AIDS cases, in general, but also disproportionally high rates of infectious disease and cancer. The basic reason is the same: a weakened immune system in general—whether produced directly by stressful living conditions or by people's reactions to them—heavy drug use, alcoholism, unsafe sex, and similar immunosuppressive life-styles.

On the other hand, some people who test positive for AIDS virus antibodies, and who must therefore be suspected of harboring the virus in their systems, never develop either ARC (AIDS-related complex) or AIDS. Their immune systems are apparently able to prevent the virus from doing any serious harm.

* January 2, 1988

189

What causes this difference? Expert opinion cites several factors, including genetic and hormonal ones, but basically, it is the *susceptibility* of a person's immune system that determines the course of the infection. And that, in turn, depends on how well we take care of ourselves, what we put into our stomachs, whether we are getting enough anti-oxidants, and, last but by no means least, how good or tough life is to us—in other words, we're back to stress. The medical histories of AIDS patients typically reveal distressing life events or debilitating illnesses just prior to the onset of the first symptoms of the disease.

In practical terms this means that everybody—but especially those testing positive who are still symptom-free—ought to take extraordinary, self-protective measures to avoid stressors of any kind. For the AIDS virus, like viruses in general, is highly opportunistic. Like any true parasite, it thrives on troubles and adversities. In other words, our *reactions* to trouble and adversity—anxiety, depression, anger, frustration, and so forth—give the AIDS virus the opportunity it needs to take hold.

Obviously, there are many life events over which we have no control. But even in a worst-case scenario—loss of job, heavy financial loss, or bereavement—we still have some control over our reactions to these events, no matter what their magnitude. In even extreme cases of adversity, we can limit the damage by proper control of our reactions. We simply can't allow, say, legitimate grief and sense of loss to suppress our immune system and thereby aggravate the problem even more.

When it comes to life-style factors such as smoking, eating fats, or drinking alcohol, we are (or can be) in control. Anyone who tests positive and still indulges in these immunosuppressive habits is literally "asking for it." But smoking, eating fats, and drinking alcohol (in *any* amount) are by no means the only activities those who test positive ought to avoid absolutely. More "innocent" pastimes (sunbathing, overworking, overexercising, not getting enough sleep) or negative emotions (anger, resentment, jealousy, envy) also help *any* virus or invading organism, including AIDS virus, to assert itself all the more.

Another medical reality is the fact that it normally takes *repeated* exposures of the weakened immune system to the AIDS virus to produce the disease. But when massive numbers of the virus are introduced, as occurs when an entire unit of contaminated blood is used in a transfusion, a single exposure will suffice for transmittal.

The same is true with regard to certain sexual practices, since the virus is present not only in high concentrations in infected blood but also in semen. Even healthy, normal semen, once introduced into the bloodstream, is highly immunosuppressive. In a study with male rabbits, rabbit semen introduced into the rectums of other male rabbits caused their immune systems to plummet to levels that laid them wide open to many kinds of infection or malignancy.[1]

While these findings might seem puzzling at first, the explanation is quite logical. Semen and spermatozoa are the richest natural sources of prostaglandins, hormone-like compounds that help to regulate many of our physiological processes, including blood pressure, body temperature, and the acid secretions of the stomach. They are also among the most immunosuppressive substances thus far discovered, if they are present in excess or in the wrong areas of the body.

Since the intestinal mucous membrane is highly permeable because of the necessity of absorbing nutrients through it, semen should not be introduced into this internal environment. Because the vaginal membrane is so much less permeable, it poses no similar risk. Ingestion also involves no comparable risk, since prostaglandins are derivates of fatty acids and are therefore digested like dietary fatty acids. Of course, in either case there is risk when the semen contains the virus. Small, undetected injuries or cracks in the vaginal, cervical, or oral mucous membranes might allow the virus to enter into the circulation.

We can't emphasize enough the preventive, immunity-enhancing effects of correct diet, a health-promoting life-style, and the cultivation of constructive, positive mental attitudes. We also suggest that anyone who tests positive for AIDS supplement his or her diet with the full spectrum of anti-oxidants and vitamin co-factors. Even though there is as yet no reliable scientific proof that anti-oxidants and vitamin co-factors indeed strengthen the immune system against AIDS, there is ample experiential and some experimental evidence for it. In fact, we personally know of one small-scale, unpublished study in which supplementation with anti-oxidants and vitamin co-factors has had at least one definite positive effect on the immune systems of a small group of ARC (AIDS-related complex) patients: In the normal, noninfected person, the ratio of T4 (helper) cells to T8 (suppressor) cells of the immune system is always in favor of the helper cells. In ARC patients, however, the ratio gets tilted in favor of the suppressor cells. During this small and admittedly inconclusive experiment, the patients took anti-oxidant and vitamin co-factor supplements for eight weeks. By the end of this period, their lymphocyte ratio had returned to a healthy one, with the T4 helper cells back in the normal, dominant position.

We mentioned earlier, in our discussion of vitamin C, that Dr. Robert Cathcart III had reportedly had very encouraging results with high-dose intravenous and oral vitamin C therapy with ARC patients and even with AIDS patients. No "miracle" cures have been claimed for such megavitamin C therapy. But it appears that some patients have been kept alive longer and in better condition with it—no small feat with a disease as serious as AIDS.

Finally, we would definitely suggest that anyone testing positive for the AIDS virus, or indeed any ARC or AIDS patient, practice one or another of several relaxation, meditation, or self-hypnotic techniques that have proven effective with other diseases, notably cancer.

UPDATE We have referred to an earlier study (1984) on the immuno-suppressive effects of semen introduced into the rectums of male rabbits. Now these findings have been confirmed in another (1985) laboratory study[2] measuring the devastating *in vitro* (test tube) effects of *human* semen on the immune system.

The researchers conclude that the high concentration of the two predominant prostaglandins in ejaculated semen "may be an important co-factor in the development of viral infections among homosexual men." They also call attention to two epidemiological (population) studies[3,4] that "have shown that the life-style factor with the highest relative risk for AIDS and sero-positive hepatitis B among homosexual men is passive anal-genital intercourse." It is especially the "repeated deposition of semen in the gut" (the sexual activity of preference among a large subgroup of homosexual men) that suppresses the protective NK (natural killer) cell activity against virus-infected and cancer cells.

We have pointed out that the vagina is much better protected against the immunosuppressive effects of prostaglandins in semen than the gut. However, the 1985 study suggests that the presence of these compounds in semen may also suppress NK-cell antitumor and antiviral activities in the vagina (maybe the old-fashioned custom of douching after intercourse was not such a bad idea, after all).

SOURCES

1. Richards, J. M., J. M. Bedford, and S. S. Witkin. "Rectal insemination modifies immune responses in rabbits." *Science,* 1984; 224:390.
2. Tarter, T. H., S. Cunningham-Rundles, and S. S. Koide, "Suppression of natural killer cell activity by human seminal plasma in vitro: identification of 19-OH-PGE, as the suppressor factor." *J. Immunol.,* 1986; 136:2865–2867.
3. Marmor, M. "Epidemic Kaposi's sarcoma and sexual practices among male homosexuals." In: *Aids: The Epidemic of Kaposi's Sarcoma and Opportunistic Infections,* A. E. Friedman-Kien and L. G. Laubenstein, eds. New York: Masson Publishing, 1985, pp. 291–296.
4. Schreeder, M. T., S. E. Thompson, et al. "Hepatitis B in homosexual men: prevalence of infection and factors related to transmission. *J. Infect. Dis.,* 1982; 146:7.

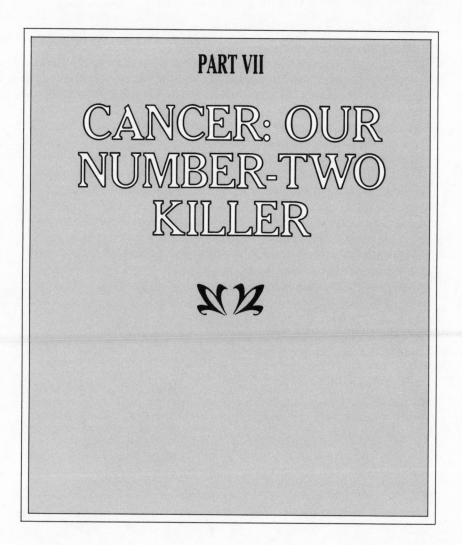

PART VII

CANCER: OUR NUMBER-TWO KILLER

CHAPTER 28

CANCER

DIET, HORMONES, AND STRESS

12 While cancer always seems to be a sudden diagnosis, in reality it develops over a period of a few decades. During this time, normal cells are being remodeled and transformed, molecule by molecule—like remodeling a building in reverse, *down*grading instead of upgrading it, until it crumbles to the ground.

The factors involved in this remodeling and transformation include the activation of silent pieces of our DNA called *oncogenes,* damage to sensitive cell parts by free radicals, and losses of immune functions. Cancer is a multifactorial disease, but it does have *predominant causes.* For example, the predominant cause of tuberculosis is the tubercle bacillus, and the associated causes are poverty, race, cold weather, and poor living conditions. So, too, with cancer we see predominant causes—smoking and drinking alcohol cause lung, mouth, and esophageal cancer; too much dietary fat and fiber deficiencies are associated with breast, prostate, colon, rectal, and other cancers.

Only one type of leukemia, and perhaps a few rare types of other cancers seem to be associated with viruses, and there are cancers that can be traced to the effects of pollution and radiation. Nevertheless, cancer is the one disease entity most directly affected by our habits, the state of our immune system, and our dietary intakes of fats, fiber, and anti-oxidants. Medical research now assumes that we all start developing malignant cells somewhere in our bodies many times during our

195

ANTI-OXIDANT AND CANCER PREVENTION

"There is no method of prophylaxis, although in the future neutral-ization of mutagen-carcinogens with vitamin C, glutathione, and anti-oxidants should be considered."—T. Sugimura, et al., in *Origins of Human Cancer* (Cold Spring, N.Y.: Cold Spring Harbor Laboratory, 1977)

lifetime, a theory first proposed by Dr. Lewis Thomas.* If our immune systems are up to par, they will either eliminate these malignancies—the PacMan-like macrophages in our bodies, for instance, might just gobble them up—or our immune defenses will at least contain them so they can't spread to other parts of the body (metastasize).

Autopsies of road accident victims reveal the presence of previously undetected cancer with surprising frequency. This evidence indicates that the immune system prevents the vast majority of new malignancies from ever progressing to the point of clinical establishment and diagnosis. In our view, life-style, diet, mental attitude, and the presence of anti-oxidants in either the diet or from supplemental sources are the crucial factors that enable (or prevent) the immune system to perform these protective functions. It is comforting for us to know from some studies that the ascorbic acid (vitamin C) on our anti-oxidant Menu may help protect us from cancer even after the invasive state has been reached: There are indications that vitamin C promotes the formation of fibrous tissue (fibroplasia), which apparently creates obstacles to the spread of cancerous tumors.[1] We also know that beta-carotene and other carotenoids in a number of vegetables and fruits, which are also well represented on our Demopoulos spectrum of anti-oxidants, protect against cancer. So do a number of other compounds in vegetables, fruits, and beans, peas, and lentils, about which we will talk later in this book.

Given the near universality of cancer and its life-threatening nature, it is only logical that, on the one hand, we avoid willful exposure to dietary and environmental carcinogens—including self-inflicted ones from smoking cigarettes or other tobacco products—and, on the other hand, maximize the anticancer factors in our diet and our total life-style. To our way of thinking, this includes the judicious, well-thought-out supplementation of dietary anti-oxidants with safe, addi-tional amounts as on the Demopoulos spectrum.

* Dr. Lewis Thomas was director of Memorial Sloan-Kettering Cancer Center in New York City, a dean of Yale University, and a dean of New York University.

We have to start, however, with correct, health-promoting nutrition. Dr. John A. McDougall,* a California physician with a vast experience in the dietary prevention and treatment of cancer, points out that by now there are many studies to convince even the most doubting Thomases that disordered nutrition not only leads to atherosclerosis, with greatly increased risk for coronary heart disease and stroke, but is also the decisive factor in a number of common cancers, including those of the colon, prostate, and breast.

Dr. McDougall emphasizes the role of the female hormones (estrogens) and their relation to diet in the prevention of breast cancer. As some studies make clear, the more fat a woman's body has, the more estrogen it will produce.[2] For some reason, the bodies of older women even learn how to convert the male hormones (androgens), of which women have a certain proportion, into estrogens. As Dr. McDougall points out, an older, overweight woman is therefore in double jeopardy, both from the extra estrogens her body produces from fat cells and from the conversion of her androgens into estrogens.

How do estrogens produce cancer (especially breast cancer) in women? Until recently, nobody had the answer. Now a medical researcher, Dr. Satyabrata Nandi and co-workers at the University of California at Berkeley have found out that estrogens cause the fat cells in a woman's body to release essential linoleic acid, which then acts on the mammary cells. In a young girl this merely leads to breast development. But in an older woman, the stimulation of the breast cells by excess linoleic acid can result in a "neoplastic transformation," that is, it produces cancer cells.[3]

Our bodies cannot make any fats properly without linoleic acid, which has to come from food. We get small amounts of it directly from grains: whole-grain breakfast cereals, whole-grain breads, corn, etc. But by far the largest portion of polyunsaturated fatty acids (PUFAs) in our diet comes from vegetable cooking and salad oils.

That's where all the trouble starts. We need only a very small amount of linoleic acid (1 to 2 percent of total calories; for children, maybe 3 percent), but our extravagant use of vegetable oils provides many times those amounts. Moreover, as explained earlier, the cooking oils are probably already well on the way to oxidation before we even start using them, and continue to oxidize inside our bodies. This process of oxidation, or rancidification, generates free radicals that can attack the DNA in the nuclei of our cells, which carry our whole genetic blueprint, and can lead to cancer. We therefore have a

* John A. McDougall, *A Challenging Second Opinion* (Piscataway, N.J.: New Centuries Publishers, Inc., 220 Old New Brunswick Rd., 08354), 1985. We recommend this book to anyone interested in alternative therapies and sound medical advice across a wide range of common diseases.

doubly good reason to be extremely careful not to exceed 20 percent of our total calories from fats, and not to allow unhealthy adipose tissue (fat cells) to accumulate.

A high-fat diet has also been shown to be a factor in the causation and promotion of prostate cancer.[4] And as with breast cancer, by the time prostate cancer is usually diagnosed—prostate cancer is practically asymptomatic—it has already been developing for many years, making it very difficult to treat.

In this connection, it is interesting to note that vegetarians develop prostate cancer about as often as do meat eaters.[5] One can only draw two conclusions from this: (1) Fat is more important than protein as far as developing prostate cancer is concerned; and (2) it is not just the saturated animal fats that are doing the damage, but all the dietary fats together, including those from butter and eggs—which many vegetarians accept—as well as the transfatty acids from margarine, and the polyunsaturates from vegetable oils that are part of a vegetarian as well as nonvegetarian diet.

STRESS AND EMOTIONAL FACTORS

In addition to dietary, hormonal, and other physical factors, stress and emotional states frequently play an important role in cancer in general and in breast cancer in particular.

A number of studies have tried to show that malignancies, including breast cancer, are supposedly associated with certain personality traits. These studies claim to have noted that a higher percentage of cancer patients demonstrated a certain "defensive stance" in their emotional orientation. They were more apt to "sit on their feelings," especially hostile or critical ones, rather than express them openly.[6]

We do not take much stock in these attempts to assign specific personality characteristics as important in the development of various diseases. Similar speculations have been made with regard to asthma, eczema, and other allergic diseases, as well as to colitis, ulcers, and so forth. While there may be a grain of truth as far as overall statistics are concerned, hypothetical connections between personality characteristics and specific illnesses simply don't hold up in individual cases. This makes them, for all practical purposes, essentially meaningless.

Take, for instance, the conclusions of a study done on a group of forty-nine English women with breast cancer: The researcher decided that these women showed "amazon" characteristics, negating "the typical female role" and seeming "quite combative, achieving, and to the point."[7] In short, this study (conducted in 1978–1979) can be interpreted as suggesting that women's liberation may lead to breast cancer!

The same study, however, pointed to some very interesting trends in the life histories of these women that may indeed relate to a weakened immune system and the development of cancer. It turned out that a high percentage of the women had lost an emotionally important person (such as a parent or beloved sibling) in early childhood. As a result they had responsibilities thrust upon them very early in life, which indeed might explain their aggressiveness—they simply had to fend for themselves.

The study indicated also that many of these breast cancer patients came from emotionally cold family environments, basic trust among their members being sadly lacking. This corroborates numerous other studies demonstrating a link between "faulty family dynamics" (including stressful marital relations) and disease, notably the "psychosomatic" ones, among which we have to count cancer. This, however, is not to say that each and every occurrence of cancer is necessarily related to stress, emotional conflict, or "negative attitudes," much less to "lack of faith," "low vibrations," and so forth. Any such implications can only be harmful rather than helpful.

CANCER OF THE COLON (COLORECTAL CANCER)

With cancer of the colon or rectum, the first sign of trouble is usually—but by no means always!—the discovery of nonmalignant polyps in the colon. In time, these polyps often become malignant, which is why a patient is advised to have them surgically removed. But if the patient does not change to a strictly low-fat, high-fiber diet, new polyps will keep developing, requiring more and more surgery. Even so, without necessary dietary and life-style changes, cancer of the colon is likely to develop.

Studies have also clearly established the connection between colon cancer and stress.[8] It would therefore be a mistake (as with *all* cancers and chronic diseases in general) to focus only on dietary changes and the elimination of chemotoxic habits like smoking and drinking alcohol. As important and fundamental as these life-style changes are, they should definitely be accompanied by attitudinal changes and the use of relaxation techniques.

MORE REASONS FOR A COMPREHENSIVE APPROACH TO CANCER

The superior effectiveness of such a comprehensive approach with cancer patients has been amply demonstrated. In particular, it has been shown that relaxation techniques—including deep abdominal breathing, tensing and relaxing of various body parts, autosuggestion, and voluntary image control—can produce significant improvements in a patient's nutritional and performance status. A combination of these techniques (preferably including hypnotic suggestions) can, as we will show in the following sections, result in considerable pain relief and make chemotherapy much more tolerable. It can also help cancer patients with their usual eating problems and result in a desirable weight reduction or maintenance.[9]

The treatment of cancer is tough on people—it hurts, it frightens, it can be physically and mentally crippling. Chemotherapy fails most often when patients give up because no one supports and encourages them. Cancer treatment absolutely requires a compassionate, comprehensive approach, including psychological and spiritual counseling.

The importance of providing such a support system to cancer patients can hardly be overemphasized. In some cases, as in breast and prostate cancers, it is also of vital importance to reduce weight. In many other types of cancer, and in the more advanced stages of cancer in general, the patient must be helped to maintain weight. In either case, the cancer patient will need psychological help, as well as *personalized* nutritional counseling, to attain these dietary goals. Just providing general nutritional guidelines is simply not enough.

A recent German review[10] of behavioral and psychological techniques with cancer patients envisions even broader applications and goals. It states that there are sufficient indications that under favorable conditions such approaches may extend survival and greatly improve the patient's quality of life.

The scientific explanation for results like these is that with the reduction of tension and anxiety, one can expect an increase of potentially helpful hormones and a corresponding decrease in potentially harmful corticosteroids. Further, the assumption is that the activity of protective NK (natural killer) cells of the immune system can be increased by psychological techniques. Clinical practice has shown that techniques like meditation do promote positive, prolife attitudes. In contrast, negative and destructive attitudes, such as denial, a sense of hopelessness/helplessness, and chronic resentments and distrust, are known to increase corticosteroid levels and suppress NK cell activity.

The review describes a comprehensive approach to cancer treatment as being able to "contribute towards an increased well-being of the cancer patient, but possibly also to positive biochemical and immuno-logical changes within the organism." For these reasons, the review suggests that specialists in psychological therapies for cancer patients (psycho-oncologists) should be included in any cancer-treatment team from the moment of diagnosis.

SOURCES

1. Kinlen, L. J., C. Herman, and P. G. Smith. "A proportionate study of cancer mortality among members of a vegetarian society." *Brit. J. Cancer,* 1983; 48:355.

2. MacDonald, P. "Effect of obesity on conversion of plasma androstenedione to estrone in postmenopausal women with and without endometrial cancer." *Am. J. Obstet. Gynecol.,* 1978; 130(448):21.

3. Hemsell, D. "Plasma precursors of estrogen. II. Correlation of the extent of conversion of plasma androstenedione to estrogen with age." *J. Clin. Endocrinol. Metab.,* 1974; 38:476; also: *American Pharmacy,* Vol. NS27, No. 8, August 1987, p. 16.

4. McDougall, John A. *A Challenging Second Opinion.* Piscataway, N.J.: New Centuries Publishers, Inc., 1985, p. 49. The studies referred to are in: Stamey, T. "Cancer of the prostate: an analysis of some important contributions and dilemmas." *Monographs in Urology,* 1982.

5. Kawasaki, H., F. Morishige, H. Tanaka, and E. Kimoto. "Influence of oral supplementation of ascorbate upon the induction of N-methyl-N-nitro-N-nitrosoguanadine." *Cancer Lett.,* 1982; 16:57.

6. Hill, P. "Environmental factors and breast and prostatic cancer." *Cancer Res.,* 1981; 41:3817.

7. Becker, H. "Psychodynamic aspects of breast cancer differences in younger and older patients." *Psychother. Psychosom.,* 1979; 32:287–296.

8. Selye, H. "Correlating stress and cancer." *Am. J. Protcol. Gastroenterol. Colon Rectal Surg.,* 1979; 30:18–20 and 25–28.

9. Campbell, D. F., et al. "Relaxation: its effect on the nutritional status and performance status of clients with cancer." *J. Am. Diet. Assoc.,* 1984; 84:201–204.

10. Baltrusch, H. J. F. "Psychosocial stress, cancer and coping." *Mitteilungen d. Gesellsch. f. Bek. Krebskrankh., Nordrhein-Westfalen,* 1984; 12:7–12. English abstract in: *Psychological and Behavioral Treatments for Disorders Associated with the Immune System,* Steven E. Locke, ed. New York: Institute for the Advancement of Health, 1986, p. 220, item No. 1221.

CHAPTER 29

PSYCHOLOGICAL FACTORS IN THE TREATMENT OF CANCER

The importance of psychological factors in the treatment of cancer has recently been brought to light by Dr. Bernie Siegel, a New Haven Hospital surgeon and assistant clinical professor of surgery at Yale Medical School.*

Dr. Siegel's basic premise is that patients must be helped to mobilize their own inner resources for healing, with or without the usual methods of surgical intervention, radiation, or chemotherapy treatments. Other people's research into the mind-body connection, together with his own practical experience as a surgeon, have convinced Dr. Siegel that "the state of the mind changes the state of the body through the central nervous system, the endocrine system, and the immune system."

To help his patients use their minds to promote healing—even in cases of what are termed "incurable" and "terminal" cancer—Dr. Siegel conducts regular group sessions with them. In these meetings, the patients share with each other and Dr. Siegel their thoughts and feelings not only about their illness, but also about any other problems in their lives. They also learn meditation, visualization, and relaxation techniques.

Dr. Siegel is very much opposed to giving cancer patients prognoses

---

* Bernie S. Siegel, *Love, Medicine and Miracles* (New York: Harper & Row, 1987).

based on life-expectancy "statistics." He admits that he used to do this, and stopped only when he saw that some patients were getting better despite the statistical odds being totally against them. But when he stopped telling his patients how long they could expect to live, he found himself in deep trouble with the medical establishment. Some doctors actually advised patients to stay away from him lest they build up "false hopes."

Dr. Siegel, however, feels that terms like "false hopes" and "detached concern" (as opposed to loving care) should be stricken from the standard medical vocabulary and practice. He demonstrates his personal caring and affection for patients by giving them hugs. Nor does he ever leave them without hope, no matter how bad the statistical odds may be. Dr. Siegel says, "If statistics say that nine out of ten people die from this disease, most physicians will tell their patients, 'The odds are against you. Prepare to die.' I tell my patients, 'You can be the one who gets well. Let's teach you how.' "[1]

There is no doubt in our minds that several of Dr. Siegel's so-called incurable patients are alive today for no other reason than that he gave them hope. Still, the "miracle" can't happen if the patient does not cooperate. As Dr. Siegel sees it, a "refusal to hope" on the part of the patient "is nothing but a decision to die."

We ourselves vividly remember an American physician in Costa Rica who was suffering from advanced colon cancer. He had already undergone all the surgery and radiation treatments feasible in his case: the medical consensus—"based on statistics"—was that he had, at most, three months to live.

Consulted by the patient's wife with regard to working out a micronutrient program his extremely delicate digestive system could tolerate, we learned that this couple had been influenced by Dr. O. Carl Simonton and his then wife, Stephanie Matthews-Simonton, early pioneers in visualization, meditation, and relaxation techniques. As a result, neither the patient nor his wife were inclined to accept the three-months-to-live verdict and give up the fight. Being a physician himself, the patient had no illusions about the seriousness of his condition. He did not exhibit the kind of denial that characterizes many "terminal" cancer patients and their families. But both he and his wife did refuse to give up all hope—even if it meant "hoping against hope."

Obviously, no two cases are exactly alike. Two people may have the same type of cancer, and the disease may have progressed to more or less the same stage. Yet one of them could be dead within a few days, and the other live on for five, ten, or more years. It all depends on many variables: genetic makeup, individual biochemistry, the degree of stress in the patient's life, and how much emotional support he or she is getting from family, friends, doctors, and nurses. And so much depends on intangibles like the person's morale, will to live, philosophy of life, belief system, and so forth.

Hope—even hope for a "miracle"—should not be confused with unrealistic denial of the facts. When people go so far as to deny the existence of a potentially life-threatening condition and as a result refuse to get professional advice, they are acting neither rationally nor responsibly. In playing such mental games with themselves, they are only worsening rather than increasing their chances of survival.

"HEALTHY DENIAL": JUST ANOTHER KIND OF OPTIMISM?

On the other hand, a certain degree of "healthy denial"—an apparent contradiction in terms—seems to be beneficial. Recent studies show that patients who don't consider their illness to be as serious as it actually is seem to do better than those who are totally realistic. Dr. Shelley Taylor, a psychologist at UCLA, observed in her work with people who have had renal transplants that failed, or with cancer patients whose tumors have recurred, that "positive illusions" sustained these patients. Another psychologist, Dr. Richard Lazarus at the University of California at Berkeley, sums up this new thinking about the relative merits of "illusion" more accurately: "You've got to distinguish . . . between what is a serviceable illusion and what is a destructive one."[2]

What all this really amounts to is that an overly "realistic" (pessimistic) outlook is bound to lead to varying degrees of depression and despondency, which have been shown over and over again to be highly immunosuppressive, cancer-promoting, and generally destructive to health.[3] In contrast, British physician and noted researcher S. Greer found that "denial" or "a fighting spirit" after surgery for breast cancer was predictive of a considerably better outcome than "stoic acceptance" and "helplessness/hopelessness."[4] Similarly, cancer researcher Dr. J. Z. Boryzenko speaks of the need for giving even desperately ill patients a "sense of control" over their illness to "immunize" them against helplessness and forestall depression.[5]

For all the above reasons, we feel that physicians like Dr. Bernie Siegel who give their patients hope are unquestionably doing the right thing. Even though such hope may turn out to be "false," in the sense that the patient ultimately dies, he or she will most likely have lived a little longer and surely more happily with that "false" hope than without it. And many cases in which the cancer is arrested or has regressed, or some other "terminal" illness has been apparently cured, would not have been possible without "hoping against hope."

We know personally of several such "miracles." In 1976 Arnold Schulman, a movie screenwriter (*The Night They Raided Minsky's*), was diagnosed as suffering from "inoperable" and "terminal" liver cancer (those were the actual terms used by his doctors). He decided on his own, without ever having read a word about it, to take up deep meditation to rid himself of the cancer. "I meditated at least four hours a day, every day, besides watching my diet and taking vitamin supplements," he told us.

"I even used visualization," he says, "like flushing out the cancer cells from the liver with all the juices I was drinking by the jugful. Later, when I read up on visualization and all these techniques, I felt rather silly—as if I had reinvented the wheel." Whatever he was doing must have worked; he beat the statistics. There's no evidence of cancer left in him anywhere.

Another friend of ours, Alan, a man in his fifties, was diagnosed as having "inoperable" lung cancer. He started attending services at a Christian Science-like church in his San Diego neighborhood and for several weeks went on a very drastic juice fast, eating no solid food. When he came off the fast he became a vegetarian, and completely changed his attitudes, becoming a different, more loving and giving person. Having, by his own admission, been "a real bastard," he is now a minister of that same church, which he credits with having put him on the right path and saving his life. He's putting in long days, and seems to be in perfect health.

There are thousands of similar "miracles" on record. Even if we don't accept the reasons given for these "miraculous" cures, there is no doubt that some so-called terminal cancer patients proceed to get well and live out productive lives. Medical science calls these inexplicable cures "spontaneous remissions." But more often than not factors other than coincidence are involved.

CANCER AND DEEP MEDITATION

The Australian physician Dr. Ainslie Meares has published several cases in which cancer was if not "cured" then at least arrested through deep meditation.[6]

He tells of a woman with "stone-hard cancer of both breasts." The skin on one of the breasts, he says, "was so tight it appeared to be about to rupture." Worse, the cancer had already spread to the spine and the liver. The woman also suffered, as is typical in advanced cases, from obstructions caused by pressure from an accumulation of serous fluids in the abdomen (ascites). In short, this was a truly "hopeless case" from every conventional medical point of view.

Dr. Meares does not indicate, but one may assume that the patient was not considered a suitable candidate either for surgery or radiation treatment. The only option left was some kind of unconventional therapy. So, under Dr. Meares's instructions, the woman started a course of deep meditation (and nothing else). Soon her breasts softened, the pressure of fluids in her abdomen went down, and before long she was able to resume a normal life.

As Dr. Meares tells it, the woman became a kind of celebrity in Australia after several TV interviews in which she revealed how she had "beaten cancer by meditation." A year later, while Dr. Meares was overseas, she changed her style of meditation and the cancer returned. Dr. Meares helped her get back on the right track with deep meditation, and she soon had a remission.

The woman remained in good health for another twelve months. Then, Dr. Meares writes, she "got involved with someone promising 'miracle cures,'" and no longer practiced deep meditation with regularity and seriousness. Shortly thereafter she relapsed again—and died within two weeks.

Dr. Meares describes many similar cases, including a woman with Hodgkin's disease who was being treated by radiation but kept deteriorating slowly over four years. She had almost given up all hope when she heard of Dr. Meares and his successes with equally desperate cases. At that point she stopped the radiation treatments and took up intensive meditation instead. Her condition began improving soon afterward and continued to improve until she was healthy again.

We could cite many more of this unusual Australian physician's well-documented accounts of cancer patients who have been "helped" (to avoid the term "cured") by nothing but intensive meditation. Dr. Meares feels strongly that it was the particular form of meditation practiced by his patients, and nothing else, that brought about their healing. He describes the meditation as "characterized by a great simplicity, a deep naturalness. It is just a profound stillness of mind."[7]

Dr. Meares's calling deep meditation nothing but a "profound stillness of mind" reminds us very much of the almost identical words Krishnamurti used to the same effect. At the deepest level, that undoubtedly is what meditation is all about. However, there exists by now a huge scientific literature about various, perhaps less "profound" but no less effective, mental techniques—from Dr. Herbert Benson's "relaxation response" (*Your Maximum Mind*) and Dr. Martin L. Rossman's "guided imagery,"* to "autogenic training," "transcendental

---

* Martin L. Rossman, *Healing Yourself, A Step-by-Step Program for Better Health Through Imagery* (New York: Walker & Company, 1987).

meditation"(TM), hypnosis, and self-hypnosis. Whatever method appeals to you and helps you mobilize your own healing resources is at least worth trying, provided it doesn't prevent you from using accepted medical treatment.

SOURCES

1. Padus, E. *The Complete Guide to Your Emotions and Your Health:* Emmaus, Pa.: Rodale Press, 1986, p. 540.
2. Coleman, Daniel. "Trying to Face Reality? It May Be the Last Thing That the Doctor Orders." *The New York Times,* November 26, 1987, p. B–12.
3. Dorian, B., and Paul E. Garfinkel. "Stress, immunity and illness—a review." *Psychological Medicine* (Great Britain, 1987; 17:393–407, cites numerous studies on the immunosuppressive effects of depression.
4. Greer, S., et al. "Psychological response to breast cancer: effect on outcome." *Lancet,* 1979; 785–787.
5. Boryzenko, J. Z. "Behavioral-physiological factors in the development and management of cancer." *Gen. Hosp. Psychiatry,* 1982; 4:69–74.
6. Meares, Ainslie. "Stress, meditation and the regression of cancer." *Practitioner,* 1982; 226:1607–1609.
7. Ibid., p. 1607.

CHAPTER 30

CAN "SUGAR PILLS" (PLACEBOS) CURE DISEASE?

12 We have already endorsed the views of Yale University's Dr. Bernie Siegel about the irrelevancy of "statistics" and the importance of never taking away hope, even for "terminal" patients. Another matter in which we totally agree with Dr. Siegel is the importance of belief ("faith") in the effectiveness of the treatment, *even if that treatment in and of itself cannot possibly cure anything.* Or, to put it another way, the importance of the lowly and much scorned placebo.

A placebo is any innocuous or neutral substance, such as a "sugar pill," that can have no physical effect whatsoever on the course of an illness in a strict medical sense. A placebo cannot do the work of, say, an antibiotic or a diuretic. But the "placebo effect" describes an oft-demonstrated improvement in patients given inactive look-alikes of the real drugs being tested.

What really works in these cases is, of course, the patients' belief (faith) that the fake pill is real and will do some good. That belief is also, we believe, the power behind the incantations of an African witch doctor or the laying on of hands by a faith healer.

Considerations such as these have led serious researchers, like Dr. Kenneth Pelletier, noted psychologist and professor at the University of California at San Francisco, to say that a "disdain for 'placebo effects' is not justified even in traditional medicine." And Norman Cousins, writer and adjunct professor at the UCLA School of Medicine, tells of an experience that taught him "holy respect" for the placebo effect.*

Cousins's story is of special interest to us because it involves a key element on our micronutrient Menu, ascorbic acid (vitamin C). A few years ago some researchers at UCLA were testing the efficacy of vitamin C against the common cold, as propounded by Dr. Linus Pauling and others. They gave one group the actual ascorbic acid; another, a placebo. "The group on placebo who thought they were on ascorbic acid," Cousins writes in *Anatomy of an Illness,* "had fewer colds than the group on ascorbic acid who thought they were on placebo."

A few years earlier, Cousins had been given intravenous infusions of ascorbic acid while getting back on his feet after a massive heart attack. Upon learning of the UCLA results, he wondered whether the considerable benefits he had ascribed to the vitamin C might have been just another manifestation of the placebo effect. We could have put Norman Cousins's mind at rest—in this particular study the daily amount of vitamin C was so small that it could not possibly have impressed the tough cold viruses. (See our discussion of vitamin C for the prevention and treatment of the common cold, pages 98–99.)

Cousins's story has features in common with the case of the American doctor in Costa Rica suffering from colon cancer. During one of our earlier visits to this cancer patient's home, the treating physician, a Harvard-trained cancer specialist, arrived to check on his patient. The patient's wife introduced us to the physician, explaining that she and her husband were consulting with us on nutritional matters. She showed him the list of micronutrients her husband was now taking on our advice.

The physician gave the list a quick glance and, with barely disguised disdain, said, "Well, it can't do him any harm." It was a remark we had heard physicians make many times before and would hear many more times in the future.

It's true that nobody can guarantee that even the best-formulated spectrum of micronutrients will be helpful in a case of advanced cancer. It's also true that both the patient and his wife had placed a certain amount of faith in the anti-oxidants and vitamins. Although they didn't expect a "miracle cure," they certainly hoped for positive results—a hope now being undermined by their physician's attitude.

As it turned out, neither the conventional cancer therapy this patient had been receiving nor the micronutrients and visualizations were ultimately able to save his life; his cancer was simply too advanced. Since in the end he was receiving no medical treatment, aside from

* In two best-selling books, *Anatomy of an Illness* (1979) and *The Healing Heart* (1983), Norman Cousins describes enlisting the help of his mind and the therapeutic effect of laughter in overcoming potentially life-threatening illnesses.

pain-killers, we feel that the micronutrients, his visualizations, and above all his positive attitude have to be credited with extending his life from the three months the doctors had given him to almost a year.

As for us, the biggest lesson we learned from this case was never to dim the light of hope for a patient. In the past we had told people to stay away from some of the popular unorthodox and unproven treatments, even if there seemed to be no harmful side effects from them. But after that experience in Costa Rica, we became more sensitive to a patient's belief system. We now try to work with it instead of against it. So long as the unorthodox therapy the patient believes in is not demonstrably harmful, we're inclined to go along with it, provided it does not exclude standard medical therapy for the specific disease.

CHAPTER 31

HYPNOSIS AND CANCER PAIN CONTROL

12 Contrary to what one might expect, the fear of death and dying is *not* the most dreaded consequence of cancer; it is pain. This may not apply to the initial stages of the disease, but later on, when metastasis has occurred, about one in three patients reports significant pain.[1] In the end stages, even medication like Demerol cannot prevent enough of the pain and allow the patient to pass the last segment of life with some dignity and peace.

Hypnosis has been of considerable benefit in this respect and able to take over where pain-killing drugs reach their limitations. Dr. Paul Sacerdote, a New York psychiatrist associated with the oncology service of Montefiore Medical Center, and now in his seventies, has spent half his life applying hypnosis to control pain to improve the quality of life of cancer patients. His status as one of the most renowned hypnotherapists in the country gives us considerable confidence in his comments on this controversial subject.

In an interview with *Science* magazine, Dr. Sacerdote said that "at a very minimum, one in four people with cancer will respond very well to hypnotherapy for relief of pain."[2] He points out that many of these "responsive" patients can do without narcotics altogether and that others can have their medications drastically reduced. He says it is possible to teach people how to become hypnotized in only a few sessions so that they can later hypnotize themselves when necessary.

Even though patients vary widely in their responsiveness to hypnosis, Dr. Sacerdote believes that almost anyone can benefit to some extent from it. He explains that the lighter trance states, which are the only level some people seem able to reach, are not much different from those mental states induced by simple relaxation techniques that are accessible to everybody.

Other researchers have pointed out that considerable pain control can be achieved with the kind of medium or even light hypnotic trance state that resembles the relaxation response described by Dr. Herbert Benson. They do, however, emphasize that work with hypnosis, on any level, should ideally be started before the pain becomes intense enough to require sedation and before a dependency on pain-killing medication develops. In perhaps the majority of cases, hypnosis can and should supplement the medication. Such a mixed regimen can often result in the patient's requiring much less pain medication.[3]

The effectiveness of hypnosis on cancer pain has been demonstrated in many controlled situations. We were especially struck by one such experiment conducted in Denmark that involved "two of the most desolate cancer patients,"[4] in which simple hypnotic *suggestion* (eliciting the relaxation response) produced significant pain reduction. Actual hypnotic techniques, including "body-mind dissociation" (out-of-body sensation), "pain-heat conversion," and so forth, produced still better results. There was even marked mood improvement—less anxiety and depression—as well as improvement in the general physical condition of these two patients. Moreover, the improvements lasted for a fairly long time.

Hypnosis has been highly successful even with children and young adolescents during very painful medical procedures (bone-marrow aspiration and lumbar puncture).[5,6] Nonhypnotic (relaxation) techniques have also met with some success in this area, though not nearly to the same extent as hypnosis. To reduce anxiety in young people, hypnosis alone was effective. (This could be because of these children's shorter attention span, which lends itself less to nonhypnotic techniques like relaxation, visualization, and meditation.)

THE WIDER USEFULNESS OF HYPNOSIS WITH ADVANCED CANCER

We cannot think of a more telling and touching case to illustrate the usefulness of hypnosis far beyond immediate pain relief than that of Maria Huxley, the first wife of the late writer-philosopher Aldous Huxley, as she was dying of cancer. In Sybille Bedford's biography of Aldous Huxley,[7] we learn that a therapist friend, Leslie LeCron, trained

Maria in self-hypnosis for relief from her agonizing cancer pains. But later her husband had to take over the hypnotic treatment himself.

We had the privilege of briefly knowing Aldous Huxley in the 1950s, shortly after publication of *Brave New World,* and we found him to have a strong spiritual presence. It therefore did not surprise us to learn from Miss Bedford's biography that he used hypnotic suggestion with Maria to protect her peace of mind and reinforce her own strong spiritual tendencies:

> I [Aldous] spent a good many hours of each day sitting with her, sometimes saying nothing, sometimes speaking. When I spoke, it was always, first of all, to give suggestions about her physical well-being. . . . I would suggest that she was feeling, and would continue to feel, comfortable, free from pain. . . . These suggestions were, I think, effective; at any rate there was little pain.

As Ms. Bedford points out, these suggestions for physical comfort "were followed each time by much longer suggestions addressed to the deeper levels of the mind." Again, she quotes from Aldous Huxley's own account of these events: "Under hypnosis Maria had had, in the past, many remarkable visionary experiences of a kind which the theologians would call 'pre-mystical.' "

Maria had been no stranger to such mystical experiences in earlier years, especially during the frequent trips she and her husband made to California's Mojave Desert. She had always lived, as Huxley put it, "with an abiding sense of divine immanence," which was the reason for her passionate love for the desert. He continues:

> In the desert and, later under hypnosis, all Maria's visionary and mystical experiences had been associated with light. . . . Light had been the element in which her spirit had lived, and it was therefore to light that all my words referred. . . .
>
> I would ask her to look at these lights of her beloved desert and to realize that they were not merely symbols, but actual expression of the divine nature; and expression of Pure Being, and expression of the peace that passeth all understanding. . . . And having reminded her of those truths. . . . I would urge her to advance into those lights. . . . Addressing the deep mind which never sleeps, I went on suggesting that there should be relaxation on the physical level and an absence of pain and nausea; and I continued to remind her of who she really was—a manifestation in time of the eternal, a part forever unseparated from the whole, of the divine reality; I went on urging her to go forward into the light . . . I told her to let go. . . . She knew what love was. . . . Now she must go forward into love. . . . And she was to forget, not only her poor body, but the time in which that body had lived. Let her forget the past, leave her old memories behind. Regrets, nostalgias, remorses, apprehensions—all these were barriers between her and the light. Let her forget them. . . . "Peace now," I kept repeating. "Peace, love, joy now. . . ."

Here, then, we have an account of a successful, compassionate comprehensive use of hypnotic suggestions. All too often the spiritual dimension is totally omitted from attempts to alleviate the suffering of dying patients. In the prevailing compartmentalization of functions, concern with matters spiritual is most often left to the presumed specialists—the priests, ministers, and rabbis. We can only hope that the Huxley example will encourage health professionals and family members of patients to utilize spiritual support more often in their ministrations. In cancer and other possibly terminal illnesses, we believe that kind of support can not only prepare the patient for death, but even, in some cases, invite remission or some degree of recovery.

SOURCES

1. Cleeland, C. S. "The impact of pain on the patient with cancer." *Cancer,* 1984; 54:2635–2641.
2. Holden, C. "Pain control with hypnosis." *Science,* 1977; 198:808.
3. Lea, P. A., et al. "The hypnotic control of intractable pain." *Am. J. Clin. Hypn.,* 1960–1961; 3:3–8.
4. Wagner, F. F. "Metastatic pain influenced by hypnotic suggestion." *Ugeskr. Laeger,* 1967;129:393–395.
5. Zeltzer, L., and S. Le Baron. "Hypnosis and nonhypnotic techniques for reduction of pain and anxiety during painful procedures in children and adolescents with cancer." *J. Pediatr.,* 1982; 101:1032–1035.
6. Zeltzer, L., and S. Le Baron. "Behavioral intervention for children and adolescents with cancer." *Behav. Med. Update,* 1983; 5:17–22.
7. Bedford, S. *Aldous Huxley.* New York: Alfred A. Knopf/Harper & Row, 1974, pp. 567–569.

CHAPTER 32

HYPNOSIS AND RELAXATION TECHNIQUES IN CANCER THERAPY

Surgery, radiation, and chemotherapy are frequently able to "cure" or at least arrest cancer. At the minimum, they usually prolong the survival of cancer patients. Yet all these therapies profoundly upset the normal physiological states of the body, which has already been traumatized by the malignancies themselves. Many a cancer patient has expressed the opinion that the "cure" is worse than the disease.

Hypnosis in its various forms and degrees of intensity—from simple suggestion and relaxation to the deeper trance states—offers relief from the difficulties caused by the "cure." Hypnotic suggestion and self-hypnosis (all hypnosis is ultimately self-hypnosis) can first of all reduce the anxiety, apprehension, and depression that almost inevitably follow a cancer diagnosis. With more advanced cancer, hypnosis may help in pain control and in maintaining such vital functions as appetite, digestion, circulation, and sleep.[1] Finally, in the terminal stages, hypnotic suggestions and guided visualization techniques may contribute greatly to the patient's ultimate peace of mind (as in Maria Huxley's case).

Hypnosis has proven to be extremely useful in helping cancer patients tolerate the often extremely unpleasant side effects of chemotherapy, notably nausea and vomiting, which affect virtually everyone to the point where they may choose to forgo treatment rather than continue suffering beyond all endurance.

Usually the nausea starts a couple of hours after the injection, and may last up to twenty-four hours. It's like being desperately seasick during a stormy ocean crossing, unable to get off the boat, only in this case there aren't even any "seasick pills" you can take to prevent it, or other medication to stop it. (There's nothing that really works, or that doesn't produce side effects almost as bad as those of the chemotherapy itself.)

Worse yet, cancer specialists admit that at least one in every three or four patients undergoing chemotherapy develops a psychologically conditioned aversion to the treatments. These poor people start retching long before they actually receive their injections. Sometimes just *thinking* about the next treatment can start the whole process going. This experience is so stressful and so counterproductive to getting well that it is, from a comprehensive point of view, totally unacceptable.

This is where hypnosis offers a way of getting around these complications so that the patient can continue with the therapy. A strong doctor-patient relationship—which borders on hypnotic suggestions—should ideally be an integral part of such an approach.

Hypnosis, however, is especially useful for the "anticipatory nausea" that many patients experience on the way to the hospital, or upon entering and being assaulted by the typical clinic odors, or from sitting in the waiting room. Others may not start vomiting till they actually get inside the treatment room and see the oncology nurse prepare their injection. Patients are even known to experience nausea and vomiting during follow-up visits, though they are aware that no more treatments await them.

Hypnosis is uniquely suited to break into this conditioned response. Psychologist Dr. William H. Redd and his co-workers write that their attention was drawn to this phenomenon almost accidentally. They had been teaching patients self-hypnosis to control cancer pain. It wasn't long before some of these people reported that, using self-hypnosis, they could also "turn off" the nausea caused by chemotherapy. This was not the first time that this possible benefit of hypnosis had been observed; it had even been reported in the scientific literature.[2] Once alerted to this welcome side effect, Dr. Redd and his colleagues began to study the matter more thoroughly and under more controlled conditions than before.

Their initial study in 1982 involved six women treated with chemotherapy at UCLA, all of them suffering from severe anticipatory nausea and vomiting. All were able to complete the entire prescribed chemotherapy course with the help of hypnosis (without hypnosis, at least one or two of the six patients would have dropped out of the chemotherapy program before completion).[3]

Furthermore, the researchers state, "hypnosis eliminated anticipatory emesis [vomiting] in all patients regardless of when during the course of chemotherapy it was introduced." Those patients who were the most highly responsive and who had become most skilled in self-hypnosis were able to cope much better with nausea and vomiting during the actual drug treatments. Other researchers (for example, Dr. Thomas Burish and co-workers at Vanderbilt University, Nashville, Tennessee) have now developed special audiotapes to help patients into a state of deep relaxation during treatment.

Some patients have learned to use self-hypnosis, with or without such tapes, to relax at home after treatment and to go to sleep before the start of any serious attacks of nausea and vomiting. This, according to the researchers, thus far has proven to be the most effective way of preventing the usual posttreatment effects. Unfortunately, only those patients who are most amenable to self-hypnosis are able to reach such a level of control, and even then it has thus far not been proven possible to control posttreatment nausea and vomiting when some of the most toxic, but effective, drugs (for example, cisplatin) have been administered.

We have seen to what a large extent emotional and, for want of a better term, "spiritual" factors enter into the course, causation, and treatment of cancer. Relaxation techniques, guided imagery, and meditation have been shown by cancer specialists like Dr. Siegel in America and Dr. Meares in Australia to play an important role in successful cancer treatment. Others have demonstrated the effectiveness of these techniques, especially that of hypnosis in controlling cancer pain and the side effects of chemotherapy in cancer treatment. Cases like that of Aldous Huxley's wife, Maria, demonstrate how hypnotic suggestion can be used as a powerful spiritual tool with a dying patient.

We have gone into all these matters to show once again how only a comprehensive, compassionate approach to cancer or, for that matter, any disease can be considered a genuine treatment of the disease itself. Anything else is merely symptomatic treatment of the disease and does not address the multiple aspects of its causation. We feel strongly that infectious diseases should be treated not only with antibiotics but also with immune-system–strengthening anti-oxidants and vitamins. The same goes for other degenerative and nutritional diseases, like atherosclerosis, diabetes, and gastrointestinal problems, all of which we shall discuss in the chapters that follow.

We shall see how nutrition, the immune system, the emotions, and life events interact either to maintain wellness or to produce illness. We cannot control life events, but we can do something about our emotions, our nutrition, and our whole life-style. And, to play it safe, we should include a well-conceived program of supplemental anti-oxidants and vitamin co-factors to give our minds and our bodies that extra boost and protection against stress.

SOURCES

1. Rosenberg, S. W. "Hypnosis in cancer care: imagery to enhance the control of the physiological and psychological 'side effects' of cancer therapy." *Am. J. Clin. Hypn.*, 1982; 25:122–127.
2. Redd et al. list several prior reports, e.g., Dempster, C. R., et al. "Supportive hypnotherapy during the radical treatment of malignancies." *Int. J. Clin. & Exper. Hypn.*, 1976; 24:1–9.
3. These particulars are discussed in the report by Redd, W. H., P. H. Rosenberger, and C. S. Hendler. "Controlling chemotherapy side effects." In: *Am. J. Clin. Hypn.*, 1982; 25:161–172.

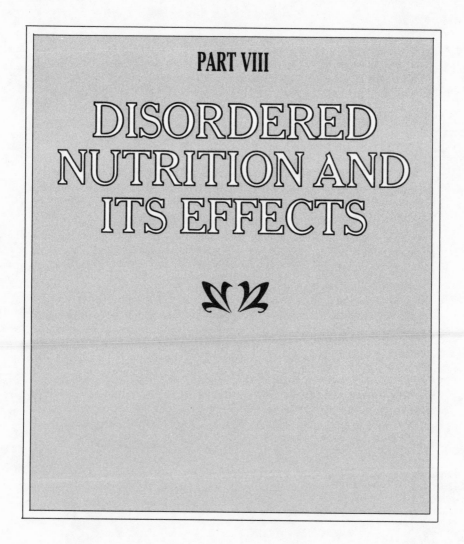

PART VIII

DISORDERED
NUTRITION AND
ITS EFFECTS

CHAPTER 33

ATHEROSCLEROSIS

THE ROAD TO HEART ATTACK AND STROKE

Let's start with some facts:

- Four out of five middle-aged American men run the risk of dying prematurely from heart disease because of unhealthy levels of cholesterol in the blood.[1]
- Health authorities predict that coronary heart disease will remain the nation's leading cause of death for the next twenty-five years. Yet studies have shown that approximately half of the population never has its cholesterol level tested, and over 40 percent have no idea what levels are desirable, and what levels will put them at risk.[2]

We would like our readers to know not only their cholesterol and triglyceride levels, but also what these terms mean. For heart disease—in spite of being near universal—is easily preventable. Put bluntly, it is strictly *self-inflicted.*

Here is what happens: High cholesterol blood levels cause a buildup of arterial plaque—better known as atherosclerosis, or hardening of the arteries. Plaque is an accumulation of fatty sludge made up of rancid (oxidized) cholesterol, thickened muscle layers in the arterial wall, rolls of stuck-together red blood cells (rouleaux) piled up like a logjam in a river, mounds of tiny, disk-shaped structures (platelets), calcium deposits, and other debris. This accumulation narrows the arteries and, as the condition progresses, forces the heart to work harder and harder to push the blood supply through the narrowed passages into vital organs; such as the heart itself, the brain, and the kidneys.

If there is too much cholesterol in your bloodstream—either from animal fats in your diet or because your liver is producing too much cholesterol, or both—some of it will separate out from the blood plasma and form deposits right underneath the *intima,* or innermost (endothelial) lining on the insides of the arteries. Since the junction between the endothelial cells that form the surface pavement of the blood vessels is not absolutely tight, these fat molecules can insinuate themselves, burrowing beneath the lining. Since these cholesterol deposits are not supposed to be there, the body reacts to them as if they were invading parasites or a foreign object, and puts the scavengers of our immune system—the PacMan-like macrophages—on red alert. The macrophages rush to the rescue and start devouring all the "garbage."

Unfortunately, whenever one of the scavengers opens its mouth to engulf invading bacteria, or a virus, or cholesterol deposits, it produces its own "ammunition" in the form of several types of superhot free radicals. These highly reactive, free radicals are not only lethal to an invading organism, but can get the better of anything else, including the macrophages themselves.

What happens in this case? Through the essential protective action of the macrophages, the cholesterol molecules become incidentally oxidized by all the free-radical activity. As the macrophages die, they liberate all those lipid (fatty) peroxides, including rancid (peroxidized) cholesterol, so that we now have these "rotting" fat molecules sitting right underneath the endothelial cells of our arteries. This interferes with the ability of the cells to manufacture a hormone-like substance called prostacyclin (PGI_2) that puts a Teflon-like coating on the insides of our blood vessels to make them nonstick.

When everything is as it should be, the various constituents of our blood—red cells, white cells, and platelets—tumble and rush along right through all the bends and loops of our arteries. If, however, the production of PGI_2 is impaired, as described above, the insides of the arteries become as sticky as flypaper. The fatty deposits produce ridges beneath the surface lining on which the platelets and everything else will stick. This is precisely the process by which plaque builds up in the arteries, a condition that can become so serious as to shut off the entire blood vessel.

We all know that clogged-up arteries often cause heart attack and stroke. But did you know that impotence in men over fifty is caused more by occlusion of the internal iliac arteries of the pelvic region, obstructing blood flow to the genitals, than by hormonal deficiency? If the main penile arteries become calcified and filled with plaque, the spongy penile matrix—the erectile tissue of the penis—becomes fibrotic too. Once that happens, there is no way enough blood can get to the area for normal functioning.

Any of a number of conditions (rancid fats in artery walls, the effects of alcohol, emotional upsets) can cause little spasms that momentarily narrow the passageways for the blood. Normally, such vasospasms are not so serious: If you have a spasm in a medium-sized artery, some blood is still likely to be able to pass through. But in an artery lined with atherosclerotic plaque that has already occluded the blood flow, a spasm can momentarily shut off the blood flow completely—producing anoxia (absence of oxygen) in the tissue or organ that is supposed to be supplied by that artery.

Vasospasms are even more likely to occur in the arterioles, much smaller blood vessels that supply our internal organs. If this happens in the brain, the result is a certain type of stroke. A vasospasm occurring anywhere else will usually go unnoticed—but repeated vasospasms in the arterioles (microscopic continuations of arteries) will cause the cells gradually to atrophy and die.

Which brings us to another direct result of atherosclerosis: the *progressive shrinkage of organs over time,* a process that accelerates from year to year—unless we do something about it! When an organ's cells atrophy, shrivel up, and die for lack of oxygen and nutrients, the organ itself eventually will shrink. If you look at internal organ tissue under a microscope, the surviving cells will show a lot of age pigment, a substance similar to the lipofuscin that produces brown "age spots" on people's skin, which are actually made up of peroxidized lipids and proteins. This pigment is the debris of cells that have died and apparently disappeared.

Organ shrinkage is one of the most drastic effects of the aging process—or, putting it another way, it is the least recognized result of atherosclerosis. The brain, for instance, shrinks from three pounds to two pounds. (Maybe it's just as well that the aged two-pound brain can't remember how much better it functioned with all of its cells still on hand and firing!)

The heart shrinks from approximately 400 grams (almost a pound) to 200 grams. Major shrinkage also takes place in the liver, the internal reproductive organs, the genitals—in short, in all our internal and external organs. Also the skeletal bone structure gets smaller and smaller with age. (There's truth behind the expressions "little old lady" or "little old man.")

One could say that *we start to disappear long before we are dead and buried.* "In my view," Dr. Demopoulos says, "aging and organ atrophy simply mean free-radical–induced vasospasms of the arterioles and a gradual dropping out of the cells over decades—a very slow, insidious process."

Most people, physicians included, do not fully appreciate how early in life atherosclerosis (hence, the beginning of the process that culminates in cell dropout and organ shrinkage) starts. A well-conducted medical study of children with atherosclerosis of the aorta (the great artery arising from the left ventricle of the heart and the main trunk from which the entire systemic arterial network originates) revealed that *all* the children in this study, three years old and up, already had "at least minimal fatty streaks, the earliest grossly recognizable lesion of atherosclerosis."[3]

Another carefully conducted study, which included 205 children in grades 1 to 6 in a Washington, D.C., elementary school, revealed that nearly three out of four children were "already at risk of developing chronic illnesses, such as cancer and heart disease, or of becoming susceptible to strokes later in life."[4]

Shocking? Yes. But not surprising in a society whose children are brought up on ice cream, hamburgers, potato chips, candy bars, soda pop, and many other atherosclerosis-promoting foods.

Researchers are finding that by the time young people reach their twenties, 90 percent—especially white males—are already well along on the way to full-blown atherosclerosis. The trouble is that the condition is hardly ever recognized—or any remedial action taken, such as necessary changes in diet and life-style—because during its early stages there are no obvious clinical symptoms.

Autopsies performed on young American soldiers killed in action in Vietnam showed that 45 percent of them had atherosclerotic lesions, and that 5 percent already had severe coronary artery blockages. These men would not have had an "average" life span, even had they not become war casualties.[5]

An earlier study (1953) of young American soldiers killed in the Korean War had already come up with similarly disturbing data: a 10 to 90 percent narrowing of the coronary blood vessels in 39 percent of the men. In 3 percent of these men (average age: twenty-two) atherosclerotic plaque had totally shut off one or more coronary blood vessels, and only 23 percent were free of "grossly visible lesions in their coronary arteries."[6] (Which is the bigger killer, war or atherosclerosis?)

The message in the results of studies like these—and there are many of them—is clear enough: Atherosclerosis is a progressive deterioration that starts very early in life. We also know that the primary causes are negative life-style factors—notably disordered nutrition, smoking, alcohol consumption, and lack of exercise—all producing excessive amounts of cholesterol, which in turn leads to a buildup of atherosclerotic plaque and the clogging up of blood vessels, which in its turn leads to . . . In short, excessive cholesterol and its twin evil, excessive triglycerides—another fatlike substance in the bloodstream that develops from eating too many fats and sweets—must be brought under control.

Any doubts? Here's one more bit of incentive: In addition to the life-threatening aspects of advanced atherosclerosis—and remember, most of us over forty are already "advanced"—excess cholesterol seriously lowers resistance to infectious diseases. In one study, for example, a high-cholesterol, atherogenic diet caused normally resistant rats to become highly susceptible to tuberculosis.[7] The oxidized cholesterol metabolites were clearly immunosuppressive in these lab animals. Finally, there is ample clinical evidence that high serum cholesterol is associated with a greatly increased risk of developing gallstones, as well as cancers of the colon, rectum, breast, prostate, and other organs.

We hope we've convinced you by now that your cholesterol level is not just your doctor's business, but also, and primarily, your own business. Although everyone has some degree of atherosclerosis, if you take charge of your health, you can improve the risk picture dramatically. With our low-fat, high-complex-carbohydrate diet, exercise, and the Demopoulos spectrum of anti-oxidants, none of us need become "little old men" and "little old women" who are gradually disappearing.

SOURCES

1. Marwick, Charles. "A nation of Jack Sprats? Cholesterol program to stress dietary changes" (Medical News and Perspectives). *JAMA*, 1986; 256:2775–2779. See also: Stamler, J., M.P.H. Wentworth, and J. D. Neaton. "Is relationship between serum cholesterol and risk of premature death from coronary heart disease continuous and gradual? (Findings in 356222 primary screenees of the Multiple Risk Factor Intervention Trial (MRFIT)." Ibid., 2823–2828.
2. Wynder, E. L., F. Field, and N. J. Haley. "Population screening for cholesterol determination—a pilot study." Ibid., 2839–2842.
3. Strong, J. P. "Coronary atherosclerosis in soldiers—a clue to the natural history of atherosclerosis in the young." Ibid., 2864.
4. Vahouny, G. V., and D. Kritchevsky, eds. *Dietary Fiber, Basics and Clinical Aspects.* New York: Plenum Press, 1986.
5. McNamara, J. J., M. A. Molot, J. F. Stremple, et al. "Coronary artery disease in combat casualties in Vietnam." *JAMA,* 1971; 216:1185–1187.
6. First reported in *JAMA,* July 19, 1953, by Maj. William F. Enos, Lt. Col. Robert H. Holmes, and Capt. James Beyer. See also: *JAMA,* 1986; 2859–2862.
7. Beisel, William R. "Single nutrients and immunity." *Am. J. Clin. Nutr.,* 1982; 35:440.

CHAPTER 34

CHOLESTEROL AND TRIGLYCERIDES: THE LESS THE BETTER

FOR FIRST TIME, CUT IN CHOLESTEROL IS SHOWN TO DETER ARTERY CLOGGING, says the front-page headline of *The New York Times* of June 19, 1987. An "aggressive, cholesterol-lowering treatment of drugs and diet," we are told, has been able to shrink the fatty deposits (plaque) in the arteries of about 16 percent of a small group of patients.

Why is this front-page news? one cannot help wondering. Well, it must be, because this little "miracle" of clogged arteries becoming unclogged has supposedly been scientifically demonstrated for the first time in medical history.

Really? Evidence that correct diet and exercise alone—without using drugs or vitamins—can and do regress arterial plaque has been around for some time. Let's just take the case of the late Nathan Pritikin: Many years ago, Pritikin had been diagnosed as suffering from advanced coronary disease (posterior wall myocardial ischemia), hypercholesterolemia (his cholesterol level was over 300), and of course advanced atherosclerosis.

Since neither mainstream medicine at that time nor the nutritionists of the day had anything to offer him, he had created his own life-saving diet and exercise program. The result: His cholesterol level dropped from over 300 to 107. And when he died some thirty years later of unrelated causes, the autopsy revealed that the clogged arteries that had formerly restricted the blood supply to his heart were whistle-clean![1]

We think an autopsy like this provides ultimate proof of plaque regression—far beyond that shown by angiograms. Moreover, there are numerous similar, well-documented cases on record, involving at least one angiogram, if not more.[2,3] Enough said. In discussing the "first-time" claim of the new study showing that diet and drugs—or diet and niacin (vitamin B_3)—are able to regress atherosclerotic plaque we only wanted to be fair to other researchers who had previously demonstrated similar results.

The fact that diet is finally being fully acknowledged as the key factor in the treatment and prevention of atherosclerosis and heart disease is to be highly applauded, however long overdue. Until now, the medical establishment's "silver bullet" against coronary heart disease has been the famous bypass operations. We don't mean to belittle them—in many cases they do save lives, at least temporarily, and win the patients precious time. And if that borrowed time is used to start a healthy diet and to stop indulging detrimental life-styles, the bypass operations may indeed have been worthwhile.

Without such drastic postoperative changes, however, the arteries tend to clog up again sooner or later. Then another bypass operation must be performed—maybe a double, a triple, or a quadruple—until finally there are no more arteries to bypass. In the end, the patient is as likely as not to succumb to a final heart attack or progressive heart failure anyway. A growing number of cardiologists and heart surgeons are following the lead of Dr. Michael DeBakey, the originator of The Living Heart Diet and author of a diet book by the same title—and actively counsel their patients along these lines.*

If the patient is not in imminent danger of heart attack, many doctors however still pay little attention to cholesterol and triglyceride levels. The same medical journal (*JAMA*) that reported on the benefits of a cholesterol-lowering diet had reported earlier that only some 30 percent of doctors believe that controlling cholesterol blood levels is as important as controlling high blood pressure or smoking. New national survey data confirm what is really a matter of common knowledge, namely that both physicians and patients still underestimate the health risks that high cholesterol levels pose.

Another article in the journal described how many physicians unintentionally lull their patients into false confidence when it comes to cholesterol. "A key and disturbing finding of our study," the report says, "was that when 300 individuals with elevated cholesterol levels were interviewed by telephone, some 70% said that their physicians told them to 'do nothing' or 'not worry.' "[4]

Physicians have by now more or less accepted the fact that the

---

* Dr. DeBakey's diet is considerably more lenient than Nathan Pritikin's, or even our own. It is, however, a feasible compromise for those who cannot accept anything else.

cholesterol levels of many of their patients are too high. But what is their first impulse? You guessed it: It is to reach for the prescription pad and order one or the other of the new cholesterol-lowering drugs. In fact, there still is a segment of the medical profession that is belligerently against those who place emphasis on a health-promoting diet rather than on medication. A *New York Times* article of July 14, 1987, headlined CHOLESTEROL: DEBATE FLARES OVER WISDOM IN WIDESPREAD REDUCTION, quotes Dr. Michael F. Oliver, a British cardiologist, complaining that health "propagandists" had unleashed a "juggernaut" of advice urging widespread dietary changes.

Dr. Marshall H. Becker of the University of Michigan School of Public Health asks, "Why are we driving people nuts about cholesterol?," suggesting that we ought to be worrying more about "things like smoking." (We wonder why these two problems should be mutually exclusive.)

The *Times* article also refers to those doctors who say that, "on an average," people who make dietary changes and lower their cholesterol don't live that much longer. However, at least one of them—Dr. William C. Taylor of the Harvard Medical School—frankly admits that "averages" and statistics don't have much meaning to the individual. "A particular person," he says, "who avoided a heart attack through cholesterol reduction would consider his personal gain enormous." And Dr. Scott M. Grundy, director of the Center for Human Nutrition at the University of Texas Health Sciences Center in Dallas, is quoted: "They say that Americans are relatively healthy and there is no reason to worry about their diet. But five out of six experts think that dietary modification would help prevent heart attacks."

The biggest controversy swirls around the issue of childhood nutrition. Many pediatricians are still convinced that children and adolescents need fats and cholesterol for proper growth and development. "Children need fat," says Dr. Laurence Finberg, chairman of the Academy of Pediatrics' nutrition committee. "If you start reducing their fat, you may introduce other problems."

Children do indeed need more calories—but not fats. Nathan Pritikin therefore told parents not to put their children on the usual low-calorie adult version of his diet. Instead, he suggested giving them larger servings of higher-calorie foods, such as whole grains, whole-grain bread, pasta, and more of the starchy vegetables like white and sweet potatoes, squash, and peas. He noted that "children usually love thick, hearty soups, with brown rice, barley, split peas, beans, potatoes, or whole wheat pasta."[5]

But at the same time, he warned that atherosclerosis starts very early in life and is cumulative. "Do everything you can," he said, "to obtain your children's cooperation, and give them the benefit of clean arteries and the superior health and functioning possible with an uncompromised circulatory system. *Limit their intake of high-cholesterol foods . . ."* (Emphasis ours.)

In our view, Pritikin was too strict in wanting the fat content of a juvenile diet to be the same low 10 percent of total calories he advised for adults. Our own diet allows 15 to 20 percent of calories from fat for relatively healthy adults, but Dr. Demopoulos and we think that growing children should get 30 percent of their calories from fat (the amount recommended for *adults* by the American Heart Association). However, we feel strongly about keeping the *cholesterol* part of fat as low as possible for adults *and* children.

Encouraging children to eat hamburgers, french fries, potato chips, butter, ham, and bacon, on the assumption that later on these cholesterol-rich foods will be on the "to be avoided" list, doesn't make sense from a psychological point of view. What *would* make sense is to help keep children from getting hooked on the kinds of rich food that make adults sick.

The way to do this is to get children accustomed as early as possible to "friendly" foods that promote health and longevity. If this can't be accomplished at an early age, then as adults most of us will find ourselves painfully unlearning wrong food habits, undoing all the conditioning of the past, and then establishing new, health-promoting habits. We advise against any kind of conditioning that will have to be undone later on. The reason is obvious: Getting rid of a habit is a thousand times more difficult than acquiring it.

Unfortunately, there is also a great deal of disagreement in the medical profession as to what constitutes an elevated cholesterol level. Many doctors consider levels of 200 and more perfectly all right; others believe that any level above 180 is cause for concern. Another group of researchers has suggested that ideal cholesterol levels for adults ought to fall between 130 and 190. With so much uncertainty among medical researchers, you can imagine the confusion of the average general practitioner.

The ideal cholesterol range depends, for one thing, on your objective. If the idea is only to maintain average health and life span, then a cholesterol level around 180 is acceptable. But if your goal is *optimum* health maintenance—a state of health well beyond what is generally considered adequate—a cholesterol range of 110 to 150 with a mean of 130 is what you should aim for.

With respect to the problem of cholesterol control one medical researcher (Grundy) put it bluntly: ". . . Many physicians at present do not have the detailed knowledge of lipoprotein [read: blood-fat] disorders required to make correct decisions about appropriate therapy for hypercholesterolemia."[6] Many doctors still treat dietary cholesterol with "benign neglect" because they feel secure in the belief that the amount of cholesterol obtained from foods isn't important since the body has a feedback mechanism to shut down the production of liver cholesterol when a lot of food cholesterol is taken in.

The problem is that this feedback mechanism does not work as perfectly as is often assumed. A moment's thought makes that quite clear: A diet low in cholesterol-rich saturated fats always results in lower cholesterol levels than a diet high in such animal fats—which means that the liver's automatic feedback mechanism cannot possibly be 100 percent effective. If it were, diet would have no effect whatsoever on how much cholesterol is circulating in your arteries.

True, some people seem to get away with eating impressive amounts of cholesterol-rich foods. If you checked their blood cholesterol level after a fatty meal, you might find only minor elevations of cholesterol. Others, having eaten exactly the same foods, may show a considerable rise in cholesterol. Why the difference? Because some people are genetically at a disadvantage in coping with cholesterol (and weight control). We will discuss this later on.

Cholesterol levels are basically controlled by certain receptors for lipoproteins on the liver cells. Until quite recently nobody even knew these receptors existed. (Their two discoverers, Dr. Michael Brown and Dr. Joseph Goldstein, received the Nobel Prize for their work in this field.) In people who have an inborn tendency to develop high cholesterol levels, there exists a not infrequent condition called *familial hypercholesterolemia,* in which the gene for these receptors is defective and the cholesterol cannot be removed from the circulation at a normal rate.[7] But this genetic abnormality, about which nothing can be done, is (as Brown and Goldstein agree) clearly aggravated by factors over which we have considerable control—diet, proper exercise, and the avoidance of contributing life-style factors, such as smoking.

Let's say that you have a cholesterol level of 200, which is about average for American adults. What does this figure mean with regard to your risk of coronary heart disease and stroke?

Pathological studies show that when about 60 percent of the surface of an artery is covered with raised plaque, the risk of heart attack or stroke becomes critical. People with a cholesterol level of 200 and no other risk factors, such as high blood pressure or smoking, do not enter a critical phase until they reach the age of seventy. With a cholesterol level of 200, it takes that long for plaque to cover 60 percent of the arterial surfaces and become life-threatening. But if the cholesterol level of a nonsmoker is raised to a range between 250 and 300, the same degree of plaque in the arteries is likely to develop by the time he or she reaches fifty or sixty.

Many people in our society, however, are smokers and/or have varying degrees of high blood pressure. What happens then?

Let's return to our hypothetical person with a level of 200: If he or she is a smoker, the critical stage is no longer postponed until the person reaches seventy, but is attained by the time he or she is sixty. And if this person is not only a smoker, but *also* suffers from hypertension (high blood pressure), the age at which the critical phase is reached drops to fifty years.

Under the same circumstances, but with a given cholesterol level of 250, the critical phase would be reached ten years earlier, at age forty. As one of the nation's outstanding cholesterol researchers put it, "Certainly it is not unusual to see myocardial infarction in a 40-year-old man who smokes and has an elevated plasma cholesterol level and hypertension."[8]

It is, however, impossible to understand how this works without knowing more about the nature of cholesterol, how it is carried around in the bloodstream, how we get rid of it, what functions its associated lipoproteins have, and how some of them interact with what is known as triglycerides (a form of fat in the bloodstream that can be used either as energy fuel, the formation of body fat, or be converted to cholesterol). Very briefly and simply, cholesterol is carried around by tiny particles called *lipoproteins*. These lipoproteins have been likened to little envelopes made up of lipids (fats) and proteins. These envelopes carry cholesterol and triglycerides around in the plasma, or serum of the bloodstream. This is important because the cholesterol and the fatty acids of the triglycerides are not water soluble by themselves and could otherwise not be transported in an essentially watery medium like blood plasma.

There are several kinds of lipoproteins, only three of which are of interest for our purposes. They are:

LDLs—*low-density lipoproteins*
HDLs—*high-density lipoproteins*
VLDLs—*very low-density lipoproteins*

The LDLs are the main carriers of cholesterol and account for 60 to 70 percent of the total. Their function is to bring cholesterol to any part of the body (where it may be needed to build cell membranes) or to the glands (where it is used to make vital hormones). The body also uses cholesterol to make the bile acids that are necessary to digestion. So, you see, cholesterol isn't all bad. The problem is that the typical American-European diet provides too much of it, loading our arteries with plaque and causing so many heart attacks and strokes.

While the LDLs carry cholesterol from the liver to the tissues, the HDLs do just the opposite: They bring the cholesterol from the tissues back to the liver. There the cholesterol can be converted into bile acids and eliminated, via the bile duct, into the intestines and, one hopes, out of the body. Unfortunately, this does not always happen. Instead, the cholesterol may be recycled back into LDL cholesterol.*

You might think of the LDLs as the "bad" guys who could kill us with heart attack and stroke, or by promoting certain cancers (for example, of the breast, prostate, and colon). The HDLs are the "good" guys, trying to protect us from LDL. High levels of HDL have actually been associated with decreased risk for coronary heart attack. Conversely, obese people and diabetics are usually short on HDL.[9,10]

One must keep in mind that HDL is, after all, part of the whole cholesterol picture and must be considered in relation to total serum cholesterol and triglycerides. For instance, there are cases in which the total cholesterol level is very high but is made up to a large extent of HDL. It would be a good idea to try to find out why this should be. Are the high HDLs the result of a healthy exercise regimen, or of unhealthy alcohol consumption, or of an abundance of polyunsaturated oils in the diet?[11]

It is only in the light of all these factors that the LDL:HDL ratio becomes meaningful. The most interesting thing about it is that we are all born with exactly the same amounts of LDL and HDL—and with a perfect 1:1 ratio between them. Only with age—or rather with disordered nutrition, to call a spade a spade—does this ideal ratio get tilted in favor of the less desirable LDLs.

Now, it is generally speaking a good sign to have an LDL:HDL ratio that is as close as possible to the original 1:1 with which we entered life. But we have seen cases where patients and doctors alike have been lulled into false confidence on the basis of an "average" serum cholesterol level (say, around 200) and a good LDL:HDL ratio, without a thorough investigation of the reasons—good or bad. Patients often tend to take such an encouraging ratio as license to indulge in less than ideal diets, usually with most unfortunate results.

Let us now consider still another important aspect of the cholesterol-triglyceride drama: the VLDLs (very low-density lipoproteins). Their main function is to carry triglycerides to our cells for immediate cellular energy, or to any part of the body for storage as body fat. The problem is that they can be broken down by enzymes in the liver and turned into the "bad" LDL cholesterol. By that circuitous route, a certain percentage of the triglycerides can wind up promoting exactly

---

* The calcium on our micronutrient Menu comes in handy to prevent this partially. The bile acids tend to bind to the calcium, which makes it much easier for the substantial fiber content of our diet to help eliminate them promptly.

CHOLESTEROL AND TRIGLYCERIDES

Most Americans and Europeans have cholesterol levels of about 200 and triglyceride levels of 150.

Ideal levels:
Cholesterol: 110–150 (average 130)

Triglycerides: 100 or less

Lipoproteins: the vehicles for the transport of fats in the blood.

Low-density lipoprotein (LDL): Carries between 60–70% of the total cholesterol in the plasma from the liver to the tissues.

High-density lipoprotein (HDL): Carries the cholesterol from the tissues back to the liver for breakdown into simpler compounds (e.g., bile acids) and thus for excretion.

Very low-density lipoproteins (VLDL): Carries primarily triglycerides, but also some cholesterol (10–15%) and phospholipids, the major construction blocks of cell membranes.

LDL : HDL ratio: At birth we have exactly as much LDL as HDL, so the ratio is 1 : 1. It is important that this ratio remains as close to this ideal equilibrium as possible.
   The higher the HDL and the lower the LDL, the better.
   The "normal" range for HDL cholesterol is 30 to 80 mg/dl. Therefore, the closer to 30 the HDL, the higher the risk for coronary heart disease; and the higher the HDL, the more protection against coronary heart disease

Example: LDL = 78 mg/dl
HDL = 70 mg/dl
Ratio: 78 : 70 = 1.1 (excellent)

Example: LDL = 150 mg/dl
HDL = 30 mg/dl
Ratio: 150 : 30 = 5.0 (high risk)

Ideal cholesterol range: 110–150 mg/dl
Ideal triglyceride range: 25–100 mg/dl

the aspect of total cholesterol that contributes most heavily to athero-sclerosis.

Considering that the triglycerides feed into our cholesterol pool, and that they come not only from simple carbohydrates (sugars) but also from saturated animal fats and unsaturated vegetable fats and oils, it's clear that simply switching from saturated animal fats to those of plant origin is not enough to solve cholesterol and triglyceride problems. Obviously, we have to cut down not only on one kind of fat but on *all* fats.

A number of studies and several decades of practical experience leave no doubt that a high-complex-carbohydrate, low-fat, high-fiber diet, coupled with regular physical exercise, definitely lowers both cholesterol and triglyceride levels.[12]

Exercise or physical work also raises the level of the "good" HDL. *Any* aerobic activity (running, fast walking, or any exercise that brings up your heart rate and speeds up your oxygen metabolism) will increase the HDL—but, oddly enough, *only in men.* Women, however, reap all the other benefits of exercise. That includes reducing their LDL concentration almost as much as men do, which is much more important than increasing the HDL. Of course, we all should exercise for any number of other reasons—strengthening the heart muscle and increasing lung capacity, for instance, not just for the cholesterol-lowering effect.

If you're overweight, your LDL:HDL ratio will greatly favor the "bad" low-density lipoproteins, and your total cholesterol is bound to be high. In that kind of situation, emphasizing complex carbohydrates in your diet and increasing your physical exercise (always in accordance with your general medical status and that of your heart in particular) will automatically improve your LDL:HDL ratio and lower your choles-terol, in direct proportion to the weight loss concerned.

SOURCES

1. Hubbard, J. "Nathan Pritikin's Heart." *N. Eng. J. Med.,* 1985; 313:52.
2. Grenoble, P. B. *Pritikin People.* New York: Berkely Books, 1986.
3. Hall, J. A., N. Pritikin, et al. "Effects of diet and exercise on peripheral vascular disease." *The Physician and Sports Medicine,* 1982; 10:90–101. Also: Wissler, R. "Studies of regression of advanced atherosclerosis in experimental animals and man." *Ann. N.Y. Acad. Sci.,* 1976; 275:363; Duffield, R. "Treatment of hyperlipidaemia retards progression of symp-tomatic femoral atherosclerosis. A randomised controlled trial." *Lancet,* 1983; 2:639; Nikkila, A. "Prevention of progression of coronary atheroscle-rosis by treatment of hyperlipidaemia: a seven year prospective angio-graphic study." *Brit. Med. J.,* 1984; 289:220; Ost, C. "Regression of peripheral atherosclerosis during therapy with high doses of nicotinic acid." *Scand. J. Clin. Lab. Invest. Suppl.,* 1967; 99:241; Bassler, T. "Re-

gression of atheroma." *Western J. Med.,* 1980; 132:474; Roth, D. "Noninvasive and invasive demonstration of spontaneous regression of coronary artery disease." *Circulation,* 1980; 64:888.

4. Wynder, E. L., et al. "Population screening for cholesterol determination—a pilot study." *JAMA,* 1986; 256:2842.
5. Pritikin, N. *The Pritikin Promise.* New York: Pocket Books, 1985, p. 159.
6. Grundy, Scott M. "Cholesterol and coronary heart disease." *JAMA,* 1986; 256:2849–2858.
7. Brown, M. S., and J. L. Goldstein. "Drugs used in the treatment of hyperlipoproteinemias." In: Goodman and Gilman, *The Pharmaceutical Basis of Therapeutics,* 7th ed., 1985. See also: Grundy, op. cit., p. 2855.
8. Kammel, W. B., W. P. Castelli, and T. Gordon. "Cholesterol in the prediction of atherosclerotic disease: New perspectives based on the Framingham Study." *Ann. Int. Med.,* 1979; 90:85–91. See also: Grundy, op. cit., p. 2851.
9. Williams, P. M. "High density lipoprotein and coronary risk factors in normal men." *Lancet,* 1979; 1:72.
10. Gordon, T., W. P. Castelli, M. C. Hjortland, et al. "High density lipoprotein as a protective factor against coronary heart disease: The Framingham Study." *Am. J. Med.,* 1977; 62:707–714. Also: Enger, S. J., I. Hjerman, O. P. Foss, et al. "High density lipoprotein cholesterol and myocardial infarction or sudden death: a prospective case-control study in middle-aged men of the Oslo study." *Artery,* 1979; 5:170–181; Gordon, D. J. (for the Lipid Research Clinics Coronary Primary Prevention Trial Investigators). "Plasma high-density lipoprotein cholesterol and coronary heart disease in hypercholesterolemic men." *Circulation,* 1985; 72:III–185; Watkins, L. O., J. D. Neaton, and L. H. Kuller (for the MRFIT Research Group). "High-density lipoprotein cholesterol and coronary heart disease incidents in black and white M.R.F.I.T. usual care men." *Circulation,* 1985; 71:417A.
11. Howard, B. V. "Obesity cholelithiasis, and lipoprotein metabolism in man." In: *Bile Acids and Atherosclerosis,* Vol. 15, Scott M. Grundy, ed. New York: Raven Press, 1986, especially p. 183. Also: Flanagan M. "The effects of diet on high density lipoprotein cholesterol." *J. Hum. Nutr.,* 1980; 34:43; Williams, P. M. "High density lipoprotein and coronary risk factors in normal men." *Lancet,* 1979; 1:72; Gordon, T. "Diabetes, blood lipids, and the role of obesity in coronary heart disease risk for women." *Ann. Intern. Med.,* 1977; 87:393; Chase, H. "Juvenile diabetes mellitus and serum lipids and lipoprotein levels." *Am. J. Dis. Child.,* 1976; 130:1113; Castelli, W. "Alcohol and blood lipids, the Cooperative Lipoprotein Phenotyping Study." *Lancet,* 1977; 2:153; Wood, P. "Plasma lipoprotein distributions in male and female runners." *Ann. N.Y. Acad. Sci.,* 1977; 301:748.
12. O'Brien, L. T., R. J. Barnard, A. J. Hall, and N. Pritikin. "Effects of a high-complex-carbohydrate, low-cholesterol diet plus bran supplement on serum lipids." *J. Appld. Nutr.,* 1985; 37:26–34. Also: *J. Card. Rehab.,* Vol. 1, No. 2, 1981; Vol. 2, No. 7, 1982; Vol. 3, No. 12, 1983; and Rosenthal, M. B., R. J. Barnard, D. P. Rose, S. Inkeles, J. Hall, and N. Pritikin. "Effects of a high-complex-carbohydrate, low-fat, low-cholesterol diet on levels of serum lipids and estradiol." *Am. J. Med.,* 1985; 78:23–27.

CHAPTER 35

FIGHTING THE FAT

THE TRUTH ABOUT OBESITY

Half of the United States is watching its weight. More than half of the women in the country, according to *The New York Times,* are on a diet. Most of these people consider themselves "a little overweight," or "chubby," or the victims of "middle-aged spread." Relatively few consider themselves "fat," and even fewer think they're "obese."

These are all labels, of course, and labels aren't important. Nor do the ten extra pounds that keep a slender woman from being slender enough to wear a French size 8 really matter. Obesity, however—which we define as being more than 15 percent over one's normal weight range—is important, genuinely health-threatening, and all too often chronic.

There is a considerable physiological and psychological difference between someone who has put on a few extra pounds and a person who is obese and has probably been obese since childhood. Specialists consider thirty-five million Americans to be technically obese. And though obesity declines considerably with advancing age, by medical standards 15 percent of white males and 30 percent of black females are still obese at the age of eighty.[1]

What this means is that tens of millions of individuals in this country alone have lives that are less healthy, less active, and, in all probability, shorter than they could be.

OBESITY AND HEALTH

As Dr. Samuel Johnson once observed to James Boswell in regard to a certain gentleman who was "much incommoded by his corpulance": "Whatever the quantity that a man eats, it is plain that if he is too fat he has eaten more than he should have done."[2]

What we know today that Dr. Johnson didn't know, is that obesity is not simply a matter of eating too much food. More important than the amount of food is the type that is eaten. Rich, calorie-dense foods like fats and sweets are the ones that do the real damage.

Fatty foods contribute readily to obesity simply because it is so easy for the body to make fat from fat. It "costs less," as Dr. Elliot Danforth, Jr., has said, "to store fat in the body from dietary fat than from carbohydrate."[3] In fact, our bodies convert dietary fats into storable triglycerides (body fat) at a metabolic cost of only 3 percent of ingested calories, while the cost of converting dietary carbohydrates is 23 percent of the calories consumed.

Besides being able to process fats more efficiently, our bodies begin to process them into body fat more quickly. The body can maintain a fairly constant balance of carbohydrates and protein, even in the face of a temporary indulgence. However, its short-term fat balance can be easily upset by excess fat intake and this leads directly to the production and storing of body fat.

Excess body fat has been found to reduce the efficiency of the immune system, causing the obese person to be vulnerable to any bacterial or viral infection that may come along, and even imposing an increased cancer risk. Excess quantities of body fat undergo a continuous process of autoxidation (rancidification).[4] These rancid fats suppress the production and activities of white blood cells (macrophages), which are a foremost defense against invading microorganisms and cancer cells. Obesity also depresses the production of growth hormone,[5] another essential part of the immune system, and the peroxidized fats themselves are both mutagenic (cause genetic mutation) and carcinogenic because of their dangerous peroxide radicals.

Another health-threatening factor of obesity is that it is frequently accompanied by hypertension (high blood pressure). Many obese people make the mistake of letting themselves be treated for hypertension only with medication without getting at the actual cause of it—their excess pounds. The trouble is, as several studies suggest, maintaining ideal weight during the third to fifth decades of life is more effective in preventing hypertension than controlling that weight once hypertension has been established.[6]

What makes this situation all the more critical is that obese people,

ACHIEVING WEIGHT LOSS AND MAINTAINING YOUR PREFERRED WEIGHT

If you follow our basic diet guidelines, you don't need to count calories. With your new knowledge about "friendly" and "unfriendly" foods, you will learn to automatically adjust caloric intake to caloric output, thereby maintaining a healthy balance.

Fewer calories = less weight = less illness = longer life span

Keys to Weight Control

1. Reduce:

   fats
   sugars
   salt

2. Eat more:

   fresh fruits
   fresh vegetables

3. Eat more (complex carbohydrates):

   whole grains
   breads
   pasta

4. Deemphasize red meat

5. Emphasize:

   white meat of chicken and turkey (cooked without the skin)
   fish (including water-packed tuna)
   wild game

6. Lower intake of sugar to a minimum. Continuing to eat sugar establishes a vicious circle:

   • sugar throws off metabolism, especially insulin production—there is a sharp rise in blood glucose with a temporary surge of energy; followed by a release of insulin to take care of the excess glucose; followed by a lack of glucose and an energy letdown with a need for "quick-fix" sugar.

   • eating too much sugar leads to cravings and food addictions—the more you eat the more you want. Eating one piece of candy leads to several pieces; drinking one sugar-laden soft drink leads to several more soft drinks.

7. Lower intake of all fats (both animal and plant). Depending on weight loss desired, reduce fats, first to 30 %, then to 20 % or less of total calories. Reduction of fats is essential to weight loss. With a lean diet, it is almost impossible to be overweight, even if you have a genetic tendency. No need to worry about not getting enough fat—all foods contain some fat (including lettuce). Adding any extra amounts of fat means you are adding calories (even "light" margarine adds calories). Also, fats oxidize (go rancid),

without necessarily giving off a detectable odor or a perceptible off taste. Oxidized (rancid) fats are highly dangerous to your health; they can initiate or promote many cancers (such as breast, colon, and prostate cancer).

As with sugar, the more fat you eat, the more you crave it. Excess fat and sugar consumption frequently go together, giving you a double whammy of fattening calories. One dish of ice cream frequently leads to eating the whole quart; a few potato chips may lead to eating the whole bag; instead of eating a few peanuts, you may find yourself eating half the bag or the whole can.

8. Eliminate as much salt as possible. Substitute spices and low-salt soya, tamari, or Chinese oyster sauce.

   If you must use salt, research shows people tend to take in less salt when they add it just before eating, rather than when adding it during food preparation. (Many people add more automatically at the table anyway!) Excess salt encourages overeating, as is true for sugar and fats. Salt addiction frequently accompanies sugar and fat addiction. Salt is often hidden in many foods, like frozen fish, and is not necessarily listed on labels.

9. Drink mainly water, and drink it frequently. Having a glass of water by your side and sipping it throughout the day is essential for good health. Drink at least seven glasses of (preferably filtered and purified) water per day.

10. Consume most of your calories during the day. Do *not* skip breakfast. Have at least a bowl of cereal (preferably oatmeal, without milk, and not the highly processed type). Eat a moderate, well-balanced lunch (not just a salad). Don't eat when you're not hungry, but don't allow yourself to get too hungry between meals; it only results in a loss of energy and a sense of frustration (chronic semistarvation can lead to serious physical problems). Also, voluntary food deprivation may become a subconscious excuse for a food binge later. Do not eat too heavy a meal in the evening. Ideally the midday meal should be the most substantial one. Do not eat later than two hours before bedtime—you will sleep better and gain less weight.

11. Keep moving whenever possible. Daily activity, whether physical work or exercise or a combination of both, is essential for weight control (it burns up calories). While many people first start exercising for weight control, most continue some form of daily exercise after having lost weight, because they enjoy it. If you are losing weight rapidly, it is essential to exercise because you may end up losing muscle mass and muscle protein. In such a stiuation, approximately one third of each pound lost would represent muscle loss! So, remember, it is essential to exercise, especially if weight loss is rapid, as for example, if you lose one pound every two days.

12. If you have a tendency to gain weight easily, do *not* sit down (e.g., to watch television) or lie down to take a nap after a meal. This puts on maximum weight because no calories are being burned. Always walk or move about after eating.

with their customary high-fat diet, not only ingest too much already peroxidized fat, but also have an excessive amount of peroxidized fats in their body tissues. This, in turn, interferes with the production of PGI_2 (prostacyclin), which keeps artery walls nonstick, inhibits platelet aggregation, and prevents the formation of dangerous blood clots that can lead to stroke or heart attack. In the presence of hypertension, this danger of course is compounded.

A complicating factor is that men tend to put on more fat around the middle (stomachs) than do women. Several studies have shown that this phenomenon is associated with greatly increased risk for heart disease, stroke, diabetes, and premature death.[7]

Women generally have more fat around their hips and extremities, a sex difference that is known to be due to the effect of hormones. However, when women do develop fat deposits around the waist and abdomen, they run the same additional health risks as men.[8]

When we encounter people of either sex with large bellies, we urge them to take immediate action to get rid of the fat deposits, not for cosmetic reasons, but because they are so imminently life-threatening. Most obese or merely overweight people with this pattern of fat distribution are seldom aware of the danger, and it generally has not been pointed out to them.

While simple carbohydrates (sugars) and highly processed carbohydrates (pasta, white bread, and bakery goods) also contribute to the production of body fats, their contribution is relatively minor compared to that of dietary fats. Nevertheless, overindulgence in sugars and processed carbohydrates produces a high level of triglycerides in the blood (hypertriglyceridemia). In turn, the triglycerides, by producing VLDLs (very low-density lipoproteins), contribute to the body's total cholesterol. These types of carbohydrates also lead to the release of insulin from the pancreas, which stimulates the production rate of cholesterol even further. Finally, as Dr. Barbara Howard of the National Institutes of Health (NIH) has pointed out, HDL (the beneficial high-density lipoprotein) can be degraded by a liver that is overtaxed by excess blood lipids derived from dietary fats and sugars. In fact, she says, "all metabolic processes in the liver may be stimulated in obese subjects."[9]

All this cholesterol produces gallstones because the cholesterol concentration in the gallbladder-bile fluid rises to saturation. When this happens, the excess cholesterol forms crystals that, under certain circumstances, can become the nuclei of gallstones. In fact, most gallstones are formed in precisely this way. Drs. Kurt Einarsson and Bo Angelin of Stockholm's Karolinska Institute have found through ultrasonography that in most gallstone patients, many of whom are obese, the gallbladder bile is a "sludge" that is the perfect environment for the formation and aggregation of cholesterol crystals.[10]

THE MIND'S ROLE
IN WEIGHT CONTROL

1. Realize that the prevailing food habits of society are hazardous to your health.

2. Accept full responsibility for weight control.

3. Commit yourself to a rational approach to nutrition.

4. Realize that no diet can succeed without a profound change in mental attitudes.

5. Work on overcoming personal food prejudices; for instance, learn to like good, nutritious, "friendly" foods like fish, fruit, vegetables, whole-grain breads and cereals, and brown rice.

6. Retrain yourself to *enjoy* healthful nutrition. Reject all self-indulgence as self-defeating, antihealth, and antilife.

7. Gain control over your intake of fats, sugars, and salt.

8. Learn to say no to "unfriendly" foods that endanger your health and may produce cancer, such as barbecued, grilled, burned, seared, overly browned, or smoked proteins (meat, seafood, cheese). Also avoid pickles, fermented foods, except for vinegar- or wine-cured sauerkraut and low-fat yogurt.

9. If you are dependent on soft drinks, work on breaking that dependency. Retrain yourself to enjoy purified water instead. (Keep telling yourself, "Water is the best drink in the house.")

10. Take one small step at a time. Many small steps take you a long way, even if you stumble sometimes.

11. Every successful step taken makes the next step that much easier. At the end of the road, you will find that you have changed

> your behavior,
> your attitudes,
> your values,
> your thinking, and
> your nutrition.

Surprise: You'll discover that you no longer have to worry about your weight!

In addition, sugars and highly processed starches have an effect on the body that is more subtly dangerous than the production of gallstones. The consumption of these carbohydrates increases the synthesis of the inhibitory neurotransmitter serotonin by increasing the brain's uptake of serotonin's amino acid precursor, tryptophan.[11] In effect, they can act just like tranquilizers. Not surprisingly, many obese people are carbohydrate cravers who snack all day on cakes, cookies, and candy bars in order to relax, reduce tension, and feel comfortable with the world and themselves. They use these "mind foods" just as others use "mind drugs" like Valium—and are even less aware of it than the pill poppers.

CHILDHOOD OBESITY

In the last fifteen years, obesity* has risen 54 percent among grade-school children (six- to eleven-year-olds) and 39 percent among adolescents (twelve- to seventeen-year-olds).[12]

There are several factors that might lead a child to become obese. Genetics is one: a tendency toward obesity can be passed on for several generations. A second is poverty and a lack of educational opportunity, as indicated by the fact that the rate of obesity among black preadolescents is almost double the average for all preadolescents. A third factor is the psychology of the child and the emotional climate of the home, which cause the child to eat for all the wrong reasons.

As important as either psychological, social, or genetic influences, however, are what Dr. Norman Kretschmer of the University of California at Berkeley calls the "subtle differences" in eating habits—ice cream with lunch, candy after school—that help create the unsubtle differences between normal-weight and overweight children. As Dr. William Dietz of the New England Medical Center Hospitals in Boston puts it: "Small imbalances can lead to obesity." Dr. Dietz points out that by eating only 50 extra calories per day a child can put on an extra five pounds a year,[13] which can amount to a serious weight problem just a few years down the road. The commonly held notion that a child can become overweight only by seriously overeating is not true.

Another commonly held conception—that obese children are less efficient in burning off calories—while not strictly true, is not far from the mark. Though obese children may use calories as efficiently as normal children, they do not get involved in the kinds of physical activities that burn off the most calories. What they get involved in instead is, without question, watching television. A study conducted in the mid-1970s (and repeated a few years later) found beyond any

---

* Childhood obesity has been defined by scientists from the Harvard University School of Public Health as a body-fat proportion that puts a child at or above the 85th percentile for all children his or her age. In other words, a child is considered obese if 84 percent of his or her age mates have less body fat and more lean mass. There is even a condition called *super-obesity*, fatness at or above the 95th percentile, as defined by the Harvard scientists, and a shockingly high percentage of American youngsters fall into that category.

reasonable doubt that for overweight children who are not yet obese, "television viewing is the strongest predictor of subsequent obesity."[14]

Television encourages obesity in children in other ways. The aforementioned study found that children who watch TV tend to munch on something, especially on the kinds of snacks advertised on the screen. And, as anyone who has watched children's programming can attest, those snacks are the most fattening and least nutritious available—candy bars, cookies, ice cream, flavored sugar in a hundred forms, or chips, salted nuts, cheese crackers, and the like, which combine salt with fat and are not much better than the fat-sugar combination.

Moreover, television can actually lower a child's metabolic rate. In an in-depth study of one twelve-year-old boy, Dr. Dietz found that during one hour of viewing, the boy's basal metabolic rate dropped by two hundred calories per hour. And yet, Dr. Dietz points out that while TV distracts children from exercise and encourages them to eat sugary, calorie-laden food, at the same time it sends children the message "You will be thin no matter what you eat." How? By showing them on the screen an almost uninterrupted stream of thin, healthy people.

Obesity among children is as unhealthy as obesity among adults. It is

CHANGE YOUR EATING HABITS

1. The number of Americans who skip lunch nine days out of ten has risen 63% in the last decade to include fifteen million people.
2. A common pattern among overweight women is to skip breakfast, eat a light lunch, and consume 80% of their calories in the evening. These women have lower metabolic rates than people who eat three meals a day. Unfortunately, the lower a person's metabolic rate, the greater the weight gain.
3. The Medical Research Council in England finds that a light 300-calorie lunch is the best choice for peak concentration. The most sensible idea is to pack a lunch—for instance, a whole-wheat sandwich made with breast of chicken or turkey, or the hard-boiled white of an egg, or water-packed canned tuna with spices (no mayonnaise), accompanied by a few raw vegetables (carrot sticks, cauliflower, or broccoli). For a change, prepare a container of cooked, short-grain whole rice with sliced fresh fruits. And be sure to *drink plenty of water during the day*!
4. Salad bars can be seductive and misleading. A study done on students at Mississippi State University found that those who chose meals from the salad bar consumed 43% of their calories from fat by adding extras like diced ham, egg, cheese, peanut butter, olives, croutons, bacon bits, and high-fat dressings to their salads.

estimated that twelve million American children already have a chronic or physically disabling ailment, and adolescents are the only sector of the population whose health status has not improved in the past thirty years. While this sorry state of affairs has a number of causes, obesity is certainly one of them. Excessive weight has been linked to a high incidence of upper respiratory infection and reduced lung capacity, early-onset hypertension and diabetes, orthopedic problems, and, perhaps most significantly, "psychosocial dysfunction."[15]

What can parents do to help their children overcome or avoid obesity and the diseases and emotional disturbances associated with it? The most obvious solution is to shift their children's diets away from rich, calorie-dense foods to those that are leaner and contain more fiber. In addition, parents should never use food for reward or punishment. This not only promotes a similar mind-set in later years, but during the adolescent years encourages the use of food to express oppositional tendencies.

Children must learn to eat for nourishment and pleasure, not for release from anxiety and stress (food as a drug), or to defy parental authority (food as a weapon), or even, out of sheer boredom (food to compensate for lack of intellectual stimulation or motivation).

THE PSYCHOLOGY OF OBESITY

Dr. Theodore B. Van Itallie, a noted obesity expert, points out that obese people are "lazy eaters." In one study, to which he refers, only one in twenty obese people ate any nuts offered to them when they had to make the extra effort of removing the shells. Half of the lean people in a control group ate the same amount of nuts whether they had to shell them or not. In a similar study, it was found that "moderately obese" subjects drank less of a thick milkshake when given a narrow straw (which was harder to use) than when given a normal straw. Nonobese subjects drank the same amount through both straws.[16] Both these studies seem to indicate that avoiding exertion is an important factor in the psychology of the obese.

This passivity can be traced back to childhood. Dr. Jean Mayer tells of a time/motion study of schoolchildren showing that obese girls not only spend less time exercising than nonobese girls, but expend far less energy in doing what exercises they do perform.[17] More recent studies show that the tendency toward inactivity develops after eighteen months of age, which indicates that it is a learned rather than inherited trait. In fact, Dr. Mayer's study seems to show that the inactive life-style is encouraged by parental attitudes that reward passivity.

PRINCIPLES OF PERMANENT, SUCCESSFUL WEIGHT LOSS

1. Appraise your body and weight realistically. Look at yourself nude in the mirror. Weigh yourself to face the facts. From then on, *do not* weigh yourself compulsively, and do not become obsessed by the number of pounds you lose. Permanent weight loss is a slow, steady process; it should involve no more than one or two pounds a week.

2. If you have a genetic tendency toward obesity, accept it as a fact of life. Love your body the way it is. This does not mean you cannot improve on what nature has given you. You can keep your weight within reasonable boundaries and learn to enjoy your fuller figure, which has its own attractions.

3. Design and take control of your own weight loss program. *Do not* follow popular diets blindly.

4. There are a few people who are unable to take control of their own nutrition. If you are one, it is better to join an organized program like Weight Watchers or Overeaters Anonymous (O.A.). O.A. is based on the same principles as A.A. (Alcoholics Anonymous). The group support such organizations provide is of great help in keeping you on the right path.

5. Educate yourself about food. Read labels on commercial products. Learn food preparation, even if you do not wish to cook, so you know the ingredients of the dishes you are eating. Ignorance about food, food preparation, and drink means:

   - lack of control over an important aspect of your life;
   - difficulty with weight control and health maintenance.

Once established, obesity and passivity feed one another in two vicious cycles. The first is purely psychological. Obese children are frequently embarrassed and sometimes even purposely humiliated because of their weight. The embarrassment isolates them from other children, and from group activities—if you're always the last one picked for games, you eventually stop playing. This isolation then leads to passivity, which leads to further obesity, and the cycle is complete.

The second cycle starts out to be psychological too, but ends up being physiological. In animal studies psychological stress has been shown to be "primarily mediated through an increase in the levels of endogenous opiates."[18] In other words, the body fights stress by producing endorphins, a type of opiate. But endorphins also stimulate overeating through a complicated mechanism within the nervous system. Again, stress leads to overeating and obesity, obesity produces more stress, which leads to more overeating, which leads to further obesity, and yet another cycle is complete.

While psychologists who have studied obesity agree that obese people on the whole are in no worse emotional shape than the nonobese, they have found certain personality traits that distinguish the former as a group. One is that most obese people have "an increased sensitivity to external cues and a decreased sensitivity to internal, physiological cues."[19] This means that as a group the obese are more susceptible to stress (and, as we have seen, often react by overeating) and are less aware of the signals from their own bodies (such as satiety signals—the feeling of being full).

The same study revealed that as a group the obese tend to be more concerned with physical-health problems, to have more muscular tension (evidence of stress), to be more impulsive, more eager to seek distractions (avoidance of monotony), and to be less sociable than others.

These findings confirm the results of an earlier study done with the MMPI (Minnesota Multiphasic Personality Inventory, a highly reliable personality test). Two groups of obese women scored significantly above average on the Psychopathic Deviate (PD) scale and somewhat above average on three psychopathy-related scales (Ma, Pa, and Sc). Despite their names, these scales do not indicate criminal tendencies. Rather, they show that on the whole the obese find it difficult to learn from experience and, rather than act on their own insights or better judgment, are more likely to act impulsively—"on the spur of the moment."[20] (Due allowance must be made for individual differences, of course.) These character traits may be responsible for the difficulty many obese people have in sticking with an effective weight-control program.

OBESITY—ANOTHER FORM OF SUBSTANCE DEPENDENCY?

It should be recognized at the outset that the genuinely obese are definitely different from other overweight people and must be helped differently. The truly obese can only achieve lasting weight loss not simply by cutting back on their food intake, but by changing their life-style and breaking many interconnected "automatic" behaviors that often have their roots in childhood.

Nonetheless, the first step in overcoming obesity is regulation of the diet. This means a shift from calorie-dense to calorie-lean foods with a greater emphasis on fish than meat, and exercising discretion in the consumption of sugars and processed starches. It also means the introduction of more and varied fiber into the diet. This is especially

AMERICA'S OBSESSION WITH ICE CREAM

- 98% of American families regularly eat ice cream.
- The average American eats 15 quarts of ice cream per year.
- "Super-premium" ice cream is preferred by most people; it has a butterfat content of 14%.

Conclusion: Ice cream eating is a major factor in heart disease, stroke, and diabetes in America.

important since obese people appear to be more responsive than lean individuals to the appetite-suppressing effects of bulking agents.[21] Fiber supplements may be the best way of introducing fiber into the diet. A noted group of British researchers treated several hundred obese patients and found they were more willing to take supplements than to eat fiber-rich foods.[22]

Sooner or later, however, the obese have to be reeducated (or reeducate themselves) to accept high-fiber foods—if for no other reason than that these foods take longer to eat. It takes time for the satiety signals in the gastrointestinal tract to go off—for the stomach, in effect, to tell the brain it's full. If you eat quickly, you can overeat before the satiety signals have a chance to reach the brain. Fiber-rich foods keep that from happening simply because they take longer to chew. In fact, even taking a sip of water between bites can prevent this type of overeating.

Regulation of eating habits may prove to be much more difficult than regulation of diet, but since such habits are learned, they can be unlearned. We find it useful to treat obesity, whether of the carbohydrate-craving or the fat-craving variety, as a form of substance abuse. Indeed, one study found that otherwise well-adjusted obese people, when placed on a stringent weight-control program, exhibited many of the physical and pyschological symptoms of drug withdrawal.[23] Consequently, we feel the treatment of choice is a group approach, such as Overeaters Anonymous, which is patterned on Alcoholics Anonymous. In such approaches the obese understand that they may have to take a hard look at their overall attitudes toward life, their fellow men, and themselves. In other words, overcoming food addictions may—as is true for alcoholism and drug addictions—involve a complete revision of one's philosophy of life and ethical value system.

NUTRITIONAL TREATMENT OF OBESITY

The necessary nutritional shift from the typical diet of the obese person to a more health-promoting one will, in this case, have to be even more gradual than usual. Obese people frequently just don't like, and are certainly not used to eating in any quantity, foods like whole grains, vegetables, and fruits, which form the basis of any health-promoting diet.

On the other hand, we have found that most obese individuals who are motivated to make the necessary dietary and life-style changes, but initially find it difficult to implement some of them, are quite willing to immediately go on our anti-oxidant program. This is doubly important in their case, as it is for others in the process of overcoming substance dependencies. First, it gives them the immediate sense that—no matter how many pitfalls they may encounter on the road to full recovery—they are already doing something about their condition. Second, the anti-oxidants and vitamin co-factors immediately start repairing some of the damage that years of disordered nutrition have produced. Third, the anti-oxidants are likely to have an energizing and mood-enhancing effect, which in turn can make it easier for obese people to break their addictive behavior patterns.

While being on an effective anti-oxidant program is very important for the obese in general, it is of special importance that they get plenty of lipid (fat)-soluble anti-oxidants, like vitamin E and beta-carotene. The reason is that the abundant fat deposits of the obese person are subject to progressive peroxidation—in plain language, they become more and more rancidified.[24] It is the lipid-soluble vitamins that are best able to inhibit or slow down this insidious and highly dangerous process.

We also recommend the use of fiber supplements—especially guar gums and pectins—which, in addition to some of the above-mentioned functions, also slow down gastric emptying time, a great help in controlling appetite.* In time, and as an increasingly fiber-rich general diet is adopted, the need for such supplements will of course diminish proportionally.

> "... the fat in the body comes mainly from fat..."—Dr. Elliot Danforth, Jr. *Am. J. Clin. Nutr.,* 1985; Vol. 41

* See boxes on pages 360, 362, and 363.

During the recovery time from obesity, we also recommend taking two more exotic micronutrients—l-carnitine and chromium GTF (glucose tolerance factor), which are not included in the basic Demopoulos spectrum for the simple reason that they are not required for the average, normal-weight person. However, in conditions like obesity (and diabetes) these micronutrients can be very helpful.

L-CARNITINE

Oral l-carnitine is easily absorbed and has been used therapeutically in daily doses of up to 900 milligrams without any apparent side effects.[25] Dr. Mark F. McCarthy, an orthomolecular physician, cites animal studies in which the blood glucose levels of rats given carnitine supplements declined by about 50 percent while those of unsupplemented rats averaged about 80 percent. Likewise, free fatty-acid levels in carnitine-treated rats leveled out well below those of unsupplemented controls.

CHROMIUM GTF

There appears to be a "glucostat" in the brain's satiety center (the ventromedial hypothalamus) that generates a signal proportional to the rate at which the body utilizes glucose. This signal in turn suppresses the brain's "hunger center," reducing the craving for food. (Since this mechanism seems to be insulin dependent, Dr. McCarthy feels that it may account for the inappropriate hunger and overeating that accompanies diabetes.) Chromium GTF has been found to amplify the effect of insulin on the hypothalamic satiety center[26,27] and thus, in effect, "turn down the glucostat." Indeed, some overweight people who have used chromium GTF have reported decreased appetite and a reduced craving for sweets.

DIETS, A FINAL WORD

You can find several diet books available in bookstores (and frequently on the best-seller lists) that will tell you how to lose weight quickly and painlessly. The diets presented in these books are usually health-endangering and always frustrating and self-defeating. Particularly dangerous are the high-protein diets and those based on appetite suppressors and starch blockers.

Let's look at the high-protein diets first. There is no doubt that they work. You can lose lots of weight with them all right, and lose it rapidly. Naturally, anybody who has been overweight and has such a marvelous thing happen feels as if they'd suddenly been transported into seventh heaven.

These people are so proud and happy to show you by their now far-too-big trousers or dresses what they looked like only a few weeks "before" the diet and how much slimmer and trimmer they are now "after" the diet. When we run into such people—as we invariably do in our health-educational work—we are always torn between two conflicting feelings: One is the obvious reluctance to throw a wet blanket on the flames of such happy excitement; the other is a powerful sense of professional responsibility to inform the recent escapee from obesedom that he or she has apparently only been darn lucky to have gotten away with a "cure" that's every bit as dangerous as the original disease.

Here's one instance where ignorance seems to be bliss. What the happy high-protein dieters don't know and are not told is that these diets pull calcium from the bones and produce serious nutritional deficiencies (no fruits, grains, or starchy vegetables with the more conservative, solid-food kinds of high-protein diets; no solid foods at all with the still more drastic liquid-protein diets). Furthermore, these diets have a dehydrating effect and overtax the kidneys' filtering system. They also force the body—by depriving it of dietary carbohydrates—to burn its own fatty acids for energy, thereby releasing massive amounts of acid substances (ketones and acetones). This can lead to *metabolic acidosis,* just as it does in untreated diabetes, and might result in fatal coma.

It doesn't help much that, in America, one type of high-protein diet, based on artificially flavored powders of amino acids that you have to dissolve in water, are—as the advertisements boast—available only under "medical supervision." We have personally checked into this

OBESE SENIOR CITIZENS

With advancing age, the percentage of obese individuals declines. Nonetheless, approximately 15% of white males and as many as 30% of black females are still considered obese at age eighty.

Older people must reduce calorie intake in proportion to their reduced energy output. After sixty or so, most people should reduce their food intake to about two thirds of what they consumed when younger. This does not apply to that minority of senior citizens who maintain a highly active life-style.

claim and have found that the expensive battery of laboratory tests given to prospective patients at the outset, and designed to screen out those at highest medical risk, usually don't eliminate countless borderline cases with lesser degrees of kidney, gout, and heart problems.

The trouble is that any damage caused by high-protein diets won't be noticeable till years later, so people don't make the mental connection. But, worst of all, all these crash diets, whether medically supervised or not, shift the focus from the need for a different permanent diet and life-style to one of quick results without basic changes in attitudes and dietary habits. This typically fragmented, quick-fix approach to a very complex and comprehensive problem totally leaves out the mental-emotional aspects of being truly obese, and includes no serious educational program that can give a patient the necessary information for implementing a different, health-promoting diet and sane life-style.

In addition to these hazardous medical reducing diets, there are, of course, the numerous over-the-counter slimming products. They are usually based on starch blockers (very dangerous!), or on appetite suppressants, containing either amphetamine-like compounds or caffeine (sometimes both). Although these products can be legally sold, they present obvious medical hazards, and many people come to serious grief from using them. Their worst aspect, however, is that they are also highly addictive, although not quite as much as products containing true amphetamines ("speed") and requiring a physician's prescription. (The addiction problem with medically prescribed reducing drugs has recently been brought to the attention of the American public by the case of Mrs. Michael Dukakis. She got hooked on them and had to be detoxified and weaned from them at the famous Hazelden Clinic in Minnesota.)

Finally, any crash diet is self-defeating because dieting increases the efficiency of the body's metabolism, "tuning" it to run on fewer calories. When the diet is over and calorie intake increases, the newly starvation-wizened body gains weight back at a much faster rate than before. It is the ability of the body to adapt to periodic semistarvation that makes weight loss more difficult at every new attempt and that has given rise to the term "yo-yo dieting," which can never lead to permanent weight control.

In fact, we are against all diets, period. Unfortunately, they have become a multibillion-dollar business, and people have become literally sold on them. What's more, they're generating hundreds of millions in advertising revenues annually. It is therefore unlikely that a simple, no-expense-involved formula like ours would fall on very enthusiastic ears in the mass media, lest it kill the goose laying all those golden advertising eggs. Nor are health practitioners who are profiting from the liquid diets likely to embrace a more comprehensive and educational approach to weight control, which is obviously more time-consuming and hence less profitable.

And yet the only safe and scientifically sound formula for permanent weight control is also the simplest and easiest one: Just beware of the fats in your diet and allow time for a minimum of daily exercise—even if it's just taking a nice long walk. You don't have to do or take anything else, and you can stop counting calories. Of course, this means not just avoiding saturated animal fats such as in meat, butter, and cheese, but also drastically cutting down on vegetable oils used in cooking, salad dressings, margarine, and shortenings (the only possible exception being olive and Canola [the same as Puritan] oils, see pages 442–446). It also means keeping a wary eye on hidden fats where one normally doesn't expect them, as in baked goods and many commercial food products. That's really all there is to it.

Perhaps it is all too simple to be believed—or so it would seem from the incredulous looks people give us when we explain that, on a low-fat diet, they can eat just about any amount of complex carbohydrates as they like. Don't hesitate, we tell them, to eat as much as you want of starchy vegetables like potatoes*—even sweet potatoes and yams, both, incidentally, rich in anticancer beta-carotene.

You can certainly have all the whole-grain brown rice (or even white rice, if you want) your heart desires. In America we ourselves have brown rice with vegetables, or vegetables and seafood, twice a day. On the farm in Costa Rica, we also eat a fair amount of potatoes and sweet potatoes (*camote*), because the local brown rice is of very poor quality.

You can even have all the bread you want, provided you are a little discriminating in the kinds of bread. Just stick with old-fashioned whole-grain bread, or at least eat whole (dark)-flour wheat or rye breads, which have always been favorites in Europe and which have in recent years also become increasingly available and popular in the United States.

The same is true for spaghetti, macaroni, lasagna, and other pastas. Use more of the whole wheat, spinach, or carrot types, but it's all right, within reason, also to eat the regular, processed pasta. But here again be careful with the sauce you intend to put on your pasta; a pesto sauce made with olive oil and sweet basil is fine—*if* not too much oil is used; *if* even the amount of basil is kept within reasonable limits (it has, surprisingly, some cancer-causing toxicities, along with natural anti-oxidants and vitamins); and *if* no Parmesan cheese has been added. Tomato or clam sauce is fine, too, but the popular meat sauce is a no-no with health-conscious diners.

We ourselves eat a lot of starchy foods, yet we never put on as much as an ounce of excess weight, and our cholesterol and triglyceride

---

* The trouble starts only if you put butter or sour cream on the potatoes (low-fat yogurt is all right), or butter, margarine, or other fats on your legumes and other vegetables (quick sautéing or using a little olive oil on them is okay).

levels are just perfect. We even snack between meals—usually just on fruit, like a banana, an apple, or whatever fruit is in season—but occasionally we have a couple of health-food cookies, a little fruit tart (if it's not too sweet), or a piece of angel food cake with fresh or frozen (but unsweetened) strawberry or raspberry sauce.

You can also rest assured that we follow our own advice and never count calories. We just watch *what* we eat, *not how much* we eat. People have been so brainwashed about calories that they are missing the basic principle of all sound nutrition—the selection on the one hand, of as wide a variety of health-promoting, "friendly" foods as possible, and the avoidance of risky, "unfriendly" foods on the other. As we mentioned before, this is also the only scientifically sound way of eating really well, not ever feeling frustrated, and yet having one's weight under perfect control.

How can we prove it? It is a matter of public record that Americans and Europeans today eat less but weigh more than they did a few decades ago. The answer is they used to eat more starchy foods and less fats. And since private and public transportation wasn't ubiquitous then, people used to move around more under their own steam, burning up excess calories.

If you still don't believe us, just look at the Chinese—in China, not in New York or San Francisco. You know how fond the Chinese have traditionally been of good food and how good they are at preparing it. In fact, they consume, on a pound-for-pound basis, 20 percent more calories than Americans (and, presumably, Europeans). But here's the secret: Only 15 percent of those calories come from fat (compared with 40 percent in the typical American-European diet).

A new study on obesity, conducted at the Stanford Center for Research in Disease Prevention, has just reconfirmed this.[28,29] The study leaves no doubt that the percentage of body fat we carry around depends entirely on the amount of daily calories we take in from fats. The more fat and the fewer starches and other complex carbohydrates—for example, from vegetables—we eat, the more of our total body mass will consist of fat. In this latest study too, the percentage of body fat was in no way related to the total calories consumed, or to the number and size of meals eaten.

So, let the days of yo-yo dieting and counting calories be nothing more than an unhappy memory. There is, as we hope to have shown, no good reason for any more pointless frustration. Just watch the fats and—eat what you want!*

---

* Eat what you want, but keep in mind that certain "unfriendly" foods are strictly off limits for anyone on a health-protecting diet. That includes seared, burned, barbecued, grilled, or broiled protein foods, whether meat, fish, or some other kind of seafood. Excluded also are salted and dried meat and fish, and all fermented and pickled foods, except no-fat or low-fat yogurt and sauerkraut made with vinegar rather than salt.

SOURCES

1. Texter, E. C., ed. *The Aging Gut.* New York: Masson Publishing USA, Inc. 1983.
2. Winich, M. *Nutrition and Exercise.* New York: John Wiley & Sons, 1986, p. 63.
3. Danforth, Elliot J. "Diet and obesity." *Am. J. Clin. Nutr.,* 1985; 41:1136–1145.
4. Ibid.
5. Hansen, "Serum growth hormone response to exercise in non-obese and obese normal subjects." *Scand. J. Clin. Lab. Invest.,* 1973; 31(2): 175–178.
6. Page, L. B. "Nutritional Determinants of Hypertension." In: *Nutrition and the Killer Diseases.* New York: John Wiley & Sons, 1981, p. 118.
7. Baumgartner, R. N., A. F. Roche, et al. "Fatness and fat patterns: Associations with plasma lipids and blood pressures in adults, 18 to 57 years of age." *Am. J. Epidemiol.,* 1988; 126:614–628. Also: Larsson, B., K. Svardsudd, L. Welin, et al. "Abdominal adipose tissue distribution, obesity, and risk of cardiovascular disease and death, etc." *Brit. Med. J.,* 1984; 288:1401–1404; Lapidus, L., C. Bengtsson, B. Larsson, et al. "Distribution of adipose tissue and risk of cardiovascular disease and death, etc." *Brit. Med. J.,* 1984; 289:1257–1261; Bjorntorp, P. "Obesity and risk of cardiovascular disease." *Acta Med. Scand.,* 1985; 218:145–147.
8. Hartz, A. J., D. C. Rupley, and A. A. Rimm. "The association of girth measurements with disease in 32,856 women." *Am. J. Epidemiol.,* 1984; 119:71–80.
9. Howard, Barbara V. "Obesity, Cholelithiasis, and Lipoprotein Metabolism in Man." In: *Bile Acids and Atherosclerosis,* Vol. 15. New York: Raven Press, 1986, especially p. 181.
10. Einarsson, K., and B. Angelin. "Hyperlipoproteinemia, Hipolipidemic Treatment, and Gallstone Disease." In: *Bile Acids and Atherosclerosis,* Vol. 15, p. 75.
11. Lieberman, H. R., J. J. Wurtman, and B. Chew. "Changes in mood after carbohydrate consumption among obese individuals." *Am. J. Clin. Nutr.,* 1986; 44:772–778. Also: Wurtman, J. J. "The involvement of brain serotonin in excessive carbohydrate snacking by obese carbohydrate cravers." *J. Am. Diet. Assoc.,* 1984; 84:1004–1006.
12. *Health and Nutrition Examination Surveys (HANES),* 1970–1980. National Center for Health Statistics, Washington, D.C.
13. Kolata, G. "Obese children: A growing problem." *Science,* 1986; 232:20–21.
14. Ibid., p. 20.
15. Blum, R., ed. *Chronic Illness and Disabilities in Childhood and Adolescence.* New York: Grune & Stratton, 1984. Also: Blum, R. "Contemporary threats to adolescent health in the United States." *JAMA,* 1987; 257:3390–3395.
16. Van Itallie, Th. B. "Dietary fiber and obesity." *Am. J. Clin. Nutr.,* 1987; 31:S43–S52.
17. Mayer, J. "Obesity." Chapter 22 in *Modern Nutrition in Health and Disease—Dietotherapy,* 5th ed. Robert S. Goodhart and Maurice Shils, eds. Philadelphia: Lea & Febiger, 1973, p. 634.
18. Morley, J. E., and A. S. Levine. "Stress-induced eating is mediated through endogenous opiates." *Science,* 1980; 209:1295–1260.
19. Björvell, H., G. Edman, S. Rössner, and D. Schalling. "Personality traits in a group of severely obese patients: a study of patients in two self-chosen weight reducing programs." *Internatl. J. Obesity,* 1985; 9:257–266.
20. Johnson, S. F., W. M. Swenson, and C. F. Gastineau. "Personality charac-

teristics in obesity: relation of MMPI profile and age of onset of obesity to success in weight reduction." *Am. J. Clin. Nutr.,* 1976; 29:626–632.

21. Van Itallie, op. cit., p. 46.
22. Krotiewski, M., and U. Smith. "Dietary Fiber in Obesity." In: *Nutrition: Dietary Fiber Perspectives.* A. R. Leed, ed. London: John Libbey, 1985, especially p. 63.
23. *Modern Nutrition in Health and Disease—Dietotherapy,* 5th ed., Robert S. Goodhart and Maurice Shils, eds. Philadelphia: Lea & Febiger, 1973, pp. 86–88.
24. Tappel, A. L. "Measurement of and protection from in vivo lipid peroxidation." In: *Free Radicals in Biology,* Vol. IV. W. A. Pryor, ed. pp. 2–47.
25. McCarthy, M. "Orthomolecular aids for dieting." *Med. Hypotheses,* 1982; 8:269–274.
26. Debons, A. F., et al. "Rapid effects of insulin on the hypothalamic satiety center." *Am. J. Physiol.,* 1969; 217:1117.
27. Mertz, W. "Effects and metabolism of glucose tolerance factor." *Nutr. Rev.,* 1975; 33:129.
28. Romieu, I., W. C. Willet, M. J. Stampfer, et al. "Energy intake and other determinants of relative weight." *Am. J. Clin. Nutr.,* 1988; 47:406–412.
29. Dreon, D. M., B. Frey-Hewitt, N. Ellsworth, et al. "Dietary fat: carbohydrate ratio and obesity in middle-aged men." *Am. J. Clin. Nutr.,* 1988; 47:995–1000.

CHAPTER 36

DIABETES

NUTRITIONAL TREATMENT FOR A NUTRITIONAL DISEASE

No doubt there exists a familial, inherited tendency toward diabetes—even of the adult-onset, "non-insulin–dependent" type known medically as *diabetes mellitus*. That's the one we will be talking most about in this chapter.

Did you know that even in the absence of such an inherited tendency, people can bring on diabetes in themselves? All it takes is eating large quantities of rich, fatty foods, lots of simple carbohydrates (sugars), and not getting enough exercise or having sufficient fiber in the diet. In other words, adult-onset diabetes—any inherited tendency notwithstanding—is basically a nutritional and life-style disease characteristic of an industrialized, affluent society.

There are eleven million diabetics in America: About four million of them are either on insulin or an oral blood-sugar–lowering medication like Diabinese. Leaving aside the side effects of all these medications, millions more Americans have what is called *impaired glucose tolerance,* meaning they are borderline diabetics. They too will eventually become fully diabetic unless they do something about it. And that "something" had better not just be a frantic reaching for another miracle drug but rather a total change in diet and life-style. From our point of view, it ought also to include a well-conceived program of anti-oxidants and vitamin co-factors—perhaps a regimen tailored especially for diabetics and including the trace element selenium, the mineral zinc, and, in some cases, yeast-free chromium GTF (Glucose Tolerance Factor).

Anti-oxidants are all the more important for diabetics since these patients are vulnerable to infections because their elevated blood sugar (hyperglycemia) suppresses the immune system[1] by impairing the function of lymphocytes and phagocytes. It has been shown over and over again that anti-oxidants, both dietary and direct, stimulate immune function.[2,3] In fact, this benefit lies at the very heart of anti-oxidant therapy: Just as uncontrolled free-radical activity depletes and breaks down the immune system, so do anti-oxidants and their vitamin co-factors replenish and build it up again.

We have repeatedly referred to the contributions that each of the anti-oxidants and vitamin co-factors on our program make to strengthening and protecting the immune system (see Part IV, "What Anti-oxidants and Vitamin Co-factors Can Do for You"). For instance, we have pointed out how beta-carotene traps singlet-oxygen radicals; how vitamin B_5 improves stamina and stress resistance; how vitamin B_6 is crucial for the proper functioning of the thymus and spleen, two vital immune-system organs; how vitamin E protects us from peroxides, especially in cell membranes;[4] and how vitamin C aides antibody production, stimulates the thymic cells to fight bacteria and viruses, and provides other benefits related to the immune system.

Additional vitamin A, indirectly provided on our program by supplementation with beta-carotene (pro-vitamin A), is also of particular importance. Diabetics not only pick up infections easily but also have very poor wound healing—as is the case with AIDS patients—and for the same reason: immune-system deficiency. Vitamin A has definitively been shown by researchers at the Albert Einstein College of Medicine in New York to be of help with regard to diabetic animals.[5] It is not yet known whether these benefits also apply to humans, but indications are that they may. In any case, people on our anti-oxidant program are known to have excellent vitamin A levels because the body's constant feedback mechanism replenishes these levels from beta-carotene. Diabetics should be among the primary beneficiaries.

Other researchers have pointed out that in diabetic blood vessel disease, a not infrequent complication of advanced diabetes, vitamin E's anti-oxidant action prevents further damage to the inner lining of blood vessels caused by all the circulating lipid peroxides. And diabetic interference with the proper metabolism of an important amino acid, tryptophan, can be reversed by pyridoxine (vitamin B_6).[6]

We have touched on all these findings to show why we feel so strongly that micronutrient supplementation is of critical importance for diabetics. It goes without saying that it is equally important for the *prevention* of diabetes.

This brings us to an important point: Many people who are already clinically diabetic don't even know that they are. They may have all the initial symptoms—increased thirst, increased frequency of urination, increased hunger, weight gain or, more rarely, weight loss—but, being used to them, consider them normal. It's only when the symptoms become more troubling—blurred vision, minor cuts that become infected and refuse to heal, weakness, and lack of energy—that they finally seek medical advice.

As with their cholesterol and triglyceride levels, most people have no idea what their blood sugar levels are. Given the high cost of laboratory fees, it's not surprising that even the more health-conscious often hesitate to have all these tests done on a regular basis. Others simply don't realize their importance, especially since so many physicians don't order them unless a particular problem is suspected.

The older we are, the more important taking responsibility for our own health becomes. With age (say, after forty), the delicate "thermostats" that keep complicated physiological mechanisms like the hormone system in perfect balance start functioning less efficiently. We have reason to believe that much of this deterioration is preventable with diet, exercise, and anti-oxidants.

One of the first systems to go out of sync is the one regulating blood sugar and insulin levels. That's why so many older people "suddenly" become diabetic, or start showing abnormal glucose-tolerance curves on lab tests. As one researcher has put it so well, "even 'normal' aging is slightly diabetic." For insulin-dependent diabetics, premature aging is even more pronounced. Immune-system biomarkers may show their bodies to be ten to fifteen years older than their chronological age.

How *does* our built-in "glucose control system" work? As you probably know, the amount of glucose in the bloodstream is controlled by insulin, a hormone produced in the pancreas. When there is too much glucose in the blood, the pancreas puts additional insulin into circulation. The insulin then gets rid of extra blood sugar (glucose) in one of several ways: by pushing it (almost literally) into the cells to be burned for energy; by stimulating the liver to convert it to *glycogen* and store it for future use; or by helping convert it to fat for storage in adipose tissue.

There is also a mechanism for putting more glucose into circulation if levels fall too low, but that need not concern us here. What *is* important to know is that overweight diabetics have fewer than the normal number of insulin receptors on the surface membranes of their cells. Since these receptors are needed to get the glucose into the cells, glucose levels rise in the bloodstream and in the urine without the cells absorbing much of it. This condition is called *intracellular glucose deficiency;* from a cell's point of view, it could be described as starvation in the midst of plenty.

Under these conditions, the sugar-starved cells start breaking down fats for energy and eventually even breaking down tissue protein. That's the reason for the progressive weight loss in a certain type of uncontrolled diabetes.

Another thing that can happen when cells are not getting their regular glucose meals—and are using fats and proteins for energy instead—is that acid particles called *ketone bodies* may accumulate, throwing off the acid-alkaline balance and producing a highly dangerous state of hyper-acidity called *acidosis.** The telltale sign for this stage of advanced, untreated diabetes is the characteristic acetone breath of the diabetic, who may not be aware of having entered this critical phase.

There is no reason why anyone on our anti-oxidant program and the right kind of diet should ever develop severe, adult-onset diabetes. Nor is there any reason why those who are already diabetic to a certain degree should not be able to control the condition by following our dietary recommendations and a slightly modified Demopoulos spectrum of anti-oxidants, if it is done under competent medical supervision.

THE RIGHT DIET FOR DIABETICS

Until fairly recently, the recommended diets for diabetics were of the high-protein, moderate-fat, low-carbohydrate type, despite the fact that it had been known in the United States since the mid-1950s (and published in the *Journal of the American Medical Association*) that diabetes is best controlled with a diet high in carbohydrates (vegetables and grains) and low in fats.[7] These findings were confirmed by other studies from India and Japan.[8–11]

The facts should have been obvious long before then. At the end of World War I, statistics clearly showed that from 1914 to 1918 the mortality rates for diabetes had fallen sharply in Germany and only slightly less in England, the countries most affected by food rationing. The most pronounced food shortages were fats, meats, and sugars, all known today to contribute to diabetes.

The same thing happened during World War II, but still nobody made the connection. Nor did anyone note the significance of another wartime dietary change: In peacetime only 70 percent of milled flour

---

* This precipitous drop in pH, together with the acute dehydration as a result of the loss of body fluids and the creation of a parallel disequilibrium in the sodium-potassium balance, sometimes leads to fatal coma in untreated diabetes.

had been used as refined flour; the other 30 percent of high-fiber "midlings" was diverted for cattle feed. During all the recent wars, however, 80 to 90 percent of a milled product was marked for human consumption. This resulted in a pronounced increase in the fiber content in bread and other flour products like pasta (spaghetti, macaroni, lasagna). In Denmark, high-fiber barley meal and rye meal further raised the fiber content of flour products during the Second World War. As a consequence, the diet of some European countries during the war years was considerably lower in fats and much higher than usual in fiber. Both fat and fiber content of the diet are, as we will show, crucial factors in the cause and control of diabetes.

Somehow all this information was not utilized for almost half a century. Even so, it was not a physician who first applied these findings experimentally to the control of diabetes but a medical layman, the self-taught nutrition expert Nathan Pritikin.

In the 1970s Pritikin began trying the high-complex-carbohydrate, low-fat, high-fiber diet on people with adult-onset diabetes that he had found earlier to be so successful with heart patients. As Pritikin suspected, it worked equally well with them—after one month on his diet, almost half of these patients no longer needed insulin or other glucose-control medication. His results encouraged Dr. James Anderson, a research-oriented physician and chief of endocrinology at the University of Kentucky Medical Center, to conduct parallel experiments with diabetic patients at his treatment center. Dr. Anderson's patients experienced the same improvement.[12,13]

Dr. Anderson succeeded in persuading the American Diabetes Association to change its dietary recommendations from the traditional high-protein diet to one based on complex carbohydrates that are slowly digested and do not raise plasma glucose levels: cereal grains, potatoes, brown rice, legumes (beans, peas, lentils), and other starchy vegetables. This low-fat, starch-based diet works, because it does not make any sudden demand on glucose tolerance and therefore does not provoke the insulin reaction some physicians had feared.

Dr. Anderson's successes with diabetics led Dr. Kelly West, at the time a professor of medicine at the University of Oklahoma College of Medicine, to state during the McGovern Senate hearings* that Dr. Anderson's work was "one of the most exciting diabetes research programs going on in the world today" and found that "2.5 million [or 62 percent] of the 4 million known adult diabetics now on drugs could be safely freed from them entirely using this diet."[14]

Nobody has as yet, to our knowledge, systematically used supple-

---

* Hearings Before the Select Committee on Nutrition and Human Needs of the United States Senate, Ninety-third Congress, 1973, U. S. Government Printing Office, Washington, 1973.

mental anti-oxidants, as in the Demopoulos spectrum, to accompany a low-glycemic, high-complex-carbohydrate diet for diabetics. Much less has anyone employed special micronutrients like dl-carnitine and chromium GTF (glucose tolerance factor), to further support such a comprehensive regimen. And yet our subjective impressions from a few individual cases that we had a chance to observe firsthand, lead us to believe that mainstream medicine may soon be treating diabetes mellitus along these lines.

Still another important factor does have to be taken into consideration—the mind-body connection, which has been shown to be so important in diabetes. There are studies that clearly show the destabilizing effect of stressful life experiences on diabetes management. The cultivation of a tranquil frame of mind is therefore of paramount importance to the diabetic. There are even indications from other studies that emotional stress can be the initiating factor in over half of all diabetic cases.

Therefore, a truly comprehensive approach to the management of diabetes should—in addition to the high-complex-carbohydrate, low-fat diet, supported by a broad-spectrum anti-oxidant regimen—include the deliberate cultivation of as serene a life-style as possible, relaxation training, and semitherapeutic educational group sessions.[15]

SOURCES

1. Baumgartner, W. A. "Antioxidants, cancer, and the immune response." In: *Trace Metals in Health and Disease,* N. Kharesh, ed. New York: Raven Press, 1979.
2. Beisel, W. R. "Single nutrients and immunity." *Am. J. Clin. Nutr.,* 1982; 35 (Suppl.):417–468.
3. Lubin, B., and L. J. Machlin. "Vitamin E: biochemical, hematological, and clinical aspects." *Ann. N.Y. Acad. Sci.,* 393:437–451. Also: Corwin, L. M., and R. K. Gordon. "Vitamin E and immune regulation." In: Kharesh, op. cit.
4. Tappel, A. L. "Measurement of and protection from in vivo lipid peroxidation." In: *Free Radicals in Biology,* Vol. IV, W. A. Pryor, ed. 1980, 2–47.
5. *Ann. Surg.,* 1981, 194:42; as discussed in: Hendler, S. *The Complete Guide to Antioxidant Nutrients.* New York: Simon & Schuster, A Fireside Book, 1984, p. 87. Also: Dice, J. F., and C. W. Daniel. "The hypoglycemic effect of ascorbic acid in a juvenile-onset diabetic." *Internatl. Res. Comm.,* 1973; 1:41.
6. "Vitamin B_6 and Diabetes." *Lancet,* 1976; 788–789.
7. Daughaday, W. H. "Dietary treatment of adults with diabetes mellitus." *JAMA,* 1955; 859–862.
8. Singh, I. "Low-fat diet and therapeutic doses of insulin in diabetes mellitus." *Lancet,* 1955; 1:422–425.
9. Patel, J. C., et al. "High carbohydrate diet in the treatment of diabetes mellitus." *Diabetologia,* 1969; 5:243–247.
10. Bush, O. B., and T. Moriwaki. "Diet and diabetes mellitus. In: *Diabetes in*

the Tropics, J. C. Patel and N. G. Talwalkar, eds. Bombay: Diabetic Assoc. of India, 1966, pp. 533–539.

11. Tsuju, S., and M. Wada. "Diabetes Mellitus in Asia." Excerpts Medica Foundations. Amsterdam, 1970.

12. Kiehm, G., J. W. Anderson, and K. Ward. "Beneficial effects of a high carbohydrate, high fiber diet on hyperglycemic diabetic men." Am. J. Clin. Nutr., 1976; 29:895–899.

13. Anderson, J. W., and K. Ward. "Long-term effects of high-carbohydrate, high-fiber diets on glucose and lipid metabolism. A preliminary report on patients with diabetes." Diabetes Care, 1978; 1:77.

14. Pritikin, Nathan. The Pritikin Permanent Weight-Loss Manual. New York: Bantam Books, 1981, p. 48.

15. Advances (International Issue), 1986; 3(4):86–87.

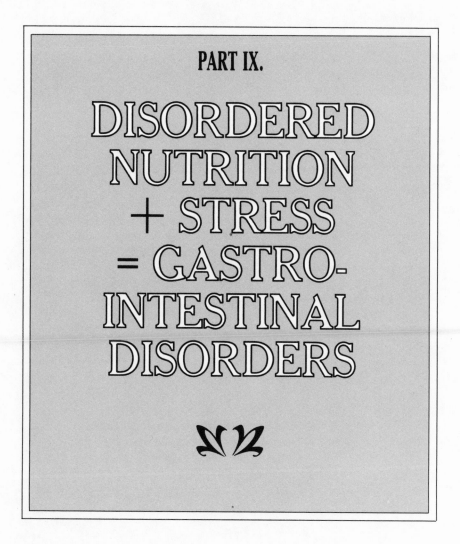

PART IX.

DISORDERED NUTRITION + STRESS = GASTRO- INTESTINAL DISORDERS

12 If you watch American TV these days, you may have seen the following commercial: A foreign couple with their children, a teenage boy and girl, obviously on a visit to the United States, appear on the screen. Smiling broadly, they tell us breathlessly, "We love America—hot dogs, fried chicken, pizza!" But the TV commercial is not selling hot dogs, fried chicken, or pizza, it is selling Kaopectate for diarrhea.

Forget the fact that those foods are more likely to give you constipation than diarrhea. The commercial illustrates the findings of a 1983 survey, conducted by Louis Harris and Associates in consultation with the National Digestive Diseases Advisory Board, that Americans know less about the nature and symptoms of digestive diseases than they do about cancer, heart disease, and a number of other major ills.

At the same time, the survey revealed that Americans do not consider digestive diseases to be very serious health problems, an astonishing fact. The reality is that up to 100 million Americans suffer from recurrent digestive problems to the tune of $50 billion per year in lost work, lost wages, and medical costs. That translates into something like 200,000 workers missing work every day because of digestive difficulties. And more Americans are hospitalized for diseases and disorders of the digestive tract than for any other group of disorders.[1]

The TV commercial we cited reflects the enormous popularity of mostly over-the-counter remedies for the symptoms of gastrointestinal disorders: a market of $1.2 billion per year and growing at a steady 10 percent rate,[2] thanks to a never-ending stream of high-powered advertisements. Most of it is wasted money because none of these medications can correct the underlying cause of the digestive problems—disordered nutrition and lack of regular exercise.

Curiously, people on the Demopoulos spectrum of anti-oxidants and vitamin co-factors do not seem to suffer from these common gastrointestinal problems, even though their diet may be far from ideal. We do not encourage dietary recklessness but, as said before, the full spectrum of micronutrients makes a certain degree of dietary permissiveness acceptable. Some of these micronutrients—for instance,

265

vitamin C and vitamin B_5—make it nearly impossible to develop constipation, even if a diet is somewhat lacking in fiber (hence little chance for getting hemorrhoids, varicose veins, or hiatal hernia).

Also, the anti-oxidants of our program detoxify the colon on a daily basis. Glutathione, for example, binds to toxic heavy metals, like mercury and lead, in the intestines, as does calcium for bile acids. At the same time, lipid-soluble anti-oxidants like vitamin E and beta-carotene (pro-vitamin A) scavenge free radicals. Thus they contribute, with other anti-oxidants, to preventing cancer of the colon or rectum, of which constipation, hermorrhoids, spastic colon, and ulcers are often the mundane forerunners. Moreover, the calming and mood-enhancing effect of the full anti-oxidant and vitamin spectrum is beneficial to all those gastrointestinal disorders caused by psychological tensions and reactions to environmental stress, such as peptic ulcer, spastic colon, and irritable bowel syndrome (IBS).

As there is a progression from the most banal digestive problems, like heartburn and hemorrhoids, to the more serious and most debilitating diseases, we shall discuss them in that sequence. We do not say, however, that ulcers, for example, are less serious than diverticulitis, or vice versa. Any of these conditions can turn nasty and all deserve medical, nutritional, and possibly psychological attention well beyond the "Band-Aid" types of popular remedies, like antacids and hemorrhoid suppositories.

SOURCES

1. Vahoney, G. V., and D. Kritchewsky, eds. *Dietary Fiber, Basic and Clinical Aspects.* New York: Plenum Press, 1986, p. 61.
2. Consumer Expenditure Study, 1983.

CHAPTER 37

HEARTBURN

12 Here's another TV commercial: A middle-aged couple are sitting in their living room. It is evening, past dinnertime. Suddenly the husband complains with a pained expression about heartburn. The wife says she's got the cure for that in the medicine cabinet. "Will it work fast enough?" asks the husband, by now in even more distress. "How fast can you get to the bathroom?" replies the wife. The husband gets up, presumably to take the "double-strength" antacid. When he comes back, the wife asks how he's feeling. All smiles, he says, "Want to go for a banana split?"

Antacid ads like this one on television and in all of the major magazines pay off because, next to constipation, heartburn is the most common digestive complaint in America and Europe, especially in Germany and the Scandinavian countries. And Japan is fast catching up with this sort of "progress" in the Western world. Huge amounts of antacids are bought and swallowed by millions of heartburn sufferers every day.

The irony of it is that while nine out of ten people suffering from recurrent heartburn regularly use antacids, only the 10 to 20 percent of cases in which the heartburn is due to peptic ulcers might find some relief from these remedies. As for all the other antacid swallowers, any relief they might receive would strictly be due to placebo effect.[1]

Actually, many antacids used for heartburn have *too much* acid-binding capacity (the much advertised "double-strength" variety!) and medical specialists say they "are probably not as safe as we have believed."[2] (These antacids can cause constipation, bind to other drugs, and be absorbed into the bloodstream.)

Dr. Gerhard Dotevall, a noted specialist in gastrointestinal diseases, explains that most heartburn sufferers who have all the symptoms of an acid stomach actually have perfectly normal or even subnormal stomach-acidity levels. He therefore advises that instead of popping more antacids, these people take a good, hard look at the internal and extrenal stressors in their lives and try doing something about them.[3]

Life-style factors may have a lot to do with developing heartburn. Smoking and alcohol increase stomach acidity, can cause the stomach contents to be propelled upward into the esophagus (as in belching), and produce the typical burning sensation of heartburn. Gulping down a meal instead of taking the time to enjoy it unhurriedly can cause heartburn. And, of course, eating greasy, hard-to-digest foods doesn't help matters either.

Since up to 30 percent of heartburn cases eventually turn into ulcer conditions or IBS, using antacids for heartburn is mostly illusionary. A good first step toward a real cure would be a low-fat diet with emphasis on seafood and lean poultry (rather than meat) and plenty of lightly cooked (steamed or sautéed but *not* raw) vegetables and noncitrus fruits. We also suggest cutting out or at least drastically cutting down on coffee and alcohol—not to mention smoking.

As far as taking anti-oxidants and vitamins is concerned, we have found no negative indications with most gastrointestinal conditions, even in cases of nonbleeding ulcers and Crohn's disease. However, such patients should start with a very low dose at first, increase it slowly to the level that feels most comfortable, and consult with their doctor.

SOURCES

1. Nörrelund, N., et al. "Ukarakteristisk hyspepsi i almen praksis: En konstrollert undersökelse med et antacidum (Aluminox)." *Ugeskr. Laeger.,* 1980; 142:1750.
2. Dotevall, G. *Stress and Common Gastrointestinal Disorders.* New York: Praeger Publications, 1985, p. 53.
3. Ibid., p. 52.

CHAPTER 38

PEPTIC ULCER DISEASE

Although the term "peptic ulcer disease" includes both duodenal and gastric ulcers, 75 to 80 percent of all peptic ulcers are of the duodenal type, that is, they occur in the duodenum, the first portion of the small intestine that is directly connected to the stomach and which seems almost to be part of the stomach.

Recent medical research has revealed certain genetic markers in people who are at risk of developing duodenal ulcers. These individuals seem to have more acid-secreting cells in their stomach walls than others.[1] However, a predisposition to any medical problem does not doom one to developing the disease. With ulcers, for instance, a high-fiber diet has definitely been shown to be "of value in the prevention of duodenal ulceration."[2]

With both duodenal and gastric ulcers, as in the case of heartburn (dyspepsia), other life-style factors apart from diet enter into the picture decisively. Smoking is one. Ulcers develop in part because of excess hydrochloric acid secretion, and nicotine prevents the proper neutralization of gastric acid by inhibiting pancreatic secretion.[3] Alcohol, *especially wine*, contributes to the formation of gastric ulcers, and prevents their healing, not so much by increasing stomach acidity directly as by damaging the mucosal lining of the stomach wall.[4] Since both alcohol consumption and smoking often increase during particularly stressful periods, a vicious circle occurs, with stress—a major psychosocial factor in peptic ulcer disease—leading to increased smoking and alcohol consumption, which in turn promotes peptic ulcers.

A number of common over-the-counter drugs such as salycilates (aspirin and salycilic-acid–containing medications for arthritis, etc.) are highly destructive to the stomach's mucosal lining and can lead to inflammation, bleeding, and ulceration.[5] Corticosteroids, commonly prescribed for rheumatoid arthritis and other painful inflammatory conditions, also produce gastric ulcers by irritating the stomach's mucosal lining, as Dr. Barbara B. Walker of the University of Michigan at Ann Arbor points out. These and other substances contribute to the formation of ulcers either by increasing stomach acidity directly (as in duodenal ulcers), or (as in gastric ulcers) by attacking the stomach's mucous lining, which is meant to buffer the acid and serve as a barrier between the stomach contents and the stomach wall.

Actually, the decisive factors in peptic ulcer disease are neither smoking, nor alcohol consumption, nor the above-mentioned drugs, but *diet* and *stress*. These two factors, above all others, can initiate ulcers and prevent their healing.

First, a few words about diet: (1) Peptic ulcer disease is extremely rare if not altogether absent in people who eat a high-fiber, low-fat diet. (2) The traditional low-fiber ulcer diet, especially one that includes milk and milk products to "neutralize stomach acidity," is dead wrong. Milk products may in fact *increase* acidity.[6]

Recently, some scientists have come to think that drinking milk can prevent stomach ulcers because of the protective E2-type prostaglandins that it contains. There is no doubt that prostaglandins do indeed have such an effect. For instance, Cytotec, a prostaglandin-containing ulcer remedy, is based on that principle. But while the pure prostaglandin E2 in Cytotec does help in curing ulcers, drinking milk does not. In fact, milk might interfere with the healing of duodenal ulcers in patients taking the anti-ulcer drug Tagamet (cimetidine).

Nevertheless, some people still suggest that milk should be drunk for ulcer prevention. We, on the other hand, feel that it is *not* a good idea to drink milk for this or any other purpose because of the allergenic and, in all probability, atherogenic *casein* and whey proteins it contains (see our chapter, "The Truth About Milk and Cheese," pages 327–334).

It has been found that patients who had been cured of duodenal ulcers had fewer relapses when they ate bread made from unrefined (whole-grain) flour rather than white flour. The same was true for people who ate whole brown rice rather than polished white rice.[7] One researcher attributed this to the fact that whole-grain bread and other high-fiber foods require more chewing, thus producing more saliva, which in turn leads to lower stomach acidity and reduced bile output. Another researcher cites evidence that wheat bran and certain water-soluble (gel-forming) types of fiber (like gums from legumes and pectins from fruit) protect against the formation of ulcers.[8,9] The delayed gastric emptying time produced by a high-fiber diet may be still another protective factor but it should be soft, soluble fiber.[10]

But apart from proper diet, the ulcer patient must learn to relax, not to take things so hard, and strive for tranquillity and serenity in his or her life. As far as peptic ulcers are concerned, what goes on in the head is every bit as important as what happens in the stomach.

We know today that ulcer patients are no more neurotic than anyone else. However, studies suggest they may differ with regard to certain personality traits. For instance, as a group, they appear to be more shy and introverted and somewhat lacking in dominance,[11] quite the opposite from high-powered Type-A individuals, often associated with developing ulcers.[12]

Do ulcer patients have more hostility toward others or do they turn more aggression against themselves, as some psychotherapists have suggested? Definitely not, at least as far as can be determined from any reliable psychological tests.[13] Nor do they appear to be any more obsessive/compulsive than the rest of us.[14] They do seem, however, to be more anxious, tending toward depression and pessimism.[15]

Anxiety-management training with ulcer patients has proven effective, both for the cure and the prevention of recurrences. One training program included the exploration and correction of "irrational, mistaken, anxiety-producing beliefs"[16] held by the patients. At the same time, they were encouraged to try to substitute more positive attitudes for habitual negative thoughts. This reeducation program also included progressive muscle-relaxation training and coping techniques for situational stress. Patients were given some assertiveness training to correct irrational beliefs, such as the notion that asserting oneself means blowing up and maybe losing a job or destroying a marriage.

This practical, semitherapeutic, but basically educational approach proved successful beyond expectations. A follow-up study, almost four years later, comparing patients who had participated in the program with those who had not showed there were many fewer recurrences among the training program participants (only one of nine in the program group, as compared with five of eight in the no-program group).

SOURCES

1. Whitehead, W. E., and M. M. Schuster, eds. *Psychophysiological Gastrointestinal Disorders.* New York: Academic Press, 1985, pp. 97–98.
2. Rydning, A., and A. Berstad. "Fiber and Duodenal Ulcer." In: *Psychophysiology of the Gastrointestinal Tract,* R. Hölzl and W. E. Whitehead, eds. New York: Plenum Press, 1983, p. 408.
3. Walker B. B. "Treating Stomach Disorders." In: Hölzl and Whitehead, op. cit., p. 213.
4. Whitehead and Schuster, op. cit., p. 106.
5. Woodbury, D. M. "Analgesic-antipyretics, anti-inflammatory agents and inhibitors of uric acid synthesis." In: *The Pharmacological Basis of Therapeutics,* L. Goodman and E. Gilman, eds. London: Macmillan, 1970.
6. Walker, op. cit., p. 221.

7. Malhotra, S. L. "A comparison of unrefined wheat and rice diets in the management of duodenal ulcer." *Postgrad. Med. J.,* 1978; 54:6–9.
8. Tovey, F. I., and M. Tunstall. "Duodenal ulcer in black populations in Africa south of the Sahara." *Gut,* 1975; 16:564–576.
9. Tovey, F. I. "Peptic ulcer in India and Bangladesh." *Gut,* 1979; 20:329–347.
10. Lawaetz, O., et al. "Effect of pectin on gastric emptying and gut hormone release in the dumping syndrome." *Scand. J. Gastroenterol.,* 1983; 18:327–336.
11. Christodoulo, G. N., et al. "Primary peptic ulcer in childhood." *Acta Psychiatrica Scand.,* 1977; 56:215–222.
12. Nolen, W. A. *Healing: A Doctor in Search of a Miracle.* New York: Random House, 1974, p. 280.
13. Lyketsos, G., et al. "Psychological characteristics of hypertensive and ulcer patients." *J. Psychosom. Res.,* 1982; 26:255–262.
14. Bellini, M., and M. Tansella. "Obsessional scores and subjective general psychiatric complaints of patients with duodenal ulcer of ulcerative colitis." *Psychol. Med.,* 1976; 6:461–467.
15. Whitehead and Schuster, op. cit., p. 107.
16. Brooks, G. R., and F. C. Richardson. "Emotional skills training: A treatment program for duodenal ulcer." *Behavior Therapy,* 1980; 11:198–207; as reported in Whitehead and Schuster, op. cit., pp. 111–112.

CHAPTER 39

CONSTIPATION

While watching television in the United States, it is not unusual to have three or more different laxative commercials during a single program. One of the commercials targets women, telling them that they suffer "three times more often" from constipation than men. Another shows a woman looking sad and listless—obviously because of "irregularity." Somebody tells her about a certain "gentle" laxative and—presto! she's all smiles and bursting with new energy. The next laxative commercial may target men, showing an unhappy, constipated gentleman who is told that all he needs to make him feel better is "MOM" (no, not his mother, but Milk of Magnesia!). So it goes, from the early morning news to the late late show.

The relentless ad campaign is paying off: Americans spend an incredible $450 million on laxatives a year, plus another $115 million on hemorrhoid preparations, which are really part of the same problem (there wouldn't be any hemorrhoids, and consequently no need for remedies, if there were no constipation producing the hemorrhoids).

To call a spade a spade, all that money for laxatives and hemorrhoid medications is essentially wasted—not to mention the lost working hours and loss of income, which runs into not millions but billions of dollars. It is a waste because nobody who eats a high-fiber diet and drinks six to eight tall glasses of water a day ever gets constipated or develops hemorrhoids. It's as simple as that. On the other hand, people on the traditional low-fiber diet generally consumed in America and most of Europe have a shockingly high incidence of constipation: between one in six among people under sixty, and one in three among people over sixty.[1]

The medical profession cannot even agree on what constitutes a "normal bowel movement," or where constipation begins. The rule of

CONSTIPATION BEGONE

Taking 1 teaspoon of pure crystalline vitamin C (ascorbic acid) upon arising and washing it down with water usually results in a bowel movement within a half hour.

In addition to eating more high-fiber foods, some wheat bran and a supplement containing a mixture of water-soluble, gel-forming fiber, like pectin, guar gum, and xanthan, could be introduced. (See Appendix C, List of Suppliers, page 596.)

Vitamin B_5 also helps in overcoming constipation by inducing peristaltic movement. The Demopoulos spectrum provides from 720 to 1,000 milligrams of B_5, depending on whether it is taken three or five times a day. But you can take 500 milligrams of additional B_5 with half a teaspoon of vitamin C in the morning.

None of these nutrients has any dangerous or habit-forming side effects, contrary to what is generally true for commercial laxatives. In fact, these vitamins (C and B_5) offer many other health benefits in addition to overcoming constipation.

thumb for the medical practitioner seems to be that constipation exists only if someone passes fewer than three stools a week (fewer than five in men). If a patient does better than that—say, has five stools per week—and still complains of constipation, many physicians will tell the patient that that's perfectly normal and not to worry about it, it's just "imaginary constipation."

Prevailing medical opinion on what constitutes proper elimination is based on national statistics. The only trouble is that our statistical averages reflect the low-fiber diet of the majority of people in our country, and ought not to be equated with a healthy and desirable standard. The result of current medical attitudes is that frequently those patients who insist on what some physicians have derisively referred to as "the magical number of one stool per day," are not taken seriously.[2] The fact that many people have a bowel movement only every second or third day, or even less often, does of course pull down the statistical averages, but it cannot mean that these are ideal conditions and that people should settle for them.

Physicians blame media advertising for giving people the idea that a daily bowel movement is a desirable and healthy goal. We, on the other hand, blame such advertising for encouraging dependency on cathartics and laxatives. Once such dependency is established, the smooth muscles of the intestines lose their ability to propel the waste materials forward by themselves. Even in such chronic cases, however, a change to a high-fiber diet often results in gradually reestablishing normal bowel function.

In addition to the wrong, low-fiber diets most people consume, inadequate water intake and lack of regular exercise are the other most decisive factors leading to a sluggish digestive system. The physical form of yoga, called *hatha yoga,* is especially effective if the intestinal musculature has lost its tone. This ancient type of total exercise works better than any other method we are aware of, not only on the skeletal muscles, but also on the internal organs, including the entire digestive system, from the stomach to the intestines. We should add, however, that just taking regular daily walks is also of considerable benefit in toning up a sluggish colon.

Atonic constipation—that is, constipation due to lack of internal muscle tone—is particularly critical in young children and the aged. In these two groups, constipation is usually associated with stool impaction. Among the elderly in nursing homes, this is a major problem. The low-fiber diet generally served in these institutions, the almost total neglect of specially designed exercise, and the routine dispensing of laxatives, enemas, and suppositories only tend to worsen and perpetuate the problem. "Soft," soluble fiber is easy to eat.

With the elderly especially, another complication often enters into the picture: When there are hard, impacted stools, painful anal fissures (cracks or breaks in the sensitive skin around the anus) may often occur. This sets up another vicious cycle: The painful fissures lead to a fear of evacuation and painful spasms of the anal sphincter, which leads in turn to further constipation and impaction. Every effort must obviously be made to prevent such a sequence from happening. If it has already occurred, no method should be left untried to break into the vicious cycle, including deep-relaxation techniques or hypnotic suggestions.

Aside from these special constipation problems of the very young and very old, most cases of bowel irregularity in the general population are primarily caused by disordered nutrition. Anthropologists tell us that constipation is practically unheard of in so-called primitive societies that consume a high-fiber diet.[3-6] Consequently, the diseases that are the direct result of bowel irregularity—diverticulitis, varicose veins, hemorrhoids, and even appendicitis—are virtually unknown among these people.[7,8]

Next to faulty nutrition, certain psychological and life-style factors are involved in the amazingly high incidence of inadequate bowel function in industrialized societies. Psychoanalysts insist that there is such a thing as an "anal-retentive" personality. Be that as it may, faulty toilet training in early childhood—especially an obsessional preoccupation on the part of the parents with the child's bowel functions—can lead to making evacuation a battleground between child and parents. If so, the stage is set for later gastrointestinal problems. Of course, the same is true if parents fail to establish a regular time for the child to defecate.

It is a generally agreed-upon psychological fact that constipation is one of the main physical (somatic) manifestations of depression. Chronic nervous strain and worry also predispose the individual toward constipation,[9] compounded by faulty life-style patterns. In societies like ours, where haste is considered a virtue, people frequently neglect the urge to move their bowels. This is just another instance of people being out of touch with their own bodies. The result is that over time the normal responses to rectal filling become dulled and chronic constipation is established.[10]

SOURCES

1. Cooke, W. T. "Laxative Abuse." In: *Clinics in Gastroenterology,* Vol. 6, No. 3, September 1977. London: W. B. Saunders & Company, Ltd., p. 659.
2. See, for instance: Schuster, M. M. "Constipation and Anorectal Disorders." In: *Clinics in Gastroenterology.*
3. Walker, A.R.P. "Effect of crude fiber intake on transit time and the absorption of nutrients in South African Negro schoolchildren." *Am. J. Clin. Nutr.,* 1975; 28:1161.
4. Antonis, A., and I. Behrson. "The influence of diet on fecal lipids in South African white and Bantu prisoners." *Am. J. Clin. Nutr.,* 1962; 11:142.
5. Burkitt, D. "Some diseases characteristic of modern Western civilization." *Brit. Med. J.,* 1973; 1:274.
6. Kelsey, J. "A review of research on effects of fiber intake in man." *Am. J. Clin. Nutr.,* 1973; 1:274.
7. Walker, A. "Appendicitis, fiber intake, and bowel behavior in ethnic groups in South Africa." *Postgrad. Med. J.,* 1973; 49:243.
8. Richardson, J. "Varicose veins in tropical Africa." *Lancet,* 1977; 1:791.
9. Krause, M. V., and L. K. Mahan. *Food, Nutrition, and Diet Therapy.* London: W. B. Saunders & Company, Ltd., 1984, p. 440.
10. Schroder, J. S. "Constipation." In: Hersh, G. *Digestive Diseases.* Boston: Butterworth Publishers, 1983.

CHAPTER 40

HIGH COLONIC IRRIGATION

We cannot close a comprehensive discussion like this on constipation without mentioning high-colonic irrigation, a practice that
is very popular in this country, especially, alas, among many of the
most health-conscious segments of the population. Many people simply
feel that they should have themselves periodically "cleaned out" or
"detoxified" through high colonics, regardless of whether they are
regular in their bowel habits or not.

The problem with this practice (and we have had personal experience
with it) is that (1) it cannot do what it is supposed to do, and (2) it is
rather dangerous on several counts. In the first place, the healthy colon
"detoxifies" itself automatically by one or more bowel movements per
day. Furthermore, an atonic colon, one which has lost its muscle tone,
is not going to get it back by high-colonic irrigation. Nor will a spastic
colon relax and become nonspastic by being filled up with water. Quite
the contrary: The injection of water under pressure into the colon can
cause more rather than fewer spasms.

The condition for which high colonics are most frequently used—
diverticular disease—is not corrected by high irrigation of the colon
either. We shall say more about diverticulosis presently; for now let us
just categorically state that the little pouches (diverticuli) that have
been blown out by internal pressure and straining during defecation
are *not* being cleaned out by any kind of enema, no matter how high up
it reaches. Dr. Demopoulos has examined colons with varying degrees

of diverticular disease and assures us that no irrigation can ever clean out the impacted material in the diverticuli.

Finally, high colonics are—notwithstanding the good intentions of their practitioners and beliefs of their aficionados—potentially health-endangering in that such prolonged enemas are literally waterlogging the entire gut. While the surface lining of the colon is highly permeable for liquids, passing large amounts of water through it for extended periods of time, as in high colonics, is almost like injecting water directly into one's veins.*

Furthermore, this water is literally leaching all the mineral salts, or electrolytes—potassium, calcium, magnesium, sodium bicarbonates, and chlorides—right out of the gut. If all the potassium were removed that way, it could actually lead to instant cardiac arrest. For that reason, colonicists try to replace the electrolytes (mineral salts in a watery solution, capable of conducting body electricity) by adding them to the water. It's like first taking the vitamins out of flour by refining it, and then putting them back in at the end. Besides, it is very difficult to get the right amounts of all these mineral salts into the solution, and few and far between are the colonicists—though there are some—who are taking this matter sufficiently seriously.

What the colonicist cannot replace, however, are the lipid-soluble vitamins in the colon, namely vitamins A, E, and K. Also, high colonics are bound to upset the bacterial flora of the gut, which is not a good thing either.

Finally, in these times of AIDS, high colonics are especially risky. Even if disposable, sterile nozzles are used, there is still a possibility of infection, because it is very difficult to sterilize equipment between patients. All in all, we strongly advise against the use of high colonics, even if you think they are making you "feel better." (Any good feelings or postcolonic highs are in all probability due to the release of the gut's own opiate endorphins under this traumatic challenge.)

---

* Medical practice takes advantage of this absorptive capacity of the gut in cases of severe dehydration resulting from prolonged diarrhea and vomiting, as in cholera and other life-threatening diarrhetic diseases. The technique consists of administering copious enemas of water and mineral salts in solution to the patient. Recently, a new oral rehydration technique has been shown to be equally effective in saving the lives of over 90 percent of cholera victims.

CHAPTER 41

DIVERTICULOSIS

12 Year after year of eating a fiber-deficient diet eventually catches up with us. One of the conditions that often develops is diverticular disease (diverticulosis). It simply means that the high pressure from small, hard stools gradually results in blowing out many little pouches (diverticuli) in the colon walls. These little pouches will of course fill up with fecal matter, which becomes trapped in them, hardens, and often leads to inflammation, a condition called *diverticulitis.*

Diverticulitis can be extremely painful, the pain being usually most severe in the lower left part of the abdomen. In a worst-case scenario, the diverticuli can start to bleed and form infectious abscesses, similar to acute appendicitis, and may require an emergency operation.

Even without the presence of an acute inflammation, the chronic pain can be so intolerable that sufferers from diverticular disease often elect to have an operation in the hope of getting rid of their distress. Unfortunately, such relief is possible only if the diverticuli are located only in one segment of the colon, which can be removed. In many cases, however, the diverticuli are present throughout the whole length of the colon. In that case, surgery is of necessity limited to a particular area in the colon where blockage or abscess may exist.

On the other hand, there is hope even for sufferers from chronic and long-standing diverticular disease merely by changing to a high-fiber diet. Diet cannot of course do away with the diverticuli, once the damage has been done. But in many cases it can bring sufficient pain relief to enable one to live with the condition.

Given the serious distress that often accompanies diverticulitis, it is a depressing thought that it is so widespread in our affluent society— affecting 5 percent of people by age fifty, 35 percent at age sixty, and 50 to 70 percent at age eighty.

279

The reason diverticulosis occurs more frequently with advancing age is that the resistance of the intestinal wall to internal pressure declines over the years.[1] This is especially true for the distal part of the colon, closer to the rectum than to the upper part of the gut. This is probably due to cross-linking of connective tissue, which gives us hope that free-radical–quenching anti-oxidants in the gut, especially lipid-soluble ones like vitamin E and beta-carotene, may offer some protection!

It is still more depressing to think that despite age-related changes in the connective tissue of the colon, diverticulosis could in most cases be avoided altogether. As one scientist, Dr. John M. Talbot of the Life Sciences Research Office, Bethesda, Maryland, put it: "Although the etiology of colonic diverticulosis is unknown, a popular hypothesis suggests it is associated with prolonged intestinal transit time, low stool weight, and increased intra-colonic pressures, which are in turn all related to inadequate intake of dietary fiber."[2] Dr. Talbot agrees that dietary changes involving increased fiber consumption by patients with symptomatic diverticulosis "seem to have alleviated symptoms in a majority of reported clinical studies."

There is also a *spastic* type of diverticulosis. In this case, spastic contractions in the arc-shaped ridges of the colon muscle can shut off small segments of the gut and thereby build up enormous pressures. This can result in similar blowouts in these segments of the colon wall, that is, create diverticuli.[3] Nervous tension and reactions to psychosocial stressors and adverse life events may well play an important role in this type of diverticulosis, as they do in spastic colon and irritable bowel syndrome, which we will discuss later on.

SOURCES

1. Almy, T. P., and D. A. Howell. "Diverticular disease of the colon." *N. Eng. J. Med.,* 1980; 302:324.
2. Talbot, J. M. "Role of dietary fiber in diverticular disease and colon cancer." *Fed. Proc.,* July 1981; 40(9):2339.
3. Painter, N. S., et al. "Segmentation and the localization of intraluminal pressures in the human colon, with special reference to the pathogenesis of colonic diverticula." *Gastroenterology,* 1965; 49:169.

CHAPTER 42

HEMORRHOIDS AND VARICOSE VEINS

Hemorrhoids and varicose veins are really not disease entities in and of themselves, but by-products of bowel irregularity (constipation). Chronic pressure from hard stools in the colon, and especially straining at stool, can cause enlarged, dilated veins of the rectal and anal passages. These hemorrhoids can be either internal, between the outer and inner anal sphincters, or external, protruding through the outer anal sphincter. The latter condition—more so than internal hemorrhoids, which are often asymptomatic and therefore often unrecognized—is what causes the distressing itching, burning, and pain we usually associate with hemorroids.[1]

The public has been conditioned, mainly by advertising, to treat this condition merely by relieving the symptoms. This is done by the insertion of suppositories and/or creams containing an analgesic to dull the pain. Some hemorrhoid preparations also contain an ingredient that temporarily shrinks the veins, giving the illusion of a "cure."

A television commercial featuring one popular brand of hemorrhoid suppositories has a man say, "My mother-in-law recommended I use [brand name] for my hemorrhoids. Why should I listen to my mother-in-law? Because my mother-in-law is also a doctor. . . . Doctors know best!" Not a word about changing one's diet, using more fiber, exercising, and drinking more water, as doctors do, in fact, advise.

Internal pressure on the colon and straining during evacuation causes the veins on the legs to become enlarged and bulge out, resulting in varicose veins. This condition is usually treated with benign neglect and regarded as no more than one of those regrettable but unavoidable signs of aging. The connection with low-fiber diet and constipation is not made by the public, even though medical research has considered a direct link between nutrition and varicose veins an established fact for many years.[2]

SOURCES

1. Thompson, W. "The nature of hemorrhoids." *Brit. J. Surg.,* 1975; 62:542.
2. Burkitt, D. "Varicose veins, deep vein thrombosis, and hemorrhoids: epidemiology and suggested aetiology." *Brit. Med. J.,* 1972; 2:556.

CHAPTER 43

HIATAL HERNIA

V2 This disease is another frequent result of wrong nutrition and consequent bowel irregularity. The condition is related to heartburn and shares with it the symptoms of indigestion; in fact, very often what passes as heartburn is in reality a manifestation of hiatal hernia.

Hiatal hernia occurs when the stomach is pushed up higher against the large membrane, or diaphragm, that separates the abdominal and chest cavities. When that happens, part of the stomach can get pushed through the enlarged opening in the diaphragm, creating a pouch on the chest side not unlike any other hernia. Usually the part of the stomach that is involved is the one that joins the esophagus (our food-intake tube). It is also the part that contains a ring of muscle fiber (sphincter) in its wall which, when contracted, closes the entrance to the stomach, thus preventing the stomach contents from being regurgitated. Under conditions of hiatal hernia, however, this sphincter can no longer work very well as a one-way "check valve" to keep the stomach contents out of the esophagus (hence the belching and burning sensations that may be mistaken for simple indigestion or heartburn). The stomach gets pushed up against the diaphragm because of pressure from straining during evacuation (and, more rarely, from extra pressure during pregnancy). A diet rich in several types of fiber* from vegetables, fruits, legumes (beans, lentils, garbanzos), and whole grains (brown rice and whole-wheat or whole-rye bread) will effectively prevent this problem.

---

* If a naturally fiber-rich diet is unavailable, we recommend taking a fiber supplement, such as Twinlab's B-Slim fiber wafers or gel-forming fiber drink, Guar Aid, or any one of the fiber supplements offered by Vitamin Research Products. (See Appendix C, List of Suppliers, page 596.)

Irritable bowel syndrome (IBS), or "spastic colon," is as common as it is mysterious. Although gastrointestinal specialists disagree as to whether it is psychological or physiological in origin, IBS takes its daily toll on millions of people and should therefore be considered seriously. As one expert put it, "Irritable bowel syndrome causes almost as much absence from work in the United States as the common cold."[1]

The symptoms are all too familiar: distension of the lower abdomen, accompanied by generalized tenderness or pain in the entire region; discomfort from gas and abnormal motility in the gut; and diarrhea or loose stools with mucus, often alternating with constipation (IBS patients characteristically complain of incomplete bowel movements, probably because the spasticity of the colon prevents more complete evacuation).

Stress of any kind or simply eating a snack or meal may trigger any or all of the symptoms. Researchers have found that the most prominent psychological factors are career worries in men and family worries in women.[2] And IBS patients show "excessive concerns about minor, routine problems" (Whitehead and Schuster);[3] in other words, they overreact to the problems of everyday living, which is another way of saying they have not developed adequate coping skills.

The validity of this theory was dramatically confirmed by a Swedish study in which one group of IBS patients received only medical and dietary treatment, while another group was treated comprehensively, including not only the same diet and medication but also psychological counseling. When the patients in both groups were checked three months later, those getting the psychological help were doing considerably better than those on the medical-dietary program alone. Another check at fifteen months showed the comprehensively treated group maintaining improvement while the others' condition gradually deteriorated.[4]

We don't mean that people who suffer from IBS are a group of hopeless neurotics. On the contrary, there is a physiological basis for their distress.[5] It's only that the nature of these physical mechanisms is not clear in our present state of knowledge.

There is also a history of childhood deprivation and traumatic life events with a majority of IBS sufferers. In one study, 61 percent reported having had unsatisfactory relationships with their parents and 31 percent indicated they had lost a parent through death, divorce, or separation before the age of fifteen.[6] It is quite understandable, against this sort of background, that IBS patients, as a group, have been found to be more anxious and depressed than others.[7]

Two additional factors seem to play an important role in IBS:

(1) People who develop it often report having received gifts of "treat" foods in childhood when ill. For some of these people, the only way of getting parental attention at all, especially in large families, was when they were sick.[8] Under those conditions, being sick has so many rewards of its own that a lifelong "illness pattern" often develops. Such a pattern may of course express itself in many forms; for instance, as asthma and other allergenic diseases, or as hypertension, and so forth. However, IBS seems to be a very frequent way of expressing this conditioned tendency toward illness. (IBS patients, in fact, report more colds and other physical problems, see a doctor more often, and are hospitalized more frequently.)

(2) IBS patients often develop a conditioned, Pavlovian kind of response to *anticipation* of potentially stressful situations. People who find their jobs particularly stressful may, for instance, develop irritable colon symptoms, such as diarrhea, while getting dressed for work in the morning.[9]

Whatever its medical causes, this debilitating syndrome is best attacked comprehensively: correcting disordered nutrition, exploring psychological factors, introducing a full anti-oxidant program, and making relaxation techniques (Benson's deep muscle-relaxation response, autogenic training, meditation) a part of the patient's daily routine. There is even an encouraging preliminary report about the use of hypnosis as part of such a program. In a recent study, fifteen IBS sufferers experienced "substantial to complete relief" with only seven hypnotic sessions over a period of three months. Better yet, these patients remained symptom-free afterward with once-a-month hypnotic follow-up sessions.[10]

HOW THE MIND AFFECTS THE GUT

We have seen that gastrointestinal disorders are to a very large extent the inevitable results of disordered nutrition and an unhealthy life-style. We have also seen that they all have a contributing and often decisive psychosomatic aspect—that is, they depend on both physical (organic) and mental-emotional factors.

There can be little doubt that stressful life events and emotional tensions can precipitate or aggravate a wide array of gastrointestinal problems, all the way from a relatively harmless "upset stomach" to spastic colon and bleeding ulcers. Today there is ample evidence that chronic anxiety is quite sufficient to produce serious and sometimes life-threatening stomach lesions or ulcerative colitis.

If chronic anxiety is part of the picture, the individual has to learn how to distinguish between realistic and unrealistic (imagined or exaggerated) fears, and learn how to deal with both. Realistic fears are easier to handle. They demand immediate action along the fight-or-flight continuum and thereby become "self-resolving." They only turn into neurotic conflict if neither one kind of action nor the other is taken.

If, on the other hand, our fears are of the imagined or unrealistic kind—and that is usually the case—we must come to understand how we created them in the first place. Once we start analyzing our fears from that point of view, it quickly becomes clear that they are produced by making the mistake of looking back at a fearful experience that happened in the past and then expecting something similar to occur now or in the future. What we have to do is shift our focus from the past and the future to what is actually happening in the here and now. It's easier said than done—but it *must* be done.

The person suffering from a gastrointestinal problem also has to understand that very often these kinds of illnesses feed on a reward mechanism that keeps them going. Sometimes the rewards are quite obvious—like the disability check coming in every month. More often, though, the rewards or "secondary gains" of the illness are much more obscure and the patient is not even aware of them.

For instance, the illness may have as a hidden agenda such unconscious motives as a wish to dominate the environment, get out of working (or, sometimes in the case of women, avoid having sex), take revenge ("punish" someone), get relief from guilt because of one's own pain and suffering, avoid feeling the full brunt of a severe underlying depression, and so on. We can see why such motives are unconscious—they are either not socially acceptable, or would be unacceptable to the patient's own ethical value system.

Quite often, gastrointestinal illnesses are associated with too hectic a life-style. We have repeatedly found this to be the case (especially with irritable bowel syndrome) in people who are overly ambitious. If that is so—and only the patient himself or herself can know—it's time to reevaluate one's value system and life goals. The question to ask oneself is: How realistic and sensible is it to sacrifice physical health and peace of mind for future rewards one might not even be able to enjoy because of chronic ill health, or for goals that, once attained, might turn out to be meaningless?

NUTRITIONAL TIPS

We cannot of course be specific in nutritional recommendations for all the gastrointestinal diseases. Some foods that are good for peptic ulcers may do nothing for a spastic colon or hemorrhoids.

Nevertheless, there are some nutritional pointers that we can give that might be equally helpful if not for all, then at least for several gastrointestinal problems. One recommendation could be to eat lightly cooked hot cereal in the morning, rather than uncooked cold cereal. Our own choice is either steel-cut or rolled oats because they are easily digested, are nonallergenic, and have a cholesterol-lowering effect. However, it is especially important for people with peptic ulcers to avoid putting milk on their cereal because milk stimulates the production of gastric acid in some instances.

Some ulcer patients have a hard time believing us when we advise them to avoid drinking milk. They often tell us, for example, that if they drink a glass of ice-cold milk when they have ulcer pains, they get immediate relief. That may very well be true. But the relief is probably due more to the cooling effect than to the milk itself. A little later on, they might experience worse pain than before because of the increase in gastric acid (milk even interferes with some anti-ulcer drugs, such as Tagamet and others that have cimetidine as the active ingredient).

As earlier mentioned, there has recently been much fanfare about the apparently protective effects of the E2-type prostaglandins in milk fat, which are said to prevent ulcers in laboratory rats that were subjected to stress.[11] Presumably the effect on humans would be identical, since the anti-ulcer drug Cytotec is based on the same prostaglandins.

However, prostaglandins are a mixed blessing; they are essential for many physiological functions, but they can also cause hormonal imbalances or become highly immunosuppressive.[12] Besides, milk is already one of the principal sources of saturated animal fats in the American diet. Also, quite aside from the fact that many people cannot digest milk because they lack the enzyme lactase to break down the

WATER IS STILL THE BEST DRINK IN THE HOUSE

You only get 1½ teaspoons of juice if you drink an 8-oz. soft drink with 10% real fruit juice. However, the drink is likely to contain a lot of sugar or a sugar substitute, caffeine, salt (sodium chloride), and artificial coloring.

Learn to like water, but use a charcoal water filter to purify your drinking water at home (see Appendix C, page 596). You'll find that even coffee (if you drink it) or tea will taste better without the chlorine taste of tap water.

milk sugar lactose, others are highly allergic to the milk proteins casein and lactoglobulin. We would therefore say that habitually drinking milk and eating milk products to prevent ulcers is not a wise strategy.

There is only one possible exception to this general rule: yogurt. For one thing, it is often better tolerated than unfermented milk, and it does seem to have a calming effect on a hypermotile colon; at least it appears to counteract diarrhea.[13,14] Most likely this action is due to the beneficial *L. acidophilus* and *L. bulgaricus* bacteria of the yogurt overwhelming the pathogenic bacteria, like *Salmonella* or *Shigella,* that are causing the diarrhea.[15] However, there may be other contributing factors, as there is some doubt whether these bacteria can actually survive and grow in the small intestine where this would have to take place to do any good.[16]

If you eat yogurt at all, we suggest a low-fat type, even though it would provide less of the alleged benefits ascribed to the higher concentration of prostaglandins in whole milk. For people who cannot normally tolerate even mildly hot, spicy foods, having yogurt with Indian-style vegetable curry, for example, would provide a welcome change in taste and not deprive them of any possible medicinal benefits of the hot spices (see pages 428–430).

We have one general recommendation: While small amounts of lean meat are permissible—though not recommended—on our regular diet, we urge anyone with a gastrointestinal problem to stay strictly away from meat, at least till the condition is well under control. The same is true for cheeses, which are not on our diet at any time because of their high fat content and the free radicals they generate (the fats in cheeses are definitely peroxidized).

On the other hand, if you do eat chicken, a lean chicken soup with brown rice would be fine for an upset stomach or diarrhea (rice is antidiarrhetic). It would also be all right to eat egg whites with perhaps one egg yolk, together with brown rice, mashed potatoes, matzoh or matzoh balls, or a low-fat type of bread.

As far as vegetables are concerned, in the case of acute gastrointestinal distress, they ought not to be eaten raw but steamed or cooked (preferably by microwave) and puréed. We have found that for this particular purpose, salads are best tolerated when they have been liquified in the blender—perhaps adding a little low-fat yogurt instead of an oil-based salad dressing—and drunk rather than eaten.

For high stomach acidity or ulcers, there is now enough scientific evidence to recommend eating cooked *unripe* (green) plantains.[17,18] Plantains contain a compound (carbenoxalone) that seems to act by stimulating the cells of the stomach lining to produce more of the protective mucus that prevents the enzyme pepsin and the stomach acids from attacking the stomach walls. In Costa Rica, where green plantains commonly replace potatoes, which are more expensive, they have always been considered medicinal in folk medicine, especially for an acid stomach.*

Some fruits, like apples and pears, should be eaten cooked and puréed, if you have acute gastrointestinal distress. Papaya is excellent because it contains a digestive enzyme, papain, as well as a high concentration of beta-carotene. All these fruits can be eaten with rice, preferably brown rice, as a complete meal; not just for weight control, but for better nutrient balance.

SOURCES

1. Almy, T. P. "Digestive disease as a national problem. II. A white paper by the American Gastroenterological Association." *Gastroenterology,* 1967; 53:821.
2. Chaudhary, N. A., and S. C. Truelove. "The irritable colon syndrome: A study of the clinical features, predisposing causes, and prognosis in 130 cases." *Quarterly J. Med.,* 1962; 31:307–323.
3. For an excellent review of studies on IBS, see: *Psychophysiological Gastrointestinal Disorders,* W. Whitehead and M. Schuster, eds. New York: Academic Press, 1985.
4. Padus, E., et al., eds. *Your Emotions and Your Health.* Emmaus, Pa.: Rodale Press, 1986, pp. 612–613.
5. Whitehead and Schuster, op. cit., pp. 179–209.
6. Hislop, I. G. "Psychological significance of the irritable bowel syndrome." *Gut,* 1971; 12:452–457.
7. Latimer, P., et al. "Colonic motor and myoelectrical activity: A comparative study of normal subjects, psychoneurotic patients, and patients with irritable bowel syndrome." *Gastroenterology,* 1981; 80:883–901.

* We have found that cooking plantains as dumplings seems to raise the concentration of the beneficial carbenoxalone; at least, they are definitely more tasty that way. You can adapt any dumpling recipe and use your favorite spices, rosemary, thyme, fenugreek, to flavor them.

8. Hill, O. W., and L. Blendis. "Physical and psychological evaluation or 'non-organic' abdominal pain." *Gut,* 1967; 8:221–229.
9. Whitehead and Schuster, op. cit., p. 200.
10. Reported in: Padus et al., op. cit., p. 613.
11. Materia, A., et al. "Prostaglandins in commercial milk preparations: their effect in the prevention of stress-induced gastric ulcer." *Arch. Surg.,* 1984; 119:290–292.
12. Richards, J. M., J. M. Bedford, and S. S. Witkin. "Rectal insemination modifies immune response in rabbits." *Science,* 1984; 224:390.
13. Niv, M., et al. "Yogurt in the treatment of infantile diarrhea." *Clin. Pediatr.,* 1963; 2:407–411.
14. Shahani, K. M., et al. "Properties of and prospects for cultured dairy foods." *Soc. Appl. Bacteriol. Sympt. Serv.,* 1983; 11:257–269.
15. Alm, L. "Survival rate of salmonella and shigella in fermented milk products with and without added human gastric juice: an in vitro study." *Prog. Food. Nutr. Sci.,* 1983; 7(3–4):19–28.
16. Robins-Browne, R. "The fate of ingested lactobacilli in the proximal small intestine." *Am. J. Clin. Nutr.,* 1981; 34:514.
17. Best, R., et al. "The anti-ulcerogenic activity of the unripe plantain banana (musa species)." *Brit. J. Pharmacol.,* 1984; 82:107–116.
18. Goel, R. K., et al. "Anti-ulcerogenic effect of banana powder (musa sapientum var. paradisiaca) and its effect on mucosal resistance." *J. Ethno-Pharmacol.,* 1986; 18:33–44.

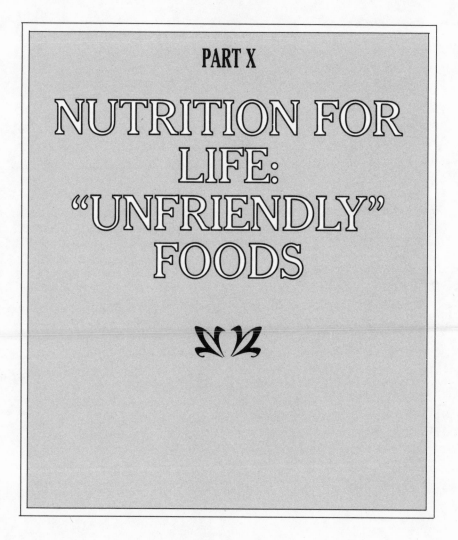

PART X

NUTRITION FOR LIFE: "UNFRIENDLY" FOODS

CHAPTER 45

SALT

THE SPICE OF THE SHORT LIFE

12 Salt is a killer. It has always been a killer. But it is only in this century that salt has begun to lose some of its historic associations with sanctity.

Salt is not only mankind's most widely used condiment, it has also served since earliest times as a preservative for meat and fish. Thanks to this use, salt came to symbolize purity and incorruptibility. A pre-Christian custom of rubbing salt on newborns to ward off evil spirits survives to this day in certain European countries in Catholic baptismal rites where a few grains of salt are put into the baby's mouth.

Salt was a scarce and precious commodity in antiquity. The ancient Greeks placed so high a value on it that a good slave was said to be worth his weight in salt, not in gold. And in Rome soldiers were often paid in *sal,* from which our words "salt" and "salary" are derived. Salt disks, in fact, were still in use as currency in Ethiopia until the early nineteen-hundreds.

A European art dealer of our acquaintance told us that as a young man, around the turn of the century, he used to travel to Japan via the then brand-new Siberian railroad to buy woodblock prints. Our friend always took along a few pounds of salt because at train stops in Mongolia, tribal horsemen would come to the stations to barter jewelry for this wonderful seasoning.

At about the same time, a German clergyman, farmer, and naturopath named Sebastian Kneipp began to suspect that salt might have some properties that were not so wonderful. In his autobiography,

Kneipp—who became known as Germany's greatest practical healer—says that he used to follow the time-honored "common wisdom" of giving his cows plenty of salt with their fodder. Eventually Kneipp noticed that the more salt he gave them, the sooner his cows died. When he stopped supplementing their feed with salt, they not only lived longer but also stopped giving birth to premature calves.

Kneipp anticipated, by over half a century, recent scientific findings that salt does indeed shorten life span. In one of many carefully conducted experiments, rats fed a 5.6 percent sodium chloride (table salt) diet had a median life span several months shorter than that of rats on a regular low-sodium diet. If the salt content of their diet was raised to 8.4 percent, there was an eight-month difference between the median rate of survival in the high-salt rats and the low-salt control rats. Translated into human terms, this difference represents a shocking thirty-two-year shortening of one's life span![1]

There is rare consensus among scientists on the health-threatening effects of the average American-European high-salt diet. Most nutritionists agree that the amounts of salt Americans eat "are clearly 10 to 20 times the minimal level compatible with health in humans."[2]

Genetic predispositions toward hypertension notwithstanding, the relationship between a high dietary intake of salt and hypertension (high blood pressure) is clearly established. Comparisons of salt use in different populations demonstrate this fact. In northern Japan, for example, an astounding 38 percent of the population suffers from high blood pressure. This figure becomes less incredible when you consider that the Japanese eat 28 grams (about six teaspoons) of salt per day.

Eskimos who have moved into towns and adopted the life-styles and food habits of their fellow urban dwellers soon exhibit the same rate of hypertension as the American norm. Alaskan natives who have not moved to the towns but have continued their traditional hunting/fishing life-style—and who usually do not add salt to their food—rarely have high blood pressure.[3] As for the average American, he or she ingests between 10 and 15 grams of salt per day, including the 3 grams or so naturally present in foods. Conservatively speaking, that amount is at least two or three times the amount we ought to be taking in. No wonder then that roughly 25 percent of American adults have high blood pressure, a main contributing factor in stroke, heart attack, and kidney failure.[4]

Among American blacks, high blood pressure (75 percent for males) is more the norm than the exception. Not only do blacks have an even higher salt intake than American whites, but recent research indicates that they have a genetic predisposition toward high blood pressure.

Dr. Clarence Grim found that identical black twins have nearly identical blood pressures. This and other factors support his hypothesis that hypertension among blacks is an inherited characteristic. Dr. Grim

"It is well known to any of us who work in the field of human nutrition that our theoretical knowledge of the biochemistry and physiology of nutrition far outstrips the application of this knowledge to the welfare of human beings."—C. M. Young, K. Berresford, and N. S. Moore, "Psychologic Factors in Weight Control," in: *Nutrition and Behavior,* Nutrition Symposium Series No. 14, J. Brozek, guest ed., 1957.

believes that thousands of years ago, blacks developed an ability to retain salt as a survival mechanism to compensate for the loss of salt due to sweating in a hot environment. Such an ability would be an advantage in a torrid climate where salt is scarce. But in an industrial society, where salt is plentiful and high intake customary, this evolutionary "advantage" is part of the reason why American blacks are two to three times as likely to have a stroke as whites, and seventeen times more likely to suffer kidney failure because of hypertension.[5]

The delicate balance in our bodies between sodium and potassium is adversely affected by excessive salt consumption. When we raise our sodium intake, we automatically deplete the potassium level in our tissues. This starts a vicious circle because potassium neutralizes some of the toxic effects of excess sodium intake.[6]

If salt is added in processing vegetables, their sodium-potassium balance is turned upside down. For example, 3.5 ounces (100 grams) of fresh raw peas contain 380 milligrams of potassium and only 2 milligrams of sodium. By canning peas and adding salt in the process, manufacturers increase the sodium content to 236 milligrams, and, at the same time, decrease the potassium content to 160 milligrams. The same applies to other common vegetables like broccoli, spinach, and Brussels sprouts.

A sodium-potassium imbalance in the human body can cause edema, an abnormal accumulation of fluid in the intercellular spaces of the body. Edema deprives the tissues of oxygen and can cause a number of other health problems, such as congestive heart failure.

Despite general agreement in the scientific community about the risks of too much salt in the diet, some authorities argue that a reduction in salt intake is "neither appropriate nor necessary" unless a person is already suffering from high blood pressure. The argument runs that hypertension is not so much a disease in and of itself as a symptom of a more general pathological condition caused by many factors, high salt intake being only one of them. Just restricting salt intake cannot therefore make much of a difference, they say.

There is some logic to this argument: Researchers at the Cornell

University School of Medicine have discovered that when a high-salt diet is teamed with a low-calcium diet, as it often is, the two together produce more hypertension than a high-salt diet alone.[7] Obviously, other factors like plaque-clogged arteries or chronic emotional tension also raise blood pressure.

The conclusion we draw from all this, however, is as follows: We must not only restrict our salt intake, but also do something about any other contributing influences to hypertension, including other dietary and subtler, psychological ones.

Another argument says, "If you are concerned about the quality of life, you don't want to impair it needlessly by restricting salt for everyone." For the life of us, we cannot see where salty foods fit into the quality-of-life equation. "Quality of life" must have a very different meaning to those who talk about it in terms of how much salt to put on food than it has to us.

When all's said and done, it still doesn't make sense to wait to go easy on the salt shaker until you develop high blood pressure or something worse. It is much easier to prevent something than to correct it later on. Furthermore, it is now known that an infant is much more susceptible to the effects of sodium chloride (table salt) than an adult. By the same token, salt restriction in later life is less effective in lowering hypertension in someone who had a high-salt diet during childhood. In other words, the later in life intervention begins, the less reversible the hypertension.[8]

Controlling hypertension by salt restriction is made even more difficult by the fact that there is a powerful *habituating* aspect to salt, one that mimics the dynamics of addiction. In the first place, salt is strictly an acquired taste. If you put a few grains on the tongue of a baby not yet used to salt, the baby will make a face and spit it out. But most babies, once accustomed to the taste, soon develop a "craving" for salt. This is why, until quite recently, baby food manufacturers added salt as well as sugar to prepared baby foods. Fortunately, this practice has come to a halt in this country, though its legacy is generations of Americans who can no longer appreciate food that is not highly oversalted by any reasonable standards.

One researcher observed that people on low-salt diets (no more than 250 milligrams per day) immediately noticed if as little as one extra gram were added to their food. In contrast, people eating 10 to 20 grams per day didn't notice if as much as 5 to 10 grams were added.[9] This same researcher noted that there was absolutely no correlation between the amount of salt people thought they were consuming and the amount they were actually consuming.[10] In other words, people build up a taste tolerance for salt that makes everything not oversalted seem bland and tasteless. We can confirm this from our own experi-

CUTTING BACK ON SALT

Flavor food as much as possible in the preparation before serving it. Use red (cayenne) or black pepper and a little salt but also herbal spices to make foods more palatable without using too much salt.

Keep a variety of hot and herbal spices, as well as low-sodium tamari, soya, or regular oyster sauce, on the table, but use them sparingly because these sauces also contain varying amounts of salt.

"Light salt"—a mixture of sodium chloride and potassium iodine—can replace regular salt if the taste is acceptable.

Cayenne pepper and hot chili flakes, as well as black pepper, help cut down on salt. However, while these spices add flavor and have medicinal qualities, they also contain toxic and potentially carcinogenic compounds. So, don't overdo a good thing!

Grated Swiss Sap Sago cheese (made from skim milk and herbal spices) can be used over pasta dishes (spaghetti, macaroni, lasagna) as a substitute for Parmesan cheese (it's too high in fat, plus it has a free-radical problem, due to its peroxidized fatty acids).

ence: Eberhard, who grew up in Germany where even greater amounts of salt are consumed than in America, could not really enjoy food that didn't taste like the Salten Sea. He thinks overcoming his "salt habit" was more of a struggle than it was to stop drinking wine—something we both thought we'd never be able to give up.

Many years ago, during experimental work with young schizophrenics that involved our sharing the same home environment, we noticed that practically all of these youngsters added large amounts of salt to their food, making our own high intake seem trivial by comparison. And almost all of them ate a lot of sweets, used large quantities of sugar in tea and coffee, and were practically addicted to sweet caffeine-loaded soda pop. It is our impression that even "normal" people who consume large amounts of salt also consume large amounts of sugar, and vice versa. One could make a fair case for this by looking at the population of Latin America, where very high consumptions of salt and sugar go hand in hand. In Latin America it is quite common to put three or four teaspoons of sugar in even a small cup of coffee. And, when we first settled in Costa Rica, we were shocked to see people salting pineapple and melon or unripe mangoes.

All this demonstrates to what a large extent food habits, particularly the use of salt and sugar, are affected by sheer habit and cultural conditioning. But just as any food habit is learned or conditioned, it can also be unlearned or unconditioned.

Once we understood all the dangers of excessive salt intake, we immediately cut down on it drastically. And it was only after kicking the salt habit that we discovered what many foods actually tasted like. All the subtle tastes that had been masked by the salt started coming into their own. Rather than feeling deprived of salt, we realized that salt had been depriving us.

Fortunately, once you have worked your way out of the salt mines, it's almost impossible to become a salt slave again. Salty food will be about as appealing to you as stale cigarette smoke is to an ex-smoker. We now sometimes have trouble eating, much less enjoying, some foods in restaurants or at the homes of friends, because they taste like pure salt to us. This change in taste perception is quite common among people who have become used to a low-sodium diet, and has now been amply confirmed by scientific studies.[11,12]

Finally, if we may pass on a little trick on how to cut down on salt without hardly noticing it: Just prepare meals with as little salt as possible but without food being totally bland. Then, at the table, everybody can add enough salt to make it more palatable to each individual taste. You'll find, to your surprise, as did the researchers of a study at the University of Pennsylvania, that because salt was put right on top of the food, much less of it was used at the table than the amount that would normally be used in the cooking.[13]

That's a neat way of weaning yourself and your family from excessive use. As time goes on, you'll see that the salt shaker will be used less and less, till you can retire it from the table altogether.

Still another way of cutting down on salt intake is to use soya, tamari, or oyster sauce, both in food preparation and at the table. These sauces, too, have quite a bit of salt in them (except Kikkoman's special "low sodium" soya sauce), but the other strong flavors in them result in less overall salt consumption. Use all the sauces sparingly, because they contain not only salt, but also small amounts of the mutagenic compound methylglyoxal (also present in roasted coffee beans).

UPDATE   The most recent research seems to indicate that only sodium chloride (table salt) is involved in raising blood pressure. Other types of sodium—sodium bicarbonate (baking soda), sodium citrate (in citrus fruits), sodium tartrate (in wine), sodium ascorbate (a form of vitamin C), or a type of sodium used in soft drinks (hence the name "soda")—are probably innocent as far as causing hypertension is concerned.[14]

It is also true, as some medical researchers keep pointing out, that so far no large-scale human studies have demonstrated conclusively that even table salt alone, without other contributing factors, is able to produce hypertension. Our concern, however, is not only with the hypertensive effect of salt. In animal studies sodium chloride has also been shown to enhance a certain type of stomach cancer (anaplastic adenocarcinoma).[15] Laboratory rats that drink water with 1 percent table salt routinely develop hypertension.

SOURCES

1. *Toxicants Occurring Naturally in Foods,* 2nd ed. Washington, D.C.: National Research Council, National Academy of Sciences, 1973, pp. 31–32.
2. *Present Knowledge in Nutrition.* Washington, D.C.: Nutrition Review, 1984, p. 446.
3. Isaacson, L. C., M. Modlin, and W.P.V. Jackson. "Sodium intake and hypertension." *Lancet,* 1963; 1:946.
4. "Primitive Society versus the Good Life." *Los Angeles Times,* December 14, 1986.
5. *The New York Times,* August 19, 1986.
6. *Present Knowledge in Nutrition,* p. 447.
7. Page, L. B. "Nutritional Determinants of Hypertension." Chapter 6 in: *Nutrition and the Killer Diseases.* New York: John Wiley & Sons, 1981.
8. As reported by science writer Gina Kolata in *The New York Times,* December 3, 1987.
9. *Toxicants Occurring Naturally in Foods,* p. 28.
10. Ibid., p. 33.
11. Bertino, M., G. K. Beauchamp, and K. Engelman. "Long-term reduction in dietary sodium alters the taste of salt." *Am. J. Clin. Nutr.,* 1982; 36:1134–1144.
12. Pangborn, R. M., and S. D. Pecore. "Taste perception of sodium chloride in relation to dietary intake of salt." *Am. J. Clin. Nutr.,* 1982; 35:510–520.
13. Beauchamp, G. K., M. Bertino, and K. Engelman. "Failure to compensate decreased dietary sodium with increased table salt usage." *JAMA,* 1987; 258(22):3275–3278.
14. Anon. "Exonerating Sodium." *Scientific American,* February 1988, Vol. 258, No. 2, p. 17.
15. Sugimura, T., M. Nagao, T. Kawachi, et al. "Mutagen-carcinogens in food, with special reference to highly mutagenic pyrolytic products in broiled foods." In: *Origins of Human Cancer,* Cold Spring Harbor Laboratory, 1977, p. 562.

CHAPTER 46

SUGAR

SWEET BUT NOT INNOCENT

Roses are red,
Violets are blue,
Sugar is sweet,
And so are you!

If salt is symbolic of purity, goodness, and preservation of the perishable, sugar is associated with comfort, love, and affection. The English language—more than any other, to our knowledge—builds this association into terms of endearment: "honey," "sweetheart," even "sugar."

The appeal of sweets is near-universal. Inhabitants of the scorching deserts, the humid tropics, and the northern wastes all love sweets. Walking through the center of Copenhagen late one night, we were not surprised to find a large, well-stocked candy store open for business next door to the all-night porno shops. Judging by the brisk business the candy shop was doing compared to its neighbors, one could only conclude that sex is definitely no competition for sweets!

The average person in the United States consumes close to a backbreaking one-hundred-pound sack of sugar or a little more per year, just through commercial foods alone. Soft drinks, ice cream, cakes, cookies, candy bars, and presweetened breakfast cereals com-

300

FRUCTOSE IN THE KITCHEN*

Breakfast cereals: Use fructose like table sugar, but a little less of it.

Lemonade, other liquids, puddings: Will take a little more to sweeten by volume (teaspoon per teaspoon) than table sugar, which is 20 to 30% less by weight.

Cakes: Use same amount of fructose by volume as for sucrose; 20% less by weight. Bake at 325°F for approximately 40 minutes. Watch for rapid browning!

Cookies: Amounts are same as for cakes. Temperature 425°F; time 10–15 minutes. Watch for rapid browning!

Drawback: May leave slick film in mouth after eating.

Advantage: Cookies keep moist in a plastic bag at room temperature for several weeks.

* Based on our own experiences and Sherrie Lynn Hardy, Charlotte P. Brennand, and Bonita W. Wise, "Fructose: Comparison with sucrose as sweetener in four products," *J. Am. Diet. Assoc.,* 1979; 74:41–46.

prise the major source of this indirect sugar consumption. But so do many foods you wouldn't expect to contain sugar: luncheon meats, pickles, many canned soups and vegetables, as well as mayonnaise, salad dressings, ketchup, and most commercial breads.

In addition to this 100-odd pounds of sugar, the average American takes in some 25 pounds a year directly from the sugar bowl. That brings the total to 125 to 130 pounds of sugar per year.

The American tooth hasn't always been so sweet. Around the turn of the century, sugar use was only about half what it is today. Earlier on, it was even less; mostly for economic reasons. But history has proved that as populations become more affluent they consume more sugar *and* more fat. In fact, the two go hand in hand: Populations that consume a lot of sugar also eat large quantities of fat—and, as a consequence, have a higher incidence of atherosclerosis, coronary heart disease, and diabetes.

As psychologists, we're aware of certain tricks our minds play on us when it comes to sweet or fatty foods. Even laboratory rats, if given a chance, will eat themselves into obesity and nausea on their favorite foods—not cheese, as you might think, but on combinations of milk, cream, and sugar,[1] the same ingredients that make up candy bars, ice creams, cakes, and cookies. What's more, researchers discovered that overweight humans, who can least afford to indulge in sweets, showed the greatest desire for ice cream, cakes, and candy bars and, just like the rats, ate them in unreasonably large quantities.[2]

Everybody is agreed that too much sugar isn't good for us, but scientists disagree as to just *how* bad it is. Some think it is worse than fat. Most specialists, however, are more afraid of fat than of sugar. The late Nathan Pritikin, for example, stated, "Sugar is less detrimental to your health than fat and cholesterol."[3]

Dr. Demopoulos agrees. "If you are metabolically and physically active," he says, "there is nothing wrong with a reasonable amount of sugar—you burn it as soon as it comes into your body."[4] He points out that simple sugars such as sucrose (table sugar), fructose (the principal sugar in most fruits), and glucose (the principal sugar in grapes and corn syrup) are very important because they are the primary energy sources for the brain.

Obviously, the effect of any sugar intake varies according to your degree of physical activity. If you're active, you'll convert the sugar into energy. If sedentary, your body will convert it into fat. It's as simple as that.

Sugar metabolism varies according to what makes up the rest of the diet. Most people on our diet—high in fiber, 70 to 80 percent of total calories from complex carbohydrates, and no more than 20 percent in fats—seem to handle small amounts of simple sugars perfectly well. In other words, it is not just the amount of sugar, but the *dietary context* in which it is consumed, that is critical.

Soluble fibers, such as pectins in fruits and gum-type fibers from oat products and legumes (beans, lentils, garbanzos), also play a major role in determining how simple carbohydrates (sugars) are tolerated. Equally important is the relative absence of fats. Under these conditions, even many non-insulin–dependent diabetics who have traditionally been placed on totally sugar-free diets can handle small amounts of sugar with ease.*[5,6]

ARE SOME SUGARS BETTER THAN OTHERS?

We are often asked whether it is better to use honey, raw sugar, turbinado sugar, brown sugar, or molasses instead of refined white sugar. The truth of the matter is that nutritionally all these forms of

---

* The paradoxical fact that diabetics have been shown to be able to handle small amounts of ice cream, which is relatively rich in fat, appears to be a result of *cold* (not fat) slowing down the glucose response. But even if this were actually the case, fat intake would still have to be highly restricted.

sugar are essentially the same. They do have advantages and disadvantages, however, so we'll take a look at each of them.

First, a quick overview of what happens in your body when you take in sugar in any form: An alarm goes off in your pancreas, which quickly releases insulin to metabolize the sugar. Unless you're diabetic, the sugar is soon gone, but the insulin hangs around in your bloodstream for hours. If larger amounts of sugar have been ingested, this can set off a "hypoglycemic rebound," a vicious circle in which the circulating insulin lowers your blood sugar above and beyond the call of duty, producing symptoms of hypoglycemia: weakness, headache, trembling, listlessness, and a feeling of general malaise. Your liver gets the signal to release glucose, which it has wisely stored in the form of glycogen. Your brain, feeling suddenly short of sugar—which it absolutely needs in order to function—sends messages that produce a craving for more sugar. Chances are, you'll eat something else sweet to make yourself feel better, which in turn, will give you another insulin jolt, thus establishing another vicious circle.

Since honey, brown sugar, and molasses all have the same quick insulin-releasing effect as plain white table sugar, there is absolutely no advantage to any of them. We stress this point because the promotion of these products, directed at the health-conscious consumer, has resulted in a great deal of confusion. Much has been made, for instance, of the fact that honey, brown sugar, turbinado sugar, and molasses contain important minerals as well as vitamins. The truth is that minerals and vitamins are present in these sugars in such minute amounts that they make no nutritional difference.

On the other hand, honey and molasses sometimes contain natural plant toxins. In honey such potentially harmful compounds might come from the nectar of toxic plants that the bees may have inadvertently picked up (it is less likely that they would not recognize man-made toxins of chemical insecticides).

Overriding these possibilities on the down side, honey seems definitely to have some medicinal properties with which it has always been credited in folk medicine. Now at least one or two of these properties have also been corroborated by scientific research.

For example, it has been found that eating honey can relieve bacteria-caused infant diarrhea,[7] comparable to the effect of streptomycin. Whatever ingredient it is in honey that has this beneficial effect, it certainly isn't the sugars (glucose and fructose), but some other, as yet unidentified compound.

As far as molasses is concerned, there is no scientific confirmation of any of the folkloric claims about its alleged medicinal virtues (whatever iron it contains can be more efficiently provided from other dietary sources or supplements). At the same time, the darker and least processed types of molasses that have the highest concentrations of iron also have the greatest amounts of contaminants from the sugar-cane or beet juice, which is eliminated in the refining process that results in granulated table sugar.

Nevertheless, honey, maple syrup, and the dark sugars, including molasses, offer an advantage over table sugar similar to that of tamari or soya sauce over salt: They taste better and sweeter so you do not have to use as much of them as you would of plain sugar.

As for the brown sugars sold in America and Europe, they are nothing but refined white sugar with some molasses added to give a darker color. They offer neither any nutritional advantage nor the interesting flavors of honey or maple syrup.

Fructose, as the name implies, is the substance that imparts sweetness to most fruits. It is also the predominating sugar in honey (38 percent), ahead of glucose (31 percent). Nutritionists often recommend fructose as a substitute for sucrose because it produces a lower serum glucose and a slower insulin response—it does not release excess insulin into the bloodstream as does sucrose (table sugar).

Fructose has the advantage of being 70 percent sweeter than sucrose, so that—at least in theory—you need less of it. In practice, however, it doesn't always work out that way because its sweetness is affected by many factors, such as temperature, acidity, and concentration.

Although ice cream and cakes made with fructose evoke lower serum glucose and insulin responses than those made with sucrose,[8] you'd be ill advised to go on a fructose binge. True, you won't get the same insulin shock as you would from sugar, or the hypoglycemic rebound effect that leaves you craving more sugar. But fructose, like sucrose, produces higher VLDLs (very low-density lipoproteins) and thus higher triglyceride levels, which in the long run contribute to your total cholesterol. The bottom line is that the advantage of fructose over sucrose is only slight—though probably still significant enough to give fructose or glucose (grape sugar) the edge over sucrose.

ASPARTAME: FOR SOME THE ANSWER TO SUGAR ADDICTION

Aspartame, unlike any of the other artificial sweeteners, is a dipeptide made up of two naturally occurring amino acids, L-aspartic acid and L-phenylalanine. Despite a lot of static from some consumer groups, it has been approved for most nutritional purposes by the FDA.

Canadian health authorities had approved it even earlier, and several years of experience of its use in soft drinks in Canada have shown aspartame to be safe for most people. As Dr. David L. Horwitz and dietitian Jeanine K. Bauer-Nehrling of the University of Illinois Medical Center, Chicago, put it: "Numerous studies have shown no potential toxicity of amounts of aspartame likely to be ingested, or even of abuse doses."[9]

Aspartame's safety should not surprise anyone, considering that its constituents are no strangers to our bodies. The L-aspartic acid of aspartame is also manufactured in the human spinal cord. In adulthood it is used by the body in several metabolic processes and, in early childhood, it is important for the development of teeth.

The other amino acid in aspartame, phenylalanine, has a role in the synthesis of certain brain neurotransmitters (catecholamines). In the L-form in aspartame, phenylalanine has a potential antidepressant and appetite-suppressing effect. But in the small amounts in those commercially prepared foods and drinks that are sweetened with aspartame, this effect is unlikely to be noticed.

For private consumption, most people in this country use aspartame only in the form of little packets marketed by the NutraSweet Company under the trade name Equal. Each little packet contains only 35 milligrams of actual aspartame, the rest being made up of a mixture of dextrose and dried corn syrup for bulk. The reason only such a small amount of the active ingredient is needed in a product like Equal is that aspartame is 170 times as sweet as table sugar—which is also why it is next to impossible to use too much of it.

In our opinion, it is these features that make aspartame the ideal sweetener for all those who cannot resist their sweet tooth, but have to watch their weight or triglyceride levels. This is especially true for diabetics, because aspartame does not adversely affect glycemic control.[10]

This makes aspartame the ideal table sweetener. Its only drawback is that it loses its sweetness at cooking and baking temperatures. That does not mean, however, that one cannot use it after cooking, once the food is at normal room temperatures.

WARNING   People who suffer from phenylketonuria (PKU), a rare genetic disease preventing the conversion of phenylalanine into tyrosine and thus leading to accumulation of phenylalanine and its metabolic products in the body fluids, should not use aspartame.

FOODS WITH HIGH GLYCEMIC INDEX

- Processed breakfast cereals (cold cereals)

- Most commercial breads

- Most root vegetables (yams, sweet potatoes, potatoes, carrots)

- Most commercially processed foods (canned foods)

FOODS WITH LOW GLYCEMIC INDEX

- Most fruits (exceptions: tropical fruits like bananas, mangoes, papayas; also fully ripened domestic fruits like sweet cherries and strawberries, dried raisins, prunes, and apricots, but not apples and pears)

- Most vegetables

- Legumes (dried beans, peas, lentils, garbanzos)

- All dark, whole-grain breads, especially pumpernickel and the Pritikin-formula breads*

- Pasta (spaghetti, macaroni, lasagna), especially whole-wheat and vegetable types

* Sources: D.J.A. Jenkins et al., "Low glycemic index carbohydrate foods in the management of hyperlipidemia," *Am. J. Clin. Nutr.,* 1985; 42:604–617; G. R. Collier et al., "Prediction of glycemic response and mixed meals in noninsulin-dependent diabetic subjects," *Am. J. Clin. Nutr.,* 1986; 44:349–352; A. W. Thorburn et al., "The glycaemic index of foods," *Med. J. Australia,* 1986; 144:580–582.

THE "GLYCEMIC INDEX" OF FOODS

The "glycemic index" you may have heard of or read about in certain diet books and magazine articles is worth noting if you are interested in sound nutrition. It is *not* a panacea for weight control. It's a ratio that measures the rise in blood sugar caused by a particular food in relation to the blood sugar rise caused by glucose. Glucose is, in essence, "blood sugar," and has therefore been arbitrarily assigned a glycemic index of 100 (similar to setting the boiling point of water at 100°C and its freezing point at zero).

Any kind of carbohydrate causes some rise in blood sugar. And sugars themselves (simple carbohydrates) cause a much greater and more rapid rise—and a correspondingly quick and pronounced insulin response—than do complex carbohydrates (rice, potatoes, pasta, vegetables, fruits, etc.).

There are indeed differences between the blood sugar rise caused by one kind of carbohydrate and another. For example, white potatoes surprisingly cause a quicker and somewhat greater blood glucose response than do sweet potatoes, rice, or corn. These differences can be expressed in terms of the glycemic index. At least 120 foods and sugars have been indexed in this manner, and we have listed in the box on page 306 some common foods with either high or low glycemic index.

The magnitude of the blood glucose response depends not only on the type of food but also on the form in which it is consumed. Spaghetti produces a much smaller rise in blood glucose than either whole-meal or white bread. This is because the glycemic index of pasta is only 40 percent that of white bread and about 60 percent that of whole-meal bread.[11]

Question: Which is better—a small piece of *cake* or a scoop of *ice cream*?

Answer: *Ice cream* is better so far as serum glucose and insulin responses are concerned. Nobody knows exactly why but it may be its coldness that makes for better glucose tolerance.

Catch 22: You are buying this advantage at the expense of the probably higher fat content of ice cream and the potential problems of its milk proteins (see pages 327–331).

Solution: Take your pick and enjoy!

Similarly, puréed vegetables and fruits generate a more pronounced blood glucose response than do whole or cut-up vegetables and fruits. A whole apple, for example, causes much less of a blood glucose response—and has a much lower glycemic index—than apple purée.

This is true also for juices. You're much better off eating whole apples, oranges, or grapefruit than drinking their juices. Plus, of course, if you eat the whole fruit, you get the full therapeutic benefit of its fiber.[12]

Natural fibers, especially the gel-forming, water-soluble pectins of whole fruits and the gumlike fibers of legumes, help to keep the glucose response of foods low. They also produce the satiety effect, so important for weight control, which signals the brain that enough food has been eaten.[13]

Cooking fruits and vegetables raises their glycemic index. For instance, cooked carrots or baked apples produce a higher blood glucose response than do raw apples or carrots.

The glycemic index, if useful in some respects, has its limitations. Nobody knows what happens to the glycemic index when several foods are eaten together, as is usually the case. Nor does the fact that honey has a higher glycemic index (75) than ordinary table sugar (60), and a still higher one than fructose (20), automatically mean that table sugar is preferable to honey. It does mean that fructose is preferable to both table sugar and honey as far as the glycemic index is concerned.

The reason the glycemic index of honey is so high is that honey is so high in glucose. But glucose being straight blood sugar, it is much more quickly absorbed and burned by our cells for energy than any other kind of sugar. Nathan Pritikin, for example, preferred glucose to fructose and used it (sparingly) in the form of grape sugar.

SOURCES

1. Doewnoski, A., and M.R.C. Greenwood. "Cream and sugar: human preferences for high-fat foods." *Physiol. and Behav.,* 1983; 30:629–633.
2. Gates, J. C., R. L. Huenemann, and R. J. Brand. "Food choices of obese and non-obese person." *J. Am. Diet. Assoc.,* 1975; 67:339–343.
3. Pritikin, N. *The Pritikin Promise.* New York: Pocket Books, 1945, p. 182.
4. Demopoulos, H. B., M.D., verbal communication.
5. *Nutritional Support of Medical Practice,* 2nd ed., H. A. Schneider, et al., eds. New York: Harper & Row, 1983, p. 311.
6. Jenkins, D.J.A., et al. "The glycaemic index of foods tested in diabetic patients: a new basis for carbohydrates exchange favoring the use of legumes." *Diabetologia,* 1983; 24:257–264.

7. Chirife, J., and H. L. Scarmato. "Scientific basis for the use of granulated sugar in treatment of infected wounds." *Lancet,* 1972; 81:560.
8. Crapo, P. A., et al. "Comparison of the metabolic responses to fructose and sucrose sweetened foods." *Am. J. Clin. Nutr.,* 1982; 35:256–261.
9. Horwitz, D. L., and J. K. Bauer-Nehrling. "Can aspartame meet our expectation?" *Research,* 1983; 83:142–146.
10. Nehrling, J. K., P. Kobe, M. P. McLane, et al. "Aspartame use by persons with diabetes." *Diabetes Care,* 1985; 8:415–417.
11. Jenkins, D.J.A., et al. "Glycemic response to wheat products: reduced response to pasta but not effect of fiber." *Diabetes Care,* 1983; 6:155–159. Also: Jenkins, D.J.A., et al. "Low glycemic response to traditionally processed wheat and rye products: bulgur and pumpernickel bread." *Am. J. Clin. Nutr.,* 1986; 43:516–520.
12. O'Dea, K., P. J. Nestel, and L. Antonoff. "Physical factors influencing post-prandial glucose and insulin responses to starch." *Am. J. Clin. Nutr.,* 1980; 33:760–765.
13. Haber, G. B., K. W. Heaton, D. Murphy, and L. F. Burroughs. "Depletion and absorption of dietary fibre. Effects on satiety, plasma glucose and serum insulin." *Lancet,* 1977; 2:679–682.

CHAPTER 47

FAT

THE ONLY "GOOD" FAT IS THE ONE YOU DON'T EAT

12 There are all kinds of fats—saturated, mostly of animal origin, polyunsaturated, like most cooking and salad oils, and monounsaturated, like olive oil. What they all have in common nutritionally is that they are not only calorie-dense, but they also involve certain serious health risks, one possible exception being the monounsaturated fats.

Saturated fats—like the fat on your steak, in your butter and cheeses, in your bacon, sausages, and luncheon meats, in the lard your hamburger is likely to have been fried in, and the baker has probably put into your bread and pastries—contribute most to your blood cholesterol level. This means you run an increased risk of cardiovascular disease like heart attack and stroke.

In contrast, polyunsaturated vegetable oils don't clog up your arteries with plaque the way the saturated animal fats do. In that sense, they are more benign. But they, too, are far from innocuous.

Monounsaturates, like olive oil, are much less prone to oxidation and don't seem to affect cholesterol levels. But they can add a lot of calories to your otherwise low-calorie salads,* thus frustrating your attempts to

---

* We discovered that we don't really need any oil on our salads, even though we're not afraid of a little olive oil. We use a little lemon or lime juice, perhaps with a tiny sprinkling of sugar to make a better acid-sugar balance, and *maybe* we add a few drops (no more than a teaspoon) of olive oil or soya sauce for additional flavor. For a change, we sometimes use fresh pineapple juice with ginger as a salad dressing. There are a number of commercial low-fat and even no-fat salad dressings like the ones under the Pritikin label. However, we found the latter too bland as is, but quite acceptable if additional spices are added.

stay slim and trim. That's why our motto is: The only good fats are the ones you don't eat.

Of course, we do need some fat in our diet, especially linoleic acid, which we cannot produce ourselves and from which our bodies produce the equally essential arachidonic acid. We need so little linoleic acid—1/10 ounce is enough to correct a deficiency—that the problem is not how to get enough of it, or any other fats, but how not to get too much. (The bowl of steel-cut oatmeal we ourselves eat in the morning, and the brown rice and whole-grain breads we eat during the rest of the day as a major part of our high-carbohydrate diet, supply more than enough of our requirements for linoleic acid and thereby also of arachidonic acid.)

To understand better the exaggerated role that fats play in the contemporary diet, it's important to view the problem in historical perspective. To begin with, our simian ancestors got most of their dietary fat from plants and fruits, although occasional lapses into carnivorous behavior may have supplied an insignificant amount of animal fat. Our Stone Age ancestors, who were hunter-gatherers, also ate very little fat because the meat from the wild animals they killed was much leaner and lower in cholesterol than most beef and pork today. Even as recently as the turn of the century, people were eating a leaner diet than is consumed today. But later on, fat consumption increased every year in the industrialized world, interrupted only by World Wars I and II.

This phenomenal increase in fat consumption, which was accompanied by a steady rise in coronary heart disease and certain cancers, finally prompted concern and action by the medical profession. In 1982, the National Academy of Sciences National Research Council issued a report titled "Diet, Nutrition, and Cancer," which helped bring about changes. Until then, most people and even some physicians simply took the typical high-fat, high-protein diets of their patients for granted.

A few years later (1988), when the Surgeon General's report on nutrition and health was published—after the American Heart Association's call for a reduction of calories from fat of about 40 to 30 percent of total calories consumed—the medical establishment had already accepted this modest goal. So too had a large segment of the American public that had become especially aware of the health dangers from eating cholesterol-rich foods. In other words, the Surgeon General's report was more of a reminder of something most people already knew, rather than the "bombshell" the government had called it.

Since most people nowadays realize, at least in general terms, the need for cutting down on saturated animal fats, particularly on cholesterol-rich foods, and since these matters were discussed earlier in the book, we won't go further into them here. Instead, we shall call attention to a little-known hazard from cholesterol—its potential for

It has been estimated that 500 million pounds of fats and oils—most of which are polyunsaturated—are used each year in the United States in the manufacture of potato chips alone.—S. S. Chang, R. J. Peterson, and C. T. Ho, "Chemical Reactions Involved in the Deep-Fat Frying of Foods," *J. Am. Oil Chem. Soc.,* 1978; 55:718.

oxidation—and why cutting down only on animal fats is not good enough.

It turns out that cholesterol is not a very stable compound. It oxidizes easily at room temperature when exposed to air. In fact, researchers have isolated as many as thirty-nine oxidation products from cholesterol and found them—in contrast to cholesterol itself—to be highly toxic to smooth-muscle cells, immunosuppressive,[1] and the real culprits behind the buildup of atherosclerotic plaque in arteries.[2]

Cholesterol oxidation products develop readily in aged meat, sausage, cheese, powdered whole eggs (widely used in commercial baking) as well as in whole milk. Consequently, as nutritionist Maria C. Linder points out, the normal human diet contains a fair amount of these potentially hazardous products. Fortunately, a reasonable diet also includes foods rich in anti-oxidants—ascorbic acid (vitamin C), tocopherols (vitamin E), the B vitamins, and beta-carotene (pro-vitamin A)—all of which prevent the free radicals generated by these oxidation products from forming tissue-destructive chain reactions. Needless to say, even more protection is afforded if we take supplemental anti-oxidants.

We hope the foregoing will make you even more aware of the dangers of eating cholesterol-rich foods and that you will avoid them like the plague, even if it means switching from bacon and eggs in the morning to cereal. And go easy even on the leanest cuts of meat, for they too—though low in fat—may still contain considerable amounts of cholesterol.

In the section that follows, we shall take a hard look at another even less-appreciated danger—the health hazards associated with the un-saturated plant-derived oils which people are urged to substitute for saturated animal fats.

HOW SAFE ARE PUFAS (POLYUNSATURATED FATTY ACIDS)?

The recognition of the health dangers posed by foods high in saturated fats and cholesterol—for the body in general and the cardiovascular system in particular—caused an abrupt shift from saturated* animal fats to unsaturated† plant oils (corn oil, safflower oil, cottonseed oil, sunflower oil, etc.).

However, there's a catch: Molecular oxygen is seven times more soluble within fats than in water, and polyunsaturated fats are even more vulnerable to attack by molecular oxygen than are saturated animal fats. In the absence of anti-oxidants, polyunsaturated fats are therefore highly subject to the formation of hydroperoxides, which develop whenever a fat molecule loses a hydrogen atom and free-radical chain reactions start.

In addition, as Dr. Demopoulos points out, molecular oxygen itself has certain properties of free radicals and can initiate free-radical chain reactions in body tissues, especially those containing susceptible fat molecules.

As we have already discussed,‡ each free radical is extremely unstable and has a high affinity for oxygen. At the same time, and to complete its electron structure, the free radical will react with another molecule, in this case a fat molecule, again removing a hydrogen atom from these "easy targets." And so another free radical is created, resulting in a chain reaction.

Remember that it is the function of anti-oxidants to provide hydrogen atoms so as to complete the electron structure of the free radical and thereby stabilize it. In this case, an anti-oxidant can replace the fat molecules as the donor of hydrogen atoms, thereby terminating the chain reaction. In that way, oxidative rancidity is retarded and the fats keep fresh longer.

Common anti-oxidants used by the food industry are ascorbyl palmitate, the fat-soluble form of vitamin C, or BHT and BHA.§ How much longer a fat can keep fresh by adding an anti-oxidant depends on how long the anti-oxidants themselves can stay fresh and active. Why? Because the loss of hydrogen by the anti-oxidant, necessarily occurring in the course of protecting the fat molecules, turns the anti-oxidant itself into a free radical.

Theoretically, that could also lead to free-radical chain reactions. But the anti-oxidant free radical assumes a more stable configuration

---

* Fatty acids that carry as many hydrogen atoms on their frame of carbon atoms as they can hold are called *saturated.*
† The carbon atoms of fatty acids can form chemical bonds with four other atoms. All along the long chain of carbon atoms that form the core of fatty acids, the carbon atoms attach to each other like a string of pearls, and each carbon atom also holds two hydrogen atoms. At either end of such a chain, they can bind to one additional hydrogen atom. When the fatty acid drops hydrogen atoms, it always drops two at a time. When only one pair of hydrogen atoms is missing, the result is a *monounsaturated* fatty acid like olive oil or peanut oil, or the oil in avocados. If more than one pair of hydrogen atoms has been dropped, the fatty acid that results is called *polyunsaturated,* which is true for most vegetable oils.
‡ See chapters on free radicals, pages 69–79.
§ The Eastman Kodak Company of Rochester, New York, has developed a series of highly effective anti-oxidant formulations for stabilizing fat-containing food products.

by an internal rearrangement of electrons, or by reacting with another anti-oxidant molecule. Sometimes two anti-oxidant free radicals combine with each other. For these reasons, we don't really have to worry about free-radical chain reactions developing from degrading anti-oxidants as long as we have abundant anti-oxidant supplies of a varied nature, that is, broad-spectrum.

Anti-oxidants should be added to the fats or oils *before* oxidation has started. We add about one teaspoon of either ascorbyl palmitate or BHT to a quart of cooking or salad oil right after opening the container to prevent oxidation from getting a start.

HOW OXIDIZED FATS AFFECT YOUR HEALTH

As molecular oxygen attacks unprotected polyunsaturated fatty acids, whether in a bottle of vegetable oil or your cell membranes, it forms many different free radicals, including the highly reactive hydroxyl radical, ·OH. Dr. Barry Halliwell of King's College, London, England, says that "the hydroxyl radical, ·OH, will attack almost any biological molecule that it is generated next to,"[3] and he goes on to explain that this free radical can cause strand breaks in DNA and the breakdown of membrane lipids and proteins. When ·OH attacks a polyunsaturated fatty-acid side chain in a fat-containing cell membrane, it removes an atom of hydrogen from the fat molecule to form water. This reaction, while removing the hydroxyl radical, leaves behind in the cell membrane another type of radical species, a carbon-centered radical. When this radical reacts with molecular oxygen, it forms a third type of radical species, the peroxy radical.

Peroxy radicals then react with another membrane fatty-acid side chain, turning it into a lipid peroxide that can trigger the radical chain reactions known as the lipid peroxidation of fats. These lipid peroxides will then produce more radicals, hydrocarbon gases, and several aldehydes, all of which are toxic to cell membranes "even in minute amounts."[4]

These oxidized fats can act as cancer-causing agents (carcinogens), and can damage the cells' DNA, leading to abnormal cell formation and functioning. Such damage to DNA is now believed to be a major factor in aging. Lipid peroxidation products have been found to collect in all the major organs as they age.[5]

As previously alluded to, the lipofuscin pigments that cause age spots on the skin are similar to those that accumulate in the aging brain, heart, and other tissues. These pigments consist mainly of oxidized lipid-protein complexes. It is noteworthy that the testes are particularly prone to lipid peroxidation, a fact largely overlooked by urologists.

The continuous production of peroxidized fats may also wear down the mitochondria, the tiny organelles within the cells that control the chemical reactions releasing energy from glucose molecules. Remember that peroxidation of fats also inhibits the macrophages, white blood cells that normally attack and eat bacteria, viruses, and cancer cells. This is why obese people, who are full of oxidized (rancid) fats, become ill more often than people of normal weight.

Multiple sclerosis (MS), a progressive central nervous system disease, has been found to be related to the intake of fat, in particular animal and butterfat. The incidence of MS is much higher in some inland areas of Norway, where more animal and butterfat are consumed, than in the coastal regions, where more fish is eaten. MS is also far more prevalent in the northern, German-speaking area of Switzerland, with its high-fat diet, than in the southern, Italian-speaking part of the country, where considerably less animal and butterfat and more olive oil are consumed. In French-speaking Switzerland, where the fat-consumption rate is intermediate between that of the German and Italian populations, the MS rate is intermediate as well.[6] These findings are paralleled by clinical experience with MS patients. Those who are on low-fat diets do better than those on high-fat diets. In fact, a single high-fat meal can initiate a relapse or intensification of symptoms in a MS patient.

Finally, the oxidation of certain fat molecules in cells can, through a series of chemical reactions, produce a family of molecules known as oxy-arachidonic acids. These substances are extremely powerful in regulating the blood flow and coagulation mechanisms, the immune system, the central nervous system, and many other processes. Overproduction of oxygenated arachidonic acids can seriously disrupt the metabolism and function of many essential life processes. Excess lipid peroxides will cause increased production of oxy-arachidonic acid and lead to major imbalances throughout the body in almost all organs.

All these destructive free-radical reactions in our bodies can be accelerated by the consumption of dietary polyunsaturates, especially if they are partially peroxidized—as they usually are. Such considerations have led medical researchers like Dr. Scott M. Grundy to say, "Although there has been a great interest in the use of polyunsaturated fatty acids, studies have shown that in laboratory animals a large intake of polyunsaturates suppresses the immune system and increases the rate of tumor formation . . ."[7] Similarly, a team of researchers at the Harold Brunn Institute, Mount Zion Hospital and Medical Center, San Francisco, has said, "Ingestion of unsaturated fats could lead to disaster as readily as ingestion of saturated fats."[8]

By taking in too many fats of any kind, we "dilute" the body's supply of anti-oxidants, especially vitamin E. A diet high in polyunsaturates creates a relative vitamin E deficiency. In fact, the routine technique for creating an artificial vitamin E deficiency in laboratory animals is simply to load their diet with polyunsaturates. Conversely, a diet low in fats will automatically lead to increases in available endogenous anti-oxidants, which will better enable cells to combat free-radical reactions.

While *any* oil can become peroxidized (become rancid), poly-unsaturated vegetable oils do so more easily than saturated animal fats. Many dietary researchers, among them Drs. Demopoulos, Levine and Kidd, and Dr. Denham Harman, have found that the peroxidation of polyunsaturates leads directly to the production of free radicals. Hence our repeated emphasis on the need for restraint in the consumption of *all* fats, and to avoid the crucial error of worrying only about the cholesterol and saturated animal fats in our diet.

Besides oxidation problems, there are other reasons to believe that unsaturated vegetable oils are as detrimental to our health as saturated animal fats. Nathan Pritikin has pointed out that blood tends to sludge and capillaries to block just as badly whether people use heavy cream (a saturated fat) or safflower oil (a polyunsaturated fat). In either case, the triglyceride levels in the blood rise; in fact, with safflower oil they remain higher much longer. Even olive oil, essentially a monounsatu-rated fatty acid—the most benign of all—causes serum triglyceride levels to rise within an hour and a half of consumption.

Polyunsaturates also seem to contribute to the formation of gall-stones and tumor growth as much as saturated fats do. Nor is this astonishing because polyunsaturates have been shown to increase the production of bile acids just as much as saturated fats, and, as we saw earlier, anaerobic bacteria in the intestines convert these bile acids into compounds that initiate or promote malignancies.

In conclusion, while polyunsaturated fats are more health-protective than saturated fats in some ways, in many other ways they are every bit as dangerous. As in the case of alcohol, a little fat causes a little damage, more fat causes more damage, and a lot of fat causes a lot of damage. We therefore recommend that all fats, polyunsaturated or not, be kept to a minimum in the diet. Remember our initial statement: The only good fats are the ones you don't eat.

LOW-FAT GOURMET DINNER

We have shown you how destructive the typical American-European diet is to health. Now we'll tell you what to do about it.

If you are a "typical" American or European, eating a typical American or European diet, at least 40 percent of your fuel for energy comes from fats. Much of that will be in the form of saturated animal fats, which clog up your arteries with plaque and cause the most heart attacks and strokes.

For this reason, the American Heart Association (AHA) wants you to cut back on fats to a total of 30 percent, of which 20 percent should come from unsaturated fats of plant origin and only 10 percent from animal fats. Exactly what does that mean in terms of actual dietary changes?

The average American male takes in 2,500 calories daily. Assuming he eats a typical diet in which 40 percent of calories come from fats, to reduce his fat intake he would have to get rid of 250 fat calories. To reach that modest goal, he would need to eat only 26 to 28 fewer grams of fat (not quite an ounce). In other words, his fat intake would have to be reduced from about 111 grams per day to 83 grams per day.

In actual practice, all our hypothetical male would have to do is eat cereal instead of bacon and eggs for breakfast, skip the butter for his rolls or bread at lunch and dinner, eliminate the two Danish or the large croissant during his coffee break, skip the hamburger on the way home, and pass up those forty or so potato chips while watching television at night. If he does this, he is already on a diet in which only 30 percent of the calories are from fat.

For the average woman, who consumes only 1,600 calories per day, it would be even less of a sacrifice to get down to 30 percent of calories from fat. She would only have to get rid of about 17 grams of fat in her daily diet. With just sensible food selection, she would be right on target. We suggest eating only the white meat of chicken instead of the richer, and admittedly tastier, dark meat, cutting back on red meat and using only lean cuts, forsaking rich pastries, and cutting in half the amount of butter, margarine, and mayonnaise.

Keeping our fat intake down becomes easier when we keep an eye on the "hidden" fats in foods. Take eggs for example: There's no visible fat on them as there is on meat, but an egg yolk is 31 percent fat and contains 250 milligrams of cholesterol.

You don't see any fat on pound cake, but it, too, is 30 percent fat. According to a survey* of 235 cakes and pastries that are sold in American supermarkets either prepared or as mixes, the five containing the most fat (48 to 63 percent of total calories) are Sara Lee "Light" French Cheesecake, Drake's Yodels, Hostess Ding Dongs, Pepperidge Farm Grand Marnier Supreme, and Pillsbury Microwave Double Chocolate Supreme Cake mix. The five with the least fat (26 to 30 percent of

* The survey identifies seven hundred products with saturated fats, listing the type and amount of fat per serving. It is available in booklet form, for $5.50, from: *Fat Attack,* The Center for Science in the Public Interest, 1501 16th St. N.W., Washington, D.C. 20036.

EGGS

Egg white is one of the most complete proteins in human nutrition, BUT:

DO NOT eat whole eggs. Egg yolk has too much cholesterol in it (250 mg per yolk—your total daily allowance).

DO NOT eat *raw* eggs in any form. Raw egg white contains a toxic protein, avidin. Generally speaking, raw egg white inhibits those human enzymes that are needed to split proteins (proteolysis). Proteins can only be properly digested by being split into smaller molecules. Raw egg white can lead to a vitamin deficiency called *egg white disease,* caused by egg white's tendency to bind itself tenaciously to biotin, forming an insoluble complex with it and making the protein inaccessible to the body.

Therefore: do not eat raw egg white in any form (not even in eggnog!). On the other hand, eating *cooked* egg white once or twice a week is a good idea since it is one of the most "complete" and most easily digestible protein foods—unless you are allergic to eggs.

CAUTION There are people who are hypersensitive to even *cooked* eggs and will suffer from allergic reactions, if they eat eggs in any form. In those cases, the egg white again seems to be the culprit because two known allergens (ovalbumin and ovomucoid) have been identified in it.*

* D. D. Metcalfe, "Food hypersensitivity," *J. All. Clin. Immunol.,* 1984; 73(6):754.

---

total calories) are Aunt Jemima Coffee Cake mix, Betty Crocker Applesauce Raisin Snackin' Cake mix, Pepperidge Farm Carrot Walnut Muffins, Weight Watchers Strawberry Cheesecake, and Weight Watchers Pound Cake with Blueberry Topping.

Nuts, consumed in great quantities by many "health nuts," are also high in fat. Almonds, for instance, are 58 percent fat. Besides, by the time you eat the nuts, they have probably been sitting around so long that their fats have become oxidized and have developed free-radical–containing compounds. The only "good nuts" are chestnuts; they are virtually fat free.

Candy bars often combine several high-fat ingredients, such as nuts (on average, about 30 percent fat), dried coconut meat (65 percent fat, much of it saturated), and sweet chocolate (35 percent fat). These are percent of "content." The percent of total calories of these fats is much higher.

Most cuts of meat are high in hidden (and often not-so-hidden) fat, mostly of the saturated variety. Prime beef, for instance, is 41 percent fat in terms of content, but about 80 percent of the total calories are from the fat. On the other hand, low-fat meats are available in this country, albeit at stiff prices.

Two other foods with plenty of hidden fat are cheeses and mayonnaise. Most American cheeses have at least a 30 to 40 percent fat content (all of them are peroxidized—rancid—which gives them their particular flavor). Some imported cheeses are even higher in fat content. As for mayonnaise, the regular types are—believe it or not—80 percent fat! That goes even for most brands that have the misleading word "natural" on the label. And even so-called low-fat mayonnaise usually has 30 percent fat. The only exception we know is a mayonnaise substitute called Nayonnaise, made from tofu (bean curd), and some mayonnaise-type products made from low-fat yogurt.

You may be surprised to find out that vegetables, too, have some fat. You needn't worry about most of them because the amount is so small. The only exception is avocados, which are 16 percent fat, some of it saturated, but most of it monosaturated.

The AHA might be more concerned about the small percentage of saturated fat in avocados than about the huge amount of polyunsaturates in mayonnaise, as long as the amount stays within 20 percent of calories from polyunsaturated fat per day. But, as we have previously stated, we consider all fats almost equally dangerous. Monounsaturated oils, as found in olive oil (oleic acid), are perhaps the safest to use.

This is also the reason why we feel that 30 percent of calories from fat is not low enough. Instead, we recommend that you eat a diet in which you get 15 to 20 percent of your calories from fats, most of them from the unsaturated kinds. Aside from the reduced cancer risk, that's the only way that keeps our own cholesterol levels in the low 130s. Nor do we feel in the least deprived by our diet. Quite the contrary, we think we are eating exceedingly well. Our diet, which has 15 to 20 percent calories from fat, even makes it possible for us to eat out if we are selective as to the restaurant and our menu choices. In our experience, the better the restaurant, the easier it is to find something to eat that's tasty and not bad for your health. We have found Japanese, Chinese, Vietnamese, Thai, Indian, and Mediterranean cuisine most compatible with our diet, but you must still choose with care and avoid oily or fried dishes.

If you try to go much below 20 percent of calories from fats, it becomes difficult to prepare tasty meals because fats carry most of the flavors of foods. Moreover, it doesn't seem necessary for most people to go below the 20 percent level. Recent animal studies have indicated that reducing fat intake from 40 to 20 percent of calories inhibits breast cancer as effectively as does a completely fat-free diet.[9] In fact, some medical experts, including Dr. Charles Kleeman of UCLA, find fault with extreme diets like Pritikin's if they are maintained over longer periods of time.[10]

We still feel that if a person is grossly overweight and has a serious cholesterol problem, he or she ought to be on a Pritikin-type diet of no more than about 10 percent of calories from fat, at least until weight and cholesterol levels have been normalized.* And anybody with a serious diabetes problem should do the same. Once the immediate crisis is past and weight, cholesterol, triglycerides, and blood glucose are all within safe limits, our maintenance diet of 15 to 20 percent of calories from fat is optimal. Not only is it perfectly safe to use, but it's relatively easy to follow because it involves little, if any, frustration. We consider this diet the happy medium between a strict Pritikin-type diet, which most people find too hard to stick to over the long run, and the American Heart Association's too lenient diet of 30 percent of calories from fat, which does not effectively reduce weight, cholesterol, or triglycerides.

MARGARINE

Margarine is made from either a mixture of highly refined vegetable and animal fats or from vegetable fats alone. The label must state the amount of each, usually expressed as the polyunsaturated:saturated (P:S) ratio. *Jane Brody's Nutrition Book* suggests that this ratio should be 2:1 in favor of the polyunsaturates, and we agree. Unfortunately, even if margarine were made only with unsaturated vegetable oils, the end product would not be polyunsaturated. To increase its stability and produce the desired degree of hardness at room temperature, margarine is hydrogenated—hydrogen atoms are added to the fatty-acid chains of the polyunsaturates.

As mentioned earlier, polyunsaturates are a mixed blessing at best, and the trans-fatty acids into which they are turned by hydrogenation pose health risks of their own. There is evidence that these trans-fatty acids can interfere with the conversion of normal linoleic acid to arachidonic acid, which can lead to higher cholesterol levels. Since trans-fatty acids behave biologically like saturated fats, and since they can raise plasma cholesterol levels, they may be atherogenic.[11]

Although this has not yet been clearly established, Drs. D. F. Horrobin and Y. S. Huang argue for "concern about the long-term effects of the consumption in large amounts of agents known to raise the cholesterol levels."[12] Margarine has also been linked, along with smoked fish and grilled sausages (the hydrocarbon effect), to

---

* It is possible to cause regression of serious atherosclerot plaques with a "10 percent of calories from fat" diet, as first shown by Pritikin and confirmed recently. But this requires a two- to three-year period and strict medical supervision.

benign skin tumors (papilloma), as well as to skin cancer and lung carcinoma.[13]

To minimize the risk of eating too many trans-fatty acids and saturated fats, Jane Brody recommends that you choose the soft tub margarines rather than the harder stick kinds, because the soft margarines are less hydrogenated and more polyunsaturated. Although we ourselves don't eat margarine, we advise our clients who do to use it sparingly and with due respect for its potential health risks.

VEGETABLE SHORTENINGS

After margarine, vegetable shortenings are the largest source of trans-fatty acids in the American diet. They are made from refined, bleached vegetable oils that have been hydrogenated and whipped or aerated to give them a semisolid consistency and a whiter appearance. They are popular for baking because they are easier to work with than solid fats or liquid oils, and because they contain small amounts of emulsifiers, which give cakes more volume and better texture.

Despite these advantages, we have found that we can substitute polyunsaturated vegetable oils of milder taste (corn oil, safflower oil, or sunflower oil) for shortening. If you do use oils, make sure they are fresh, that they have not sat around too long on supermarket shelves, and that you have added a fat-soluble anti-oxidant like BHT, BHA, or ascorbyl palmitate (a form of vitamin C) into the bottle (½ to 1 teaspoon per quart or liter).*

Fats from completely hydrogenated (and therefore saturated) soybean oil, containing 90 percent of *stearic acid,* do not seem to raise plasma cholesterol or lower the high-density lipoproteins. Researchers therefore suggest that fats high in stearic acid could advantageously replace other fats in some foods, for instance in margarines and shortenings. These fats would provide better texture, a characteristic of saturated fats, in such foods without raising cholesterol levels.[14] While lower cholesterol levels are an advantage, the trans-fatty acids produced during hydrogenation would still exist. Also, the researchers themselves urge that their findings not be "extended unreservedly to common fats rich in stearic acid, such as beef fat and cocoa butter, without further evidence." They call special attention to the fact that

---

* Since light can accelerate the oxidation process, cooking and salad oils should not be kept in the translucent bottles in which they are usually sold, but put into a metal or crockery container that can be tightly closed. Plastic bottles are not good because they also allow air to pass through the walls.

these other fats also contain palmitic acid, which is notorious for raising cholesterol levels.

COCONUT OIL AND PALM OIL

Coconut oil is one of the most highly saturated fats not of animal origin. Coconut oil is used to make the popular nondairy creamers many people put in coffee or tea to avoid the saturated butterfat of whole milk or cream. But that's like switching from Scotch to bourbon to get away from alcohol.

Palm oil, also highly saturated, may not be as undesirable as had earlier been thought because of its relatively high content (40 percent) of the same monounsaturated oleic acid present in olive oil, along with 10 percent of linoleic acid. Animal experiments and human studies indicate that although palm oil contains about 50 percent of saturated fatty acids, it does not actually behave as a saturated oil.

In addition, one fraction of palm oil is very rich in alpha tocopherol (active vitamin E) and several carotenoids, which are all free-radical scavengers, help prevent blood clotting, and have anticancer properties. In other words, palm oil contains respectable amounts of protective anti-oxidants that may also, as some scientists believe, affect membrane fluidity and function when taken up in plasma membranes.[15,16]

This is good news, considering that palm oil is the second most common vegetable oil produced in the world today, about 90 percent of it used for nutritional purposes.[17] The only trouble is that so much of it is consumed in the form of semisoft products, such as Crisco, made from partially hydrogenated palm and soybean oils, that it results in the formation of possibly harmful trans-fatty acids. The firmer *manteca,* used for almost all frying throughout Latin America, consists of totally hydrogenated palm oil and presents even more of a problem.

Our recommendation: Don't use manteca and similar totally hydrogenated oils at all, and partially hydrogenated products like Crisco only sparingly. Whenever possible, use substitutes.

SOURCES

1. Beisel, W. R. "Single nutrients and immunity." *Am. J. Clin. Nutr.,* February Supplement, 1982; 35:417–468.
2. Linder, M. C. *Nutritional Biochemistry and Metabolism.* New York: Elsevier, 1984, p. 338.
3. Halliwell, B. "Free radicals and metal ions in health and disease." *Proc. Nutr. Soc.,* 1987; 46(1):13–14.

4. Ibid.
5. Levine, St. A., and P. Kidd. *Antioxidant Adaptation, Its Role in Free Radical Pathology.* San Leandro, Calif.: Allergy Research Group, 1985, p. 38.
6. Swank, Roy Lave. *A Biochemical Basis of Multiple Sclerosis.* Springfield, Ill.: Charles C. Thomas, 1961.
7. Grundy, S. M., G. L. Vega, and D. W. Bilheimer. "Causes and treatment of hypercholesterolemia." In: *Bile Acids and Atherosclerosis,* S. M. Grundy, ed. New York: Raven Press, 1986, 15:22.
8. Friedman, M., S. O. Byers, and R. H. Rosenman. "Effect of unsaturated fats upon lipemia and conjunctival circulation." *JAMA,* 1965; 193:882–886.
9. Kalamegham, R., and K. K. Carroll. "Reversal of the promotional effect of high-fat diet on mammary tumorigenesis by subsequent lowering of dietary fat." *Nutr. Cancer,* 1984; 6:22–31.
10. Kleeman, C., personal communication.
11. Krichevsky, D. *Fed. Proc.,* 1982; 41:2813.
12. Horrobin, D. F., and Y. S. Huang. "The role of linoleic acid and its metabolites in the lowering of plasma cholesterol and the prevention of cardiovascular disease." *Int. J. Card.,* 1987; 17:241–255.
13. Furihata, C., and T. Matsushima. "Mutagens and carcinogens in foods." *Ann. Rev. Nutr.,* 1986; 6:67–94.
14. Bonanome, A., and S. M. Grundy. "Effect of dietary stearic acid on plasma cholesterol and lipoprotein levels." *N. Eng. J. Med.,* 1988; 318:1248.
15. Berger, K. G., and S. H. Ong. *Oléagineux,* 1985; 40:613–624.
16. Qureshi, A. A., et al. *J. Biol. Chem.,* 1986: 261:10544–10550.
17. Anon. "New Findings on Palm Oil." *Nutrition Reviews,* 1987; 7:205ff.

CHAPTER 48

HAMBURGERS AND CAVIAR

12 The hamburger has long been an American obsession, one might even say an addiction. And recently, hamburger has even become politicized.

During the 1986 congressional elections, actress Jane Fonda backed a certain Democrat who was campaigning for a seat in the South Dakota Senate. The press had a field day when the Republican the man was running against charged that his opponent was being supported by someone opposed to the consumption of red meat.

Don't laugh—an accusation like this is serious business in a state where livestock is the economic backbone. This was dirty politics, all right, but Fonda nevertheless printed a disclaimer saying that she was by no means a strict vegetarian and had at times even been known to down a Big Mac. This incident reminded us of a drive we took through Texas some time ago where we saw bumper stickers with the message NOT EATING STEAK IS UN-AMERICAN! To this day we have not been able to figure out whether this was meant as a sick joke or as a sick political statement.

We have news for those who consider vegetarianism un-American or, by implication, pro-Communist. As it happens, most Soviet populations are heavy meat eaters—a tradition in Eastern European cuisine. In fact, having to stand in long lines to buy meat (of which there never seems to be enough) is one of the standard gripes of people living in Soviet-bloc countries.

Long before the advent of communism in either China or Vietnam, the cuisines of these countries were semivegetarian. Asian cooking has traditionally used meat more as a condiment to flavor rice and vegetables than as the principal focus of a meal—the way it is used almost everywhere else, unfortunately.

One can also make the case that vegetarianism is very American. Consider the Seventh-day Adventists, a totally American Christian denomination, one of whose basic tenets is that a "real" Christian does not eat meat. For this reason, Seventh-day Adventists are often used as control groups in scientific studies that examine the relationship between diet and certain diseases such as cancer.

Prince Charles of England, who certainly ought to be above suspicion of being a Communist, confesses a leaning toward more or less vegetarian fare. He gets understandably exasperated when queried on this point. "If you only ate meat and no vegetables at all," he is quoted as saying, "nobody would complain at all."

How true. It is absolutely amazing how deep feelings can run on matters as trivial as dietary preferences. But let's get back to the big, fast-food hamburger. We don't need to remind you that it is literally dripping with saturated animal fats and is super-high in cholesterol. So let's go right to the heart of the matter and talk about the *real* problem with hamburgers, a problem most people are completely unaware of.

Hamburgers, as well as hot dogs and sausages, are made from ground meat, and ground meat is particularly prone to self-oxidation. The meat-grinding process greatly increases the surface area exposed to oxygen. Grinding also breaks up the red blood cells, releasing copper and iron molecules that when mixed with fat act as catalysts to speed up the oxidation (peroxidation) of the fats.

It is this peroxidation that is so worrisome. You can actually watch it happening as the ground meat turns gray when exposed to the air.

The peroxidation is enhanced by the high heat of frying or grilling. In grilling, fats and proteins in the browning meat change into mutagenic or cancer-causing compounds. Any fat that drips onto the hot coals, or onto an electric heating element below the grill, compounds the problem by returning as carcinogenic smoke loaded with highly toxic, mutagenic, and carcinogenic chemicals called *polynuclear aromatic hydrocarbons,* and free radicals.

Now that more and more people are waking up to the dangers posed by the high-fat and high-cholesterol content of hamburgers (realizing the cancer risks from peroxidized fats and grilling may take a few more years), the meat industry is fighting back with ads and television commercials with such themes as "real food for real people." (People who don't eat red meat are, by inference, "unreal.")

One television commercial is particularly offensive. It features pencil-slim Hollywood actress Cybill Shepherd giving the following message: "People have an instinctive, primeval craving for hamburgers," she says with a meaningful expression. "I know there are people who don't eat 'burgers'—but I wouldn't trust them!" Well, the meat industry may regard us as "unreal" and "untrustworthy," but we simply cannot recommend eating hamburgers under any circumstances.

So much for hamburger—"the poor man's poison." Let's turn now to "the rich man's poison," caviar.

Another episode involving Jane Fonda comes to mind: a story in the *New York Daily News* of October 21, 1986, describing her lunch at the Russian Tea Room. There, we are told, she ate "a simple dish of beluga caviar" and nothing else—presumably, the article suggests, "for reasons of fitness."

Now, Jane Fonda, who is almost as famous a physical-fitness guru as she is a movie star, is inarguably health-conscious. If indeed she eats caviar, she must assume it is a good choice for health-conscious diners. She may also assume that whatever cholesterol content the caviar might contain (a great deal) would be more than offset by the cholesterol-fighting, omega-3 marine oils in which caviar also happens to be rich.

So far so good. The trouble is, even experts can overlook important little details. In caviar, those cholesterol-lowering fish oils are almost certain to be rancid (peroxidized), and hence full of free radicals, unless anti-oxidants are added.

Caviar is also very salty, both naturally and as a result of the salt added in processing. Now, Beluga caviar may not be a temptation for most of us, who can't afford it. But please keep in mind that everything we have said about genuine caviar (sturgeon roe) applies equally to its less expensive substitutes—black lumpfish roe, which looks like a miniaturized version of caviar, and the larger, pink-colored salmon eggs—both of which are often used in hors d'oeuvres in the United States.

The moral of the story? For Jane Fonda, it would seem, the next time she's at the Russian Tea Room, she'd better have the borscht. It's an excellent soup and has no cholesterol, provided you leave out the sour cream traditionally served with it.

CHAPTER 49

THE TRUTH ABOUT MILK AND CHEESE

*M*ilk is, and probably always will be, a controversial food. To some it is the "elixir of life"; to others, it's sheer poison. With such polarization of views, the truth has to be somewhere in between.

ON THE UPSIDE

Many nutritionists maintain that milk is a very complete, nearly perfect food. Milk contains thiamine (vitamin B_1) and niacin (vitamin B_3) in moderate amounts, and tryptophan, an amino acid that can act as a substitute for niacin, in very large amounts. Milk is also a good source of vitamin B_2, vitamin A, and vitamin D, though the latter vitamin is usually added during processing. A cup of cow's milk contains 8 grams of well-balanced protein, including the amino acid lysine. (Since lysine is not present in grains, milk forms a major part of the "nutritious breakfast" so familiar through advertising.) Because milk contains these other nutrients, it provides a better source of protein than meat.

A few years ago, much more sensational health claims were made for milk, and by highly reputable researchers at that. One of these studies, conducted by Dr. Cedric Garland and colleagues at the University of California at San Diego, analyzed the dietary histories of two thousand men over a twenty-year period and found that "risk of colorectal cancer was inversely correlated with dietary vitamin D and calcium" supplied from milk.[1]

Comparative studies from Scandinavia—where milk is not routinely fortified with vitamin D and where the vitamin D content therefore varies considerably, depending on the seasonal availability of sunshine—show that the apparent anticancer effect of milk remains fairly constant throughout the year. We cannot help but assume from this that any anticancer effect of milk must be mainly due to its calcium content and only to a lesser extent, if at all, to its vitamin D content. It is fairly well established, as said earlier, that calcium can bind to the free bile acids in the colon and convert them to insoluble calcium soaps,[2] which can be eliminated with the feces.

Precisely for these reasons, the Demopoulos spectrum of anti-oxidants and vitamin co-factors provides just the right amounts of calcium and vitamin D, and does so in a reliable, steady manner. That's how we prefer getting these nutrients, without having to worry about the negative properties of milk.

It has also been claimed by some researchers that certain E2-type prostaglandins have a protective effect on gastric ulcers[3] (see our discussion in the chapter on gastrointestinal disorders, page 270). However, one would have to judge each case on its own merits, weighing the possible anti-ulcer benefits of the prostaglandins against the atherosclerotic liability of the saturated milk fat and possible allergy problems caused by milk proteins. Remember, too, that some prostaglandins can suppress the immune system.

Very interesting, too, are the findings of Dr. Robert Yolken, a medical researcher at Johns Hopkins University Medical School, Baltimore, that cow's milk contains antibodies that can protect infants and young children against common gastroenteritis and dangerous diarrhea caused by rotavirus infections.[4] The good news is that such antibodies were found in both raw and pasteurized milk, the form in which it is usually sold to prevent contamination with harmful microorganisms. The bad news is that young infants usually have trouble digesting cow's milk and may get violent diarrhea from it. Yogurt, on the other hand, is much better tolerated and has even higher antibacterial activity, a matter to which we shall return presently.

It is because so many infants cannot digest either whole or low-fat milk that soya-milk–based infant formulas were developed. But, as is well known, many infants cannot tolerate soya-milk–based formulas either and must be put on still other formulas.

It would be good if all those infants who can tolerate milk-based formulas could benefit from the antibodies aimed at harmful bacteria and viruses. Unfortunately, Dr. Yolken discovered that the heat used in processing milk for the formulas is too high for the antibody molecules to survive, and, therefore, the formulas provide no such protection. For this reason, Dr. Yolken suggests that "efforts should be directed at the production of milk preparations suitable for human infants that contain sufficient levels of anti-rotavirus antibody."[5] This, he says, could be accomplished either by changing the processing methods, or by adding antibodies with rotavirus activity to infant formulas.

ON THE DOWNSIDE

It's good to know that milk can provide various health benefits. Unfortunately, milk also poses a number of very serious health hazards to both children and adults.

First, a large percentage of the world's population (5 to 20 percent of whites, 80 to 100 percent of nonwhites[6]) cannot digest milk because the enzyme lactase is not present in the small intestine. Lactase is used to break down lactose, the carbohydrate of milk sugar, into simpler sugar molecules that the body can absorb. In the absence of lactase, consumption of milk and cheese can lead to gastrointestinal infections and inflammatory bowel disease. Lactase deficiency can be acquired over time, leading to "mysterious" gastrointestinal problems later in life.

Whole milk is the single largest source of saturated fat in the American diet. That problem can be circumvented by substituting the popular low-fat types of milk, but a rabbit study showed that the cholesterol-raising effect of skim milk approximately equals that of whole egg.[7]

Skim milk also has more allergenic proteins than whole milk. In fact, one medical scientist, Dr. James S. Koopman, at the University of Michigan's School of Public Health, thinks that a sizable percentage of infant gastroenteritis is due to mothers giving their children low-fat milk[8] in the mistaken belief that what is good for adults must be good for children as well. Worst affected, he says, are one- to two-year-olds—an age group where concerns about high-fat and cholesterol content are certainly misplaced!

What many people don't realize is that reducing the fat content of milk raises its concentrations of casein and other allergy- and atherosclerosis-causing proteins proportionately. And although casein and the other hard-to-digest milk proteins are not present in great quantities in whole milk (only 2.8 percent casein), they can still cause allergic reactions and even to contribute to atherosclerosis.[9]

True, there is a Japanese study on rabbits that led the researchers to feel that skim milk has a "preventive effect" on high blood cholesterol and atherosclerosis.[10] However, the overwhelming body of scientific evidence is to the contrary. For example, a group of Australian researchers, who also used rabbits for their study, observed that when the animals were fed a diet containing casein as the only protein, they developed excessively high cholesterol levels and atherosclerosis.[11] Similarly, Dr. David Kritchevsky has pointed out that casein has been found to be more atherogenic for rabbits than soy protein (regardless of what kind of fiber is included in the diet).[12] Further, casein seems to accelerate the kinds of changes in lipid metabolism that normally occur with aging.[13,14] Therefore, it is highly unlikely that the casein in milk would behave differently from the pure casein used in the cited studies.

So much for the controversy about the effect of milk on blood lipids (fats). Among the allergic reactions that milk can provoke are diarrhea, vomiting, and abdominal pain. (The abdominal pain often starts as much as an hour after milk has been drunk and is therefore usually attributed to other causes.) Other allergic reactions can affect the respiratory tract in ways ranging from inflammation of the nasal mucous membrane to bronchitis and pneumonia. Some children are so allergic to milk that their lips and tongues swell within minutes of taking a drink, while others may break out in hives (urticaria).

In these dramatic cases, it is easy to make the connection between cause and effect. In most instances, however, the link is far less obvious. Many parents—even highly intelligent and sophisticated ones—often tell us they frankly never thought of milk allergies being the cause of their baby's prolonged crying spells and typical flexing of the thighs during the first three months of life. Even fewer parents guess that an older child's frequent "tummy aches," which seem to come out of nowhere, could actually be due to drinking milk.[15]

Other reactions to milk may involve the respiratory tract—rhinitis (inflammation of the nasal mucous membrane), excess mucus in the throat and nasal passages, difficulty in breathing during sleep, chronic cough and throat-clearing (as in "smoker's cough"), frequent attacks of bronchitis, or even pneumonia, as well as such typical allergies as sinusitis and asthma. Here, again, milk is usually not suspected as being the culprit by the parents, by the affected people, or by physicians.

The principal cause of these allergic reactions is the milk protein beta-lactoglobulin, although casein and albumin and a couple of rarer proteins also play a part. But lactoglobulin, not easily broken down by either heat or the body's enzymes, is now definitely considered "the most allergenic of the milk proteins."[16]

It has been our experience that many asthmatics have fewer and less severe attacks if they abstain from milk and milk products. While not saying that all cases of severe and persistent bronchitis in children are due to milk allergies, we have seen "miraculous" cures by taking them off milk, cheeses, and ice cream.

In addition to problems inherent in the milk itself, even pasteurized milk can often contain contaminants. Dr. Dean D. Metcalfe, of the National Institutes of Health, Bethesda, Maryland, has found milk from cattle to be contaminated with bacitracin, penicillin, and tetracycline used to treat bovine diseases.[17] Cattle can sometimes feed on a common, toxic bracken fern. Milk from these cattle can produce moderate to severe symptoms, depending on how much the toxic substance is concentrated in the milk. This contamination is less of a problem in the United States, where most milk comes from large dairy farms on which cattle do not graze wild. But the problem can be significant in rural areas of Europe, Central and South America, Africa, and other third-world areas. In Costa Rica, for example, we do occasionally have cases of cattle dying from eating too much bracken fern, which grows abundantly at higher elevations, and of people getting violently ill from drinking milk containing significant levels of the toxic compound in this plant.

THE BOTTOM LINE

Milk can, for the first two years of life, provide a good source of nutrients for those children who are able to digest milk properly and are not subject to milk allergies. However, we do not recommend using either whole milk or skim milk in adult nutrition. There is only one shining exception: yogurt. We shall discuss this matter in Chapter 58.

THE TROUBLE WITH CHEESES

Because cheese is a highly concentrated form of milk (about ten pounds of milk go into one pound of cheese), all the problems associated with milk are present in exaggerated form in cheeses. For example, the fat content of whole milk is only 3.8 percent, while that of Cheddar cheese is 38 percent, or ten times that amount. Some cheeses have an even higher butterfat content as well as potentially troublesome milk proteins.

Nevertheless, many people seem to be able to digest cheeses without any apparent difficulty; others may have all kinds of problems. Most affected are those using antidepressant drugs of the monoamine oxidase inhibitor (MAOI) type.[18] They tend to develop hypertensive attacks, sometimes after eating only small amounts of cheese. The reason is that tyramine, a compound in cheese, steps up activity of the sympathetic nervous system and stimulates the same neurotransmitters that these drugs stimulate. The resulting overstimulation of the nervous system can lead to headaches, palpitations, nausea, and dangerous rises in blood pressure that can produce stroke.*[19]

* People on MAOI medication should be aware of other foods with a high tyramine content, such as pickled herring, chicken livers, broad beans, Chianti wines, and beer. Even without the presence of MAOI, cheeses have been known to trigger headaches, but because the

Cheeses are subject to contamination by *Listeria* bacteria, though this is less prevalent with common processed cheeses. The problem becomes much greater with hand-produced gourmet cheeses, which are generally made from raw, unpasteurized milk. Especially vulnerable seems to be a velvety, soft variety called Vacherin Mont d'Or, which we remember well, and not without a touch of nostalgia, from our days in France.

But Vacherin Mont d'Or is not the only fine cheese to occasionally be found contaminated by *Listeria*. In 1987, the Swiss discovered these bacteria in two dozen other types of cheeses. That's not good news because *Listeria* attacks the central nervous system. And even though such contamination occurs only very rarely, this would be of little comfort to those who become affected.

Quite aside from such special problems, cheeses in general have too many drawbacks to be included on any truly health-conscious diet: There are the high-fat and high-salt problems, the casein, the possible contaminants and, last but not least, the fact that the fatty acids in cheese are likely to be peroxidized and loaded with free radicals as a result of the aging that gives different cheeses their specific flavors.

HUMAN MILK VERSUS COW'S MILK

Breast-feeding has been growing more popular in recent years. The number of newborns who start breast-feeding at the hospital is now 60 percent, almost twice as many as in 1970. But encouraging as this statistic is, almost half of all babies are still being given formulas from birth. By two months, more than half (55 percent) are on either straight formula or a combination of formula and mother's milk; and by six months this figure rises to 75 percent. Similar trends are found throughout the rest of the world (except for Israel, the Soviet Union, and China) and for many of the same reasons—working mothers, beauty consciousness, shame over nursing in public, and a lack of awareness that breast-feeding is superior to formulas.

For although formulas have grown increasingly sophisticated through the years, they are still not fit substitutes for mother's milk unless the mother is ill, or is malnourished, as in some underdeveloped countries. Breast milk contains less saturated fat and more bile acids than cow's milk and formulas, which makes it easier to digest. Breast-fed children also receive an enzyme (lipase), not present in formulas, that helps

headaches often occur many hours after the consumption of the cheese, the connection between the two is missed.

break down the fats in the milk and make them more easily digestible.[20] Breast milk also contains more cholesterol than cow's milk or formulas—an advantage because the only time high cholesterol levels are needed is in the early stages of growth.

Breast milk contains higher concentrations of vitamin C, several B vitamins, and a special, water-soluble form of vitamin D, which is otherwise soluble only in fats. It also contains two important natural antibiotics—lactoferrin and immunoglobulin A, which help protect the infant from disease. A breast-fed baby also automatically receives all its mother's antibodies against a large number of harmful bacteria and viruses. Furthermore, breast-feeding leads naturally to the development of a benign intestinal flora due to the *Lactobacilli bifidi* in mother's milk, which keeps undesirable bacteria at a minimum.[21]

Another recently discovered nutrient, taurine, is present in appreciable amounts in mother's milk. Taurine, naturally synthesized in the body from cystine, has been found useful in synthesizing bile acids. The effects of a shortage of taurine, while not fully understood, are known to include several shifts in metabolism, which may have an adverse effect on vision.[22]

However, it's not only what is *in* mother's milk that makes it so superior, but also what is *not* in it—like the allergenic beta-lactoglobulin of cow's milk.

Finally, breast milk seems to adjust its composition incredibly to the changing nutritional needs of the infant from shortly after birth to weaning. The mother's body even adjusts the composition of the milk during a single feeding: The first milk is much more watery, containing less fat and protein, than at the end of a feed. That means the breast-fed baby is getting the right amount of nutrients at the right time. This neat mechanism functions even as a built-in appetite control—something impossible to duplicate in any other way.

Despite all the well-established advantages of breast-feeding, the majority of pediatricians passively acquiesce to many mothers' wishes not to breast-feed their babies, regardless of the fact that there are valid medical reasons for doing so. Nor, in most instances, are the advantages of breast-feeding thoroughly explained to mothers.

And yet anthropologists like the late Margaret Mead[23] who have observed breast-feeding in other societies have told us for the last thirty or more years about the physical and mental-emotional benefits of breast-feeding well beyond the first year of life. One can only hope that more women in the industrialized world will wake up to these facts.

SOURCES

1. Garland, C., et al. "Dairy vitamin D and calcium and risk of colorectal cancer: a 19-year prospective study in men." *Lancet,* February 9, 1985, 307–309.

2. Newmark H. L., M. J. Wargovich, and W. R. Bruce. "Colon cancer and dietary fat, phosphate, and calcium: a hypothesis." *J. Natl. Cancer Inst.*, 1984; 72:1323–1325.
3. Materia, A., et al. "Prostaglandins in commercial milk preparations: their effect in the prevention of stress-induced gastric ulcer." *Arch. Surg.*, March 1984; 119:290–292.
4. Yolken, R. H., et al. "Antibody to human rotavirus in cow's milk." *N. Eng. J. Med.*, 1985; 312(10):605–610.
5. Ibid., p. 609.
6. Metcalfe, D. D. "Food hypersensitivity." *J. Allergy and Clin. Immunol.*, June 1984; 73(6):755.
7. Texter, E. C., Jr. *The Aging Gut.* New York: Masson Publications, 1983.
8. Koopman, J. S. "Milk fat and gastrointestinal illness." *Am. J. Pub. Health.* December 1984; 74:1371–1373.
9. Kanhai, J., D. D. Kitts, and W. D. Powrie. "Temporal changes in serum cholesterol levels of rats fed casein and skim milk powdered diets." *J. Food Sci.*, 1987; 52(5):1410–1412.
10. Kiyosawa, H., et al. "Effects of skim milk and yogurt on serum lipids, development of atherosclerosis and excretion of fecal sterols in cholesterol-fed rabbits." *Sapporo Med. J.*, 1984; 53(5):493–504.
11. Allotta, E. C., S. Samman, and D.C.K. Roberts. "The importance of the non-protein components of the diet in the plasma cholesterol response of rabbits to casein." *Brit. J. Nutr.*, 1985; 54:87–94.
12. Kritchevsky, David. "Fiber, lipids, and atherosclerosis." *Am. J. Clin. Nutr.*, October 1978; 31:S65–S74.
13. Carroll, K. K., and R.M.G. Hamilton. "Effects of dietary protein and carbohydrate in plasma cholesterol levels in relation to atherosclerosis." *J. Food Sci.*, 1975; 4018–4023.
14. Terpstra, A.H.M., R.J.J. Hermus, and C. E. West. "Dietary protein and cholesterol metabolism in rabbits and rats." In: *Animal and Vegetable Proteins in Lipid Metabolism and Atherosclerosis,* J. J. Gibney and D. Kritchevsky, eds. Also: *Current Topics in Nutrition and Disease,* 8:19–49. New York: Alan R. Liss, Inc., 1982.
15. Kulczycki, A., Jr., and Richard P. MacDermott. "Adverse reactions to food and eosinophilic gastroenteritis." In: *Gastrointestinal Immunity for the Clinician.* New York: Grune & Stratton, 1985, p. 132.
16. Metcalf, op. cit., p. 754.
17. Ibid., p. 755.
18. *Present Knowledge in Nutrition.* Washington, D. C.: The Nutrition Foundation, Inc., 1984, p. 808.
19. Gettis, A. "Serendipity and food sensitivity." *Headache,* February 1987, 27(2):74.
20. Linder, M. C. *Nutritional Biochemistry and Metabolism.* New York: Elsevier, 1985, p. 269.
21. Nutrition Committee of the Canadian Paediatric Society and the Committee on Nutrition of the American Academy of Pediatrics. "Breast-Feeding." *Pediatrics,* 1978; 62(4):594.
22. Hayes, K. C., R. E. Carey, and S. Y. Schmidt. "Retinal degeneration associated with taurine deficiency in the cat." *Science,* 1975; 188:949–951.
23. Mead, Margaret. *From the South Seas; Studies of Adolescence and Sex in Primitive Societies* and *Coming of Age in Samoa.* New York: William Morrow & Company, 1939.

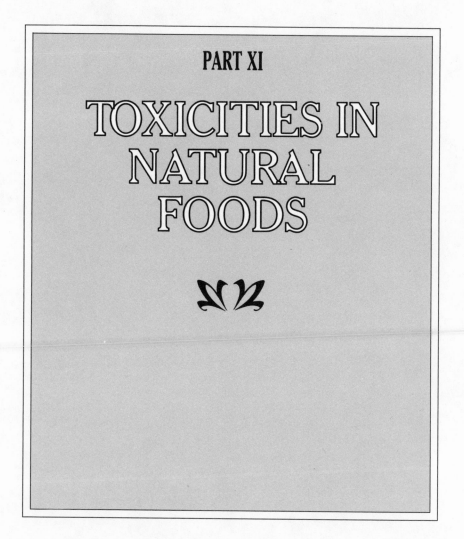

PART XI

TOXICITIES IN NATURAL FOODS

12 There is a growing movement among health-conscious people towards natural foods—those grown, preserved, and prepared without man-made chemicals. The movement is most visible in the proliferation of health-food stores, magazines devoted to organic gardening, and even in the (often misleading) use of the word "natural" in advertising processed foods. It may shock members of the natural-foods movement to find out that even the most pesticide-free, organically grown foods produce chemicals that are, in many instances, as toxic, mutagenic, or carcinogenic as any man-made pesticide and herbicide residues in foods—in fact, sometimes many times more so.[1] These "homemade" chemicals are the plants' own natural pesticides, produced by them as a defense against insects, fungi, and even small predators.

Do not be unduly alarmed: Dr. James Duke, chief of the Germplasm Resources Laboratory of the U.S. Department of Agriculture (USDA), thinks that our immune systems must have built up a tolerance to most of these naturally occurring toxins over millions of years of evolution.[2] Since man-made toxins have only been around for a few decades, they may therefore, Dr. Duke persuasively argues, pose a larger risk simply because of their novelty,* even though, in the usual concentrations in which they are found in foods, they may be no more and often much less potentially harmful than the natural toxins.

Even Dr. Bruce Ames, head of the Department of Biochemistry of the University of California at Berkeley, who has, perhaps more than anyone, warned us against toxicities in natural foods, also stresses that the carcinogenic, mutagenic, or otherwise toxic effects of certain compounds in natural plant foods are, in all probability, free-radical–mediated and can therefore be counteracted by anti-oxidants. For one thing, we would say, the natural anti-oxidants that abound in these plant foods should to a large extent be able to neutralize and

---

* Keep in mind, though, that some common foods, like potatoes, which were introduced into the American-European diet only a couple of hundred years ago, or coffee (introduced about four hundred years ago), have hardly been around long enough for our bodies to have gotten used to or develop adequate defenses against their known toxicities.

override the carcinogens or toxic effects. If not, how has the human race survived?

Furthermore, one has to keep in mind that the toxic or carcinogenic effects of potentially harmful substances in many vegetables, herbs, spices, and fruits is strictly dose-dependent. In other words, the anti-oxidants and our own bodies' defenses should be able to neutralize them if we ingest them in relatively small quantities.* Nevertheless, we feel that the health-conscious public should be forewarned about any inadvertent overconsumption of these substances.

Let us then take an unbiased look at some natural foods that contain substantial amounts of toxins—or carcinogens, as the case may be—and that you have probably never suspected of being anything but benign.

MUSHROOMS

Of course, everybody knows that some wild mushrooms are highly poisonous. But who would have thought that even the white *champignons* you buy in the supermarket—to say nothing of the many delicious edible wild mushrooms sold in Europe—have powerful toxins too?†

Practically all mushrooms—particularly the ones most popular in America, the white champignon (*Agaricus bisporus*) and the "false morel" (*Gyromitra esculenta*), and probably the ones that are most popular in Europe too—have varying amounts of toxic and usually mutagenic or carcinogenic compounds in them. Foremost among these substances are the mushroom hydrazines, including a compound called *agaritine.* These substances have been studied in great depth by University of Nebraska scientist Dr. Bela Toth, who is considered the world's leading expert in this field.[3]

Fortunately, Dr. Toth tells us, most of the hydrazines—but only 50 percent of the agaritine—are destroyed by cooking. The latter finding is important, for agaritine is present in appreciable amounts of 45 milligrams per mushroom, in the white champignon. The worrisome part about all of this, as Dr. Bruce Ames says, is that when agaritine is eaten, it is distributed in the body tissues, where it is converted to a highly reactive, mutagenic metabolite (a diazonium compound) that studies have found caused stomach tumors in mice at disturbingly low doses.

---

* Those who are on an effective anti-oxidant program need be even less concerned about the possible carcinogens and other toxic substances in natural foods.
† In a personal communication, Dr. Toth told us of a Swedish researcher who analyzed forty-eight edible European mushroom varieties and found two thirds were mutagenic.

HOW SAFE ARE JAPANESE *SHIITAKE* MUSHROOMS?

What about those expensive Japanese *shiitake* mushrooms that are supposed to have antiviral effects and protect their happy eaters from certain cancers, as some Japanese scientists claim?* Don't they contain carcinogenic hydrazines too? Dr. Toth tells us an interesting story about these mushrooms, of which the Japanese are so fond. The shiitake that are grown commercially in Japan in the traditional manner (that is, on logs), and take eighteen months to mature, do indeed have hydrazines. However, those experimentally grown in a totally different manner by researchers in California, and which take only six months to mature, do not seem to contain any hydrazines. So there's hope that in the near future we may be able to enjoy safe, California-grown shiitake!

What then are we to make of the alleged anticancer properties of shiitake in view of the fact that they also contain cancer-promoting hydrazines? Well, the fact that they contain dangerous hydrazines does not necessarily mean that these potentially cancer-causing substances cannot also attack cancer cells, as do many highly toxic man-made chemicals used for cancer treatment.

WHAT ABOUT THE CHINESE BLACK TREE FUNGUS?

There is research on the Chinese black or brown tree fungus (*Auricularia polytricha*), popularly called *mo-er* or *mok yhee* ("tree ear") in Chinese, showing that its ingestion inhibits blood platelet aggregation. In Chinese cuisine, especially Cantonese, it is used in many dishes, particularly in a Cantonese specialty, a hot spicy bean-curd dish called *Ma-po dou-fu*.

It is undoubtedly because of its inhibiting effect on platelet aggregation that this tree fungus has gained its reputation in Chinese folk medicine for being "good for you," for extending life, and that "it thins the blood." For the latter reason, it has been used traditionally by Chinese women to prevent postpartum thrombophlebitis

* One group of scientists is from the Department of Microbiology, Kobe University School of Medicine, and the Mushroom Research Institute of Japan in Kiryu City (M. Takehara et al., "Isolation and antiviral activities of the double-stranded RNA from Lentinus edodes [Shiitake]," *Kobe J. Med. Sci.*, 1984; 30:34–35). Another group, from the Faculty of Pharmaceutical Sciences, Toyama Medical and Pharmaceutical University, Sugitani, Toyoma, Japan, studied this mushroom and found that extracts from shiitake suppressed cell proliferation in liver tissue of experimental rats and "significantly raised the survival rate" of rats with liver cancer (N. Sugano et al., "Anticarcinogenic actions of water-soluble and alcohol-insoluble fractions from culture medium of Lentinus edodes mycelia," *Cancer Lett.*, 1982; 17:109–114).

(blood clots).* By the same token, mo-er can be expected to have a protective effect with regard to stroke, atherosclerosis, and heart disease.†

What we don't know—and even Dr. Bela Toth cannot tell at this point—is what medical risks might accompany the apparently protective effects of the tree fungus with respect to cardiovascular diseases. The problem is that it is still not known whether mo-er contains carcinogenic hydrazines and, if so, in what concentrations.

We would also like to remind the reader of the similarly "blood-thinning" effect of hot chili peppers (Capsicum), which have both protective and carcinogenic effects. The Chinese bean-curd dish Ma-po dou-fu therefore would combine the blood-thinning effect of a substance (adenosine?) in the tree fungus with the capsaicin from the hot chili peppers, a fact which seems to have been overlooked.

Do we ourselves eat Chinese tree fungus? Sure, occasionally we do put a few into a salad, soup, or vegetable dish—just as we like to spike up our food with cayenne or hot chili peppers. But we don't do it to thin our blood—for that, we take pure liquid vitamin E and anti-oxidant–protected fish oils—but for purely culinary reasons.

OTHER EXOTIC MUSHROOMS

Nobody knows for sure what properties are contained in the white, stringy Japanese mushroom *enoki,* which has aficionados also in the United States, and is reputed to "strengthen the immune system." Or take the Japanese oyster mushroom (*Pleurotus sajor-caju*), which apparently has a scientifically established hypotensive (blood-pressure-lowering) effect, as well as the ability to improve kidney function.[4] If such is the case—and indications are that it is—it would be extremely important to know about any coexisting toxicities or

---

* Scientists Amar N. Makheja and J. Martyn Bailey of George Washington University have suggested that the inhibition of platelet aggregation following ingestion of the Chinese black tree fungus is probably due to the presence of *adenosine,* which they isolated in extracts of the fungus, and which is known to inhibit platelet aggregation (*N. Eng. J. Med.,* 1981; 304(3):175).

† Dr. Dale E. Hammerschmidt of the University of Minnesota School of Medicine, who first researched mo-er, feels that its inhibiting effect on platelet aggregation might be partly responsible for the low incidence of coronary artery disease in China in general and the southern Chinese provinces in particular (*N. Eng. J. Med.,* 1980; 302(21):1191–1193). However, as we pointed out elsewhere, the Chinese diet is relatively low in overall fat content and high in complex carbohydrates, for which reason alone it is less likely to clog arteries than the typical American-European diet.

carcinogens in the oyster mushroom as it is more nutritious than most others.* However, as of this writing, there is no such information.

THE BOTTOM LINE ON MUSHROOMS

Where does this leave us with respect to eating or not eating mushrooms? We asked Dr. Bela Toth whether he was still eating them. "Well," he answered. "I happen to be very fond of white champignons. But after seeing the huge tumors, including tumors of the bones, in our experimental mice that were fed these mushrooms, I'm too scared to eat them anymore. The worst thing," he added, "is that in the United States people eat these mushrooms raw in salads, while in Europe, they are mostly eaten cooked, which is, of course, much safer." He also won't eat the other most widely eaten mushroom in the United States, the "false morel." The reason? He has found eleven hydrazines in the false morel, three of which are known carcinogens.†

As for us, we certainly won't put white champignons into our salads like we used to. On the other hand, when we eat at friends' homes or in restaurants, we won't make a fuss over a few cooked champignons in the sauce. Another thing we won't do anymore is to devour a whole plate of wild mushrooms, as we used to do frequently in France during the fall mushroom season. And we won't fly to Tokyo to eat fresh shiitake for their possible antiviral and cancer-preventing effects, or to give our immune systems a boost—there are better, safer ways of doing that with anti-oxidants.

However, we don't mind using small quantities of any dried mushrooms, whether Chinese, Japanese, or European, to flavor a dish and make it more interesting. The point is that, fortunately, we can get all these exotic mushrooms here only in dried form. They first have to be soaked for some time, after which the water is discarded, hopefully carrying with it some of the hydrazines. More hydrazines will subsequently be destroyed in cooking or sautéing the mushrooms, so that the final count of these hazardous natural chemicals is probably too low to pose much of a risk. But we don't kid ourselves that they would

---

* *Pleurotus sajor-caju* contains substantial amounts of protein, carbohydrate, fat, minerals, and vitamins.

† Gyromitrin, present in large amounts in these mushrooms (500 parts per million, dry weight), is not only a particularly potent carcinogen in mice but, Dr. Bruce Ames tells us, has recently been shown to "massively alkylate" the genetic code-carrying DNA of rats. Alkylation is the substitution of a certain (alkyl) type of free radical for an active hydrogen atom in an organic compound—in this case, the rat's DNA—suggesting equally massive, free-radical–initiated genetic mutation.

add a single day to our life span, strengthen our immune system, or "cure" anything.

TOMATOES

Tomatoes are rich in vitamin C, have some of the B vitamins, and, while not particularly high in beta-carotene, seem to be high in another carotenoid called *lycopene*, which may have the same anticancer properties beta-carotene has. While all this makes tomatoes basically highly desirable and health-promoting, you should be aware that they also contain the same mutagenic compound (dicarbonyl aldehyde methylglyoxal) that has been isolated in coffee.[5,6]

Still, eating raw or cooked tomatoes in the small quantities in which they are normally consumed should cause no problems; rather the opposite. There is, however, one thing to keep in mind: The mutagen methylglyoxal is present in much higher concentrations in tomato purée than in whole tomatoes. When using tomato purée for sauce, you should take care not to use too much of it, otherwise the health-endangering properties of tomatoes might overpower the health-protective ones.

CELERY

Celery belongs to a family of plants (umbelliferae) that produce potent, light-activated chemicals called *psoralens*. Psoralens have been shown by Dr. Ames to be potential carcinogens and mutagens.[7] Fortunately, healthy celery plants contain them in such low concentrations that they do not pose a health risk. However, if the celery is injured or attacked by fungus, the psoralen level can rise a hundredfold, to the point where it does become a problem (plenty of celery on the market is already over the hill or damaged).

As in the case of the toxins in mushrooms, those in celery are leached out by cooking. But this does not help the thousands who eat celery raw, often as part of a high-fiber, low-calorie diet. Choose only healthy, unbruised celery and eat only moderate amounts. Those seeking a vegetable high in fiber and low in calories may want to substitute raw carrots for celery, since carrots are not only free of psoralens but they are also lower in sodium.

POTATOES

Potatoes are, on the whole, a healthful and highly nourishing food, well deserving of their historic place in human nutrition (see Chapter 57, pages 440–444). However, potatoes contain two potent glyco-alkaloids, solanine and chaconine, both well-known toxins (cholinesterase inhibitors) that can interfere with the transmission of nerve impulses. Moreover, according to Dr. Bruce Ames, they are present in high enough concentrations as not to leave much safety margin for humans.[8] In fact, there have been isolated cases of serious potato poisoning among people and farm animals. Furthermore, solanine and chaconine are not destroyed by cooking, and, as in the case of celery, damaged or diseased potatoes may contain unacceptable levels of these toxins.

Above all, do not eat the potato skins, since they contain high concentrations of the toxins. We wish especially to stress this point, since many dietitians and dieters are under the impression that the skin is the healthiest part of the potato, rich in vitamins and minerals. There are even restaurants that serve fried potato skins to customers who are anxious to lose weight. In fact, the vitamins are not in the skin but right underneath it, and the only mineral present in high concentrations is selenium, which we can get from other sources. The risks involved in eating potato skins simply outweigh the advantages. Fried potato skins with sour cream and bacon filling is a real "time bomb." Many restaurants serve them with a variety of other dangerous fillings.

Sweet potatoes, normally full of vitamins and rich in beta-carotene, can also be highly toxic if moldy or damaged. Even minor blemishes or discolorations below the skin can lead to the development of at least four toxins, including the potent liver toxin ipomeamarone.

Should you stop eating yams and sweet potatoes then? By no means. These highly nutritional starchy vegetables also contain proven health-promoting and cancer-inhibiting substances like beta-carotene, vitamin C, and B vitamins. Their beneficial effects in healthy, undamaged sweet potatoes far outweigh any negative factors. The only thing is, be careful to use only healthy, unblemished potatoes and sweet potatoes. If you do, you'll have nothing to worry about.

CANCER-CAUSING SUBSTANCES IN NATURAL FOODS

Dr. Bruce N. Ames and co-workers at the University of California at Berkeley have devised a way of judging the relative toxicities of many foodstuffs. Their index is based on the known cancer-causing potential of these substances with laboratory animals. They then transposed their findings to reasonable estimates of the effects of the toxins if applied to humans. The toxicity rankings are expressed in terms of so many HERP; the higher the HERP value, the greater the expected cancer risk for humans.

HERP (%)	SUBSTANCE	CARCINOGEN
0.001	Tap water, 1 quart	Chloroform
0.03	Comfrey herb tea, 1 cup	Symphytine
0.06	Diet cola (12 ounces)	Saccharin
2.7	Regular cola (12 ounces)	Formaldehyde, etc.
2.8	Beer (12 ounces)	Ethyl alcohol
4.7	Wine (8 ounces)	Ethyl alcohol
0.003	Bacon, cooked (3½ ounces)	Dimethylnitrosamine
0.03	Peanut butter (1 ounce)	Aflatoxin
0.1	Basil (1 gram of dried leaf)	Estragole
0.1	Mushroom, 1 raw	Hydrazines
0.09	Shrimp (3 ounces)	Formaldehyde
0.06	Fish (or, anything else, cooked in gas oven)	Nitropyrenes and nitrosamines from the gas

ALFALFA SPROUTS

Ask the average person to name the first health food that comes to mind and chances are it will be alfalfa sprouts. To our, and probably many other people's, minds, the name conjures up images of vegetarian sandwiches piled high with them, and falling off faster than you can get them into your mouth.

We can't get very excited about alfalfa sprouts, because of the way they clump together in salads and the fact that they don't have much taste. But they do contain a good mixture of micronutrients, such as vitamins A, C, and E, and the anti-oxidants ferulic acid and quercetin. Unfortunately, they also contain a highly mutagenic arginine analog, canavanine,[9] which makes them somewhat less of a perfect health food than many people think. For instance, when monkeys are fed alfalfa sprouts, they develop a severe lupus erythematosus-like syndrome for which scientists think canavanine is responsible.[10] Since lupus in man is considered a typical immune-deficiency disease, it is thought that the canavanine in the sprouts is producing oxygen radicals, which are known to alter and suppress the immune system.[11]

Aside from all that, besides being a protective anti-oxidant the quercetin in alfalfa is also a mutagen, according to Dr. Ames. He cites a study on two strains of laboratory rats that makes one suspect it is a carcinogen too, although other studies provide contradictory evidence.[12] (Here's a good example of how the same compounds can sometimes have both desirable anti-oxidant and undesirable toxic, mutagenic, or carcinogenic characteristics, depending largely on the quantities involved.)

On the other hand, Dr. Jim Duke of the USDA says that alfalfa leaves also contain the anti-oxidant and detoxifier glutathione, as do soybean leaves.[13] In fact, Dr. Duke seems to agree with our earlier observation that stressed or injured plants produce higher concentrations of glutathione, which we think is the reason why insects flock to such plants and gorge themselves on them. In some cases, however, as with bruised or damaged celery, potatoes, and sweet potatoes, the alfalfa plants simultaneously produce even more insect and fungus-repellent toxins than glutathione, thereby making them undesirable for human consumption.

COMFREY

Many health-conscious people have in recent years switched from coffee and black tea to herb teas. That's something to be applauded—not just because of the caffeine in coffee and similar compounds, theophylline in tea and theobromine in cacao—but especially because coffee contains methylglyoxal, which has been shown to be mutagenic and carcinogenic in mice.

The only trouble is that far too many people are drinking herb teas like comfrey tea, which is every bit as bad as, if not worse than, coffee. (Another dubious alternative to coffee is sassafras tea, drunk traditionally in parts of the American South.)

Comfrey, however, is by far the worst offender. Dr. Bruce Ames laments that the health-conscious public is so obsessed with man-made pesticides that some of the more dangerous natural compounds in plants like comfrey are not recognized for the poison weeds they are. The comfrey plant contains symphytine and symglandine, which are pyrrolizidine alkaloids that have been shown to produce lesions in the liver and malignant tumors in animals.[14]

If you drink a cup or two of comfrey tea, it's probably no worse than drinking the same amount of coffee. The real problem is that many people have been sold on taking comfrey pills or capsules, which are sometimes made from the leaves and sometimes from the roots of the comfrey plant, and the concentration of these toxins is many times higher in pills that are made from comfrey roots than in those made from comfrey leaves. Dr. Ames assigns a cancer-risk factor (HERP) of 6.2 for a daily dose of nine tablets made from comfrey roots, by far the highest of any of the many potentially carcinogenic substances in natural foods he has tested.[15]

Let us repeat: The alkaloids in comfrey leaves and the roots are toxic to the liver, where they are metabolized, as well as carcinogenic (cancer causing) in all animal studies done so far. There have even been reported cases of a rare venocclusive liver disease resulting from taking comfrey tablets in regular daily dosages. In one well-documented case, a woman had been taking two comfrey-pepsin tablets, prepared from comfrey leaves, per meal for four months and came down with serious liver disease.[16] At that point, the medical experts estimated, she had taken a total of 85 milligrams of comfrey alkaloids—the equivalent of taking the same number of tablets made from comfrey *roots* for only nine days, instead of the four months with the weaker leaf preparation.

We cannot resist relating a personal incident involving comfrey tablets. While shopping in a large New York health-food store, we overheard a salesperson counsel a customer to take comfrey pills. We waited till the sale had been made and the customer was gone to approach the young man who had so enthusiastically recommended the comfrey preparation. We told him briefly about the health hazards involved in taking comfrey pills, and, to make him take us more seriously, identified ourselves as health professionals who had studied these matters in some depth.

None of that impressed this young man. Not even our offer to let him read several scientific studies on the subject so he could see for himself that what we were saying was backed up by serious research.* This

---

* In addition to Dr. Bruce Ames's more general research studies on toxicities in natural foods, the following are some of the specific studies we would have recommended that the young man read: J. Brauchli et al., "Pyrrolizidine alkaloids from *Symphytum officinale L.* and their percutaneous absorption in rats," *Experientia,* 1982; 38:1085–1087; C.C.J. Culvenor et al., "Structure and toxicity of the alkaloids of Russian comfrey (*Symphytum uplandicum Nyman*), a medicinal herb and item of human diet," *Experientia* 1980; 36:377–379; I. Hirono et al., "Carcinogenic activity of *Symphytum officinale,*" *J. Natl. Cancer Inst.,* 1978; 61:865–869; I. Hirono et al., "Induction of hepatic tumors in rats by senkirkine and symphitine," *J. Natl. Cancer Inst.,* 1979; 63:469–471.

didn't cut any ice either. What science had to say about these things didn't matter to him, he said. He "knew" he had a "personal affinity" for comfrey, drank several cups of comfrey tea every day, and "could just feel its detoxifying power." That's when we decided to give up. How can you reason with so much un-reason?

MOLD-PRODUCED TOXINS

In addition to toxins produced by vegetables themselves, several potent carcinogens (mycotoxins and aflatoxins) are produced by molds that can attack vegetables and grains. Wheat, corn, beans, lentils, and rye are all subject to a variety of *Aspergillus* molds, which produce a powerful liver carcinogen, mycotoxin B_1. This mycotoxin presents a larger problem than usual because it is not destroyed by cooking. Wheat, rice, and corn are subject to contamination by the *Fusarium* fungus to the extent that cases of *Fusarium* poisoning have been reported throughout the world.[17]

Peanuts are another common foodstuff susceptible to molds. This problem is not serious in the United States, where cultivation and storage conditions are advanced enough to keep the mold infections to a bare minimum.* However, mold contamination is far more widespread in the third world, especially in the tropics. Indonesia, where peanut butter is a main flavoring in many dishes, has one of the highest liver cancer rates in the world, possibly because of mycotoxin B_1 from contaminated peanut supplies.

When talking about the problems of peanut production, we speak from experience, having once grown some of the finest peanuts in Costa Rica. But no matter how hard we tried, we could not keep the crop free from mold and eventually had to give it all up.

Sprouts, especially those grown at home, can also present a problem. Make sure that the seeds and grains are free from mold when you buy them from the health-food store.†

---

* While American peanut butter may have minute amounts of mold-producing carcinogens, there are other, equally compelling reasons for not eating it. The peanut butter and jelly sandwich, so popular with American children, should be replaced, if for no other reason than for its high fat content and the danger from the peroxidation of these unsaturated fatty acids.
† When sprouting the seeds, change the water in the jars three to five times a day, rinsing the seeds each time to ensure that no molds will develop. With these precautions, sprouts can provide a healthy addition to your diet.

OTHER TOXICANTS IN NATURAL FOODS

There are other naturally occurring chemicals that, while not proven carcinogens or mutagens, are still harmful in too large amounts. Spinach, rhubarb, and beet leaves all contain appreciable quantities of oxalites that are not destroyed by cooking, and chocolate and almonds contain high levels of oxalic acid. These oxalites bind to the calcium and other minerals in food, preventing the body from metabolizing them. When these foods are eaten in small quantities, the amount of calcium lost does not present a problem. However, those who drink large amounts of vegetable juice made from spinach or beet leaves run the risk of depleting their dietary calcium to the point where their bodies will begin to remove calcium from the bones.

CONCLUSIONS

In this chapter we have seen that even the most natural foods contain proven carcinogens, sometimes in concentrations several hundred times greater than those of man-made carcinogens. What can we conclude from this fact?

The first conclusion is that there is no cause for alarm. We have no patience with professional anxiety peddlers in the nutrition world and have no desire to join their ranks. As one scientist quipped, "If we were to avoid all foods that have one potentially harmful substance or another, we'd probably starve to death." (About the only natural food that would qualify as being almost totally wholesome and without great risk is carrots—but even rabbits want a change of diet once in a while.)

The second conclusion is to try to minimize those risks, partly through the use of supplemental anti-oxidants, and partly through simple common sense. If we cannot avoid eating some carcinogens or otherwise hazardous substances, even with the most prudent of prudent diets, we can certainly avoid piling one risk factor upon another: for example in salads using raw mushrooms and a mustard dressing (mustard contains the carcinogen allyl isothiocyanate), spicing heavily with black pepper (which contains piperine), and adding loads of basil (estragole). All we'd have to do would be to drink some strong coffee (containing caffeine, methylglyoxal, and other pyrrolization products from the roasting) afterward—a not unlikely event—and we'd have an accumulation of carcinogenic risk factors, the combined effect of which might indeed be a realistic health hazard. (The reader may be thinking of similar "worst-case scenarios" from his or her own experience in combining foods!)

In our view, one should take a reasonable attitude with regard to man-made pesticides and other agrochemicals. As in the case of the raw-food fanatics, there are those extremists who want to have all chemical pesticides banned forever. Though perhaps well-meaning, proponents of such radical measures reveal their ignorance of the fact that some of the natural plant toxins in our most healthful foods literally can be thousands of times more dangerous than residues from the man-made chemicals in them.

But let there be no mistake: We do not defend the pollution of the environment. Clean air and water are the natural birthright of mankind and we should all do whatever is necessary to "clean up our act" so future generations will have no reason to curse our selfishness and greedy indifference. On the other hand, based on our own farming experience in Costa Rica, we cannot but agree wholeheartedly with Dr. Ames that banning a chemical fungicide like EDB, which has a very low toxicity, while developing much more dangerous, though perfectly "natural" aflatoxins in some most basic foodstuffs, like corn, beans, and other grains and legumes, errs in the opposite direction. As in so many other matters, extreme answers are no answers at all.

SOURCES

1. Ames, Bruce N. "Ranking possible carcinogenic hazards." *Science,* 1987; 236:271–280.
2. Duke, J. *Father Nature's Farmacy.* HerbelGram No. 12, Spring 1987.
3. Toth, B., in: *Carcinogens and Mutagens in the Environment,* F. H. Stich, ed. Boca Raton, Fla.: CRC Press, 1984, pp. 99–108. See also: Lawson, T., and B. Toth, *Am. Assoc. Cancer Res. Abstr.,* 1983; 24:77.
4. Tam, S. C., et al. "Hypotensive and renal effects of an extract of the edible mushroom *Pleurotus sajor-caju." Life Sciences,* 1986; 38:1155–1161.
5. Fujita, Y., et al. *Mutation Res.,* 1985; 144:227.
6. Petro-Turza, M., and Szarfoldi-Szalma. *Acta Alimentaria,* 1982; 11:75.
7. Ames, B. N. "Dietary carcinogens and anticarcinogens—Oxygen radicals and degenerative diseases." *Science,* 1983; 221:1256.
8. Ames, B. N. "Ranking possible carcinogenic hazards." *Science,* 1987; 236:271–280. See also: Jadhav, S. J., et al. *CRC Crit. Rev. Toxicol.,* 1981; 9:21ff.
9. Malinow, M. R., et al. *Science,* 1982; 216:41ff.
10. Ibid.
11. Emerit, I., et al. *Hum. Genet.,* 1980; 55:341.
12. Ames, B. N. "Dietary carcinogens." *Science,* 1983; 221:1257.
13. Duke, J. "Herbs as Anti-aging Agents." In: *Health Foods Business,* August 1985, 31(8):38–40.
14. Ridker, P. M., et al. "Hepatic venocclusive disease associated with the

consumption of pyrrolizidine-containing dietary supplements." *Gastroenterology,* 1985; 88:1050–1054.

15. Ames, B. N. "Ranking possible carcinogenic hazards." *Science,* April 17, 1987; 236:272–273.
16. Huxtable, R. J. "Toxicity of comfrey-pepsin preparations." *N. Eng. J. Med.,* 1987; 315:4095.
17. *Toxicants Occurring Naturally in Foods.* Washington, D.C.: National Academy of Sciences, 1973, p. 400.

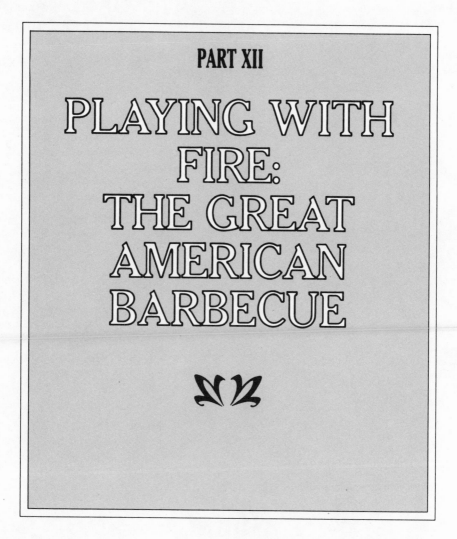

PART XII

PLAYING WITH FIRE: THE GREAT AMERICAN BARBECUE

12 Every Fourth of July, as Americans celebrate Independence Day, private barbecue grills are stoked up in gardens and backyards, and on rooftops all across the land. Tons of ribs, pork, chicken, hamburgers, and hot dogs are roasted to a crisp over smoldering, red-hot embers of charcoal, hickory, mesquite, or whatever other kind of wood happens to be on hand.

In temperate areas of our country, like the West Coast and the Deep South, America's passion for barbecued food continues full blast all year round—"These ribs want to make your tongue want to slap your brains out," a woman staff member from the University of Alabama is quoted saying while wiping some sauce from her chin, we are told in a full-length article, "Barbecue from Coast to Coast," in *The New York Times*. With passions for barbecued ribs running so high, who needs the special excuse of a holiday to stop at any one of the famous barbecue places in the South and indulge?

So, what's wrong with an innocent pastime like that? Everybody enjoys a barbecue, it's a great tradition, and a lot of pleasant socializing takes place around it. It's a pity we can't give this time-honored national ritual a clean bill of health.

Forget about the far too large amounts of meat on the average barbecue plate. Forget also about all the saturated fat in barbecued meat. Forget about the loads of salt and sugar in the typical barbecue sauce. Forget about all of these things. Realize instead that a two-pound, well-done steak, broiled over charcoal, can contain as much cancer-causing benzopyrene as six hundred cigarettes.[1] Fortunately, this carcinogenic effect in the digestive tract is not equivalent to that of cigarette smoke in the respiratory system, or the consequences would be even worse.

The problems start with the indisputable fact that any kind of browning reaction during cooking—even the toasting of bread or the caramelizing of sugar, but especially the browning or burning of proteins—can produce mutagenic substances in these foods.* As one group of Swedish researchers, investigating the effect of diet on pancreatic cancer, stated: "The risk [for pancreatic cancer] increased with higher consumption frequency of fried and grilled meat." They also found associations of cancer with other fried or grilled foods, "but not with meat other than fried or grilled."[2]

These scientists confirmed earlier findings that burned or browned proteins are highly mutagenic. For instance, people who have eaten fried pork or bacon "excrete detectable levels of mutagens in their urine." It is clear that several mutagenic chemicals isolated from fried or grilled meat (chemically speaking, pyrolized amino acids) do cause cancer in laboratory rats and mice.

The higher the temperatures, the more pronounced these pyrosynthesis reactions that can turn an essentially nutritious food—say, a piece of white-meat chicken—into a veritable accumulator of free radicals. These radicals can undergo further dehydrogenation and, via a complicated biochemical route, eventually wind up as highly cancer-causing polycyclic aromatic hydrocarbons (PAH).

However, the trouble with meats broiled over an open flame, hot coals, or wood cinders doesn't end there. It doesn't matter whether the intense heat is generated by organic materials or by gas or electricity. The fat drippings come into contact with the heat source—the burning charcoal or the red-hot heating element—and deposit more mutagenic hydrocarbons on the meat surfaces as the smoke rises.

Dr. Bruce Ames compares the effect of three carcinogenic compounds (nitropyrenes) in diesel exhaust to those ingested from grilled chicken and concludes that the concentration of these compounds in the chicken is much higher than in air pollution. "The total amount of browned and burnt material eaten in a typical day," says Dr. Ames, "is at least several hundred times more than that inhaled from severe air pollution."[3] So, as you can see, the "innocent" fun of the Great American Barbecue turns out to be not quite as innocent as we would like to believe.

But don't dump your barbecue grill yet. There is one way to continue using it and keep on socializing around it: Just put plenty of spices on skinless chicken breast halves, or anything else you want to fix on the grill, and wrap the pieces in aluminum foil. True, the foil touching the food directly is not ideal either, but it's no worse than cooking in aluminum pots and pans. And it's sure a whole lot safer than letting the smoke with all its cancer-causing compounds get onto your food.

---

* Typical mutagens, noted biochemists Drs. Charles Zapsalis and R. Anderle Beck say in their authoritative work on the subject, are "pyrazines, imidazoles, and other nondescript amino acid reaction products including polymers." A. Zapsalis and R. A. Beck, *Food Chemistry and Nutritional Biochemistry* (New York: John Wiley & Sons, 1985).

OTHER COOKING HAZARDS

As we said before, heating fats and oils by any method always speeds up the oxidation process. However, some types of cooking are worse than others in this respect, the worst being, of course, deep frying. Not only does the high heat in deep frying break down the fatty acids of the fats or oils and destroy a large percentage of the heat-sensitive nutrients in the foods, but it also produces a dangerous browning reaction as, for example, that in french fries, potato chips, and so forth. To some extent this also applies to panfrying, although it is the lesser of the two evils. Quick sautéing is one way out of the dilemma. The use of Teflon-coated frying pans and other cookware obviates the need for oils and butter to prevent food from sticking. Cooking with low heat, and with the pan covered, allows for thorough cooking while minimizing the dangerous browning. Microwave cooking, poaching, and steaming are excellent ways to cook without browning.

Remember, too, that the high heat involved in frying red meat, poultry, or fish does the same thing to the proteins and fats in these foods that it does to the fats or oils in which they are being fried.[4,5] If a significant amount of your food is deep-fried, panfried, grilled, or broiled, you are consuming huge amounts of mutagens and carcinogens. And yet much regional cooking in America favors these cooking techniques, resulting in many of these areas having much higher rates of colorectal and other cancers.

COOKING WITH GAS OR ELECTRICITY?

Most professional chefs and devoted home cooks prefer to cook with gas, for the very good reason that the heat is easier to regulate and faster to turn up or down. The problem, however, is that when you cook food in a gas oven, the flames generate nitrogen oxide (NO), which, as Dr. Ames and others have pointed out, can form both carcinogenic nitropyrenes and potentially carcinogenic nitrosamines in food.[6,7] On the other hand, it is not known at this point how significant a risk this represents. To be on the safe side, we cook at home on a professional electric Vulcan range, or with a microwave oven, whenever possible.

SMOKED FOODS

Smoking meats, fish, and game was historically one of the basic means of preserving food. In the smoking process a layer of antibacterial soot is deposited on the food that, at the same time, seals off the food and thus prevents its further invasion by microorganisms.[8]

The problem is that smoking foods involves the same dangerous PAH (polycyclic aromatic hydrocarbons) that make barbecuing and grilling meats so hazardous. The smoking also accelerates lipid peroxidation of unsaturated fats in fish and the oxidation of cholesterol in meats. Artificial "liquid smoke" reduces but does not eliminate these free-radical–induced changes in smoked fish and smoked meats. They should not be on anyone's diet.

SOURCES

1. Zapsalis, C., and R. A. Beck. *Food Chemistry and Nutritional Biochemistry.* New York: John Wiley & Sons, 1985, p. 1061.
2. Norell, S. E., A. Ahlbom, R. Erwald, et al. "Diet and pancreatic cancer: a case-control study." *Am. J. Epidem.,* 1986; 124:914–915.
3. Ames, B. N. *Science,* 1983; 221:1256; ibid., 1984; 224:668.
4. Shorland, F. B., et al. *J. Agric. Food Chem.,* 1981; 29:863.
5. Simic, M. G., and M. Karel, eds. *Autoxidation in Food and Biological Systems.* New York: Plenum Press, 1981.
6. Ames, op. cit.; *Science,* 1984; 224:668,757.
7. Ohgaki, H., et al. *Cancer Lett.,* 1985; 25:239.
8. Linder, M. C. *Nutritional Biochemistry and Metabolism.* New York: Elsevier, 1985, p. 252.

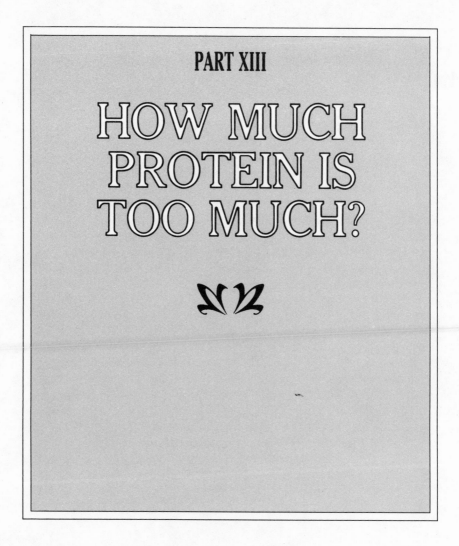

PART XIII

HOW MUCH PROTEIN IS TOO MUCH?

12 The average American or European eats two to three times the recommended amount of proteins, as is true for fats. But the body cannot store excess proteins the way it stores excess fats in the form of adipose tissue (body fat). Instead, the body has to get rid of protein quickly, which is the job of the liver and kidneys. The problem is that if you eat too much protein, your kidneys have to excrete such large amounts of urea (nitrogen) that it puts a heavy burden on them. In our youth, that's not so noticeable, but as we get older, the progressive loss of kidney tissue and function becomes more and more serious.[1-3] As Dr. John A. McDougall puts it, "The damage can be so serious that, in an otherwise healthy person, half the functional capacity of the kidneys can be destroyed after spending seven or eight decades living on the high-protein American diet."[4]

Fortunately for us, our kidneys are real marvels of engineering that can stand quite an overload. But if protein abuse continues year after year, eventually there comes a day of reckoning. When that happens, a person has to be put on a kidney machine, if life is to be sustained. With some people, who have a tendency toward kidney disease (nephritis), or those with only one kidney, that day can come sooner rather than later. They have therefore all the more reason to go easy on meats, which have a much higher concentration of protein than legumes, cereal grains, and vegetables (even fruits have small amounts of protein).

Another group of people who have to be very careful about not eating too much protein are those who have or have had an extremely dangerous skin cancer called *pigmented malignant melanoma* (see pages 527–531), or who have a familial tendency toward developing it. The reason is that tyrosine, one of the amino acid building blocks of proteins, will feed the skin cells (melanocytes) that synthesize the dark pigment (melanin) of the skin, hair, and eyes, as well as of certain tumors, like melanoma, which often occurs in light-complexioned, sun-exposed people.

We only need about 1,000 milligrams of tyrosine per day, but the average American-European diet contains about 5,000 milligrams of tyrosine and phenylalanine, another amino acid in protein, from which the body produces additional amounts of tyrosine. As important as tyrosine is for health and energy—we shall come back to this presently—5,000 milligrams are far too much, especially in the presence of melanoma. Dr. Demopoulos, who has studied melanoma in some depth, points out that tyrosine is the "principal fuel supplier" for this potentially deadly skin cancer. He explains that one therefore has to restrict melanoma patients to no more than 1,000 milligrams of tyrosine per day, maximum. He found that such tyrosine restriction works like a charm in controlling this fast-growing tumor, which can otherwise metastasize and kill within a few months or weeks. But, as Dr. Demopoulos soon discovered, the only way one can drastically reduce one's intake of protein in general, and of tyrosine in particular, is to go on an absolutely strict vegetarian diet—a point many other health professionals seem to have ignored.

Still another group who have to reduce their protein intake to about ½ gram per kilogram of body weight per day are people with Parkinson's disease, because dietary amino acids interfere with the absorption and transport into the brain of the drug levodopa (a precursor of catecholamines), which they have to take in order to control the condition.[5] We frequently encounter Parkinson patients who have not been given this important piece of dietary guidance.

A similar situation prevails even with regard to asthma. It is a known

---

GUAR GUM

Guar gum occurs naturally in the Indian cluster bean; it is also present in other beans. It is made into a food supplement to provide additional soluble fiber and to control obesity.

Studies have shown guar gum moderately lowers serum cholesterol. Moreover, it tends to lower the "bad" LDL fraction of cholesterol without affecting the "good" (protective) HDL fraction.

Studies to determine whether guar gum also lowers serum triglycerides have been inconclusive; some showed significant reduction, others none.

It is the most effective fiber known to lower blood glucose and insulin.*

CAUTION Guar gum can produce gastrointestinal symptoms such as (in descending order) flatulence, diarrhea, excessive full feeling, nausea, upper abdominal pain, loss of appetite, and heartburn.

* D.J.A. Jenkins et al., "Dietary fiber, fiber analogues, and glucose tolerance: importance of viscosity," *Brit. Med. J.*, 1978; 1:1392.

medical fact that the drug theophylline, which many asthmatics have to take, doesn't work well with a high-protein diet. In fact, one can say that high-protein diets interfere with the effectiveness of most drugs. One gains this impression from the clinical observation that drugs like antipyrene (an ingredient in many popular analgesics and deconges- tants) and other medications have shorter half-lives, that is, their serum levels drop very rapidly with high-protein diets.

There is even some evidence from animal studies that high protein consumption—or a high intake of methionine, a main amino acid in meat—over time encourages vascular aging, that is, the deterioration of blood vessels. It was observed that under these conditions, there occurs a premature thickening of the intima (the innermost lining of the arteries) and of the media (the midsection of the artery lining), along with the formation of fibrous tissue and other degenerative processes. None of this was sufficient to make the animals clinically ill or kill them, but, in the words of the researchers, it indicated "advanced arterio- sclerotic changes" and "accelerated vascular aging."[6]

On all these counts, therefore, the prudent course is not to go overboard on protein—especially since it is very likely that a protein- cancer link exists, which we will discuss presently in some detail. Meanwhile, we would like to point out that while caution is clearly indicated, there are some people—for example, the very poor and strict vegetarians ("vegans")—who are not getting enough protein and thus may be deficient in tyrosine and phenylalanine. Chronic shortfalls of these important amino acids can have far-reaching consequences. Adrenaline production depends entirely on tyrosine, as does thyroid hormone synthesis; other neurotransmitters in the nervous system, like noradrenaline and dopamine, are also largely dependent on it. These are all stimulatory body chemicals, which keep the locus ceruleus— our brain's mental alertness center—loaded. This may be why strict vegetarians and most noncarnivorous animals are far more placid than carnivores.

Many people who are concerned about not getting enough protein don't understand that it doesn't take much to produce enough cate- cholamines or neurotransmitters to keep them perfectly energized and more than sufficiently "aggressive." If you eat a small amount of fish, or some egg white (one of the most complete and best-utilized proteins), or a combination of legumes, cereal grains (rice, whole-grain bread, etc.), and vegetables, and maybe some no-fat yogurt, you need nothing more to get sufficient amounts of phenylalanine and tyrosine. The problem with tyrosine—as with all the other single amino acids like arginine and ornithine, the darlings of bodybuilders, or amino acids like tryptophan, which many people take *in lieu* of sleeping pills—is that when you load up on them, this increases their concentrations not only in the brain, but throughout the whole body. It is this systemic (whole

---

PSYLLIUM HUSKS (METAMUCIL)

1. Is a water-soluble, gel-forming plant fiber.
2. Relieves constipation.
3. Used as basis in many laxatives.
4. Significantly decreases plasma cholesterol, particularly LDL.*

* Z. D. Abraham and T. Mehta, "Three-week psyllium-husk supplementation: effect on plasma cholesterol concentrations, fecal steroid excretion, and carbohydrate absorption in men,"[1-4] *Am. J. Clin. Nutr.*, 1988; 47:67–74; "Popular laxative also effective," *Am. Pharm.*, 1987; NS27(7):480.

---

body) effect which, as Dr. Demopoulos points out, can have such detrimental effects as heart arrhythmias and neurotransmitter imbalances.

The other side of the coin is that there are at least nine amino acids—phenylalanine, from which the body produces tyrosine, being one—that we can only get from eating protein. Protein molecules, however, are too large to be absorbed through the intestinal membranes, so the body has to break them up into smaller amino acid molecules, which can get absorbed. This digestion of proteins begins in the stomach with the action of hydrochloric acid and pepsin and continues in the upper small intestine, where pancreatic and intestinal juices (proteases) turn the proteins into free amino acids and small peptides.

Since plant foods, on which some of us rely primarily for our protein, are not as complete in amino acids as animal protein, we have to be careful to eat them in combinations that make their amino acid content more complete.* For instance, rice is low in methionine, as are lentils and most other legumes, which are relatively high in lysine. Eating bread made from wheat, like papadums or chapatis, with rice and lentils as is customary in India brings up the methionine content. So does eating rice and beans with corn tortillas as is done in Latin America. Similarly, if green vegetables, which are high in practically all the other essential amino acids, are eaten along with these grain-legume combinations, as is more characteristic of American and European vegetarian diets, a complete amino acid balance is obtained that compares very favorably to meat protein—and without the latter's problems.

---

* The amino acid complementation does not necessarily have to be simultaneous, that is, in the same meal; it is sufficient if it takes place within a few hours.

GLUCOMANNAN

Glucomannan is a water-soluble, gel-forming fiber, similar to pectin, made from the Japanese *kojac* root. It has exceptionally high water-holding capacity, and is the basic ingredient in some fiber supplements.

Glucomannan helps reduce calorie intake and postmeal energy expenditure, thus creating a helpful pattern for weight control.

On the downside: Glucomannan is expensive and (in pure form) difficult to obtain outside of Japan. In some people it can produce the same gastrointestinal problems guar gum does.

In contrast to these traditional maximally nutritious amino acid combinations, some contemporary foods are much less satisfactory. Take the popular peanut butter sandwich to which we have referred previously: Here we get a combination of proteins that are deficient in exactly the same essential amino acids, lysine and threonine. All the body can do if it does not get some additional complementary protein soon is burn the protein as fuel. This involves a process called *deamination* (splitting off the nitrogen of the protein), which, as we mentioned earlier, puts an extra burden on the liver and kidneys in getting rid of the nitrogen (urea).

About the only plant protein that doesn't need to be complemented from another source is that of soybeans. It's almost as complete as the best animal protein. Nonetheless, it's best to eat soy protein in the form of bean curd (tofu) with green vegetables, not to improve amino acid balance, which is close to ideal, but to add anti-oxidants, vitamins, minerals, and fiber.

Some popular writers (for example, Harvey and Marilyn Diamond in *Fit for Life*) have been insisting that it is wrong to combine proteins with starches in the same meal. We believe this is dead wrong because free (pure) protein is very rare in nature; egg white is the only exception. As a rule, most protein is thoroughly mixed with or closely surrounded by other substances, mainly carbohydrates and lipids (fats).[7] Legumes are typical examples of this kind of linkage between proteins and starches in a single food. But starches and proteins coexist in various combinations and concentrations in all plant foods.

Second, roughly one quarter of the cells lining the gastrointestinal tract are sloughed off daily, and the protein in these cells is digested, just as if it were food protein, and the amino acids are absorbed.[8] So the digestion of proteins and starches proceeds simultaneously in any case, regardless of whether we only eat foods from one group or another. Nor does our digestive system have the least problem with the simultaneous digestion of proteins and starches.

The only foods that are *not* advisable to mix simultaneously are proteins and sugars. Table sugar and most other sugars contain varying amounts of glucose; and there are studies showing that the ingestion of glucose plus protein is followed by a very large increase in plasma insulin. In fact, the surge of circulating insulin that occurs after eating a combination of proteins and sweets—as, for instance, with a sweet-and-sour dish—is, some scientists say, "of such magnitude as to suggest synergism between glucose and amino acid with respect to insulin release."[9]

There is also the question whether excess protein in the diet can produce certain human cancers. There are studies that suggest such a connection.[10,11] In various animals a link between high protein intake and liver cancer has been definitely established.[12] There are indications from rat studies that high protein consumption may be "causally associated with a high incidence of bladder cancer."[13] Of course, one cannot draw any definite conclusions from these animal studies and apply them to the human situation. However, there is a strong suspicion that when protein intake in humans reaches a threefold multiple of the RDA (Recommended Daily Allowance)—which is not uncommon in some diets—it can promote cancer.

These clinical findings are strengthened by epidemiological (population) studies that consistently suggest that excessive beef consumption and low vegetable consumption are somehow causally related to colon cancer. This does not mean that beef—or, for that matter, a high per-capita consumption of other protein-dense foods like pork, eggs, and milk—is directly responsible for any cancer, but it may "provide a microenvironment favorable to the actions of carcinogens."[14]

Animal and population studies have also shown similar correlations between high protein intake and the development of breast tumors. One study discovered the connection between breast cancer and a high-protein diet almost accidentally, not by following the diets of the women themselves but of their husbands. The men who were married to women with breast cancer consumed conspicuously more beef, butter, cheese, and hot dogs than those who were married to women without breast cancer. Assuming that spouses eat pretty much the same kinds of food, the researchers concluded that these diets had something to do with the women's breast cancer.[15]

It is obvious that the apparently cancer-related foods, mentioned above, are not only high in protein but are also high in fat. In other words, the association between these foods and cancer might be due as much to oxidized fats as to excessive protein, especially since most animal carcasses are routinely "aged" to tenderize the meat, a practice that enhances free-radical oxidation of fats in the carcasses. The researchers did, in fact, demonstrate the existence of such a protein-fat interaction with regard to breast cancer. What they found was that with protein intake at 16 to 32 percent of calories (the average U.S. and Japanese protein intake is approximately 11 percent), any increase in dietary fat also increased the incidence of tumors.[16] In layman's language, breast cancer seems to be related as much to excessive fat as to excessive protein in the diet. By "excessive" we mean three times, or more, of the RDA for protein.

With cancer of the bowel, however, research strongly suggests that along with high dietary fat, low fiber intake, and low anti-oxidant consumption, "meat protein is probably the single most important factor associated with its etiology [causation]."[17]

The role of dietary proteins in the causation of cancer is strongly suggested by still another, albeit indirect consideration: We refer to the protease inhibitors—compounds in certain plant foods that block the enzymes responsible for digesting proteins (proteases). Research seems to indicate that when protease inhibitors come into play and prevent the digestion of proteins, the cancer risk is being decreased.[18,19] Even if this is so, other dietary factors, such as excessive fat and a deficiency of fiber, must be considered, as many other studies have demonstrated.

In assessing the role of excess protein in the causation of human cancer, we have to consider still another important factor: how the food was prepared, specifically, to what temperatures was the protein subjected before being ingested. In a Swedish study about the association of pancreatic cancer and dietary factors, it was found that the risk increased with high consumption frequency of *fried* and *grilled* meat, but not with meat per se.[20]

Japanese researchers also found that when proteins or their amino acid building blocks are heated to temperatures high enough to char the food surfaces, several extremely potent mutagens are formed.[21–25] Other research has determined that any cooking method may be unsafe if food, especially protein, becomes overcooked, charred, or burned.[26] There are studies showing that up to one third of the potentially cancer-causing mutagens from fried bacon or pork were still active in the urine excreted by those who had eaten them.[27] Even eggs, fried at too high temperatures (as is frequently the case in fast-food restaurants), contain a major mutagen (benzo(a)pyrene) plus a mixture of suspicious but unidentified compounds.[28]

Scientists in Japan have found exactly the same connection between cancer and protein foods that have been subjected to high heat during cooking. Broiled fish is a very common dish in Japan. It is considered one of the major sources of mutagenic compounds (pyrolyzates) created by the conversion of proteins through exposure to the intense heat of grilling. Not surprisingly, the mortality rate from *all* cancers among those consuming broiled fish twice weekly or more was found to be 1.33 times that of those who eat broiled fish less often or not at all; and the rate was 1.67 times higher for *stomach* cancer. In terms of overall mortality statistics in Japan, broiled fish makes the fourth largest contribution to deaths from all cancers, and the third largest contribution to deaths from stomach cancer.[29] This is a shocking example of the impact that a single unfriendly food can have on the health of a whole nation.

Briefly, what all this amounts to is that (1) many Americans and Europeans (and, increasingly, Japanese) are consuming too much rather than too little animal protein; (2) their favorite methods of cooking animal protein by barbecuing, grilling, and frying involve excessively high temperatures that often produce searing, scorching, and even direct burning of the proteins. All research has also shown that methods of food preparation that "involve direct contact with a hot metal surface or radiant heating, and associated with rapid, partial dehydration of the exterior portions of the meat, lead to greater mutagen formation than methods utilizing lower temperatures and the continued presence of water and steam."[30] Stewing, simmering, steaming, poaching, and microwave cooking have all been shown to be considerably safer.[31,32]

One group of researchers has summed it up neatly: "Generally speaking, cooking acts as a *detoxification* process but here is an example of *toxification.*"[33] (Italics ours.) Therefore, relying more on plant proteins—such as legumes—and the most easily digested animal proteins—seafood, poultry, and egg white—recommends itself to reason. So does changing traditional cooking methods. These are not opinions that reflect personal or philosophical prejudices: They are signals that science is giving us loud and clear. The rest is up to us.

SOURCES

1. Brenner, B. "Dietary protein intake and the progressive nature of kidney disease: the role of hemodynamically mediated glomerular injury in the pathogenesis of progressive glomerular sclerosis in aging, renal ablation and intrinsic renal disease." *N. Eng. J. Med.,* 1982; 307:652.
2. Kennedy, G. "Effects of old age and over-nutrition on the kidney." *Brit. Med. Bull.,* 1957; 13:67.
3. Baldwin, D. "Chronic glomerulonephritis: nonimmunologic mechanisms of progressive glomerular damage." *Kidney Int.,* 1982; 21:109.
4. McDougall, J. A. *A Challenging Second Opinion.* Piscataway, N.J.: New Century Publishers, Inc., 1985, p. 260.
5. *Nutrition and Diet Therapy,* 5th ed., S. R. Williams, ed. Mosby/Times Mirror, 1985, p. 92.

6. Fau, D., J. Peret, and P. Hadjiisky. "Effects of ingestion of high protein or excess methionine diets by rats for two years." *J. Nutr.,* 1988; 118:133.
7. *Modern Nutrition in Health and Disease: Dietotherapy,* 5th ed., R. S. Goodhart and M. E. Shils, eds. Philadelphia: Lea & Febiger, 1973.
8. *Nutritional Biochemistry and Metabolism.* M. C. Linder, ed. New York / Amsterdam / Oxford: Elsevier, 1985, p. 57.
9. Rabinowitz, D., et al. "Patterns of hormonal release after glucose, protein, and glucose plus protein." *Lancet,* August 27, 1966; 454–456.
10. Armstrong, B., and R. Doll. "Environmental factors and cancer incidence and mortality in different countries, with special reference to dietary practices." *Int. J. Cancer,* 1975; 15:617–631.
11. U.S. National Academy of Sciences, National Research Council. *Diet, Nutrition and Cancer.* Washington, D.C.: National Academy Press, 1982.
12. Bailey, G., et al. "Mechanisms of dietary modification of aflatoxin B_1 carcinogenesis." In: *Genetic Toxicology,* R. A. Fleck and A. Hollaender, eds. New York: Plenum Press, pp. 149–165.
13. National Research Council. *Recommended Dietary Allowances,* 9th ed. Washington, D.C.: National Academy Press, 1980.
14. Correa, P. "Epidemiological correlations between diet and cancer frequency." *Cancer Res.,* 1981; 41:3685–3690.
15. Nomura, A., et al. "Breast cancer and diet among the Japanese in Hawaii." *Am. J. Clin. Nutr.,* 1978; 31:2020–2025.
16. *Nutritional Aspects of Aging,* Vol. I, L. H. Chen, ed. Boca Raton, Fla.: CRC Press, 1986, p. 93.
17. Cummings, J. H., et al. "The effect of meat protein and dietary fiber on colonic function and metabolism. I. Changes in bowel habit, bile acid excretion, and calcium absorption." *Am. J. Clin. Nutr.,* 1979; 32:2086–2093.
18. Troll, W., and R. Wiesner. "Protease inhibitors: possible anticarcinogens in edible seeds." *Prostate,* 1983; 4:345–349.
19. Yavelow, J., et al. "Bowman-Birk soybean protease inhibitor as an anticarcinogen." *Cancer Res.* (Supplement), 1983; 43:2454s–2459s.
20. Norell, S. E., et al. "Diet and pancreatic cancer: a case-control study." *Am. J. Epidemiol.,* 1986; 124(89):894–902.
21. Nagao, M., et al. "Mutagenicities of smoke condensates and the charred surface of fish and meat." *Cancer Lett.,* 1977; 2:221.
22. Nagao, M., et al. "Mutagenicities of protein pyrolysates." *Cancer Lett.,* 1977; 2:335.
23. Matsumoto, T., et al. "Mutagenic activity of amino acid pyrolysates in Salmonella typhimurium TA 98." *Mutation Res.,* 1977; 48:279.
24. Sugimura, T., et al. "Mutagen-carcinogens in food, with special reference to highly mutagenic pyrolytic products in broiled foods." In: *Origins of Human Cancer,* H. H. Hiatt, J. D. Watson, and J. A. Winsten, eds. Cold Spring Harbor, N.Y.: Cold Spring Harbor Laboratory, 1977.
25. Matsumoto, T., et al. "Mutagenicities of the pyrolysates of peptides and proteins." *Mutation Res.,* 1978; 56:281.
26. Plumlee, C., L. F. Bjeldanes, and F. T. Hatch. "Priorities assessment for studies of mutagen production in cooked foods." *J. Am. Diet. Assoc.,* 1981; 79:446–449.
27. Baker et al., cited in: Serres, F. J., et al. "Future directions and research priorities for food mutagens." *Environmental Health Perspectives,* 1986; 67:153–157.
28. Serres et al., op. cit., p. 155.
29. Kuratsune, M., M. Ikeda, and H. Takaharu. "Epidemiologic studies on possible health effects of intake of pyrolyzates of foods, with reference to

mortality among Japanese Seventh-day Adventists." *Environmental Health Perspectives,* 1986; 67:143–146.

30. Hatch, F. T., J. S. Felton, and L. F. Bjeldanes. "Mutagens from the cooking of food: thermic mutagens in beef." Chapter 12 in: *Carcinogens and Mutagens in the Environment,* Vol. I, *Food Products,* H. F. Stich, ed. Boca Raton, Fla.: CRC Press, 1982.

31. Dolara, P., et al. "The effect of temperature on the formation of mutagens in heated beef stock and cooked ground beef." *Mutation Res.,* 1979; 60:231.

32. Nader, C. J., L. K. Spencer, and R. A. Weller. "Mutagen production during pan-broiling compared with microwave irradiation of beef." *Cancer Lett.,* 1981; 13:147.

33. *Naturally Occurring Carcinogens of Plant Origin, Bioactive Molecules,* Vol. 2, I. Hirono, ed. New York: Elsevier, 1987.

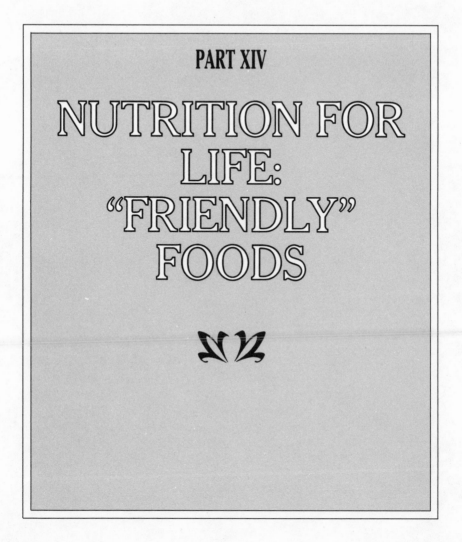

PART XIV

NUTRITION FOR LIFE: "FRIENDLY" FOODS

12 We consider foods that cause disease and accelerate aging "unfriendly" foods. Foremost among them are those with a high fat content (especially animal fat), salt, sugars, milk and dairy products (including cheese), as well as barbecued, fried, grilled, smoked, and pickled foods (the only exception being low-salt sauerkraut). In contrast, "friendly" foods promote health and slow down the aging process. We know that's saying a lot, but there is a growing body of research showing that this is actually so.

Basically, all vegetables and fruits, with few exceptions, are "friendly" foods. Some, like carrots and others, are rich in beneficial carotenes; others, like cabbage, cauliflower, and Brussels sprouts, are high in compounds called *indoles,* which, like the carotenes, can protect us against cancer; still others, like spinach, exert their protective effect more by their high chlorophyll content. And all of them, including the most commonly eaten fruits, contain significant amounts of vitamins, minerals, and enzymes. Last but not least, all vegetables and fruits provide different types of fiber, which has a protective effect on colon and rectal cancer and helps control weight, serum cholesterol, and triglycerides.

In the chapters that follow we shall take a closer look at how various types of vegetables and fruits can promote our health and why, despite certain toxicities they all contain, most of us ought to eat more of them than we do now.

CHAPTER 50

CARROTS

THE POOR MAN'S GINSENG?

12 Among the "friendly" foods, we rate very highly those that are not only rich in vitamins and minerals, but also in the anti-oxidant beta-carotene and other carotenoid compounds. Scientists have barely begun to identify and study these compounds, but it has already transpired that some may be even more important than beta-carotene itself. However, beta-carotene, as a lipid-soluble anti-oxidant—like lipid-soluble vitamin E—is well established as a first-class free-radical interceptor and natural anticancer "drug."

Carrots are so very high in beta-carotene that the latter derives its name from them. Also rich in beta-carotene and, one can safely assume, in other carotenoids as well, are sweet potatoes and dark yellow-orange vegetables (yellow squash and pumpkin). One might have expected this, however, because of the color. It therefore does come with some surprise that dark green vegetables are also excellent sources of beta-carotene (the yellow-reddish beta-carotene is covered up by the vegetables' green chlorophyll).

Another great source of carotenoids is red bell peppers, as is paprika. As far back as 1962, a scientist identified thirty-one different carotenoids in red bell peppers. Recent analysis showed their major constituent to be capsanthin (60 percent), followed by capsorubin (20 percent), beta-carotene (11 percent), lutein (3 percent), and the rest are unidentified compounds.[1] We don't yet know much about the medicinal properties of carotenoids other than beta-carotene, but we may assume that some of them may turn out to rival beta-carotene in importance.

Red bell peppers and paprika are also high in vitamin C, thus combining the free-radical–quenching effects of both beta-carotene and ascorbic acid. Unfortunately, in the United States, green but not red bell peppers are generally eaten. There's nothing wrong with green bell peppers—they are good sources of vitamin C and chlorophyll, and they do contain a fair amount of beta-carotene—but they're lower in beta-carotene than red peppers and are practically devoid of any other carotenoids. Most recently, however, we have noticed that red bell peppers are appearing in supermarkets more often. In Costa Rica, we eat them almost daily, as sweet red peppers (*chile dulce*) are a must in Latin American cooking; besides, we find them easier on the stomach than green peppers.

Some fruits are very high in beta-carotene and other carotenoids, among them yellow melons and cantaloupe, apricots, papayas, and mangoes (see table on page 374). It was recently discovered that even the stamens of some flowers contain important carotenoids. Thus far only saffron and the stamens of gardenias are known to contain the carotenoid crocetin, which is known to oxygenate the blood and carry extra oxygen to the heart, brain, and other internal organs. It therefore seems to be an important natural anti-aging compound.

Most studies on carotenes have been done either on vitamin A or beta-carotene (known as provitamin A). All the above-mentioned vegetables contain both, and both have been shown to be protective against several types of cancers. The way each acts to produce its protective effect seems, however, to be quite different. Vitamin A appears to act more in the promotion stage of already established cancers. There is evidence that vitamin A can actually induce malignant cells to differentiate back to normal.[2] That, of course, has enormous practical implications, especially for people who by dint of their occupations are exposed to chemical carcinogens or radiation—farmers using carcinogenic pesticides and herbicides, workers in chemical factories, uranium miners, and others. Since such individuals are constantly at risk for the development of malignant cells, it is comforting to think that the vitamin A they get from the vegetables in their diet can prevent these abnormal cells from turning into malignant tumors. The way they do this is by apparently stimulating the production of T4 lymphocytes and NK (natural killer) cells, the two foremost defensive players of our immune system.[3,4]

Beta-carotene, on the other hand, works more in the beginning stage of cancer. Cancer initiation may, as we have pointed out, be the result of free-radical and singlet-oxygen activity. We have also called attention to the fact that free radicals and singlet oxygen can be caused by many factors and are among the by-products of lipid peroxidation in our fat-containing cells; these free radicals result in damage to the genetic-blueprint–carrying DNA and RNA. You may recall that this internal,

FOOD SOURCES OF CAROTENE*

	μG/100G SERVING
Carrots	12,000
Spinach	6,000
Sweet potatoes	4,000
Broccoli	2,500
Cantaloupe	2,000
Apricots	1,500
Pumpkin	1,500
Mangoes	1,200
Papaya	1,200–1,500
Lettuce	1,000
Tomatoes	600
Peaches	500
Brussels sprouts	400
Cabbage	300
Oranges	50
Yams	12

* Source: A. H. Smith and J. W. Sullivan, "Should Dietary Changes Be Recommended to Workers at Risk of Occupational Cancer?" In: *Cancer Prevention, Strategies in the Workplace,* C. Becker, and M. E. Coye, eds. (Washington, D.C.: Hemisphere Publ. Corp./Harper & Row, 1986).

cell-destructive process of free-radical reactions is greatly encouraged when we inadvertently eat partially peroxidized (rancid) fats in aged meats and cheeses, leftover food, unrefrigerated cooking oils, and so forth. The anti-oxidant properties of beta-carotene exert their protective effect by intercepting the destructive lipid peroxidation processes and other free radicals right at the beginning.

There is a great deal of evidence from epidemiological (population) studies—comparing the dietary habits of national, religious, or other groups of people and their differing cancer rates, indicating that both vitamin A and beta-carotene play a role in reducing the incidence of lung, prostate, pancreas, breast, and other cancers). Most dramatically, beta-carotene can cut the risk of lung cancer in smokers from fifty times greater to "only" fifteen times greater than in non-smokers.[5]

Another study also confirmed that individuals with higher blood levels of beta-carotene from their diet had some protection against lung cancer in general, but four times more protection against squamous-cell carcinoma of the lung than people who had lower blood levels of beta-carotene.[6] In other words, people who eat more beta-carotene–containing vegetables and fruits develop somewhat less generalized lung cancer, but four times less squamous-cell lung cancer, which kills more smokers than any other type of this malignancy.

We would like to think that after reading our book, smokers who cannot or do not want to give up the habit will at least increase their consumption of carotenoids and perhaps take additional supplemental beta-carotene. Such positive action will mitigate some of the damage smoking has done to their bodies.

The protective effects of carotenoids extend far beyond the special health problems of smokers. For example, it has been amply documented that people whose regular diet includes fresh fruits and vegetables, particularly carrots and citrus fruits, on an almost daily basis more rarely develop pancreatic cancer than others do.[7] That may be due as much to the vitamin A as to the beta-carotene and other carotenoids in the vegetables and fruits that contain the highest levels of these substances.

Several other studies have found that people who eat more beta-carotene–containing vegetables and fruits develop less cancer of the larynx, bladder, breast, cervix, and prostate.[8]

A strong protective effect of beta-carotene has already been found against chromosome breakage in the oral mucosa of betel nut and tobacco chewers in the Philippines.[9] (An unhealthy and unpleasant pastime, betel nut chewing is practiced by Indian men, too. We vividly remember having to avoid the bright red juice being directed our way on Indian streets by unconcerned betel nut chewers.)

Now it has been shown that fresh carrot juice protects against chromosome damage in laboratory mice, if given immediately after they have been exposed to a strong mutagen and carcinogen. The protective effect was especially marked when the mice were given an additional "dose" of carrot juice a couple of hours before exposure to the mutation-causing substance.[10] On the strength of these findings, we would think that drinking a tall glass of fresh carrot juice both before and after exposure to any mutagenic action—for instance, before and after chemotherapy—might be a good idea. It should be fresh though, because the carotenoids oxidize rapidly and turn brown when the juice has been sitting around. (We ourselves like to use carrot juice to wash down some extra glutathione, which appears to have a similar protective effect against radiation-induced chromosome breakage.)

All these recent findings about carrots and carotenes make earlier medicinal claims sound almost prophetic. Carrots, carrot juice, and carrot tea (including even the greens) have been considered helpful for a wide variety of human ills since ancient times in India, Greece, and Rome. Dr. James Duke says that botanist J. L. Hartwell devoted three whole pages to the carrot in his monumental *Plants Used Against Cancer.** According to Dr. Duke, Hartwell said that folk medicine has traditionally considered carrots a remedy for cancers, cancerous ulcers, tumors, degeneration of the spleen and liver, in such diverse areas as Belgium, Chile, California, Connecticut, England, Germany, Indiana, Ohio, Oregon, Russia, and Washington.

Dr. Duke's own studies actually convinced him that the lowly carrots from North America have considerable medicinal potential, comparable to Siberian or Korean ginseng (see table on facing page comparing the medicinal substances in carrots and ginseng).

Since we all have finally become aware of the importance of keeping cholesterol levels down, it is not just oat bran—as many people seem to think—that can help bring them down, but a lot of other foods too, among them carrots. In a study from the Wolfson Gastrointestinal Laboratory of Western General Hospital, Edinburgh, Scotland, people who ate 200 grams of ground raw carrots at breakfast for three weeks had a serum cholesterol decrease of 11 percent on average. Moreover, this and other beneficial changes persisted three weeks after stopping the experiment.[11] Of course, nobody can reasonably be expected to eat so many carrots every day. But good cholesterol-lowering results have ben obtained with much smaller quantities. The main reason for this effect is carrot fiber's considerable capacity (thanks mostly to its high pectin fraction) to absorb bile acids and carry them out with the stools, thus preventing reabsorption and recycling into new cholesterol. (We shall see that legumes, like beans and lentils, and fruits also exert a cholesterol-lowering effect.)

Most of the studies on carrots and carotenes in general have been done with raw carrots. However, scientists consider that the carotenoids in fruits and vegetables remained stable under normal cooking procedures. Even when frozen vegetables were used, there was complete retention of the beta-carotene with microwave or conventional cooking methods (only dehydration destroys beta-carotene).[12] In some respects, cooked carrots may even be nutritionally better than raw ones. It is therefore advisable to eat both raw and cooked carrots with some regularity.

We like to carry a couple of raw carrots with us to munch on for snacks when doing library research, and we almost always put carrots in salads, or include them in cooked meals. Moreover, for a highly nourishing, quick-energy drink that's full of concentrated carotene and

---

* *Plants Used Against Cancer: A Survey* (Lawrence, Mass.: Quarterman Press, 1982).

COMPARISON OF CARROTS AND GINSENG (ZMB)*

	Average[1] Root	Carrot[1]	Korean[2] Ginseng Root	Korean[3] Ginseng Root	American[3] Ginseng Root	American[3] Ginseng (Leaf/Stem)
Calories	365	356	375	—	—	—
Protein	8.9	9.3	13.6	9.0	8.7	10.3
Fat	1.5	1.7	1.1	0.8	0.6	1.4
Carbohydrate (total)	85.2	82.2	82.5	84.6	86.1	79.8
Fiber	4.9	8.5	4.7	5.9	6.4	24.0
Ash	4.4	6.8	2.9	5.6	4.6	8.5
Calcium	158	314	260	320	250	1,080
Phosphorus	266	305	240	310	270	330
Iron	4.9	5.9	5.4	40.7	36.6	10.8
Sodium	69	398	—	—	—	—
Potassium	1,966	2,890	—	—	—	—
B-Carotene	2,798	55,932	< 111 IU	—	—	—
Thiamin	0.44	0.51	0.11	—	—	—
Riboflavin	0.25	0.42	0.12	—	—	—
Niacin	3.9	5.1	5.2	—	—	—
Ascorbic acid	89	68	< 1.1	—	—	—

[1] Duke and Atchley (1985) average of 10 roots; ZMB = Zero Moisture Basis
[2] Duke (1981) converted to ZMB by multiplying fresh weight by 100/100-10, where 10 is the moisture basis of the as-purchased material
[3] Jhang, Staba, and Kim (1974); dry basis assumed to be ZMB

* Source: James A. Duke, Ph.D., "Carrots Are Cheaper Than Ginseng," unpublished paper, 1984. By permission of the author.

tastes absolutely delicious, there is nothing quite like a glass of freshly squeezed carrot juice.*

Seeing how good carrots and other carotene-containing vegetables are for us, it is truly distressing to learn from a recent study by researchers at the National Cancer Institute of dietary customs among a cross-section of nine hundred white New Jersey men that thirty-two percent of them never ate carrots alone, either cooked as a side dish or

* The Champion juicer is ideal for this purpose, but carotenes, once exposed to oxygen and light, oxidize quickly so the juice should be drunk without much delay and the residual pulp kept in a tightly closed container and refrigerated to use in making carrot cake, bread, soups, etc.

raw as a snack (as carrot sticks). The only way they ate them was mixed with other vegetables or in salads or stews, and 13 percent never ate them at all. Similarly, many of these men did not eat any other vegetables and fruits with a high carotene content. Twenty-seven percent never ate green leafy vegetables of any kind; 25 percent never ate broccoli; 63 percent never ate green leaf lettuce, which is much richer in carotene and chlorophyll than iceberg lettuce; 50 percent never ate summer squash; and 22 percent never ate cantaloupe. The researchers comment with fine official understatement that people who habitually avoid eating such healthful foods may thereby "possibly be jeopardizing their health." Can there be any reasonable doubt about it?

SOURCES

1. Gregory, G. K., et al. "Quantitative analysis of carotenoids and carotenoid esters in fruits by HPLC: red bell peppers." *J. Food Sci.,* 1987; 52:1071–1073.
2. Blaun, R., and A. Belson. "Can vitamin A keep cancer away?" *Medical Month,* 1983; 1:53.
3. Watson, R. R., and S. Moriguchi. "Cancer prevention by retinoids: Role of immunological modification." *Nutr. Res.,* 1985; 5:663.
4. Watson, R. R. "Regulation of Immunological Resistance to Cancer by Beta-carotene and Retinoids." In: *Nutrition, Disease Resistance, and Immune Function.* New York: Marcel Dekker, Inc., 1984.
5. Watson, R. R., and T. K. Leonard. "Selenium and vitamins A, E, and C: Nutrients with cancer prevention properties." *Perspectives in Practice,* 1986; 86:505–510.
6. Menkes, M. S., et al. "Serum beta-carotene, vitamins A and E, selenium, and the risk of lung cancer." *N. Eng. J. Med.,* 1986; 315:1250–1254.
7. Norell, S. E., et al. "Diet and pancreatic cancer: A case-control study." *Am. J. Epidem.,* 1986; 124:895–901.
8. Hennekens, C. H., et al. "Vitamin A , carotenoids, and retinoids." *Cancer,* 1986; 58:1837–1841.
9. Stich, H. F., M. P. Rosin, and M. O. Vallejera. "Reduction with vitamin A and beta-carotene administration of the proportion of micronuclear buccal mucosal cells in Asian betel nut and tobacco chewers." *Lancet,* 1984; 2:1204–1206.
10. Abraham, S. K., et al. "Inhibitory effects of dietary vegetables on the in vivo clastogenicity of cyclophosphamide." *Mutation Res.,* 1986; 172:51–54.
11. Robertson, J., et al. "The effect of raw carrot on serum lipids and colon function." *Am. J. Clin. Nutr.,* 1979; 32:1889–1892.
12. Park, Y. W. "Effect of freezing, thawing, drying, and cooking on carotene retention in carrots, broccoli and spinach." *J. Food Sci.,* 1987; 52:1022.

CHAPTER 51

DO CABBAGE PATCH BABIES REALLY LIVE LONGER?

12 The family of cruciferous* vegetables includes not only all cabbages themselves, like the common green and red varieties, but also Brussels sprouts (really miniature cabbages), cauliflower, turnips, kale, and broccoli. In the same family are also Chinese broccoli, Chinese cabbage, and bok choi, as well as some other exotic Oriental varieties of them.

Cabbage itself has been grown for thousands of years as a food crop in many parts of the world. It has a long history in folk medicine and has been credited with being able to cure a large variety of ills. Many of these folkloric claims are of course devoid of any scientific basis. Over the past twenty-some years, however, cabbage and its family of related vegetables have been scientifically researched and found to be protective of human health, especially with regard to various cancers.

On the other hand, it has transpired—as is so often the case—that cabbage is not always and in every form benign. There is evidence from Japan that if cabbage is eaten in the form of the popular highly salted and pickled vegetables collectively called *hakusai* or *tsukemono*, it ceases being friendly. In fact, it seems to turn decidedly unfriendly and is suspected of causing rather than preventing cancer.[1] The same, most

---

* The term "cruciferous," used for vegetables of the cabbage (*Cruciferae*) family, derives from the fact that they all have four-petaled flowers; they are also classified as plants of the *Brassica* family.

unfortunately, appears to be true for sauerkraut, so beloved by Germans and Alsatians. It is featured prominently on many health-oriented diets, including the macrobiotic diet. Nonetheless, a 1987–1988 study by two Dutch researchers (P. J. Groenen and E. Busink), supported by the Netherlands Cancer Foundation, discovered that sauerkraut contains high-nitrate compounds that are definitely geno-toxic, that is, they are able to attack our genetic-blueprint–carrying DNA, and can cause cancer. In the opinion of these scientists, there exists the distinct possibility that "sauerkraut is a kind of Western-world equivalent of some of the oriental-style pickled vegetables."[2]

The only friendly sauerkraut may be the kind made with wine vinegar instead of by adding salt to the shredded cabbage to extract the water. We cannot be sure at this point whether using vinegar instead of salt really does make the difference between sauerkraut being an unfriendly (mutagenic) food or a friendly one. The studies conducted until now have not distinguished between the two types. However, there are indications that salt may be the main problem with sauerkraut, as it seems to be with Japanese salted and pickled vegetables. So at least we are led to believe from studies done by Japanese scientists from the Faculty of Medicine at Kyushu University.[3]

Let's just hope, for the sake of all sauerkraut lovers, that sauerkraut made with vinegar instead of salt is safe. Leaving this question aside for now, we can definitely say that the consumption of cabbage and all the rest of the cruciferous vegetables is positively health-promoting. Early studies have shown that they have a healing effect on stomach ulcers and are useful in the control of blood sugar levels, an important point for diabetics and diabetes-prone individuals. More recent studies indicate that they may exert an antibacterial and antiviral effect by strengthening the immune system.

However, the most important medicinal function of cabbage and the other cruciferous vegetables is their proven ability to exert a protective influence on cancers of the digestive system. First indications to this effect came from population studies. In 1978 Dr. Saxon Graham and colleagues, at the State University of New York at Buffalo, published a study based on dietary interviews with hundreds of patients with diagnosed cancer of the colon or rectum and a matching sample of people without cancer. These scientists found a definite increase in risk for colorectal cancers in those individuals who were eating the lowest amount of vegetables in general. But, more important, there was a marked decrease in cancer risk for those who ate vegetables most often, especially cabbage, Brussels sprouts, and broccoli.[4]

What lent even more credence to these findings was that previously conducted laboratory studies with animals had produced similar findings. Several years earlier Dr. Lee W. Wattenberg, professor of pathology at the University of Minnesota Medical School, had found that cabbage, broccoli, and Brussels sprouts were able to stimulate an enzyme system in the intestines of rats that inhibits the development of cancer.[5] In a subsequent study, Dr. Wattenberg and his colleagues discovered that certain compounds (indoles) in these vegetables were able to induce the same kind of protective enzyme activity in the liver and intestines of the rats.[6]

Many confirmations of these findings in the United States, Europe, and Japan were to follow. In 1983 Dr. Graham found that cruciferous vegetables were related to a reduced risk of not only cancer of the colon and rectum, but also of the bladder.[7] That same year, an Italian study with laboratory mice showed that cauliflower juices could inhibit the mutagenic activity of (N-nitroso) compounds that would otherwise set the stage for cancers.

Also in 1983, Greek researchers, analyzing the previous diets of one hundred colorectal cancer patients, discovered that what these patients had in common was that they had been eating more meat and fewer vegetables, including less cabbage. Those who had eaten vegetables the least were at eight times greater risk for cancer, as compared with a matched group that did not develop colorectal cancer.[8]

A study from Norway showed that people who eat fewer cruciferous vegetables and don't get enough vitamin C are more likely to develop polyps of the colon, which frequently turn into cancer.[9]

Dr. Wattenberg discovered that if laboratory animals were given cabbage, cauliflower, or Brussels sprouts to eat before being exposed to cancer-causing substances, they were better protected than others who had been fed these vegetables after such exposure. Not surprisingly, animals who had received such protective foods before *and* after exposure to carcinogens fared the best. Dr. Wattenberg found that just giving the animals the active anticancer compounds in cruciferous vegetables (indoles, isothiocyanates, or dithiolthiones) rather than the vegetables themselves had the same protective effect.[10-14]

Another study (1986), this one by scientists at Johns Hopkins University, used only biochemicals called *dithiolthiones,* which are present in cabbage and other cruciferous vegetables, to see whether they would protect laboratory mice from chemicals that induce liver cancer, such as aflatoxins (mold poisons). It turned out that the dithiolthiones did protect the animals by stimulating protective enzyme systems in their bodies (glutathione transferases) and by raising tissue levels of the anti-oxidant glutathione (a constituent of our full spectrum of micronutrients). In fact, the mice that had been given the vegetable compound were four to eleven times better protected against liver cancer than those who had only been eating regular laboratory chow.[15]

A second study, also by investigators at Johns Hopkins, on the protective effects of dithiolthiones on the liver when attacked by mold toxins, confirmed the results of the earlier work. Levels of aflatoxin B_1

bound to the liver's DNA molecules, and therefore able to cause genetic damage and abnormal cell growth (cancer), were reduced between 40 to 80 percent, depending on the amounts of dithiolthiones used.*[16]

A third study, this one by scientists at Cornell University in Ithaca, New York, came up with very similar findings, using extracts of Brussels sprouts to supplement the standard laboratory chow of rats before they received liver carcinogens. These researchers found that the rats who had been given the Brussels sprouts extract had stepped-up anticancer enzyme activity and consequently produced fewer tumors.[17]

It had been known since the 1930s that rabbits fed cabbage leaves in addition to their usual diet survived a normally lethal dose of radiation from uranium.[18] A later study (1959) with guinea pigs by two U.S. armed forces researchers (H. Spector and D. H. Calloway) found that feeding the animals raw cabbage significantly reduced their mortality from exposure to X radiation by 52 percent on average. Feeding the animals broccoli turned out to be even more effective than cabbage in reducing radiation mortality. As in the Wattenberg tests, if the guinea pigs were given the cabbage or broccoli only *after* exposure, the protection was very much less than if they had been fed with them *before* getting zapped by the X rays. Prefeeding the animals not only delayed the onset of death, but actually enabled some of them to survive. The greatest number of survivors, however, again were among the group that had been given protective prefeeding *and* were fed cabbage or broccoli afterward, too.[19]

These repeated findings, including his own research, caused Dr. Wattenberg later on to refer to "chemoprevention" with regard to the protective effects of vegetables in general and the cruciferous vegetables in particular.† However, to apply all these encouraging animal experiments to the human case, we have to keep in mind that a genuinely protective effect of natural anticancer plant compounds can only be achieved by consuming the protective, friendly vegetables and fruits on a *regular basis,* not just once or twice a week. At the same time, you have to avoid the less friendly or decidedly unfriendly foods to benefit the most.

The large-scale study done of white New Jersey males, mentioned in our preceding discussion of the carotene-containing vegetables, exemplifies this important point. Another, even more recent study (1988) of Wisconsin residents with two different types of colon cancer and a matched control group of people without colon cancer bears out the

---

* In this experiment, the natural dithiolthiones in cabbage and Brussels sprouts were replaced by a synthetic equivalent (oltipraz) in order to avoid the unavoidable fluctuations in natural compounds.
† We would like to include in this very appropriate term, "chemoprevention," the full Demopoulos spectrum of anti-oxidants and vitamin co-factors. We believe that only by such a comprehensive approach can cancer prevention be expected to work.

same conclusions. As this study established, only vegetable consumption over lifetime was consistently protective for both types of colon cancer. On the other hand, those who regularly consumed more processed luncheon meat and panfried foods had a three to four times greater risk for colon cancer than those who ate more cruciferous vegetables.[20]

Having sung the praises of the cabbage family, we have to add some qualifying words of caution. Some of the same substances in these vegetables that provide cancer protection (for instance, indole-3-carbinol) have been shown also to be cancer promoters.[21,22] In addition, since the 1960s it has been known that potentially carcinogenic hydrocarbons, which occur in small quantities in many natural substances, are present in the leaf cells of banana leaves (the original subject of the study), but, unfortunately, also in cabbage and Brussels sprouts.[23]

Also, there are population studies that seem to contradict the protective effects noted by the numerous earlier studies. One of those investigations seemed to show that women who ate more cabbage, coleslaw, and turnips developed more cancer of the cervix rather than less. On the other hand, women who ate more broccoli, which contains besides the indoles, dithiolthiones, and isothiocyanates present in all cruciferous vegetables, substantial amounts of beta-carotene, did prove to have significant protection against cervical cancer.[24]

Frankly, we don't know what to make of the results of this study, finding that only broccoli was protective and that all the other cruciferous vegetables were associated with an *increased* cervical cancer risk. It might be, as the researchers suggest, that the cruciferous vegetables, especially the cabbage, were eaten more frequently by the less affluent women in the study. In that case, the result would not be so surprising: It would merely reflect the fact that these women had fewer preventive medical checkups, less adequate health care, and were affected by generally poorer living conditions than others in the study; all these factors would put them at greater risk of cervical cancer. It could also be that pure random chance produced the contradictory results because of the "multitude of comparisons" that were made in this study, as the researchers also thought was possible.

Random chance or otherwise faulty study design might have been responsible for similarly contradictory findings in a Japanese population study (1985). In this study, higher consumption of certain vegetables, including cabbage, was associated with higher risk for colon and stomach cancers, contrary to the vast majority of previous studies.[25]

Frequently the effect of plant compounds is somewhat ambiguous rather than clear-cut and uniformly protective, as some popular writers want us to believe. Depending on quantities and circumstances, the compounds may be either protective or destructive, as Drs. H. F. Stich and W. D. Powrie, two noted specialists, point out. Take, for instance, the plant phenolics present in cruciferous vegetables. Their reaction with nitrites, which are ubiquitous in foods and even in our own saliva, seems to explain their inhibitory effect on the formation of carcinogenic nitrosamines. However, under certain conditions, phenolics suddenly start acting as catalysts for potentially health-endangering nitrosation reactions. Some phenolics, coumarins and flavonoids, both of which are present in cruciferous vegetables, are actually "potent genotoxic agents," that is, they are able to damage the genetic code of cells. But they can also be protective of the genetic code and inhibit mutagenesis, depending on the presence or absence of other compounds in the interior of cells. As Drs. Stich and Powrie say, "Once we leave the simplicity of studying the reactions of single compounds, we must be prepared to find this kaleidoscopic pattern."[26]

We must also mention the most recent (1988) long-term population study by Dr. Saxon Graham and colleagues on the effects of different dietary habits with regard to cancer of the colon.[27] In that study, involving people living in and around Buffalo, New York, the researchers no longer found that cruciferous vegetables had a protective effect. Instead, they found such an effect only with celery, carrots, green peppers, onion, and tomatoes. The researchers themselves were puzzled by these contradictory results, compared with those of their own earlier studies. They suggested that the contradiction was probably due to the fact that the American diet has changed considerably over the past three decades, the period covered by the studies, especially with respect to eating different vegetables. Today, for example, cabbage and turnips are eaten less, and bell peppers, tomatoes, and broccoli are being eaten more. The later findings therefore do not necessarily mean that cruciferous vegetables are less protective of colon cancer than the earlier studies seemed to indicate.

One more point: Cabbage, turnips, and kale also contain two antithyroid compounds—goitrin and thiocyanate—which are potent goitrogens, that is, they are able to induce goiters (enlargement of the thyroid gland in the neck). On the other hand, cabbage (but not the other members of the cabbage family) seems to contain mucin-like compounds that some researchers credit with being able to heal stomach ulcers.[28] In the 1950s an American physician, Dr. G. Cheney, recommended that peptic ulcer patients drink a quart of cabbage juice a day. Similar recommendations continue in the popular, health-oriented media to this day. However, it is obvious that such quantities of cabbage juice—it takes between four to eight pounds of raw cabbage to produce a quart of juice!—may well tip the scale in favor of the goitrogens and even turn potentially anticancer compounds, like the indoles and dithiolthiones, into carcinogenic substances.

For all these reasons, most people should probably eat more cabbage (except salt-cured sauerkraut), Brussels sprouts, and especially broccoli* than they generally do. We totally agree with Drs. J. P. Whitty and L. F. Bjeldanes of the Department of Nutritional Sciences, University of California at Berkeley, who, after a careful review of all the pros and cons about cabbage and other members of the Cruciferae family, said: "The recommendation for a *moderately increased intake* of these vegetables seems valid, on the basis of evidence from epidemiological studies and carcinogenesis assays, but *high-level consumption* of the vegetables, their extracts or substances that they contain is *clearly not advisable* at present because of the potential hazard of such regimens."[29] (Emphasis ours.)

SOURCES

1. Tajima, K., and Tominaga, S. "Dietary habits and gastrointestinal cancers: a comparative case-control study of stomach and large intestinal cancers in Nagoya, Japan." *Japan. J. Cancer Res.*, 1985; 76:705–716.
2. Groenen, P. J., and Busink, E. "Alkylating activity in food products— especially sauerkraut and sour fermented dairy products—after incubation with nitrite under quasi-gastric conditions." *Fed. Chem. Toxicol.*, 1988; 26:215–225.
3. Endo, H., et al. "An Approach to the Detection of Possible Etiologic Factors in Human Gastric Cancer." In: *Recent Topics in Chemical Carcinogens*, S. Odashima et al., eds. Baltimore & Tokyo: University Park Press, 1975, pp. 17–29.
4. Graham, S., et al. "Diet in the epidemiology of cancer of the colon and rectum." *J. Natl. Cancer Inst.*, 1978; 61:709–714.
5. Wattenberg, Lee W. "Studies of polycyclic hydrocarbon hydroxylases of the intestine possibly related to cancer." *Cancer*, 1971; 28:99–102.
6. Loub, W. D., L. W. Wattenberg, and P. W. Davis. "Aryl hydrocarbon hydroxylase induction in rat tissues by naturally occurring indoles of cruciferous plants." *J. Natl. Cancer Inst.*, 1975; 54:985–988.
7. Graham, S. "Results of case-control studies of diet and cancer in Buffalo, New York." *Cancer Res.* (Supplement), 1983; 43:2409s–2413s.
8. Manoulos, N. E., et al. "Diet and colorectal cancer: a case-control study in Greece." *Int. J. Cancer*, 1983; 32:105.
9. Hoff, G., et al. "Epidemiology of polyps in the rectum and sigmoid colon." *Scand. J. Gastroenterol.*, 1986; 21:199–204.
10. Wattenberg, L. W. "Effects of dietary constituents on the metabolism of chemical carcinogens." *Cancer Res.*, 1975; 35:3326.
11. Wattenberg, L. W. "Environmental carcinogenesis: occurrence, risk evaluation and mechanisms." *Proc. Int. Conf. on Envir. Carcinogenesis*, Amsterdam, 1979; 401.

* The stalks of broccoli contain too much copper for most people, who do not generally suffer from a copper deficiency. In fact, too much copper can become toxic to liver cells, and is only useful in proper balance with other minerals and trace elements. We therefore recommend that you cut off and discard the stalks of broccoli and use only the tops, which contain most of the carotenes, vitamins, and chlorophyll as well as small amounts of copper and other minerals.

12. Wattenberg, L. W., and W. D. Loub. "Inhibition of polycyclic aromatic hydrocarbon-induced neoplasia by naturally occurring indoles." *Cancer Res.*, 1978; 38:1410.

13. Wattenberg, L. W., et al. "Dietary constituents altering the responses to chemical carcinogens." *Fed. Proc. Fed. Am. Soc. Exp. Biol.*, 1976; 35:1327.

14. Wattenberg, L. W. "Inhibition of neoplasia by minor dietary constituents." *Cancer Res.* (Supplement), 1983; 42:2448s–2453s.

15. Ansher, S. S. "Biochemical effects of dithilthiones." *Fed. Chem. Toxicol.*, 1986; 24:405–415.

16. Kensler, T. W., et al. "Mechanism of protection against aflatoxin tumorigenicity in rats fed 5-(2-pyrazinyl)-4-methyl-1, 2-dithiol-3-thione (oltipraz) and related 1,2-dithiol-3-thiones and 1,2-dithiol-3-ones." *Cancer Res.*, 1987; 47:4271–4277.

17. Godlewski, C. E., et al. "Hepatic glutathione S-transferase activity and aflatoxin B_1-induced enzyme altered foci in rats fed fractions of brussels sprouts." *Cancer Lett.*, 1985; 28:151–157.

18. Eisner, G. "The lifesaving action of portions of plants and the juices removed from them in the case of otherwise fatal subacute uranium intoxication." *Biochem. Z.*, 1931; 232:218.

19. Spector, H., and D. H. Calloway. "Reduction of x-radiation mortality by cabbage and broccoli." *Soc. Experim. Biol. and Med.*, 1959; 100:405–406.

20. Young, T. B., and D. A. Wolf. "Case-control study of proximal and distal colon cancer and diet in Wisconsin." *Int. J. Cancer*, 1988; 42:167–175.

21. Bailey, G., et al. "Indole-3-carbinol promotion and inhibition of aflatoxin B_1 carcinogenesis in rainbow trout." *Proc. Meet. Am. Assoc. Cancer Res.*, 1985; 26:115.

22. Pence, B., et al. "Multiple dietary factors in the enhancement of dimethylhydrazine carcinogenesis: main effect of indole-3-carbinol." *J. Natl. Cancer Inst.*, 1986; 77:269.

23. Nagy, B., et al. "Hydrocarbons in the banana leaf, musa sapientum." *Phytochemistry*, 1965; 4:945.

24. Marshall, J. R., S. Graham, et al. "Diet and smoking in the epidemiology of cancer of the cervix." *J. Natl. Cancer Inst.*, 1983; 70:847–851.

25. Tajima, op. cit.

26. Stich, H. F., and W. D. Powrie. "Plant phenolics as genotoxic agents and as modulators for the mutagenicity of other food components." In: *Carcinogens and Mutagens in the Environment*, Vol. I, Food Production, H. F. Stich, ed. Boca Raton, Fla.: CRC Press, 1982, pp. 140–141.

27. Graham, S., et al. "Dietary epidemiology of cancer of the colon in Western New York." *Am. J. Epidemiol.*, 1988; 128:494–503.

28. Singh, G. B., et al. "Effect of brassica oleracea Var. Capitata in the prevention and healing of experimental peptic ulceration." *Ind. J. Med. Res.*, 1962; 50:741–749.

29. Whitty, J. P., and L. F. Bjeldanes. "The effects of dietary cabbage on xenobiotic-metabolizing enzymes and the binding of aflatoxin B_1 to hepatic DNA in rats." *Fed. Chem. Toxicol.* 1987; 25:581–587.

CHAPTER 52

THE UNDERRATED LEGUME FAMILY

When we say legumes are underrated in human nutrition, we mean mostly by North Americans and Europeans. In contrast, the people of Latin America, from the Mexican border all the way down through Central and South America, could not survive without the ubiquitous red and black beans. In fact, rice and beans (*arroz y frijoles*) are about all the poorer classes in that part of the world eat day in and day out, breakfast, lunch, and dinner.

In Asia, too, legumes play an important role in the diet. In India the almost daily staple is not rice and beans, but one form or another of lentils (*dal*) with rice. Under more favorable economic conditions, the rice-and-lentil mixture will be supplemented with breads (*chapatis* or *papadums*) made from whole wheat flour, and maybe a vegetable, meat, or fish curry, depending on religious dictums.

In the traditional Japanese diet, several kinds of beans (the small brown azuki beans and a larger, perfectly round variety of black beans) are eaten with rice. In both Japanese and Chinese cooking, soya beans form the base of bean curd and soya sauce.* The Chinese and Japanese use bean curd in many different ways, from hot and spicy to sweet and sour. Many of their sauces are based on fermented black beans and

---

* Remember that there are problems with soya sauce, not only because the regular variety has a high salt content (contrasted with a more recently available low-salt version), but most important, because it has relatively high concentrations of carcinogenic methylglyoxal, also present in roasted coffee beans. (Apparently, methylglyoxal is not much of a problem in coffee made by the drip method, compared with the perculator method in which the ground beans come into direct contact with constantly boiling water.)

they like to put different kinds of beans into steamed dumplings. Sweet bean paste is also used in various desserts. In Japan *miso,* a soup made from a special kind of bean paste, is eaten at least once, if not twice, a day by most people.

In Latin America, centuries of practical experience seem to have taught people that rice and beans are highly nourishing and life sustaining (as are rice and lentils in India and bean curd and other bean-rice combinations in China and Japan).

In contrast, in North America, where the majority of the population lives in large urban centers and is almost totally divorced from the land and nature, many people no longer even realize that dried beans, peas, and lentils represent the dormant seeds of leguminous plants. Therefore, we had better mention that what all the leguminous plants have in common is that they can fix nitrogen from the air and store it up in little nodules on their roots. For that reason, they need less or, if need be, no commercial fertilizer. Of course, the seed yields are not what they would be if commercial fertilizer or compost were used. That, however, is not a consideration for the poor survival farmer in the third world who's only interested in feeding himself and his family, and couldn't afford commercial fertilizer anyway.

The reason legume seeds are so nourishing is that the concentration of protein in them is two to five times that in nonleguminous cereal seeds like wheat, rye, or oats. The more we learn about them, the more they also look like the "champions of fiber sources."[1] Most people are probably not aware of this because they think of fiber mostly in terms of television cereal commercials, rivaling each other in the percentage of "bran" they contain. That means mostly wheat bran and—more recently—oat bran, touted these days as a "magic bullet" to cure dangerously high cholesterol levels. We shall come back to these misleading notions, but first a word about the different classes of fiber.

The fibers you hear about most are the bran, or the ground outer layers of cereals, from wheat and oats. But there are big differences in the way these two types of fiber function in our digestive system. Wheat bran, for example, like most other cereal brans (except oat bran), is insoluble. It was therefore thought that it would pass intact through the whole alimentary canal. We now know, however, that this is not quite the case: The hemicellulose and lignin, which form the large part of insoluble fiber, gets broken up by the gut bacteria, and some of it is absorbed as volatile fatty acids. What insoluble fiber like wheat bran is mainly good for is to increase stool mass and weight, which is why it helps to keep a person's bowel habits regular.

Oat bran, on the other hand, dissolves in water, meaning it is soluble. That's also true for the fiber in barley, though not in other cereal grains. Fruits, carrots, and okra have a soluble fiber called *pectin* that doesn't help much with constipation, but swells up like a sponge in the stomach and small intestine, giving one a feeling of satiety and fullness. This obviously helps with weight control. Pectin does still another thing: It slows down food absorption in the gut. This is particularly important for diabetics, who have to avoid a sudden surge in blood sugar and the consequent strain on insulin production to counteract it that occurs when too many sugars in one form or another have been ingested. We'll return to that. At this point we only want to call attention to the fact that the legumes have pectin too. Beans, for instance, have only one tenth of 1 percent less pectin than apples, and peas have actually one tenth of 1 percent more pectin than apples.

Admittedly, carrots have twice as much pectin as beans. Beans, however, are rich in certain gums that are water soluble and capable of doing what pectin does, especially in slowing down food absorption. While that makes beans even more important for diabetics than sweet fruits, they have also turned out to be highly effective in bringing down cholesterol levels—every bit as much as oat bran. This is all the more important since oat bran has been shown to promote potentially dangerous cell proliferation in the colons of laboratory animals, a precondition for cancer.[2] Nobody knows whether this applies to humans, but we wouldn't want to put all our eggs into the oat bran basket.

We feel the risk is all the greater, since rather large quantities of oat bran are necessary as a sole means of bringing down cholesterol: You'd have to eat a serving of cooked oat bran for breakfast plus five oat bran muffins—every day! Moreover, oat bran muffins won't do you any good unless they have been made without whole egg because of the high cholesterol content of the yolk, and without saturated or hydrogenated vegetable fats like Crisco or margarine. It's not easy to produce muffins that way that don't taste like warmed-over cardboard and don't fall apart. (All the commercial ones we have checked out have too much fat and cholesterol, as well as too much sugar.) You'd have to make your own muffins, if that regimen is supposed to work.

Fortunately, there is no good reason for going to all this trouble. In the first place, whole (steel-cut) oats or unprocessed rolled oats are as effective as oat bran in lowering cholesterol.[3] Secondly, as shown by Dr. James W. Anderson of the University of Kentucky, one of the pioneers in lipid research, almost identical results can be had from either oat bran or any kind of beans: Oat bran diets resulted in reductions in serum LDL cholesterol concentrations that averaged 23 percent; bean diets resulted in average reductions of 24.4 percent. True, bean diets knocked down the "good" HDL cholesterol fraction more than oat bran diets, but that's not a serious drawback. Much more important is that bile acid secretion averaged 65 percent higher on oat bran diets than on control diets. In contrast, bean diets resulted in an average *decrease* in fecal bile acids of 30 percent, compared with control diets.[4] This again means a lesser cancer risk because bile acids are considered to promote cancer in the gut.

The well-established cholesterol-lowering effect of legumes is not their only health-promoting property. It is a fact that foods rich in gel-forming fibers like beans, lentils, and chick peas (garbanzos) do not raise the glucose (blood sugar) and insulin levels as much as other foods.[5] Dr. David Jenkins of the Faculty of Medicine at the University of Toronto, Canada, and a foremost diabetes specialist, reports on even more sensational findings on the role of legumes in diabetes management. In a recent experiment with low-glycemic-index foods for non-insulin–dependent diabetics, he and his colleagues found that not only oat bran, but legumes too were "most consistently useful in the dietary management of diabetes and hyperlipidemia."[6]

Dr. Jenkins also found the nonleguminous cereal grain barley and its soluble fiber were very useful in the control of diabetes mellitus. But other researchers discovered that the most underrated and most underused legume—the soya bean—is perhaps the most effective single food in the control of both cholesterol and triglyceride levels. In 1983 another famous specialist in cholesterol control, Dr. Scott M. Grundy, called attention to studies showing that if soy protein was substituted for animal protein in the diets of such diverse animals as chickens, rabbits, rats, and pigs, the result was always the same: a dramatic drop in cholesterol levels. None of these animals showed any fatty streaks in their arteries, which are the first signs of atherosclerotic buildup of plaque.

"Do humans show a similar response?" he wondered. Searching scientific literature worldwide to answer his own question, he found plenty of affirmative evidence, especially in a series of studies from Italy. These researchers found that if patients with dangerously high cholesterol levels were placed for three weeks on a diet in which textured soy protein replaced animal protein, their plasma cholesterol levels dropped a sensational average of 31 percent. This average was somewhat reduced in later experiments with larger numbers of patients in Italy and Switzerland, but it still hovered around an impressive 23 percent in men and 25 percent in women.[7–9] But even these results are better than those achieved with the highly publicized prescription drugs that are being used to lower cholesterol levels—and with these natural foods there is no worry about possible side effects, as with the drugs.

Dr. Grundy confirmed these findings with studies of his own in the United States. He arrived at a very important conclusion, namely that "soy protein is effective in reducing cholesterol only when it is combined with other cholesterol-lowering factors."[10] That is true not only for soya beans (unfortunately too few people have caught on to this possibility) but also for the faddish and one-sided oat bran diet that many Americans are following. Oat bran cannot possibly "cancel out the fat and cholesterol in a steady diet of prime steaks and french fries, fettucini Alfredo and chocolate sundaes," food columnist Marion Burros writes in *The New York Times*.[11] Also, as already mentioned, too much oat bran in the daily diet can cause harmful intestinal cell proliferation and a tremendous increase in equally risky bile acid secretion.

The only sensible course of action therefore is to use *several* of the known cholesterol-lowering foods in your regular diet. That's what we do: We have a bowl of whole, unprocessed steel-cut or rolled (NOT the fast, precooked oatmeal) oats in the morning. We don't even add oat bran to our cereal, feeling that it already contains enough bran of its own. We also recommend eating soya beans, maybe once a week, as a vegetarian chili. It's also good sometimes to eat the delicious Middle Eastern dish known as *hummus*. Hummus is traditionally made from mashed chick peas and sesame seeds to complement its amino acids and make it a more complete protein. We have a very good reason to favor this dish, since chick peas lower cholesterol and triglyceride levels as effectively as beans and are the least gas-producing of all the legumes.

We eat plenty of black and red beans—both as bean soup, whole

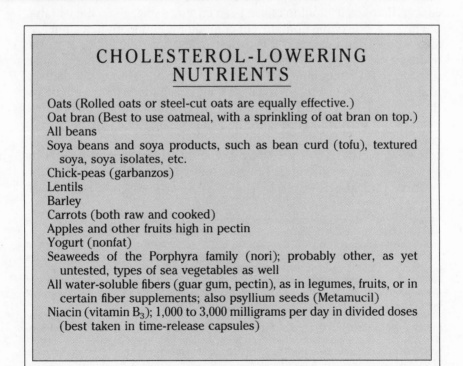

CHOLESTEROL-LOWERING NUTRIENTS

Oats (Rolled oats or steel-cut oats are equally effective.)
Oat bran (Best to use oatmeal, with a sprinkling of oat bran on top.)
All beans
Soya beans and soya products, such as bean curd (tofu), textured soya, soya isolates, etc.
Chick-peas (garbanzos)
Lentils
Barley
Carrots (both raw and cooked)
Apples and other fruits high in pectin
Yogurt (nonfat)
Seaweeds of the Porphyra family (nori); probably other, as yet untested, types of sea vegetables as well
All water-soluble fibers (guar gum, pectin), as in legumes, fruits, or in certain fiber supplements; also psyllium seeds (Metamucil)
Niacin (vitamin B_3); 1,000 to 3,000 milligrams per day in divided doses (best taken in time-release capsules)

beans, or bean paste—especially when we are on our farm in Costa Rica.* We also love barley, which has a similar cholesterol-lowering effect, in soups and stews to get away from the monotony and implicit health risks of overemphasis on any single cholesterol-lowering food like oat bran.

NEWLY DISCOVERED HEALTH BENEFITS OF LEGUMES

Over the past few years it has been discovered that some of the "antinutrients" in legumes (lectins, saponins, phytates, tannins, and protease inhibitors), which were traditionally thought of mainly as problems and health risks, are in general friendly too. For one thing, it is now clear that these nonnutrient compounds are as much as or more responsible than fiber for the low glycemic index of beans, peas, and lentils. It is this property that, as we pointed out earlier, makes legumes especially protective for diabetics and others who have to watch their blood sugar.[12]

However, who would have ever thought that beans, lentils, and chick peas could protect us from cancer? And not only from colorectal cancer. Perhaps it shouldn't have been so surprising, given the fact that phytic acid, one of the nonnutrient compounds abundant in legumes, is also a potent anti-oxidant. It is an especially effective inhibitor of the hydroxyl radical (OH)[13] that plays such an important role in oxidative damage to fat-containing cell membranes. By preventing cell damage from this destructive free radical, the phytic acid in legumes might, on that account alone, stop some mutagenic chemicals from the environment or the diet from getting to the genetic material in the interior of cells.

In other words, phytic acid may indirectly protect us from cancer by preventing fat-containing cell membranes from being attacked by the hydroxyl radical.† However, that's not all: Beans, peas, lentils, and peas

---

* Many city dwellers will see these combinations of beans offered at the now popular salad bars in restaurants and grocery stores. But the trouble is that usually these prepared bean dishes are swimming in oil, so they should be drained before being consumed. Just as Southerners in our country smother black-eyed peas in pork fat, so do present-day Latinos prepare bean dishes by adding generous amounts of manteca, made from hydrogenated palm oil. All these dishes should be drained of oil, too. In all these cases, many of the health-promoting effects of the legumes are nullified by the addition of health-endangering ones of fats.

† Dr. Ernst Graf, a food scientist with the Pillsbury Company in Minneapolis, feels that phytate from legume seeds holds tremendous promise as an "effective and nontoxic food preservative," because of its important anti-oxidant properties. In fact, phytic acid is already being produced in commercial quantities for use by the food industry (*Phytic Acid,* Tsuno Rice Fine Chemicals Co., Wakayama, Japan, 1986).

also contain compounds, collectively called *protease inhibitors*, which have only recently been investigated and have definitely been found to protect laboratory animals from skin, breast, and liver cancers.[14–16] Also, there are human population studies that suggest the same effects for breast and prostatic cancers.[17]

Let's back up for a moment to explain what medical scientists mean when talking about these mysterious-sounding "protease inhibitors." As the name implies, these compounds in leguminous seeds prevent certain enzymes, called *proteases*, without which we could not digest any proteins, from functioning. In other words, the proteases are able to split protein molecules so we can digest them. Scientists suspect, however, that cancer cells use them for their own ends in order to proliferate and spread in the body. The protease inhibitors apparently prevent them from doing so.

Another way in which protease inhibitors seem to protect us from cancer is by quenching oxygen radicals, thus preventing tissue injury as occurs in ionizing radiation, for example, thereby stemming an "oxygen cascade" that would otherwise proceed unchecked.[18] Still another way in which protease inhibitors may prevent cancer is, as Dr. Walter Troll of the New York University School of Medicine says, by preventing the oncogenes, which reside in the DNA of every normal cell, from becoming activated and turning into cancer-promoting genes. Here again the "common pathway," in medical language, by which the protease inhibitors seem to provide this cancer protection is by intercepting free radicals that could cause oncogenes to "switch on" the process of wild cell proliferation that produces malignant tumors.[19]

Dr. Ann Kennedy of the University of Pennsylvania who, together with Dr. Troll, is undoubtedly one of this country's greatest experts on protease inhibitors, thinks that these substances actually "have a selective toxicity for transformed cells."[20] If that is so, it means we have in these plant compounds, which abound in soya beans and other leguminous seeds, nature's own guided-missile system, which is able selectively to home in on only those cells with chromosomal, precancerous abnormalities while ignoring normal, healthy cells.

If that is nothing short of sensational, Dr. Kennedy also discovered that the protease inhibitors are able to perform even greater feats: They can *reverse* damage to the genetic-blueprint–carrying DNA inside the cells and turn those damaged cells back to normal—something thought completely impossible until now.[21]

Dr. Kennedy showed that protease inhibitors in soybean extract are able to suppress oral and colorectal cancers in laboratory hamsters and mice—and do so without any noticeable ill effects on the health, weight, and normal life span of these animals. In fact, her research suggests that these nonnutrient substances, which had been considered useless at best and dangerous at worst, might be able to inhibit *all* cancers, except stomach cancer.[22–32] This exception, she explained in a personal communication, is based on the fact that protease inhibitors are pH-dependent and cannot work within the acidic environment of the stomach. They do, however, definitely get into the intestinal tract and are able to block cancer there, as Dr. Troll and Dr. Kennedy have amply demonstrated.

Furthermore, even though all these studies were conducted with laboratory animals, there is every reason to believe that protease inhibitors can prevent human cancers. Dr. Kennedy, for instance, points out that the oral cancer artificially induced in the experimental hamsters resembles in every respect the most common form of human oral cancer, squamous-cell carcinoma. She therefore feels that "human oral carcinogenesis might respond to BBI [a particularly effective type of protease inhibitor in soya beans] in a comparable manner."[33] (Bracketed text is ours.)

Notwithstanding all this positive news about protease inhibitors, some researchers are still very wary of them because they have been found to *cause* rather than prevent cancer in some laboratory animals. Here, as in the case of indoles and the other nonnutrient compounds in cruciferous vegetables discussed earlier, the ultimate nature of the protective or destructive effect might depend on the quantities involved and the presence or absence of other compounds. Evidence from population studies indicates as clearly for legumes as for cruciferous vegetables that the overall effect of these vegetables is predominantly protective: People who regularly consume more of them develop less colorectal and other cancers than those who consume less or none of them.[34]

DO BEANS HAVE TO BE SO "GASSY"?

Finally, we have to face the delicate topic of gas-producing properties of beans and other legumes, like lentils. It is undoubtedly this unfortunate feature that prevents many of us from eating these foods as much as we should.

Well, let's look at this problem. It is a very realistic one, to be perfectly candid. First of all, let us be clear on one point: Intestinal gas is not a health problem—at least not in most cases—but a social problem. The famous Greek physician Hippocrates taught that passing gas was necessary for one's well-being.[35] Today we know that the average healthy person passes varying amounts of gas at least twelve to fifteen times over a twenty-four-hour period. This group includes kings, presidents, popes, and beauty queens. It has nothing to do with morals or good and bad manners—it's just a fact of life, like it or not.

Some great minds with a healthy sense of humor have even tried to help us over our embarrassment about this socially taboo matter. No less than one of the founding fathers of our country, the brilliant and eccentric Benjamin Franklin, actually wrote a tongue-in-cheek, pseudo-scientific essay on the subject. In it he proposed with mock seriousness that scientists should experiment with various chemical substances that people could take and which would produce an infinite number of perfumed scents for every occasion.

Mark Twain, probably the greatest humorist in American literature, wrote an absolutely hilarious essay on the subject entitled "Fireside Chat at the Court of Queen Elizabeth I." In this little-known work, Twain used the technique of "reversal of affect"—described in Freud's *The Psychology of Humor*—by having the participants in the "fireside chat," including Sir Walter Raleigh among other dignitaries, apologize to the queen not for breaking wind in her presence, but for not doing so loudly and forcefully enough! There are even counterparts in the visual arts as well.

We thought it useful to begin with this social and psychological review of the intestinal gas that, like it or not, busy bacteria keep producing day and night in our alimentary tract. Our purpose in doing so is to remind people that this is a perfectly natural and morally neutral phenomenon, and to suggest that an overconcern with it is perhaps not in the best interests of one's health and well-being.

Nor are beans and other legumes the only foods that can cause intestinal gas. Cereal grains, for instance, can do the same thing, but people don't generally complain about it. (Do cereals have better PR than beans?) Yet in one study* it was found that the popular breakfast cereal All-Bran definitely caused more intestinal gas than any other sample of cereal grains tested.[36] Fruits, too, can cause intestinal gas. Apples and bananas are notorious for it; nonetheless, they are among the healthiest, friendliest foods you can eat.

What causes the gas with beans, lentils, and other legumes are certain sugars (oligosaccharides)[37] rather than skins,[38] as had been thought previously. Since the human small intestine does not produce an enzyme to hydrolize (digest) these complicated sugars, they are being acted on and eagerly consumed by anaerobic gut bacteria, in the process of which gas is formed.[39] Of course, other foods—onions and garlic as well as cabbage and other high-fiber foods—produce intestinal

---

* Ralston Purina (dark farina with 5 percent added wheat germ) and Cream of Wheat (light farina) were the only other commercial breakfast cereals studied; the others were milling fractions, which are not consumed by themselves.

gas by other chemical processes, but fermentation by intestinal bacteria is always the key element.

One thing, however, is clear: Many of the most health-promoting foods, not only beans and the other legumes, happen to be "gassy." The question then arises, would you rather be sick or put up with some intestinal gas?

In that connection, it is interesting to note, as Dr. Demopoulos points out, that chemically, hydrogen gas is an important component of intestinal gas, and that such molecular hydrogen is an incredibly powerful free-radical scavenger. As health-conscious people eat more fresh fruits, vegetables, grains, and legumes, the bacterial flora in the intestines change, resulting in the production of greater amounts of hydrogen and methane gases. Hydrogen produced this way may be among the specific chemical reasons for the decreased risk of colo-rectal cancer in people who are on this kind of diet. In other words, the hydrogen scavenges free radicals that might otherwise convert choles-terol and other fecal fats into dangerous cancer-causing substances (so, while intestinal gas may not have any redeeming social value, it certainly has plenty of redeeming medical value!).

To get back to practical considerations: It is a fact that individuals react differently to foods and micronutrients that are potentially gassy. It depends primarily on one's bacterial flora, which may differ even within the same individual from one time to another. You may have heard that beans produce gas only the first time you eat them and that if you keep eating them regularly, there will be no recurrences. Unfortunately, that is a mistaken notion. Beans do not gradually stop producing intestinal gas, either on a short-term or a long-term basis. What does happen is that people who regularly eat beans and other gas-producing foods gradually develop a greater subjective tolerance to the gas.[40,41] Earlier researchers of this unfortunate side effect of legume consumption were misled by the fact that their test subjects reported more discomfort only during the first twelve to forty-eight hours of a heavy bean diet, and that this discomfort quickly disappeared as far as their subjective experience was concerned.

However there are things you can do to minimize the gassiness of legumes. Let the beans soak overnight and discard the water the next morning. Then pour boiling water over them, or cook them for a few minutes, and let them sit in the water for another four hours or so. Discard the water and cook the beans in fresh water until they are tender. We have found that doing this eliminates some of the gas problem.

It also seems that mashing the cooked beans in a food processor to make bean paste also renders them less gassy. We usually add either a little salt or soya sauce and black or red pepper to the bean paste, plus finely chopped red bell peppers (chile dulce), and some cumin, turmeric, fenugreek, or whatever seems to go well with beans. On the other hand, we do not advise using other gas-producing foods like onions or garlic with any legume dish because this compounds the problem.

One thing is certain: We would never forgo the well-established health-promoting effects of beans and other legumes—or, for that matter, of any other beneficial foods—just because they may produce gas. To our minds, there can be no doubt about the priorities in matters like these, even if it means putting up with some discomfort or small adjustments in life-style—like taking a short walk after the meal, something we should do anyway. We also noticed that if we eat a cup of low-fat yogurt* for dessert after an otherwise especially gassy meal, there's not much of a problem left.

SOURCES

1. Slavin, J. L. "Dietary fiber: classification, chemical analyses, and food sources." *J. Am. Diet. Assoc.,* 1987; 87(9):1164–1168 and 1171.
2. Lupton, J. R., and L. R. Jacobs. "Fiber supplementation results in expanded proliferative zones in rat gastric mucosa." *Am. J. Clin. Nutr.,* 1987; 46:980–984.
3. Degroot, A. P., et al. "Cholesterol lowering effect of rolled oats." *Lancet,* 1963; 2:303–304. Also: Judd, P. A., and S. Truswell. "The effect of rolled oats on blood lipids and fecal steroid excretion in man." *Am. J. Clin. Nutr.,* 1981; 34:2061. Also: Roth, G., and C. Leitzmann. "Long-term influence of breakfast cereals rich in dietary fibers on human blood lipid values." *Aktruel Ernahr,* 1985; 10:106–109. Also: Van Horn, L. V., et al. "Serum lipid response to oat product intake with a fat-modified diet." *J. Am. Diet. Assoc.,* 1986; 86:759–764.
4. Anderson, J. W. "Hypocholesterolemic effects of oat bran or bean intake for hypercholesterolemic men." *Am. J. Clin. Nutr.,* 1984; 40:1146–1155.
5. Ryttig, K. R. "Dietary Fiber Supplements and Weight Reduction." In: *Dietary Fibre Perspectives—Reviews and Bibliography,* Part I, A. R. Leeds and A. Avenell, eds. London/Paris: John Libbey, 1985, p. 65.
6. Jenkins, D.J.A., et al. "Low-glycemic-index starchy foods in the diabetic diet." *Am. J. Clin. Nutr.,* 1988; 48:248–254.
7. Sirtori, C. R., et al. "Soybean-protein diet in the treatment of type-II hyperlipo-proteinnaemia." *Lancet,* 1977; 1:275–277.
8. Sirtori, R. R., E. Gatti, et al. "Clinical experience with soybean protein in the treatment of hypercholesterolemia." *Am. J. Clin. Nutr.,* 1979; 32:1645–1658.
9. Descovich, G. D., et al. "Multicenter study of soybean protein diet for outpatient hypercholesterolaemic patients." *Lancet,* 1980; 2:709.
10. Grundy, Scott M., and J. J. Abrams. "Comparison of actions of soy protein and casein on metabolism of plasma lipoproteins and cholesterol in humans." *Am. J. Clin. Nutr.,* 1983; 38:245–252.

* See also our discussion of yogurt (pages 465–470) in which we explain that yogurt should contain at least two cultures, *L. acidophilus* and *L. bulgaricus;* ideally it should also have *L. thermophilus.*

11. Burros, Marian. "Eating Well," *The New York Times,* July 27, 1988.
12. Jenkins et al., op. cit.
13. Graf, E., et al. "Phytic acid: A natural antioxidant." *J. Biol. Chemistry,* 1987; 262:11647–11650.
14. Goldstein, B. D., et al. "Stimulation of human polynuclear leukocyte superoxide anion radical production by tumor promoters." *Cancer Lett.,* 1981; 11:257–262.
15. Goldstein, B. D., et al. "Protease inhibitors antagonize the activation of polymorphonuclear leukocyte oxygen consumption." *Biochem. Biophys. Res. Comm.,* 1979; 88:854–860.
16. Hatcher, V. B., et al. "Characterization of chemotactic and cytotoxic proteinase from human skin." *Biochem. Biophys. Acta,* 1977; 483:160–171.
17. Correa, P. "Epidemiological correlations between diet and cancer frequency." *Cancer Res.,* 1981; 41:3685–3690.
18. Yavelow, J., et al. "Bowman-Birk soybean protease inhibitor as an anticarcinogen." *Cancer Res.* (Supplement), 1983; 43:2454s–2459s.
19. Troll, W., et al. "Protease inhibitors: Possible anticarcinogens in edible seeds." *Prostate,* 1983; 4:345–349.
20. Kennedy, A., and J. B. Little. "Effects of protease inhibitors on radiation transformation in vitro." *Cancer Res.,* 1981; 41:2103–2106.
21. Kennedy, A. "The conditions for the modification of radiation transformation *in vitro* by a tumor promoter and protease inhibitors." *Carcinogenesis,* 1985; 6:1441–1445.
22. Kennedy, A. R., and P. C. Billings. "Anticarcinogenic Actions of Protease Inhibitors." In: *Anticarcinogenesis and Radiation Protection,* P. A. Cerutti, O. F. Nygaard, and M. G. Simic, eds. New York: Plenum Publishing Corp., 1987; pp. 285–295.
23. Chang, J. D., et al. "C-MYC expression is reduced in antipain-treated proliferating C3H 10T½ cells." *Biochem. Biophys. Res. Comm.,* 1985; 133(2):830–835.
24. Weed, H. G., et al. "Protection against dimethylhydrazine-induced adenomatous tumors of the mouse colon by the dietary addition of an extract of soybeans containing the Bowman-Birk protease inhibitor." *Carcinogenesis,* 1985; 6(8):1239–1241.
25. Yavelow, J., et al. "Nanomolar concentrations of Bowman-Birk soybean protease inhibitor suppress x-ray–induced transformation in vitro." *Proc. Natl. Acad. Sci.,* 1985; 82:5395–5399.
26. Kennedy, A. R., et al. "Protease inhibitors reduce the frequency of spontaneous chromosome abnormalities in cells from patients with Bloom syndrome." *Proc. Natl. Acad. Sci.,* 1984; 81:1827–1830.
27. Baturay, N., and A. R. Kennedy. "Pyrene acts as a carcinogen with the carcinogens Benzo[a]pyrene, β-propiolactone and radiation in the induction of malignant transformation in cultured mouse fibroblasts: soybean extract containing the Bowman-Birk inhibitor acts as an anticarcinogen." *Cell. Biol. and Toxicol.,* 1986; 2(1):21–32.
28. Kennedy, A. R., and J. B. Little. "Protease inhibitors suppress radiation-induced malignant transformation in vitro." *Nature,* 1978; 276(5690): 825–826.
29. Kennedy, A. R. "Antipain, but not cycloheximide, suppresses radiation transformation when present for only one day at five days post-irradiation." *Carcinogenesis,* 1982; 3(9):1093–1095.
30. Billings, P. C., et al. "A serine protease activity in C3H/10T½ cells that is inhibited by anticarcinogenic protease inhibitors." *Proc. Natl. Acad. Sci.,* 1987; 84:4801–4805.

31. Chang, J. D., and A. R. Kennedy. "Cell cycle progression of C3H 10T½ and 3T3 cells in the absence of an increase in c-myc RNA levels." *Carcinogenesis,* 1988; 9(1):17–20.
32. Billings, P. C., et al. "Potential intracellular target proteins of the anticarcinogenic Bowman-Birk protease inhibitor identified by affinity chromatography." *Cancer Res.,* 1988; 48:1798–1802.
33. Messadi, D. V., et al. "Inhibition of oral carcinogenesis by a protease inhibitor." *J. Natl. Cancer Inst.,* 1986; 76:447–451.
34. Correa, P. "Epidemiological correlations between diet and cancer frequency." *Cancer Res.,* 1984; 40:3685–3690.
35. Bouchier, I.A.D., "Flatulence." *Practitioner,* 1980; 224:373–377.
36. Hickey, C. A., et al. "Intestinal-gas production following ingestion of commercial wheat cereals and million fractions." A publication of the American Association of Cereal Chemists, Inc., St. Paul, Minn., 1972.
37. *Nutritional Support of Medical Practice,* 2nd ed., H. A. Schneider et al., eds. New York: Harper & Row, 1983, p. 14.
38. Hellendoorn, E. W. "Intestinal effects following ingestion of beans." *Food Technology,* 1969; 23:87–91.
39. *Nutritional Support of Medical Practice, op. cit.*
40. Fleming, S. E., A. U. O'Donnell, and J. A. Perman. "Influence of frequent and long-term bean consumption on colonic function and fermentation." *Am. J. Clin. Nutr.,* 1985; 41:909–918.
41. O'Donnell, A. U., and S. E. Fleming. "Influence of frequent and long-term consumption of legume seeds on excretion of intestinal gases." *Am. J. Clin. Nutr.,* 1984; 40:48–57.

CHAPTER 53

VEGETABLES OF THE SEA ("SEAWEED")

12 "The supply of food for the increasing population of the world is a very serious problem."[1] These are the words of scientist Dr. Heinz A. Hoppe, an outstanding German specialist on marine algae, or in layman's language, "seaweeds." He goes on to say that "seaweeds," or vegetables of the sea—as we prefer to call these most underrated and underused plant foods in the Western world—are so rich in all the basic nutrients that they would go a long way to solving the increasingly severe food crises in the third world.

Not only could marine algae as food nicely fill in the protein and vitamin gap that exists in large parts of Africa and Asia, "seaweed meal" could also be the answer to the shortage of affordable livestock feed. Equally important could be the role played by those seaweeds that are most plentiful but less suitable for human nutrition, such as kelps, as a cheap constituent of fertilizers. Although most seaweeds have little nitrogen and therefore cannot be used as complete fertilizers, they are rich in ideally balanced minerals and trace elements, which are lacking or poorly represented in commercial fertilizers.

Seaweeds are highly valuable as raw material for many industrial products, as emulsifiers and stabilizers in the food industry, for example; for a wide variety of foods, from ice cream to whipped cream, yogurt, cheese, milk powder, toppings, puddings, fruit syrups, icings, cake mixes, confections, jams, marmalades, sauces, pickles, and salad dressings. These are about the only times most of us ever get to "eat" seaweed—without, of course, being aware of it.

There are many uses for seaweed constituents (alginates) in the pharmaceutical industry. Alginates are often used as fillers and stretchers in tablets, or as stabilizers in suppositories, and as suspensions. Most important, perhaps, they are used in slowly dissolving, gelatin-like coatings on "time-release" medications.

A gelatinous substance in seaweed called *agar* is also used by medical laboratories around the world as an ideal neutral medium in which to grow bacteria, fungi, and viruses. When suffering from an infectious disease, you have probably benefited from this use of seaweed when your doctor ordered a laboratory test to culture the bacteria or other microorganisms that were giving you trouble and find out to what antibiotics they were most sensitive.

What interests us, however, most about edible marine algae—vegetables of the sea—is the fact that they are one of the most "friendly," highly nutritive, and health-protecting—and yet almost totally neglected —foods around. At least, that is true in America and Europe. In other parts of the world, notably China, Japan, Malaysia, and Hawaii, sea vegetables have for centuries, if not millennia, been recognized and appreciated for their many nutritional and medicinal properties.

The lore of sea vegetables goes back to the dawn of human civilization. In the Babylonian *Epic of Gilgamesh,* which is considered the source of the biblical story of the great flood, the hero brings up from the depths of the sea a "plant," said to bestow eternal youth and immortality on the eater. Similarly, about 3000 B.C., Shen Nung, venerated in China as the "Father of Medicine," prescribed "plants of the sea" to all those desiring a long life. The ancient Chinese *Book of Poetry* also extols the nutritional and medicinal virtues of sea vegetables, as did Confucius (c. 551–479 B.C.). Interesting, too, is the Chinese character for edible sea plants, revealing in its elegance and delicate composition the high esteem in which they were held.

But ancient China and Japan did not have a monopoly on appreciation of sea vegetables. The oldest law book of Iceland, dating back to 961 B.C., includes detailed regulations about coastal property rights to be respected in the collection of sea vegetables. And there are early records of sea vegetables being collected and eaten by the coastal populations of northern Europe, as well as by the people around the Mediterranean and Aegean seas.

With such an illustrious history, it is hard to understand why sea vegetables should have fallen in such low esteem in more recent times, except in Japan, China, and the rest of the Pacific basin. Was it because the Roman historian Cicero wrote about them as "vile" and unfit for civilized people's food? Coming from as renowned a historical personage as Cicero, perhaps this statement did prejudice the creators of French cuisine (from which all Europe took its cues) against this important food group.

Whatever the reasons, the almost total neglect of sea vegetables in American and European culinary practices is most regrettable. In contrast, estimates are that in China's coastal regions, the average household (four persons) consumes sea vegetables about two or three times a week. And not just as a condiment or a minor side dish, but to the tune of more than one pound being eaten each time.[2] These figures are recent, and we are told by researchers that sea-vegetable consumption in China, along with other foodstuffs, has been boosted in the last few years, since the government started encouraging individual farmers and fishermen to sell their produce and catches in numerous open markets that instantly sprang up everywhere.

It strikes us as strange that the Japanese should be eating somewhat lower, though still substantial, amounts of sea vegetables, since in restaurants in Japan, one is likely to be served sea vegetables in one form or another, either as a thin, green wrapping around rolls of rice with pieces of raw fish inside (sushi), or in miso soup, in which they are basic (although invisible) ingredients, or in some other form. In contrast, in Chinese restaurants about the only way sea vegetables are featured is as "seaweed soup," and even then the egg drops in the soup usually predominate.

ANTICANCER EFFECT

In the West we are more familiar with Japanese than with Chinese studies about the various medicinal properties of sea vegetables, although this may merely reflect better communications between our two societies. While from earliest times to the present, "seaweed" decoctions have been used in Chinese herbal medicine for cancer, unfortunately we know of no current scientific Chinese data, and therefore have to rely only on the many cancer/seaweed studies from Japan.

The average per-capita consumption of sea vegetables in Japan varies from 0 to 5 grams per day among those who do not seem to care for them so much, to 65 to 70 grams (about 2 ounces) per day for aficionados, with a daily across-the-board average of 7.3 grams per person.[3] This finding led researcher Dr. Jane Teas, formerly of the Harvard University School of Public Health, to think that this still relatively large consumption might partly account for the much lower breast cancer rate among women living in Japan, especially those who live in certain coastal areas, like Sago prefecture and Hokkaido, where more sea vegetables are eaten than elsewhere in the country and where breast cancer rates are correspondingly the lowest.[4]

Actually, sea vegetables' protective effect against breast cancer had already been observed by the ancient Egyptians, as the famous *Ebers Papyrus* suggests. Of course, the Egyptian physicians of the time had no idea what factor in sea vegetables to credit for this peculiar anticancer effect. Originally, it was thought that it was the high iodine content of marine algae that was responsible for protecting against breast cancer.[5] In fact, for women with breast cancer who also have thyroid dysfunction there is a poorer prognosis than for those with normal thyroid function. But, as Dr. Teas points out, this theory is contradicted by the fact that, due to the use of iodized salt, goiter rates have gone down in the United States, while breast cancer mortality rates have not. She therefore feels that other factors must account for the anticancer effect.[6]

Whatever the mysterious factor or factors are, that such protection does exist was demonstrated again by a subsequent (1984) study by Dr. Teas and colleagues. This study was important in that, contrary to earlier studies, it did not use highly concentrated sea-vegetable extracts, but a dried *Laminaria*—or *kombu,* commonly eaten in Japan—to supplement the diet of experimental rats. Moreover, the amount used was compatible with that normally consumed in the typical Japanese diet. Again it was found that rats that were fed the *Laminaria* took longer to develop breast tumors and got fewer of them than rats not fed sea vegetables. The researchers therefore concluded that "to the Japanese population, seaweed may be an important factor in explaining the low rates of certain cancers in Japan."[7] These findings become all the more impressive in light of the fact that breast cancer has a threefold lower rate among premenopausal women and a ninefold lower rate among postmenopausal women in Japan than for women in the United States.[8]

Other animal studies from Japan—for example, those of Dr. Ichiro Yamamoto of Kitasato University—conducted over a period of fifteen years, confirmed the antitumor effect of several sea vegetables in breast cancer, leukemia, and other types of cancer.[9–11] These studies attempted to shed more light on the biochemical reasons for this protective effect. Dr. Yamamoto, as late as 1987, still stated: "The antitumor action mechanism of dietary seaweeds has not yet been clarified." However, he and his co-workers suggest that the anticancer action of certain brown sea vegetables like *wakame (Undaria)* may be due to a substance called *fucoidan.** The Japanese scientists found that this chemical compound in marine algae acts by stimulating the immune system in animals with malignant tumors, thus producing an antitumor effect.

---

* The compound fucoidan, unique to brown sea algae such as *wakame,* is chemically a polysaccharide sulfate ester, concentrated in the cell walls of these sea plants.

In Japan there is available a seaweed-based health-food product, Viva-Natural.* In tests on mice at the University of Hawaii in Honolulu, this product was found to be therapeutically active against lung cancer. This extract seems to work by enhancing immune-system activity, and may therefore protect against other types of cancer as well. Best of all, it does not seem to produce any of the side effects that are, alas, common to most cancer-fighting synthetic chemicals, such as loss of appetite and weight, baldness, and so forth.[12]

Fucoidan can then logically be expected to have an immune-system–strengthening and thereby an antitumor effect on cancer in general, and specifically on cancer of the bowel. Sea vegetables have also been found to have antitumor effects on cancers of the alimentary canal, due to at least three other factors:

1. The alginic acid content of the fiber in sea vegetables has an incredible swelling capacity in the alkaline intestinal secretions.[13] This makes it an ideal diluter of potential carcinogens in the intestine. Like other vegetable fibers, it is also known to bind intestinal bile acids and enhance their elimination, thereby decreasing cancer risk.[14]

2. Several popular red members of the *Porphyra* family—from which the familiar thin sheets of nori are made to wrap around rice for *sushi*—contain a compound called *beta-sitosterol*† that is credited with protecting against colon cancer.[15]

3. Still another protective factor could be the reported antibiotic activity of certain compounds in sea vegetables that have been found to inhibit the growth of several species of Gram-positive and Gram-negative bacteria which can produce cancer-causing substances in the colon.[16–18]

A fourth protective factor, which applies not only to colon cancer but to all cancers, is an anti-oxidant activity in sea vegetables. They contain small amounts of highly unsaturated fatty acids, which can normally be expected to oxidize when these plants are dried and stored. Yet experience shows that a rancid odor is not detectable even after long storage. Scientists in the Department of Food Chemistry at Tohoku University, Sendai, recently took note of this strange phenomenon and tested dried purple laver (*Porphyra tenerra*), or nori, to discover why these lipid (fat)-containing plants are so resistant to spoilage.[19]

What they found first was that the lipids in nori are enclosed in

* Viva-Natural is a lyophilized natural product, extracted from spore-producing organs of the *Undaria pinnantifida* (*wakame*), a popular sea vegetable in Japan. It is produced by the Corona Shoji Company, Tokyo, Japan.
† Sitoserol is a white, waxy substance, similar to cholesterol, but made only by plants. It competes with the latter for absorptive sites in the small intestine, thereby effectively blocking cholesterol from being abosrbed (*The Nutrition and Dietary Consultant,* June 1985). This may be the reason for the alleged cholesterol-lowering effect of sea algae.

double cell membranes that do not allow molecular oxygen easy access to them; second, and more important, the various sterols and phospholipids in nori showed a strange synergism between them that resulted in an anti-oxidant effect, similar to that of the synthetic food anti-oxidant BHT (butylated hydroxytoluene). It is therefore possible that marine algae of the *Porphyra* family (and, by inference, other sea vegetables) have a mild anti-oxidant effect similar to that of beta-carotene and vitamin E (present also in sea vegetables) and other anti-oxidants in land plants.

ANTIBIOTIC EFFECTS

As early as 1917, the German scientist R. Harder called attention to the presence of inhibitory substances on the proliferation of bacteria in marine algae.[20] Perhaps this was not surprising, considering the antibacterial properties of the seawater in which algae live, a fact that had been known since even earlier times.* It was not until 1959, when the American scientist J.M.N. Sieburth noticed a curious lack of bacteria in the intestines of Antarctic penguins, and showed that this lack was due to the antibiotic effect of marine algae found in shrimp eaten by the penguins, that the scientific community got really excited.[21]

Another observation helped to focus scientific attention on this antibiotic effect of marine algae: In one study a brown seaweed (*Ascophyllum nodosum*) was fed to one of each of seven pairs of monozygotic (identical) twin cows over a seven-year period. To everyone's surprise, there was only one incidence of mastitis (an inflammation of the udder that occurs because of unhygienic conditions) in this group of cows compared with nine cases among other cows that had not been given supplemental seaweed. Even skeptics could find no other explanation for this curious phenomenon than to ascribe it to what they grudgingly called the "mild" antibiotic properties of seaweed. As an additional bonus, the seaweed-supplemented cows yielded a great deal more milk than the other cows.[22] No wonder farmers along the seacoasts of Europe had traditionally encouraged cattle to graze on seaweed along the shore.

* The antibacterial nature of seawater is undoubtedly why humans have been getting away for such a long time with so relatively little serious contamination of the oceans. However, even seawater has its microbe-fighting limits; nor are microorganisms the only contaminants to worry about. Toxic heavy metals like mercury, cadmium, and lead are even more dangerous to our health, and seawater has no mechanism of getting rid of them.

Since 1959, numerous studies have identified several antibacterial, antiviral, and antifungal substances in a large variety of sea vegetables, including some most commonly eaten by humans. As in the case of land plants, the antibiotic substances in sea plants—for instance, halogenated compounds—provide toxic defenses against the rapacious plant-eating sea creatures that abound in subtropical and tropical waters. These chemical defenses are crucial for delicate marine algae, which have no protection like the thorns and thistles some land plants have developed in the course of evolution.

Some antibiotic substances in sea vegetables compare favorably with the most commonly used antibiotics, like penicillin, terramycin, streptomycin, and so forth. They have been found effective in the test tube against a wide variety of pathogenic bacteria and fungi, among them *Staphylococcus aureus* (Gram-positive bacteria), *Eschericia coli* (Gram-negative bacteria), *Candida albicans* (fungi), *Streptococcus pyogenes* and facecalis (Gram-positive bacteria), and *Klebsiella pneumonia* (Gram-negative bacteria).[23,24]

Marine algae possess antiviral substances that have been proved to work against influenza B virus, polio virus, herpes simplex virus, and encephalomyocarditis virus. Scientists credit certain sulfated saccharides in sea algae for this effect.[25,26] But let's not be deceived—you can't fight off the next cold or flu just by eating miso and sushi—although it might help!

SEA VEGETABLES AND TOXIC METALS

It has been shown that as a group sea algae can bind certain toxic metals and prevent their intestinal absorption. Among these are included radioactive strontium, cadmium, and lead. We need not tell you how important this is in a time when water- and air-pollution have reached health-threatening heights, and radioactive fallout from nuclear tests and accidents, like the one at Chernobyl, must be reckoned with also, along with radon gas in our homes and other buildings.

Cadmium, like radioactive strontium, is considered one of the most hazardous pollutants. In Japan cadmium poisoning has resulted in painful disorders in bone metabolism, and it is suspected of causing kidney damage.[27,28] (The reader may recall the terrible medical consequences of mercury poisoning through contaminated seafood that occurred a few years ago in Japan.) The best news of all is that Dr. Jerry F. Stara of the Toxicology Laboratory, Environmental Protection Agency in Cincinnati has demonstrated in cats that the amount of radioactive strontium already deposited in the bones can be reduced by the continuous administration of alginate from marine algae.[*][29] This shows that, in the long run, alginate from sea vegetables can function not only in the prevention but also in the treatment of poisoning by radioactive strontium.

OTHER PROTECTIVE EFFECTS

It has always been accepted in Japan that eating sea vegetables like nori and wakame will prolong life. Now, Japanese and other scientists have demonstrated that such assumptions are not so far-fetched, given the proven ability of sea vegetables to lower both blood pressure and cholesterol, as well as thinning out the blood.

Traditionally, sea vegetables, especially of the *Laminaria* family, have been regarded in Japanese folk medicine as hypotensive (blood-pressure-lowering). For that purpose, usually hot water extracts of these plants are being used, and apparently with some success. Commercial products from the basal parts of the blades of plants belonging to the *Laminaria* family ("ne-kombu") are being widely used there for the same purpose.

When scientists first started getting interested in this alleged hypotensive property of these sea vegetables, they thought that it was the amino acid laminine in them that was responsible for it.[30,31] More recently (1981), however, it was shown that laminine was *not* able to lower blood pressure in experimental animals. On the other hand, another substance in them, histamine, was indeed capable of doing so, and not just a little, but to a "significant" extent.[32] Unfortunately, at the same time it turned out that of the seven commercial "ne-kombu" preparations analyzed only two contained the therapeutically active histamine, the other five being totally useless (It's like only two out of seven brands of penicillin doing any good!).

During the 1960s and 1970s also, studies on edible sea vegetables showed that some had a definite cholesterol-lowering effect. It was found that *Porphyra* was most effective in rats, resulting in the reduction of plasma cholesterol by an astonishing 40 percent over a thirty-day period.[33–36] Scientists who have given the question of how sea vegetables lower cholesterol the most thought, feel that this salutary effect is due basically to the observed fact that the acidic polysaccharide in sea vegetables forms an indigestible solution (lyophilic colloid) in the gut that inhibits cholesterol absorption.[37]† This

---

* As Dr. Tanaka comments, the radioactive strontium is resecreted into the intestine, where it is bound by alginate and then excreted in the feces.
† See also our footnote regarding the cholesterol-absorption–blocking role of sitosterol, p. 404.

effect, added to their demonstrated blood-thinning and blood-pressure–lowering properties,[38] would be enough fully to justify their life-extending reputation in Japan and China.

Certain green algae also seems to be therapeutic in cases of gallstones and other stones.[39,40] Sea lettuce (*Ulva lactuca*) has been used in folk medicine for gout and podagra (a gouty pain in the big toe).[41] Folk medicinal sources also universally credit sea vegetables with antidiarrhetic and antiulcer properties.[42]

While some of the foregoing claims are not scientifically well documented, sea vegetables in general and dried and powdered kelp extracts are helpful as natural laxatives. They have been found to be vastly superior to other fiber laxatives, as well as quicker-acting but irritant medications. The biggest advantage of kelp-derived laxatives is not that they are tasteless and economical, but that their ability to swell in the intestines is superior to that of virtually all other water-soluble fibers. Furthermore, with algae-derived laxatives, swelling does not take place in the stomach, only in the intestines, and therefore does not interfere with appetite.[43] This is an important point in relieving constipation in geriatric patients where reduction of food intake and weight loss must often be avoided.*

Scientifically verified are folk medicinal claims about the effectiveness of *Undaria pinnatifida* (wakame) against intestinal parasites such as roundworms and pinworms.[44,45] In fact, in South China adults and children take a popular worm remedy, TSE Ko-tsoi, made from marine algae (*Digenea simplex*).[46]

We would like to mention one more documented but largely ignored benefit of wakame. This plant contains a compound that strongly counteracts the harmful effects of nicotine.[47] It seems to us that a natural substance like this deserves further exploration as a possible help in overcoming nicotine addiction (in the absence of a pharmaceutical product that has this compound as the active ingredient, perhaps smokers who want to quit should try chewing on dried wakame when they have the urge to reach for a cigarette, or while smoking).

THE BOTTOM LINE ON SEA VEGETABLES

With all the medicinal benefits that sea vegetables can offer, we should not look upon them as just something that is "good for us"—never a good motivation for eating anything—but as highly palatable and nutritious foods that can enhance the taste and nutri-

---

* In the United States, laxatives prepared from marine algae are produced by Wallace Laboratories, Inc., New Brunswick, New Jersey, and Carter Products, Inc., New York City.

tional value of many a dish. To begin with, the protein content of sea vegetables accounts, on average, for about 25 percent of their dry weight, paralleled only by that of soy beans among plant foods. Furthermore, these proteins have a digestibility factor greater than 75 percent, are extraordinarily well balanced, and about as complete as any animal protein. Present in high concentrations in wakame, for example, are the amino acids alanine, arginine, glutamic acid, glycine, isoleucine, leucine, proline, threonine, and tyrosine. Nori, hijiki, and kombu are especially high in a number of other important amino acids. If therefore you regularly eat several kinds of sea vegetables, not necessarily at the same meal, you get not only a rich variety of different tastes—no marine alga tastes just like another—but you also benefit from a very complete protein intake.

Sea vegetables are very high in calcium, potassium, and phosphorus, and reasonably high in iron.[48] They are high in all the trace elements of the sea.[49] Moreover, most of the minerals and trace elements are in a highly available form.

We don't expect that consumption of sea vegetables in the United States and Europe will ever come anywhere near the popularity that they enjoy in parts of Japan and China. However, sea vegetable consumption is definitely on the rise in the Western world, with more and more health-conscious people catching on to their culinary and nutritional potentials.

We are embarrassed to admit that it took us so long to see their value in making our far from monotonous diet even more varied and exciting. We now eat small amounts of different sea vegetables almost daily, either as ingredients in soups and vegetable dishes, or with fish and other seafood.

Admittedly, to appreciate sea vegetables fully involves an acquired taste, as with so many other foods. Their taste properties defy easy comparisons. Some of them tend more toward the sour and some more toward the sweet end of the spectrum. Some have a mildly fishy but not at all disagreeable taste, and therefore go especially well with other seafood. Others have more of a nutty or "beany" taste, actually not unlike that of truffles. For the experimental cook, there are many interesting possibilities of creating new taste sensations and giving the most commonplace, traditional dishes a new dimension.

SOURCES

1. Hoppe, H. A. "Marine Algae and Their Products and Constituents in Pharmacy." In: *Marine Algae in Pharmaceutical Science.* H. A. Hoppe et al., eds. New York: DeGruyter, 1979, pp. 90–91.
2. Xia, A., and I. A. Abbott. "Edible seaweeds of China and their place in the Chinese diet." *Economic Botany,* 1987; 41:341–353.

3. Toyokawa, H. "Nutritional status in Japan from the viewpoint of numerical ecology." *Social Science and Medicine,* 1978; 12:517–524.
4. Teas, J. "The consumption of seaweed as a protective factor in the etiology of breast cancer." *Medical Hypotheses,* 1981; 7:601–613.
5. Loeser, A. A. "Hormones and breast cancer" (Letters to the Editor). *Lancet,* 1956; 2:961.
6. Teas, op. cit., p. 603.
7. Teas, J., et al. "Dietary sea weed (*Laminaria*) and mammary carcinogenesis in rats." *Cancer Res.,* 1984; 44:2758–2761.
8. Reddy, B. S., et al. "Nutrition and its relationship to cancer." *Adv. Cancer Res.,* 1980; 32:237–332.
9. Yamamoto, I., et al. "Antitumor effect of seaweeds, I." *Japan. J. Exp. Med.,* 1974; 44:543–546.
10. Yamamoto, I., et al. "Antitumor effect of seaweeds, II." *Japan. J. Exp. Med.,* 1977; 47:133–140.
11. Yamamoto, I., et al. "The effect of dietary seaweeds on 7, 12-dimethyl-benz(a)anthracene-induced mammary tumorigenesis in rats." *Cancer Lett.,* 1987; 35:109–118.
12. Furosawa, E., and S. Furosawa. "Anticancer activity of a natural product, Viva-Natural, extracted from *Undaria pinnatifida* on intraperitoneally implanted Lewis lung cancer carcinoma." *Oncology,* 1985; 42:364–369.
13. Mulinos, M. G., and B.B.J. Glass. "The treatment of constipation with a new hydrosorbent material derived from kelp." *Gastroenterology,* 1953; 24:383–393.
14. Story, J. A., and D. Kritchevsky. "Bile acid metabolism and fiber." *Am. J. Clin. Nutr.,* 1978; 31:S199–S202.
15. Raicht, R. F., et al. "Protective effect of plant sterols against chemically induced colon tumors in rats." *Cancer Res.,* 1980; 40:402–405.
16. Mautner, G. G., G. M. Gardner, and R. Pratt. "Antibiotic activity of seaweed extracts." *J. Am. Pharm. Assoc.,* 1953; 42:294–296.
17. Pratt, R., et al. "Report on antibiotic activity of seaweed extracts." *J. Am. Pharm. Assoc.,* 1951; 40:575–579.
18. Vacca, D. D., and R. A. Walsh. "The antibacterial activity of an extract obtained from *Ascophyllum nodosum.*" *J. Am. Pharm. Assoc.,* 1954; 43:24–26.
19. Kaneda, T. H. Ando. "Component lipids of purple laver and their antioxygenic activity." *Proc. 7th Internat. Seaweed Symp.* New York: John Wiley & Sons, 1972; published by the Science Council of Japan, Tokyo, pp. 553–557.
20. Harder, R. A. Oppermann. "Über antibiotische Stoffe bei den Grünalgen *Stichococcus bacillaris* und *Protosiphon bombyoides.*" Arch. Microbiol., 1953; 19:398–401.
21. Sieburth, J.Mc.N. "Acrylic acid an 'antibiotic' principle in *Phaeocystis* blooms in Antarctic waters." *Sciences,* 1960; 132:676–677.
22. Teas, J., op. cit., p. 605.
23. McConnell, O. J., and W. Fenical. "Antimicrobial Agents from Marine Red Algae of the Family Bonnemaisoniaceae." In: *Marine Algae in Pharmaceutical Science,* H. A. Hoppe et al., eds. Berlin/New York: Walter DeGruyter, 1979.
24. Pesando, D. M. Gnassia-Barelli. "Antifungal Properties of Some Marine Planktonic Algae." In: Ibid.
25. McConnell and Fenical, op. cit., p. 424.
26. Ehresmann, D. W., E. F. Deig, and M. T. Hatch. "Anti-Viral Properties of

Algal Polysaccharides and Related Compounds." In: *Marine Algae in Pharmaceutical Science,* H. A. Hoppe et al., eds. Berlin/New York: Walter DeGruyter, 1979, op. cit. pp. 294–295.

27. Tanaka, Y. "Algal Polysaccharides: Their Potential Use to Prevent Chronic Metal Poisoning." In: Ibid.

28. Tanaka, Y., et al. "Application of Algal Polysaccharides as *in vivo* Binders of Metal Pollutants." In: *Proc. 7th Internat. Seaweed Symp.* New York: John Wiley & Sons, 1972; published by the Science Council of Japan, Tokyo.

29. Stara, J. F. "Metabolism of internal emitters—repressive action of sodium alginate on absorption of radiostrontium in kittens." *Abstr. Symp. Nuc. Med.,* Omaha, Nebraska, 1965.

30. Takemoto, T., et al. "Studies on the hypotensive constituents of marine algae." *J. Pharm. Soc. Jap.,* 1964; 84:1176–1179.

31. Tagaki, N., et al. "Studies on the hypotensive constituents of marine algae, V." *J. Pharm. Soc. Jap.,* 1970; 90:899–902.

32. Funayama, S., and Hikino, H. "Hypotensive principle of laminaria and allied seaweeds." *Planta Medica (Journal of Medicinal Plant Research),* 1981; 41:29–33.

33. Kaneda, T., et al. "Studies on the effects of marine products on cholesterol metabolism, V." *Bull. Japan. Soc. Sci. Fish.,* 1965; 31:1026–1029.

34. Kaneda, T., et al. "Studies on the effects of marine products on cholesterol metabolism, I." *Bull. Japan. Soc. Sci. Fish.,* 1963; 29:1020–1023.

35. Abe, S., and T. Kaneda. "The effect of edible seaweeds on cholesterol metabolism in rats." In: *Proc. 7th Internat. Seaweed Symp.* New York: John Wiley & Sons, 1972; published by the Science Council of Japan, Tokyo, pp. 562–565.

36. Kimura, A., and M. Kuramato. "Influences of seaweeds on metabolism of cholesterol and anticoagulant actions of seaweed." *Tokushima J. Exp. Med.,* 1974; 21:79–88.

37. Ito, K., and Y. Tsuchiya. "The effect of algal polysaccharides on the depressing of plasma cholesterol levels in rats," op. cit., No. 34.

38. Elsner, H., et al. "Tierversuche mit einen gerinnungshemmenden Algenstoff aus *Delesseria sanguinea* (L.) *Lam. Naunym-Schmiedebergs Archiv f. exp. Pathologie und Pharmakologie,* 1938; 190:510–514.

39. Bonotto, S., et al. "Recent advances in research on the marine alga *Acetabularia.*" Adv. Mar. Biol., 1976; 14:123–250.

40. *Biology of Acetabularia,* J. Brachet and S. Bonotto, eds. New York and London: Academic Press, 1970.

41. Schneider, W. *Lexikon der Arzneimittelgeschichte. Pflanzliche Drogen V/1–3.* Govi-Verlag GmbH.–Pharmazeutischer Verlag, Frankfurt a. M., 1979.

42. Ibid.

43. Mulinos, M. G., et al. "The treatment of constipation with a new hydrasorbent material derived from Kelp." *Rev. Gastroenterol.,* 1953; 24:385–393.

44. Takemoto, T., and T. Sai. "Studies on the constituents of *Chondria armata.*" Yakugaku Zasschi, 1965; 85:33–37.

45. Takemoto, T., et al., ibid; 83–85.

46. Yosisige, K. "Present status and development trends of the plant drugs in Japan." *Herba Polonica,* XVI, 1970; 1:96–103.

47. Watanabe, Y. "Harmful effects of nicotine can be prevented by intake of *Undaria.*" General Meeting of Nippon Dietetical and Food Technological Society (1968). In: *Advance in Phycology in Japan,* Hirose Tokida, ed. Jena: VEB Gustav Fischer Verlag, 1975.

48. Johnston, H. W. "Detailed chemical analysis of some edible Japanese seaweeds." *Proc. 7th Internat. Seaweed Symp.* New York: John Wiley & Sons, 1972; published by the Science Council of Japan, Tokyo.
49. Yamamoto, T., and M. Ishibashi. "The content of trace elements in seaweeds." Ibid.

CHAPTER 54

THE SPICES OF LIFE

12 Just to give you an idea of how complicated things can get when you think seriously about the chemical nature of the most commonly used herbs and spices, take a look at the list of spices on page 414. Only some of the most important chemicals in these innocent-sounding herbs are listed. The actual number of chemicals these herbs contain may well exceed a hundred or more compounds, some beneficial and medicinal, others potentially harmful and possibly cancer-causing, if they are ingested in quantities too large for our bodies to handle.

Before going into our discussion of individual herbs and spices, we would like to make a couple of general remarks that pertain to all of them. First, the aromatic compounds they contain are highly volatile and perishable and lose much of their potency rather quickly. Moreover, the substances that give each spice or herb its particular fragrance and flavor are suspended in the plants' own essential oils—which means they are subject to oxidation, just like fats or oils.

It is therefore important to prevent, or at least slow down, the degradation of the spices, which are so important for the flavor they add to our foods—and all the more so in a health-conscious diet where salt is kept to a minimum. All of that is quite apart from the medicinal properties of spices, which are also subject to the same degradation as their flavors, and are often one and the same.

For these reasons we are often greatly chagrined when we observe spices in people's kitchens neatly arranged on little shelves or revolving plates, but exposed to both light and heat. Sometimes the spices are on shelves right above the stove, or on windowsills, where daylight and sunlight hasten their deterioration.

Spices should be kept in a kitchen cabinet, away from heat and light.

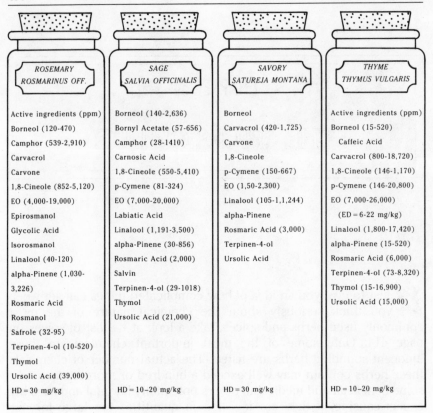

ROSEMARY ROSMARINUS OFF.	SAGE SALVIA OFFICINALIS	SAVORY SATUREJA MONTANA	THYME THYMUS VULGARIS
Active ingredients (ppm)	Borneol (140-2,636)	Borneol	Active ingredients (ppm)
Borneol (120-470)	Bornyl Acetate (57-656)	Carvacrol (420-1,725)	Borneol (15-520)
Camphor (539-2,910)	Camphor (28-1410)	Carvone	Caffeic Acid
Carvacrol	Carnosic Acid	1,8-Cineole	Carvacrol (800-18,720)
Carvone	1,8-Cineole (550-5,410)	p-Cymene (150-667)	1,8-Cineole (146-1,170)
1,8-Cineole (852-5,120)	p-Cymene (81-324)	EO (1,50-2,300)	p-Cymene (146-20,800)
EO (4,000-19,000)	EO (7,000-20,000)	Linalool (105-1,1,244)	EO (7,000-26,000)
Epirosmanol	Labiatic Acid	alpha-Pinene	(ED = 6-22 mg/kg)
Glycolic Acid	Linalool (1,191-3,500)	Rosmaric Acid (3,000)	Linalool (1,800-17,420)
Isorosmanol	alpha-Pinene (30-856)	Terpinen-4-ol	alpha-Pinene (15-520)
Linalool (40-120)	Rosmaric Acid (2,000)	Ursolic Acid	Rosmaric Acid (6,000)
alpha-Pinene (1,030-3,226)	Salvin		Terpinen-4-ol (73-8,320)
Rosmaric Acid	Terpinen-4-ol (29-1018)		Thymol (15-16,900)
Rosmanol	Thymol		Ursolic Acid (15,000)
Safrole (32-95)	Ursolic Acid (21,000)		
Terpinen-4-ol (10-520)			
Thymol			
Ursolic Acid (39,000)			
HD = 30 mg/kg	HD = 10-20 mg/kg	HD = 30 mg/kg	HD = 10-20 mg/kg

* Reproduced by permission from James A. Duke, Ph. D., *Father Nature's Farmacy: The Mint Family* (Fulton, Md.: Herbal Vineyard, 1987).

In addition, let us pass on to you a little trick we learned from Durk Pearson and Sandy Shaw. They taught us to preserve dried herbs and spices by putting them into glass bottles that can be tightly sealed and that are large enough to accommodate a little cheesecloth bag containing a teaspoon of BHT, which we use to protect cooking oils (BHT is readily available from many health-food stores). It is best to put the little bag of BHT at the bottom of the bottle so that when it slowly vaporizes, it permeates the spice above it. In that fashion, you'll be able to keep the full aroma of your spices many times longer than you would otherwise.

Best of all, of course, is to use fresh herbs and spices. Once you've tried the fresh kind, you'll no longer like dried ones at all, unless you have no choice. There is no good reason why you can't plant at least a few herbs like rosemary, thyme, parsley, and dill (just to mention some that lend themselves well to being potted) on your windowsill. It is even worthwhile to invest in a plant light so the herbs can be kept away from the window in winter, protected from cold drafts or frost and independent of sunshine (very attractive and relatively inexpensive metal shelves and overhead lights are available in the United States, Europe, and Japan).

Last of all, if you are among those who are unused to herbs and spices, or think you don't like them, try to reeducate yourself to use and enjoy them. As usual, it's just a question of habit and conditioning. There is plenty of reason to make the effort to like them, because you'll be rewarded by tastier food and you'll probably get considerable medicinal benefits from them into the bargain.

ROSEMARY AND THYME

Rosemary and thyme are two of our most favorite herbs, and we cannot urge you enough to grow them yourself either in the garden or on the windowsill. You will enjoy the superior taste of the fresh leaves. They even make very attractive houseplants and, according to Dr. James Duke, the famous herbalist and botanist, some rosemary cultivars are good candidates for homemade bonsai and hanging gardens.

Both herbs, rosemary in particular, are so strongly flavored that they must be used with great care lest they overpower the milder flavors of the food. For instance, both are fine with strongly flavored meats like mutton and venison. Used very sparingly, rosemary goes well with chicken, but not with fish, whereas a sprinkling of thyme, especially lemon thyme, is quite all right with fish and chowders. Both herbs are excellent with eggplant and indispensable for the Provençal vegetable dish ratatouille, in which eggplant is one of the main ingredients. Besides, we can hardly imagine a vegetable soup or mixed salad without some rosemary and thyme.

In folk medicine, rosemary is said to enhance memory and "clear the mind." There is even a reference to this reputed property of rosemary in Ophelia's soliloquy in Shakespeare's *Hamlet*. Since rosemary has now been shown to contain no fewer than a dozen or so powerful anti-oxidants, its traditional reputation for memory enhancement no longer appears so far-fetched.

Rosemary contains numerous compounds, credited in folklore with various medicinal properties (antitumor, anti-allergic, anti-inflammatory, antipruritic, antibronchitic, anti-asthmatic). The more general and numerous rather than specific the medicinal claims for any plant are, the less likely it is that they are based on fact. However, rosemary and thyme do contain a number of compounds that might justify such a reputation. Besides, if only one tenth of all the folkloristic claims for these two herbs were ultimately confirmed, they could be considered a whole natural pharmacy on their own.

Rosemary and thyme appear to share many of the same compounds, including some of the anti-oxidants. But since rosemary has been more thoroughly researched than thyme, let's just consider the remarkable story of the anti-oxidants in rosemary, keeping in mind that much of it probably also pertains to its sister herb, thyme.

The natural anti-oxidant rosmaridiphenol has been known and recognized as a food preservative for some time.* However, in 1984 Japanese scientists discovered two more anti-oxidants, epirosmanol and isorosmanol, in rosemary.[1] Both were discovered to be about four times more active than the two man-made anti-oxidants, BHT and BHA, widely used by the food industry. More recently (1987), scientists found that two more anti-oxidants in rosemary (carnosol and ursolic acid) did at least as well as BHT and BHA in preventing microbial spoilage of foods, and in some instances did even better.[2]

Thyme has among its active ingredients a compound called *thymol,* which is known to have antiseptic activity and is therefore present in some mouthwashes. Infusions (teas) of thyme are also known to be antispasmodic—that is, they relieve cramps and relax the throat (singers and public speakers take note!). Dr. Duke says he drinks a thyme tea (*tisane*) when his lower back pain flares up, and it seems to help. But no folk remedy, or any of the synthetic steroids often prescribed for back pain, is a substitute for regular exercise to strengthen back and stomach muscles and develop correct walking and sitting posture.

CUMIN

Cumin, too, has toxic compounds, but it is a wonderful spice and without it there would be no curry powders, of which it forms the base. In Costa Rica we use cumin almost daily especially with black bean paste and soup. Cumin goes well with lentils, white and red bean dishes, chicken, fish, and many vegetables.

* Extracts of rosemary are marketed in the U.S. not as anti-oxidants but as flavor additives, because of the costly process of having to get USDA approval for that purpose. In fact, the food industry has not woken up as yet to the remarkable anti-oxidant potential of rosemary extract.

At this writing, rosemary extract is available only in larger quantities to the food industry (we hope this will change in the near future). Meanwhile, a tip to our friends in the food industry: We found the liquid extract of rosemary from one particular supplier far superior to any other because the bitter, camphorous compounds have been eliminated and the level of anti-oxidants has been held constant. (The extract is available from Kalsec, Inc., P.O. Box 511, Kalamazoo, Mich. 49005; Tel.: (616) 349-9711.)

PARSLEY AND CORIANDER (CILANTRO)

Green parsley is the most commonly used kitchen herb in the United States and Europe, and its cousin, cilantro, permeates Latin American and Asian cooking. In French cuisine especially, large quantities of parsley are used with abandon. There's hardly a French sauce recipe that doesn't call for bouquets of chopped green parsley.

We like parsley, but it has a rather strong flavor and, like rosemary or oregano, can easily overpower rather than enhance the subtle taste of food. For that reason alone it should be used more sparingly than it usually is. All of this is quite aside from the fact that parsley—being a member of the umbelliferae family—contains furocoumarins, such as psoralen derivatives that are potent light-activated carcinogens and mutagens.[3] Parsley also contains myristicin,[4] a problematic compound that's present also in black pepper and a number of other members of the carrot family, including carrots, celery, and dill. (Still, we much prefer carrots to celery because carrots do not have furocoumarins, but do contain plenty of the anti-oxidant and anticancer substance beta-carotene.)

At the same time, the toxic compound myristicine in parsley, along with another compound, apiol, are also scientifically proven uterine stimulants. In fact, parsley concoctions have for that very reason been used in folk medicine to bring on menstruation and even to induce abortions (in the high concentrations in which parsley must be used for the latter purpose, it is as likely to cause cancer as to bring on abortion).

On a lighter note, the chlorophyll, which is abundant in parsley, has been credited with combating halitosis. However, scientific tests have shown that this is not so. This does not mean that other compounds in parsley don't have such an effect, because studies have been conducted with pure chlorophyll only, rather than with the whole parsley plant.

We now don't use parsley very frequently. This is not so much because of the potentially carcinogenic compounds it contains (many other herbs, spices, and vegetables have them too), but because other herbs and spices go better with the kinds of food we eat. For example, when we lived in Europe we used to eat more potatoes than rice, and parsley is, of course, ideal with potatoes, but doesn't do anything for rice. Occasionally, however, we do enjoy the flavor a persillade of finely chopped parsley and shallots gives to certain dishes, like minestrone, vegetable stews, and fish soups, if added at the end of cooking. With soups, sauces, and stews of all kinds, it is a good idea to follow the French custom of adding a *bouquet garni* of parsley, rosemary, and thyme, all tied together and easy to remove before serving the dish.

We have become very fond of parsley's exotic cousin coriander (cilantro), but must confess that it is definitely an acquired taste. Many years ago, when we first encountered it in food served to us in Mexico and Thailand, we used to complain that it was ruining our favorite dishes. We actually carefully picked it out of our food as much as possible. Now we enjoy the taste and often miss it in American and European cooking.

Like parsley, cilantro has carcinogenic as well as medicinal compounds. For example, it is reputed to lower blood sugar, which would make it useful in a diabetic diet. It is also said to break down triglycerides, which would make it doubly useful for diabetics. But to our knowledge, none of these claims has been sufficiently established where we can recommend eating cilantro for those specific purposes. However, it goes well with tomato salad, as a change from using sweet basil. Providing you like it, cilantro can add a lot of flavor to steamed fish, fish soup, and, of course, all the obligatory Latin American black bean dishes, like black bean soup and purée.

BASIL AND TARRAGON

Dr. Ames rates basil about one third more carcinogenic than chlorinated tap water because of its estragole content. This sounds bad enough to make you wonder whether it might not be better to give up altogether eating spaghetti with pesto sauce, one of our favorite pasta dishes. But to put all this into perspective, 250 milliliters of wine (about two glasses) would be 4,700 times more carcinogenic than tap water. Dr. James Duke figures that one gram per day of basil (and probably oregano), though more of a cancer risk than tap water, is only one twenty-eighth as carcinogenic as a twelve-ounce can of beer. This estimate is based on the carcinogenicity of beer's alcohol (ethanol) content—to say nothing of the dozens of other chemicals in it, some of which are almost certainly carcinogenic.[5]

That's why we don't mind occasionally having pesto sauce, since we make it with monounsaturated olive oil, which at least doesn't raise one's cholesterol. Basil has, as Dr. Duke says, a long, historic pedigree in both folkloric and scientific herbal literature. The Roman naturalist Pliny praised it for relieving gas pains, nausea, and dysentery.[6] However, if you don't make your own pesto sauce, beware of the fact that commercial pesto sauces are often liberally laced with Parmesan cheese, a definite no-no on any health-conscious diet (grating cheese, like grinding meat, increases the surface area exposed to oxygen and thereby hastens the food's rancidification).

We frequently use fresh or dried basil in tossed green salads or in tomato salad, with a standard vinegar and olive oil dressing. It also goes well with cooked red beets and in potato salad. We often use basil or tarragon in sauces with fish or chicken. However, for sauces and soups, it is best to use whole-leaf basil and tarragon, sold only in specialized herb stores, rather than the ground herbs that are generally used in the United States.

DILL

To us, who have spent considerable time in Scandinavia where dill is used as an accompaniment to almost everything, dill is very familiar and well liked. Dill is, as Dr. Duke says, a "cool, relaxing, stomach settling herb." It is a fact that, in animal experiments, dill oil has worked as an antispasmodic, relieving smooth-muscle cramping of the intestines. But nobody knows for sure whether it might have the same effect in humans, although dill has that reputation in folk medicine. According to Dr. Duke, dill has been shown, in other animal experiments, to lower blood pressure, dilate blood vessels, and stimulate respiration. Dill oil, diluted with water, has apparently been helpful with infant colic and with dyspepsia in older children.

Be that as it may, dill contains the toxic compound myristicin,* which is present in other herbs, spices, and carrots. While this is not alarming, we cannot help wondering whether dill is not slightly overused in Scandinavia and should perhaps be treated with more respect for the inherent toxicities which, alas, coexist with its medicinal properties.

MARJORAM AND OREGANO

In any dish where you can use marjoram, you could also use oregano; in fact, they are frequently teamed together for a more rounded flavor bouquet.

In folk medicine marjoram has been used for ages as a tea to cure abdominal cramps and upset stomachs. We now know that this time-honored custom is based on scientific fact, for marjoram's antispasmodic properties have been demonstrated in guinea pig experiments.[7]

The active ingredient in oregano is the compound carvacrol, which

---

* Nutmeg and mace (the outer layer of the seed kernel that is the nutmeg proper) contain substantial amounts of myristicin. Nutmeg is used more often than mace for the good reason that it is much cheaper and more readily available. However, nutmeg, which also contains another compound, elemicin, has narcotic and hallucinogenic effects if it is ingested in larger quantities than normal. Fortunately, its aftereffects (headache, cramps, nausea) are so unpleasant as to make it unattractive for repeated usage.

is responsible for its specific flavor with which most Americans are familiar from its use on pizza. Back on our farm in Costa Rica, we have two large bushes of Italian oregano growing right outside the house, and we use the fresh leaves, as well as the tiny white flowers (sparingly because of their strong flavor), to spice many soups and sauces. Also, for a sore throat or bronchitis, we recommend following the old folk remedy of making a tea from the fresh or dried leaves and drinking it with milk and honey. It seems to soothe the throat and definitely works in this combination as an expectorant, though not nearly as well without the added milk and honey. There is, however, some scientific basis for using oregano for this purpose. Carvacrol is now known to have antiseptic and antispasmodic properties that might well explain oregano's throat-relaxing effect.

SAGE

Dr. James Duke assures us that sage contains strong anti-oxidants and that even now it is being tested for use as a natural anti-oxidant in salad oil and for potato chips (this still wouldn't make the chips fit to eat because of their high fat content and the browning effect, which alone makes them a hazardous food).

In folk medicine sage is used for bleeding gums, sore throat, and tonsillitis—in the first case, perhaps for its antiseptic effect; in the latter two instances, probably because of its antibiotic compound, salvin, which has been proved *in vitro* to act against *Staphylococcus* bacteria.

On the downside, sage contains a highly toxic compound, thujone, which is a major component of oil of wormwood, the principal flavoring ingredient of the infamous French liqueur absinthe, banned in 1915 after some serious cases of absinthe poisoning.[8] When sage is used as a flavoring only, its small thujone content is, of course, nothing to worry about.

FENNEL, ANISE, AND CARAWAY SEEDS

If we follow Dr. Duke's and other experts' advice, what fennel, anise, and caraway have in common is a carminative effect, that is, they counteract stomach gas. In fennel seed it may be the antispasmodic thiol that produces this welcome effect. In folk medicine an infusion (tea) made from fennel seeds has long been a remedy for colicky babies, and has been recommended for stomach cramps in adults as well. The same is true for anise and caraway, with carvacrol, one of the active ingredients in oregano, being credited for this effect (anise liqueurs have long been used in Europe to settle upset stomachs and help digest heavy meals).

But let there be no mistake—although Dr. Ames has not yet analyzed these seeds for carcinogenicity, one cannot reasonably expect them to be exempt. Use these interesting spices in moderation and not in such strong concentrations that they could possibly become harmful.

SAFFRON, THE QUEEN OF SPICES

Saffron's worth its weight in gold,
As it was in days of old.
   But it takes a million flowers,
   And about that many hours,
For 10 kilograms, I am told.*

The saffron plant is a crocus and grows from bulbs or corms that can survive several seasons. It grows readily in the right climate, a dry, Mediterranean one being ideal. However, according to Dr. James Duke, it takes about a ton of small bulbs to plant one acre. When the plants bloom, the flowers are hand picked, and the stigma on their stems, carrying the yellow pollen, are removed and quickly dried to make commercial saffron. About 100,000 flowers have to be picked to yield one kilogram (about two pounds) of saffron. No wonder its price—as in the case of glutathione—is almost the same as for gold (the same being true for the man-made triple amino acid glutathione on the Demopoulos spectrum of anti-oxidants and vitamin co-factors).

Which brings us to our point: Saffron not only gives white rice a lovely golden color and adds a sophisticated flavor for which it has been famed for centuries—it has recently been shown to be a first-class anti-oxidant. The reason for that is that saffron contains a carotene derivative, crocetin, a substance chemically similar to our old friend beta-carotene. However, crocetin has quite different functions and properties from those of beta-carotene, making these two carotenoids ideal complements to each other.

* Poem by Dr. James A. Duke from *Living Liqueurs* (Lincoln, Mass.: Quarterman Publications, Inc., 1987). By permission of the author.

While beta-carotene is mainly known for its free-radical chain-breaking ability and anticancer functions, crocetin lowers cholesterol levels and enhances the diffusion of oxygen into tissues.[9] Crocetin's ability to deliver oxygen becomes all the more important in view of the well-known fact that atherosclerosis accompanies diminished oxygen supplies in the bloodstream. Atherosclerosis is widespread in our country, and it increases with age. Therefore, anything, like crocetin, that can counteract this pernicious process and increase oxygen diffusion in the blood, must be more than welcome.[10]

There is evidence that crocetin improves the oxygen supply to the brains of hemorrhaged rats.[11] Without jumping to conclusions from such preliminary findings, it does offer hope that crocetin might, in synergy with other anti-oxidants, help prevent the frequent mental deterioration of aging, as well as stop ischemic cerebral accidents (resulting from a lack of oxygen to the brain) and aid in recuperation from strokes. At any rate, this ability of crocetin to increase oxygen transport from the lungs to the brain and other internal organs is its unique feature. One can say this because other carotenoids, even those with a close chemical structure such as beta-carotene, have not been found to have this effect.[12]

In view of crocetin's properties, it is obvious that we should be using saffron wherever its color and flavor enhancement are desirable. Unfortunately, most of us are limited by the justifiably high prices genuine saffron demands (and the saffron substitutes commonly available in food stores cannot provide the same benefits). Likewise, pure crocetin, extracted from saffron, would be an exorbitantly expensive supplement that only the wealthiest could afford. We are therefore pleased to learn that crocetin can apparently also be extracted from gardenia flowers,[13] which would be much cheaper. Meanwhile, we will have to be content with flavoring white chicken meat or fish with precious saffron when we can afford to do so. And we are definitely looking forward to the day when either an even cheaper natural source for crocetin than gardenias has been found, or that synthetic crocetin becomes available.

GINGER

Ginger contains two potent anti-oxidants, shogaol and zingerone, both of which are lipid soluble and hence able to protect our lipid (fat)-containing body tissues from oxidation and free-radical damage. By the same token, shogaol and zingerone (and perhaps other anti-oxidants that have not yet been isolated and studied) are the real reasons why the ancient Chinese practice of preserving pork by liberally lacing it with ginger actually works.*

It is also true that ginger helps us digest proteins, as for example in Chinese pork and fish dishes, in which liberal amounts of fresh ginger root are traditionally used. The reason for that sensible custom is that ginger (like papaya and pineapple) contains a proteolytic (protein-splitting) enzyme that works as a meat tenderizer, breaking up protein molecules and thus making these foods more easily digestible. At the same time, ginger adds an agreeable flavor or seasoning to many dishes, as well as providing other medicinal benefits.

One of the additional benefits of ginger is that it helps keep blood platelets from sticking together, as has been demonstrated in a recent Danish experiment[14] (the anticoagulant factors in ginger are probably certain compounds, called *gingerols,* which it contains in high concentration). In fact, in animal experiments, ginger was even more effective in preventing platelet aggregation than extracts of garlic and onion.†

Several Japanese studies have shown that, in addition to its blood-thinning property, ginger has even more directly protective effects on the heart: It slows down the heart rate while increasing the force of contractions in the upper (atrial) chamber of the heart,[15,16] similar to the effect of the drug digitalis.

Another medicinal property of ginger root, for which it has long been reputed in folk medicine, is that it is an antidote against motion sickness. Chinese fishermen in rough seas are reported to chew on it to combat seasickness. While none of this is of any scientific significance, in 1982 a study[17] from Brigham Young University (Utah) and Mount Union College (Ohio) found that people taking capsules of powdered ginger root were better protected from motion sickness than by the popular antinausea drug Dramamine. The researchers concluded that ginger probably works against motion sickness by "interrupting the feedback between the stomach and the nausea center of the brain."[18] It is believed to bind gastric acids. Other researchers, continuing these investigations in Denmark a few years later, obtained similar results,

* That ginger helps preserve pork has now been scientifically established in experiments at the University of California at Davis. Food technologists there compared what happens to pork patties if they are mildly spiced with ginger, more strongly spiced, or not spiced with ginger. The results showed that the two ginger-spiced batches stayed fresh up to one third longer than the patties without any ginger.

† Aspirin is touted these days for a similar blood-thinning effect and is therefore taken by millions of people as insurance against future heart attacks and strokes. However, aspirin can have nasty side effects. It increases stomach acidity and can make latent ulcers bleed, just to mention the most common complications. We consider ourselves at no risk on the cardiovascular front, yet we take a teaspoon of Twinlab's anti-oxidant–protected, emulsified cod liver oil, and eat fair amounts of garlic and hot, spicy food. We get plenty of pure liquid vitamin E from the Demopoulos spectrum of anti-oxidants plus ½ teaspoon of HMP's vitamin E at bedtime. While we don't believe we are at any "special cardiac risk," if we were, we might take a tiny amount of aspirin weekly—no more than ¼ to ½ tablet—which is all that Dr. Demopoulos recommends, because in most cases larger amounts are neither safe nor needed.

but found that ginger may also work by affecting the nerve centers in the inner ear on which our sense of equilibrium depends.[19]

Folk medicine ascribes many other virtues to ginger, the most believable of which are its alleged ability to aid digestion, relieve stomach gas, and combat nausea (probably for the same reason that it might be effective against motion sickness). On the other hand—and folk-remedy enthusiasts like to overlook this—the same gingerols (together with the shogaols) that seem to account for blood thinning and other medicinal effects can become toxic if certain thresholds are crossed. We think that if ginger were submitted to Dr. Ames's test for cancer-causing substances, it might rate an impressive score, maybe on the order of that of hot chili peppers or black pepper. Again, moderation seems to be indicated, even despite ginger's many proven benefits.

A 1987 study on ginger from Taiwan[20] mentions that the activity of fresh ginger is closer to its constituent compound, gingerol, and that dried ginger is closer to shogaol. Thus, it is perfectly logical that in Chinese herbal medicine, dried ginger is used quite differently from fresh ginger. However, if we may assume that Chinese sailors and fishermen do indeed fight seasickness by chewing on fresh ginger root, and since we know from the Brigham Young University study that dried ginger root is able to control motion sickness, we must conclude that both are effective. Perhaps the reason is because all three of the active compounds in ginger—zingerone, shogaol, and gingerol—contribute to the effect. Or perhaps it is because there is enough of the most important compound (shogaol?) in both fresh and dried ginger to inhibit motion sickness.

We look forward to trying this ginger trick on our next ocean excursion, and we'll make sure to have both fresh and dried ginger on board. Eberhard should make a particularly good guinea pig, since even Dramamine can't help him much if the going gets rough. Stay tuned for an update!

GARLIC

Garlic has a long and venerable history as a food and it is well known for its medicinal properties. Contemporary Indian researchers like to remind us that in ancient India, garlic was used for prophylaxis and treatment of a variety of diseases. Charak, the father of Ayurvedic medicine (which combines material and nonmaterial aspects of health and disease), wrote as early as 3000 B.C. that "garlic helps in maintaining the fluidity of the blood, strengthens the heart and prolongs life." If it weren't for its unpleasant odor, he said, "garlic would be costlier than gold."

Contrast this with the *Oxford English Dictionary*'s nose-holding comment about garlic's "very strong smell" and "acrid, pungent taste." No wonder that *Allium sativum* is not much used in English cookery, a fact that some researchers associate with the high incidence of atherosclerosis and coronary heart disease in England and northern Europe, where garlic is used with the greatest restraint. A ten-year Seven Countries Study[21,22] of twelve thousand men, comparing heart disease rates in northern Europe with those of the Mediterranean area, considered the presence or lack of garlic in the diet as one of several other factors that probably account for much lower heart disease rates among southern European populations (among other dietary factors cited were drinking wine rather than milk and beer, using olive oil instead of butter, eating small versus large portions of meat, as well as an abundance of green, leafy vegetables in the southern European diet contrasted with their scarcity or lack in the northern European diet).

In the United States, garlic of course is not eaten much either except by some ethnic groups (Italian, Greek, Chinese, Near Eastern). Thus far, however, nobody has said anything bad about garlic here, or raised any warnings about any toxicities it might contain. Perhaps that is because some of garlic's scientifically proven medicinal assets far outshine any potential liabilities. Garlic—or, more precisely, the extract of its essential oil—has been shown to:

1. prevent the cholesterol-raising effect of high-fat foods;
2. prevent a rise in triglyceride levels, due to sucrose-rich foods;
3. slow down the body's production of fibrin, a blood-clotting compound; and
4. inhibit (in the test tube) the clumping of blood platelets (platelet aggregation).[23]

In addition, there are other claims about garlic's probable antibiotic and antifungal activity and immunity-strengthening effect. We shall return to these matters presently, but first let us look at garlic's heart-protective properties. There is no doubt that they are for real. The trouble is that most experiments have not been done with actual garlic but with garlic extracts. That means you would have to eat enormous quantities of garlic to arrive at the same therapeutic dosages used in these studies. For instance, to improve your body's ability to dissolve blood clots, a person weighing no more than 120 pounds would have to eat eighteen cloves of garlic a day (heavier persons would have to eat even more than that).[24,25]

Nor can we imagine that people would voluntarily eat nine cloves of garlic daily, even if they were assured that in 60 to 70 percent of cases this would lower their LDL blood cholesterol in favor of the protective HDL fraction.[26] In one experiment, the patients were actually taking only 1 gram of Kyolic garlic extract from Japan, a more feasible proposition except it is almost impossible for the average person to obtain this product. (Incidentally, garlic pills and capsules do not have the same concentration of the active principle in garlic, allicin, as does the essential oil of garlic, although pills and capsules may be quite useful for other purposes.)

Nor is it realistic to expect that Americans or Europeans would comply with drinking ⅛ to ½ cup of liquified garlic every day, even if assured that it would significantly lower their cholesterol levels if they only stuck with it for a couple of months.[27,28]

Similarly, we don't think many Americans or Europeans would be willing even to eat "just" five cloves of garlic and some onions every day for about a month which another study found adequate to reduce cholesterol levels, and follow this up with eating two cloves daily.[29] This study was done with members of the strictly vegetarian Indian Jain sect, for whom eating such large amounts of garlic might seem not nearly as out of the ordinary as it surely would for most westerners.

We can now return to some of the earlier-mentioned therapeutic properties of garlic, such as its antibiotic activity. An early study (1969) had already shown that garlic (and onion) is effective in test tube experiments against *Salmonella* and *Escherichia coli* bacteria.[30] Another test tube study, conducted about ten years ago, found that low concentrations of aqueous (water) extract of garlic killed all of eighteen strains of a dangerous microorganism, *Cryptococcus neoformans,* which is more a yeast than a bacterium, and which likes to attack the central nervous system and sometimes the lungs, bones, or skin. This was not an inconsequential discovery, since this parasite is being diagnosed more and more on a worldwide scale.[31] It is therefore comforting to learn that garlic's ability to kill dangerous mycobacteria was fully confirmed in more recent tests.[32]

Dr. Irwin Ziment, a renowned specialist in respiratory diseases and associate professor of medicine at the UCLA School of Medicine at Los Angeles, is enthusiastic about the ability of garlic along with hot chili peppers, black pepper, and curries, to help relieve the chest and sinus congestion that usually accompanies upper respiratory infections. But, more than that, he believes that the sulfhydryl compounds in garlic quench the free radicals that seem to cause much of the damage caused by emphysema* and other lung diseases, as well as in bronchitis.[33–35]

---

* Emphysema is essentially the result of the cross-linking of protein molecules due to oxidation—by definition, a free-radical–generating process.

Another study found that *local* application of garlic's active ingredient, allicin, has a positive, therapeutic effect on fungal lesions of the skin. So strong was this effect that the researchers flatly stated, "We can suppose that fungal skin diseases can be effectively cured by [garlic] extract."[36] We shall certainly try this next time one of our German shepherds has fungus infection (a frequent occurrence in the tropics), which sometimes does not yield to even the most sophisticated fungicidal creams and powders, till local treatment is combined with internal (systemic) drugs that can have side effects.

There is no doubt that garlic (and probably also onion) has a protective effect against cancer of the colon, stomach, and breast, and there is every reason to feel that this is due to the same free-radical–quenching effect of the sulfhydryl groups that help in respiratory diseases. This effect was recognized twenty years ago by two Japanese researchers, Motonori Fujiwara and Toshikazu Natata, who reasoned that their good results with pretreating cells with garlic extracts to strengthen their immunity against cancer were due to the allicin, which reacts with sulfhydryl groups of tumor cell proteins.*[37]

TURMERIC

Turmeric, a spice widely used in Asia for its color, flavor, and medicinal properties, is unfortunately almost totally neglected in Western cuisine. The only time Americans and Europeans ever get to eat it at all is in curries, perhaps at an occasional visit to an Indian restaurant.

Yet yellow-pigmented turmeric (*Curcuma longa*) is a delicious-tasting spice that can improve the flavor of many dishes. This alone may be good enough reason to use it in salads and vegetable stews or soups. But now we also know that turmeric is a potent natural anti-oxidant (similar to rosemary) and that it can inhibit the mutagenicity of many carcinogenic agents in our environment and food.

A recent study by Indian medical scientists at the Cancer Research Institute, Tata Memorial Center, Bombay, shows that turmeric can, for instance, neutralize the cancer-causing compounds in cigarette smoke and other standard mutagen-carcinogens. The researchers comment that the Indian people not only smoke a lot but are also exposed (as we are) to several mutagen-carcinogens in the diet and from occupational sources. At the same time, they also consume considerable amounts of

---

* Taking garlic in combination with glutathione, which also reacts with sulfhydryl groups, might provide even better immunity.

powdered turmeric (amounting to gram quantities per day) in their diet. This may be one of the reasons, the scientists speculate, why the Indian people do not have higher rates of certain cancers than one might otherwise expect.[38]

BLACK PEPPER AND HOT CHILI PEPPERS

You may have read the advice of some diet counselors to use more black pepper, red pepper (cayenne), and hot chili peppers to make up for cutting down on salt. But neither is it advisable to pour on the black pepper or the hot chili pepper flakes to spike up low-salt dishes. The reason is that black pepper and hot red pepper both contain compounds that are carcinogenic at high dosages. Fortunately, both these spices have certain protective medicinal and anti-oxidant properties alongside their more sinister ones—a statement that can be made for almost every herb, spice, or vegetable, as Dr. James Duke points out. And if these spices are used correctly, we agree with Dr. Duke that their health-promoting effects probably far surpass their potential for trouble. Let moderation, again, be the key!

First, let's talk about the bad news about peppers and other common spices. Black pepper contains, as Dr. Bruce Ames points out, small amounts of safrole and large amounts of a closely related compound, piperine. When laboratory mice were given extract of black pepper equivalent to 4 grams (about 1 level teaspoon) per day for three months, they promptly developed tumors all over their bodies. While it's true that in the case of humans, a person would have to eat the enormous amount of 140 grams per day—something quite unimaginable—to produce the same effect,[39] still, it's a factor you cannot just entirely discount.

We are not particularly happy writing about this, for we actually grow a small amount of pepper in Costa Rica and every month we send fresh green peppercorns to the Culinary Institute of America and a number of the finest restaurants in the United States. So we are taking double comfort from the fact that black pepper has antiseptic, antidiarrhetic, and other medicinal properties. We hope that these benefits will make up for some of the discomforting aspects of black pepper.

The story about hot red peppers—from paprika and the milder jalapeño peppers, to cayenne powder and red chili peppers—is very similar. Dr. Bela Toth of the University of Nebraska, best known for his research on the dangerous hydrazines in mushrooms, has also studied capsaicin, the pungent material present in all red peppers, but which is most highly concentrated in hot chili pepper, and, sure enough, he found capsaicin to be carcinogenic in mice.[40]

Here again, there are important redeeming features. Capsaicin, which can cause cancer at higher concentrations, also has decided medicinal qualities if used in normal quantities. It has a long history in folk medicine as an effective analgesic.* A drop or two of hot chili extract applied on cotton to a sore tooth was recommended by the *Dublin Medical Press* as early as 1850 as an instant remedy for toothache.[41]

More important, however, it has recently been discovered that the capsaicin in hot chili peppers also has an antiblood-clotting effect, which may explain the relatively low incidence of thromboembolism† among certain ethnic groups like the Thais, in whose diet hot peppers are an integral part, and where incidence of postoperative embolism is rare.[42]

There is some scientific evidence that red pepper has a hypocholes-terolemic (cholesterol-lowering) property.[43] Even if this effect is not in itself as substantial as, say, that of niacin (vitamin B_3), the combined blood-thinning and cholesterol-fighting effects of the capsaicin in red pepper makes regular spicing of food with it especially recommendable to anyone with cardiovascular problems. In fact, if one regularly eats several foods and spices with these characteristics—preferably at least two or three in the same meal, or at least during the same day—their synergistic effect should be considerable.

Dr. Duke talks about Russian scientists having reported "high antioxidant activity from capsicosides found in pepper seeds."[44] We assume that any such anti-oxidant activity would be greatest in fresh rather than dried chili peppers. It would not be surprising if similar anti-oxidant activity is discovered someday in fresh green peppercorns (from which dry black and white pepper derive).

More good news is that neither black pepper nor hot chili peppers seem to cause any harm to the gastric mucosa (stomach lining) in the amounts in which they are normally used, even in hot, spicy dishes. This has been established by both Thai researchers[45] and American investigators, who found that "the ingestion of highly spiced meals by normal individuals is not associated with endoscopically demonstrable gastroduodenal mucosal damage."[46,47]

Dr. Irwin Ziment also recommends both black and red pepper to

* The chemical structure of capsaicin is similar to that of eugenol, which is the active ingredient in oil of cloves. It is therefore not surprising to find that chewing on cloves has for centuries been recommended in folk medicine as a toothache remedy.
† The anticlotting element in hot peppers seems to be due to the neutralization of fibrin, an insoluble protein essential to blood clotting. This appears to be a different mechanism from that involved in the blood-thinning effect of the Chinese tree fungus *mo-er,* whose inhibition of platelet aggregation is probably due to adenosine activity (see pages 339–340).

clear up stuffed sinuses and relieve bronchial congestion in chest colds.[48] Strongly spiced vegetable or chicken soup, also containing copious amounts of garlic or onion, are Dr. Ziment's standard dietary prescription for colds and bronchitis, and we heartily agree. A good vegetable or chicken soup with some extra hot spices and garlic or onion certainly beats swallowing the risky and not very effective over-the-counter cold remedies one sees every day on countless TV commericals.

BROWN MUSTARD AND HORSERADISH

Dr. Bruce Ames rates 5 grams (about 1 teaspoon) of brown mustard more than twice as carcinogenic as a cup of comfrey tea.[49] That sounds bad, but in reality it does not represent any serious risk. However, it is true that allyl isothiocyanate, a major flavor ingredient in oil of mustard and horseradish has, as Dr. Ames observes, been shown to cause chromosome aberrations in hamster cells, even at low concentration[50] and to be a carcinogen in rats.[51] On the other hand, mustard and horseradish have been used, both internally and externally, for centuries in folk medicine for their alleged medicinal properties.

We don't like the common American-type mustard, but frequently use French Dijon mustard for salad dressing, thinning it out with either small amounts of water or wine vinegar, unless the tomatoes in the salad provide sufficient liquid of their own. In that way we avoid adding any more oil to the dressing than is already in the mustard. We don't think that the weak concentration of the carcinogen in mustard presents any realistic risk.

Horseradish can be used for a low-fat or no-fat salad dressing, which, to our way of thinking, is safer by far than most commercial salad dressings. Sometimes we use either mustard or horseradish to flavor white wine sauces for breast of chicken or turkey. We do it as a change from our usual routine of baking half breasts of chicken, generously spiced with rosemary, thyme, and garlic, in a casserole or wrapped in foil so the flavor of the spices goes into the meat and the juice.

SOURCES

1. *J. Agric. and Bot. Chem.,* 1984; Vol. 48.
2. Collins, M. A., and H. P. Charles. "Antimicrobial activity of carnosol and ursolic acid, two antioxidant constituents of rosemarinus officinalis L." *Food Microbiol.* (London), 1987; 4:311–316.

3. Ames, B. N. "Dietary carcinogens and anticarcinogens." *Science,* 1983; 221:1256.
4. *Toxicants Occurring Naturally in Foods.* Washington, D.C.: National Academy of Sciences, 1973, p. 456.
5. Duke, J. A. "Biting the Biocide Bullet." Draft memorandum, January 13, 1988.
6. Duke, J. A. "Spice Medicine: Parsley, Sage, Rosemary and Thyme." *Am. Health,* September 1987; 91–106.
7. Duke, J. "Spice Medicine: Parsley, Sage, Rosemary and Thyme." *Am. Health,* September 1987; 91–106.
8. *Toxicants Occurring Naturally in Foods.* Washington, D.C.: National Academy of Sciences, 1973, p. 458.
9. Kesden, D. (Correspondence). *JAMA,* 1987; 258:909.
10. Gainer, J. L., Jr., and J. R. Jones. "The use of crocetin in experimental atherosclerosis." *Experientia,* 1975; 31(5):548–549.
11. Seyde, W. C., et al. "Carotenoid compound crocetin improves oxygenation in hemorrhaged rats." *J. Cereb. Blood Flow Metab.,* December 6, 1986; 703–707.
12. Gainer, J. L., Jr., and G. Nugent. "Effect of increasing the plasma oxygen diffusivity on experimental cryogenic edema." *J. Neurosurg.,* 1976; 45: 535–538.
13. Dr. Daniel Kesden, Fort Lauderdale, Florida, personal communication.
14. Srivastava, K. C. "Effects of aqueous extracts of onion, garlic and ginger on platelet aggregation and metabolism of arachidonic acid in the blood vascular system: in vitro study." *Prostaglandins, Leukotrienes, and Medicine,* 1984; 13:227–235.
15. Suekawa, M., et al. "Pharmacological studies on ginger zingiber-officinale. 1. Pharmacological actions on pungent constituents G. gingerol and G. shogaol." *J. Pharmacobio-Dyn.,* 1984; 7(11):836–848.
16. Shoji, N., et al. "Carciotonic principles of ginger (zingiber officinale roscoe)." *J. Pharmaceut. Sci.,* 1982; 71(10):1174–1175.
17. Kasahara, Y., et al. "Pharmacological actions of pinellia ternata tubers and zingiber-officinale rhizomes." *Shoyakugaku Zasshi,* 1983; 37(1):73–83.
18. Mowrey, D. B. "Motion sickness, ginger, and psychophysics." *Lancet,* March 20, 1982; 655–657.
19. Grontved, A., and E. Hentzer. "Vertigo-reducing effect of ginger Zingiber-officinale root: a controlled clinical study." *ORL (Oto-Rhino-Laryngol),* Basel, 1986; 48(5):282–286.
20. Hsien-Chang Chang, et al. "A comparative study of Chinese herb drugs (1)—ginger." *Oriental Healing Arts International Bulletin,* 1987; 12(3):139–146.
21. Keys, A., ed. "Coronary heart disease in seven countries." *Am. Heart Assoc. Monograph,* 1970; No. 29.
22. Keys, A., et al. *Seven Countries: Death and Coronary Heart Disease in Ten Years.* Cambridge, Mass.: Harvard University Press, 1980.
23. Srivastava, K. C. "Evidence for the mechanism by which garlic inhibits platelet aggregation." *Prostaglandins, Leukotrienes, and Medicine,* 1986; 22:313–321.
24. Bordia, A. K. "Effect of the essential oil (active principle) of garlic on serum cholesterol, plasma fibrinogen whole blood coagulation time and fibrinolytic activity in alimentary lipaemia." *J. Assoc. Phys. Ind.,* 1974; 22:267.
25. Bordia, A. K., et al. "Effect of essential oil of garlic on blood lipids and

fibrinolytic activity in patients with coronary artery disease." *Atherosclerosis*, 1977; 28:155.

26. Lau, B.H.S., et al. "Allium sativum (garlic) and atherosclerosis: A review." *Nutr. Res.*, 1983; 3:119–128.
27. Bordia, A. K. "Effect of garlic on blood lipids in patients with coronary heart disease." *Am. J. Clin. Nutr.*, 1981; 34:2100.
28. Bordia, A. K. "Effect of essential oils of garlic and onion on alimentary hyperlipemia." *Atherosclerosis*, 1975; 21:15–19.
29. Sucur, M. "Effect of garlic on serum lipids and lipoproteins in patients suffering from hyperlipoproteinemia." *Diabetol. Croatica*, 1980; 9:323.
30. Johnson, M. G., and R. H. Vaughn. "Death of *salmonella typhimurium* and *escherichia coli* in the presence of freshly reconstituted dehydrated garlic and onion." *Appld. Microbiol.*, 1969; 17:903–905.
31. Fromtling, R. A., and G. S. Bulmer. "In vitro effect of aqueous extract of garlic (allium sativum) on the growth and viability of *cryptococcus neoformans.*" *Mycologia*, 1978; 70:397–405.
32. Delaha, E. C., et al. "Inhibition of mycobacteria by garlic extract (allium sativum)." *Antimicrobial Agents and Chemotherapy*, April 1985; 27(4): 485–486.
33. Dr. I. Ziment, personal communication.
34. Ziment, I. *Respiratory Pharmacology and Therapeutics.* Philadelphia: W. B. Saunders Company, 1978.
35. Ziment, I. *Practical Pulmonary Disease.* New York: John Wiley & Sons, 1983.
36. Amer, M., et al. "The effect of aqueous garlic extract on the growth of dermatophytes." *Int. J. Dermatol.*, 1980; 19:285–287.
37. Fujiwara, M., and T. Natata. "Induction of tumor immunity with tumor cells treated with extract of garlic (allium sativum)." *Nature*, 1967; 216:84.
38. Amonkar, A. J., and S. V. Bhide. "In vitro antimutagenicity of curcumin against environmental mutagens." *Fed. Chem. Toxicol.*, 1987; 25:545–547.
39. Ames, B. N. "Dietary carcinogens and anticarcinogens." *Science*, 1983; 221:1256.
40. Toth, B., and E. Rogan. *Fed. Proc. Am. Soc. Exp. Biol.*, 1984; 43:593.
41. Anon. "Hot peppers and substance P." *Lancet*, May 28, 1983; 1198.
42. Visudhipan, S., et al. "The relationship between high fibrinolytic activity and daily capsicum ingestion in Thais." *Am. J. Clin. Nutr.*, 1982; 35:1452–1458.
43. Sambaiah, K., et al. "Hypocholesterolemic effect of red pepper and capsaicin." *Ind. J. Exp. Biol.*, 1980; 18:898–899.
44. Duke, J. "Herbs as anti-aging agents." *Health Foods Business*, August 1985; 31(8):38–40.
45. Ketsusink, O., et al. "Influence of capsicum solution on gastric acidities. A preliminary report." *Am. J. Proctol.*, 1966; 17:511–515.
46. Graham, D. Y., and J. L. Smith. "Effect of spicy food on the gastric mucosa: videoendoscopy" (Abstract). *Am. Gastroenterol. Assoc.*, May 15–18, 1988.
47. Myers, B. M., et al. "Effect of red pepper and black pepper on the stomach." *Am. J. Gastroenterol.*, 1987; 82:211–214.
48. Dr. I. Ziment, personal communication; *Pratical Pulmonary Disease*, I. Ziment, ed. New York: John Wiley & Sons, 1983; Ziment, I. *Respiratory Pharmacology and Therapeutics.* Philadelphia: W. B. Saunders Company, 1978; Ziment, I. "Mucokinetic Agents." Chapter 5 in: *Current Topics in*

Pulmonary Pharmacology and Toxicology, Vol. 3, M. A. Hollinger, ed. New York: Elsevier, 1987.

49. Ames, B. N. "Ranking possible carcinogenic hazards." *Science,* 1987; 236:271–280.
50. Kasamaki, A., et al. *Mutat. Res.,* 1982; 105:387.
51. Dunnick, J. K., et al. *Fundam. Appld. Toxicol.,* 1982; 2:114.

CHAPTER 55

RICE

"SUSTAINER OF THE HUMAN RACE"

Starches or complex carbohydrates can provide readily available calories from molecules made up of long chains of sugars. They differ from the simple sugars (sucrose, fructose, and glucose) in that they contain other nutrients such as protein, essential fat, fiber, vitamins, and minerals, the rest being water. Of the most commonly consumed starches, rice is undoubtedly the most important one, worldwide. We shall therefore take it up first.

The historical importance of rice to the entire Asian half of humanity is reflected in the name of the sixth-century B.C. king of Nepal—Suddhodana, or "Pure Rice"—the father of the Gautama Buddha, and in the ancient name of Japan—Mizuho-no-kuni, "The Land of Luxuriant Rice Crops." To this day traditional Japanese housewives refer to meals as *asa gohan* (morning rice), *hiru gohan* (midday rice), and *yoru gohan* (evening rice). And in India the Hindi word for rice, *chawal,* means "sustainer of the human race."

Over the past few years we personally have joined the Asians in using rice as our main source of starch. We eat whole-grain brown rice rather than the polished white rice consumed almost without exception throughout the Far East and preferred by most Americans and Europeans. Actually, many people are not even aware of the existence of any other kind of rice than the white, polished kind. They have never had occasion to compare white rice with whole-grain brown rice and therefore have no way of knowing which one they might like best.

The principal reason we prefer brown rice is because in milling, only the indigestible outer husk is removed, leaving all the vitamins minerals, and fiber intact.

Here's a quick comparison between brown and white rice:

434

VITAMIN CONCENTRATION
(IN MICROGRAMS PER GRAM)*

	THIAMIN	RIBOFLAVIN	NIACIN	PYRIDOXINE
Brown rice	3.4	0.5	47	10.3
Polished rice	0.7	0.3	16	4.5

* Data from M. C. Linder, *Nutritional Biochemistry and Metabolism* (New York: Elsevier, 1985).

Compared with polished rice, brown rice contains about five times as much thiamine (B_1), three times as much niacin (B_3), and more than twice the amount of pyridoxine (B_6). You would have to eat between 1,000 and 5,000 grams (1 to 5 kilograms) per day of fully milled white rice, but only 400 grams per day of brown rice to meet the Recommended Daily Allowances (RDAs) of thiamine, riboflavin, and niacin.[1] And compared with white rice, brown rice contains five times as much zinc, twice as much manganese, and more than twice the calcium.

If despite the difference in amounts of nutrients, you still prefer white rice, we suggest using *parboiled* ("converted") rice. The raw rice is first briefly steamed or boiled before milling, a process that drives a percentage of the micronutrients into the interior of the grain where they cannot be removed by milling or polishing.

The protein content of brown rice is only slightly higher (4.9 percent) than that of white rice (4.1 percent). Some authorities claim that the protein in white rice is somewhat more available than that of brown rice,[2] but the protein quality of either rice is among the highest of cereal proteins.[3]

If consumed in mixed diets sufficient to meet caloric needs, rice seems to meet protein needs very well. In Latin America this is accomplished by eating the rice together with beans and perhaps some corn tortillas. In India the same result is achieved by eating rice with dal (yellow or red lentils) and chapatis, flat breads made from whole wheat. In the United States, on the other hand, the protein in some commercial rice products has been rendered less available by dry heat, the amino acid lysine having been altered in the process. Gun-puffed rice, produced by subjecting rice simultaneously to high heat and high air pressure, is an extreme case in point.

Unlike white rice, brown rice still retains the inner bran layer—only the indigestible outer husk is removed. It is therefore that much richer in a very good type of fiber, in addition to having retained most of the micronutrients that are removed by further milling to produce white rice.

Eating whole-grain rice is all the more advisable for people who have a tendency to produce urinary calcium stones. A study conducted by the Department of Urology at Wakayama Medical College, a major medical teaching and research center in Japan, found that people treated with rice bran for one to three years developed fewer stones than the untreated control group. The rice bran apparently reduces the intestinal absorption of calcium. These medical researchers therefore concluded that "rice bran treatment should be effective for prevention of recurrent urinary stone disease."[4] A later study, also from Japan, confirmed that with rice bran "the frequency of stone episodes was reduced dramatically," that the patients tolerated the bran very well, and that there were "no serious side effects."[5] There is no reason why brown rice, with most of its bran still present, shouldn't do as well.

One type of white rice should especially be avoided—the talc-coated brands. Manufacturers often coat white rice with a layer of glucose and talc in order to give it a high sheen and possibly help protect it against spoilage and insect damage. We have not found any convincing proof of this last claim, and we do not like the idea of eating talc powder.

Unfortunately, in some parts of the world it isn't all that easy to find white rice that is *not* talc-coated. In Hawaii, for instance, 75 to 80 percent of all white rice—most of it imported from California—is talc-coated, and only talc-coated rice is readily available in Puerto Rico. Even on the American mainland, you will find talc-coated rice sitting next to non-talc–coated rice on many supermarket shelves, and the labels don't necessarily inform you about the presence or absence of talc.

How do you tell the difference? For one thing, the uncooked coated rice looks shinier and whiter. For another, the cooking directions on a package of talc-coated rice usually recommend washing the product before using it.

Of course, the entire issue can be avoided by simply using brown instead of white rice. Aside from all these health reasons, we ourselves prefer the rich, nutty flavor of brown rice to the much blander, less interesting taste of white rice. But, if given the choice between *any* kind of rice and potatoes as the primary source of starch in our diet, we would opt for rice. This is not because we don't like potatoes, which we eat with some frequency, but because rice requires 50 percent less insulin production in our bodies than potatoes do. Though neither of us is diabetic, we don't like to make our bodies work harder than necessary. This factor is very important in our type of diet, which has no restrictions on the amount of fresh fruit one can eat and therefore makes greater demands on glucose tolerance than, for example, the Pritikin diet.

A ten-year follow-up study from Japan appears to show that eating rice (even white rice!) has a cancer-protective effect. The study shows that people who eat more rice have less stomach cancer than those who eat smaller amounts. Best protected are those who eat six cups of rice or more per day, with the protection factor declining in proportion with the lesser amounts consumed.[6]

Rice has, however, one nutritional disadvantage compared with potatoes: It does not contain any vitamin C, whereas potatoes do contain a fair amount of this crucial vitamin/anti-oxidant—50 percent of the U.S. RDA. For people who eat a lot of other vegetables, as well as the 6,000 to 10,000 milligrams of vitamin C on the daily anti-oxidant program—rice's lack of vitamin C is not of any serious concern. It explains, however, why people have been known to subsist on practically nothing but potatoes, as has been historically true for the Irish. If, on the other hand, rice is one's basic starch food, vegetables and fruits containing vitamin C should definitely be an important part of the diet.

COOKING RICE

First, it is neither necessary nor advisable to rinse or wash rice before cooking it. In the United States, Europe, and Japan, rice is mechanically cleaned and foreign particles are removed prior to packaging. All you accomplish by washing it is to leach out valuable nutrients.

Second, the amount of water used in cooking rice is crucial. If you use too much water, you will have to drain some of it, thereby losing nutrients just as you would with washing the rice. A good rule of thumb in cooking is two parts of water to one part of whole-grain rice.

Bring the water to a boil before adding the rice, to avoid excessive stickiness, then lower the heat as much as possible. From then on, the trick is to stir the rice only once—when it comes to a boil again—and then to leave it alone. Stirring the rice during cooking can break the grains and make them stick together. The water should boil gently throughout the cooking process. When the water is all absorbed, you will see numerous holes in the rice where the final steam has escaped, at which point you turn off the heat and cover.

We never fry rice—or anything else, for that matter, although we do occasionally quick-sauté food Chinese style. However, we see no reason at all for frying rice—boiled brown rice has sufficient taste by itself. Besides, the heat necessary for frying encourages the oxidation of the fat or oil, and, in addition, destroys a certain percentage of vitamins (as much as 70 percent of the B_1, for example). Unfortunately, there is no other way of frying foods without using some kind of oil or fat. But when sautéing rice, a small amount of chicken, fish, or vegetable stock can be substituted for the oil. You can make pilaf just by adding more chicken or fish broth to the rice, depending on whether you intend to serve the dish with poultry or seafood. We actually prefer a pilaf cooked with some kind of fish, chicken, or vegetable stock to avoid the otherwise unavoidable oily taste of preparing it in the traditional method.

DIFFERENT TYPES OF RICE

There was a time—and not so long ago!—when most people thought of rice in only one way: as sticky white stuff that didn't have much taste. But that perception has changed over the past few years. More and more people every year come to realize that there are different kinds of brown and white rice, with one type more suitable for a certain kind of dish, and another type best used for something else.

Each type has its own characteristics: The long-grain varieties tend to cook up drier and fluffier, the grains remaining more separate. The shorter-grain varieties tend to be more cohesive, which may affect appearance, although it does not affect the taste.

One very fine type of rice called *basmati* comes from the Himalayan foothills and, like other superior kinds of rice, is imported by some of the best specialty food stores in America and Europe. The Hindi word *basmati* translates poetically as "queen of fragrance," and well it might: As basmati rice cooks, it gives off a rich fragrance quite unlike that of ordinary rice.

There is also a rice that is a cross between basmati and American long-grain rice named Texmati. We have not tried it yet, but according to Jenifer Harvey Lang, a well-known American writer on food, it is particularly suitable for variations on classic Spanish *paella*—sautéed

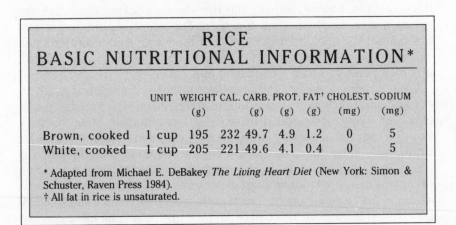

RICE
BASIC NUTRITIONAL INFORMATION*

	UNIT	WEIGHT (g)	CAL.	CARB. (g)	PROT. (g)	FAT† (g)	CHOLEST. (mg)	SODIUM (mg)
Brown, cooked	1 cup	195	232	49.7	4.9	1.2	0	5
White, cooked	1 cup	205	221	49.6	4.1	0.4	0	5

* Adapted from Michael E. DeBakey *The Living Heart Diet* (New York: Simon & Schuster, Raven Press 1984).
† All fat in rice is unsaturated.

rice with a mélange of seafood or chicken, or both together, or a version using only vegetables.

Another exceptionally tasty rice is grown by the Lundberg Family Farms in Richvale, California. It is called Wehani. This rice is a bit chewy perhaps, even after being properly cooked, but by the same token it lends itself especially well to dishes where you want a firmer texture—for instance, when it is served with soft-textured vegetables like squash, cooked oysters, or fish.

Quite the opposite is true for the oval-shaped Arborio rice that ends up—if you have the patience—in the velvety consistency that Italian chefs prefer for risotto.

Finally, for special occasions because of its exorbitant price, there is the royal rice of Indian maharajahs, called *calmati,* which beats even its aristocratic cousin basmati for its rich aroma and subtle flavor. But if basmati rice is hard to find, you'll have to look even harder for calmati, or settle for one of the finer, home-grown varieties like Texmati.

For most purposes, we use a good short-grain brown rice, preferably the one from the Lundberg farms—if we can find it. Short-grain rice is perhaps a little stickier than some of the long-grain varieties, but this is not a major problem if it has been cooked properly. We use it all across the board, from soups to accompanying vegetables, chicken, or seafood. We find it suitable even for rice pudding and French-style *gâteau de riz* (rice cake). Sometimes we even put a little of it in our mixed green salads, as much to give them better texture as to create a better nutritional balance, or just to reduce the acidity of a lemon or vinegar dressing. However, for serving, say, sliced breast of chicken or fish on brown rice, it would be better for appearance to use a firmer, long-grain variety.

SOURCES

1. Saunders, R. M., and A. A. Betschart, "Rice and Rice Foods." In: *Tropical Foods: Chemistry and Nutrition,* B. E. Inglett and G. Charalanbous, eds., Vol. I. New York: Academic Press, 1979, p. 209.
2. Cullumbine, H. "Nitrogen balance studies on rice diets." *Brit. J. Nutr.,* 1950; 4:129–134.
3. Saunders and Betschart, op. cit., p. 208.
4. Ohkawa, T., S. Ebisuno, M. Kitagawa, et al. "Rice bran treatment for patients with hypercalciuric stones: experimental and clinical studies. *J. Urol.,* 1984; 132:1141–1145.
5. Ebisuno, S., S. Morinoto, T. Yoshida, T. Fukatani, et al. "Rice-bran treatment for calcium stone formers with idiopathic hypercalciuria," *J. Urol.,* 1987; 138:224.
6. Hirayama, T., "Changing Patterns of Cancer in Japan with Special Reference to the Decrease in Stomach Cancer Mortality." In: *Origins of Human Cancer,* Book A, R. Doll, ed. Cold Spring Harbor, N.Y.: Cold Spring Harbor Laboratory, 1977, p. 60.

CHAPTER 56

POTATOES

THE OVERLOOKED GOLD IN THE GROUND

When the Spanish conquistadors under Francisco Pizarro overran Peru in the 1530s, they carried off shiploads full of gold stolen from the vanquished Incas and Aztecs. Little did they realize that in the blood-soaked ground under their feet there lay another kind of gold: potatoes (named after the Spanish *papas*), which the Indians of the high Andes were—and still are—cultivating as their staple food. Compared with the tubers' commercial value in future centuries, "all the gold of Peru becomes small potatoes," as anthropologist Robert Rhoades, who has studied the impact of potato cultivation on human civilization, has so pointedly remarked.[*]

Even though wild potatoes have been found as far north as Nebraska, they have not always been as popular in America—or, for that matter, in Europe—as they are today. In fact, it took a lot of doing on either side of the Atlantic to have people accept them.

If the lowly potato hadn't found some pretty high-placed friends in both the Old and New Worlds, things might have turned out quite differently, so much resistance was there against this new kind of food. But some of the more dictatorially inclined potentates of Europe, like Frederick the Great of Prussia and Catherine the Great of Russia, didn't even bother trying to persuade their farmers to plant them—they simply ordered them to do so.

[*] Reference is to an article, "The Incredible Potatoe," by Robert E. Rhoades, in *National Geographic,* May 1982.

In more democratic England, Sir Walter Raleigh became the official champion of potatoes and convinced English farmers to cultivate them. Ironically, it was he, an Englishman, who introduced the potato to Ireland, where it soon became the primary food crop—the rest, including the Irish potato famine which lasted from 1845 to 1851 and during which about a million people died of starvation, being history (since it caused the mass exodus of hundreds of thousands of the Irish to America, it also became part of our country's history).

In France the potato found another enthusiast in the famous chemist Antoine Auguste Parmentier. While a prisoner of war in Germany in 1757, Parmentier and many of his captured fellow Frenchmen had been fed practically nothing but potatoes. Nonetheless, they all survived remarkably well. Today we know why: Potato starch forms up to 80 percent of the tuber's dry weight. But that is not a negative—starches are our fuel for cellular energy. In addition, the protein content of potatoes may be small in quantity, but high in quality. It is said to be nutritionally even better than the protein of soya beans. Last but not least, potatoes can provide up to 50 percent of the U.S. RDA of vitamin C. This was undoubtedly the reason why the explorer Captain Cook insisted on having plenty of potatoes on board, having learned from experience that during long voyages they helped prevent outbreaks of scurvy.*

When M. Parmentier was released and back in France after the war, he went on a one-man mission to get potato cultivation started in his own country. He had convinced King Louis XVI that only potatoes could feed the poorly nourished masses of Paris and prevent social unrest or worse. But the conservative peasants wanted nothing to do with something so untried and unfamiliar to them. Besides, didn't the potato plant belong to the family of deadly nightshades, such as the hallucinogenic mandrake that had figured prominently in medieval witchcraft? (The fine point that mandrake belongs to the genus *Podophillum* and potato to *Solanum* was, of course, lost to the populace!)

At that point, Parmentier had a brilliant idea: The government would plant an acre or so of potatoes just outside of Paris, all of which was then farming area. There would be soldiers posted during the day to guard the plot, but discreetly withdrawn at nightfall. Parmentier, who was not only a chemical scientist but also a practical psychologist, figured that when the peasants saw that if the government considered the crop so precious that it had to protect it with soldiers, it must be worth stealing.

And sure enough, the trick worked: It wasn't long before potato plots sprang up all around Paris. Even Queen Marie ("Let them eat cake") Antoinette got into the act, glamorizing the humble spud by wearing

---

* To this day, an antiscurvy dish, a specialty of the seaport city of Hamburg, Germany, called *Lapskaus,* has survived from earlier seafaring times. It consists of mashed potatoes, onions, and pieces of cured ham, all items that could be kept on board for extended periods of time.

potato blossoms in her hair. This act wasn't enough to stave off the revolution, which came anyway, or save her own pretty head and that of her husband, the king. But it is doubtful that the revolution could have ultimately succeeded, or the subsequent Napoleonic wars been fought, without potatoes providing the basic foodstuff.

As far as the introduction of potatoes in the American colonies is concerned, it was again Auguste Parmentier who had a lot to do with it. At a banquet he arranged in honor of Benjamin Franklin, then American commissioner to France, no fewer than twenty different potato dishes were served—including what has since become known as french fries!

No wonder Benjamin Franklin was duly impressed and, upon his return to America, became an avid potato advocate himself. But it was not until President Thomas Jefferson served them at a White House dinner that potatoes became more widely accepted.

Today Americans consume incredible amounts of potatoes—for the most part, unfortunately in the nutritionally least desirable forms. In 1980, the last year for which production figures are available, Americans ate five billion pounds of french fries and one billion pounds of potato chips, largely because of the fast-food chains that push them on people. As the American Potato Board, an industry organization solemnly intoned, "What is a hamburger without french fries? Breakfast without hash browns?"

What indeed? Never mind the high-cholesterol and high-fat content of these types of potatoes—or the free radicals that are generated by superheated frying oils. But the profits are just too big to expect reason, prudence, and honesty.

If reason should ever prevail, there would be other uses for potatoes. We could switch to eating more boiled and baked potatoes. With respect to the future, it looks as though we willl be using all the potatoes we can possibly grow—not as much for eating as for producing alcohol to run our cars on. Henry Ford had always thought that this would happen someday when the planet's finite oil reserves ran out. He actually started planting potatoes in confident anticipation of it—only he was off by a century or so.*

SHOPPING FOR POTATOES

When shopping for potatoes, avoid those with greenish areas—an indication that the potato has been exposed to too much light and is likely to contain extra amounts of two toxic substances called *solanine*

* Corn and, of course, sugarcane may also play a role.

and *chaconine.* Since these carcinogenic substances are most concentrated in the skins, we strongly advise—contrary to what you may have heard or read—not to eat them.*

We also recommend that you not use potatoes that have soft dark areas or have been bruised or cut into during harvesting. Remember, a plant that has been attacked by disease or is injured produces more defensive, toxic substances than normal. Even if you can't find "perfect" potatoes, cut out any blemishes before cooking them. Also stay away from potatoes with wilted or wrinkled skins; they have probably been stored too long. Chances are they have already started to get moldy (which is not easy to detect) and contain aflatoxins (mold toxins), in addition to solanine and chaconine (see also our chapter "Toxicities in Natural Foods," page 347, about these potato toxins).

STORING POTATOES

If you have to store potatoes, be sure to put them in a dark, cool place. The refrigerator is not a good choice because potatoes tend to develop a sweet taste below 50°F, and to look darker when cooked. The lower the temperature, the more starch is converted into sugar.

PREPARING AND COOKING POTATOES

Since it's best to cook potatoes whole and in their skins to conserve the most nutrients, we prefer simply to clean them with a vegetable brush or cellulose sponge. If you do peel and cut up the potatoes before cooking, make the peelings as thin as possible, since, as with fruits and other vegetables, the greatest concentration of micronutrients lies just beneath the skin.

Once potatoes have been peeled they should be cooked right away. Otherwise they start turning dark as quickly as peeled and cut apples

---

* It has even been suggested in the popular media to eat potato skins on the basis that they contain chlorogenic acid, a polyphenol, which a German study claims to be able to prevent cell mutations *in vitro* (in the test tube). Well, maybe so. But we know from careful assays of Dr. Bruce Ames, head of biochemistry, University of California at Berkeley, that there can be no doubt about the carcinogenic nature of solanine and chaconine.

It has also been asserted that potatoes have antiviral properties. Such claims are based on studies showing that extracts from *raw* potatoes contain certain compounds called protease inhibitors (see pp. 393–394) which have, indeed, antiviral and anticancer properties. It is, however, misleading to suggest that such benefits can be gained by eating cooked potatoes.

do, and for exactly the same reason: oxidation. If you can't cook them right away, sprinkle them with a little ascorbic acid (vitamin C) powder or squeeze some lemon juice over them to stop the oxidation process. Don't soak potatoes in cold water, as some cookbooks recommend, because soaking will only leach out more nutrients.

We cook our potatoes in a heavy (nonaluminum) pot in just enough water to cover them. No matter what your cookbook says, *don't* add salt to the water (the potatoes don't need it, and neither do you). Be careful not to overcook them, and if you mash them, do not overwork them. If the cell walls of a potato rupture, a multitude of tiny starch granules will be released and will make your mashed potatoes pasty rather than fluffy.

When baking potatoes, pierce the skin deeply with a fork in three or four places before putting them into the oven. If you don't, they may explode and will certainly turn out to be soggy. Do not bake them in aluminum foil; this produces steamed rather than baked potatoes.

Baking potatoes in a microwave oven retains the most nutrients. A single potato can be pierced and put in the center of the oven on a double layer of paper toweling. If you are baking several potatoes at a time, arrange them spoke-fashion, with the smaller ends pointing toward the center. Cooking times vary depending on the type of microwave oven; a good average is about four minutes for one medium-to-large potato, and one to two extra minutes for each additional potato.

Mealy potatoes, high in starch and low in sugar, are best suited for baking and mashing. The outstanding varieties in this category are Russet, Bake-King, and Idaho potatoes. The waxy type of potato—the Maine variety, for example—is best for boiling as well as slicing for salads and for scalloped potatoes.*

New potatoes are especially good for salads and stews. Harvested before reaching full maturity, they have firmer flesh than do starchier, mature potatoes. Since they also contain more moisture, they absorb less of the cooking water or salad dressing.† Their firmer flesh makes them less likely to break when you mix or serve the salad. An additional convenience to the cook is that their skins have not yet set and can be easily slipped off.

---

* For those not satisfied with merely following recipes, but who wish to understand the rationale behind them, we highly recommend the following books: H. Hillman, *Kitchen Science* (Boston: Houghton Mifflin, 1981); Gladys C. Peckham and Jeanne H. Freeland-Graves, *Foundations of Food Preparation,* 4th ed. (New York: Macmillan, 1979).

† Since the customary mayonnaise dressing is out of the question for health-conscious dieters because of its extraordinarily high oil content, we recommend a vinaigrette dressing made with high-quality vinegar and cold-pressed olive oil, or a low-fat yogurt dressing with dill or other herbs and spices.

CHAPTER 57

"FRIENDLY" OILS

OLIVE OIL

Olive oil is undoubtedly the first choice of health-conscious gourmets. It is rich in monounsaturated *oleic acids,* while most other vegetable oils are polyunsaturated and hence more readily oxidizable, especially upon heating.

Some researchers, including Scott M. Grundy of the Health Sciences Center in Dallas, have claimed that olive oil actually lowers blood cholesterol levels. However, that has been categorically denied by other authorities, such as Ancel Keys of the University of Minnesota School of Public Health.

Those who say it does lower cholesterol and LDL levels base their argument largely on the indisputable fact that Mediterranean peoples who use large amounts of olive oil are known to have low heart attack rates. However, this may simply be because the less harmful olive oil is replacing highly atherogenic animal and dairy fats in their diet, rather than due to any health-protective virtues in the olive oil itself.

The few clinical studies thus far conducted with actual patients are just as ambiguous in their results and cannot settle this long-standing argument among experts. We would, however, like to mention Nathan Pritikin's insistence that olive oil raises triglyceride levels, just as any other fat does.

Leaving all these scientific arguments aside, it is clear that if olive oil is used in a diet that is definitely low in cholesterol and animal fats, its effect on cholesterol levels (though not on triglycerides) is basically neutral. In other words, it neither raises nor lowers serum cholesterol and LDL levels.

It is also true that the rate of breast and colon cancer is lower in Spain, Crete, and Greece, areas where olive oil largely replaces other fats in the diet. Nor is this unexpected, given the lesser oxidizability of the monounsaturated oleic acid of olive oil, which translates into fewer toxic peroxidation products and hence less cancer-initiating and promoting free-radical activity.

HOW TO USE OLIVE OIL

Keep in mind that olive oil is not a uniform product like corn or safflower oil, which are always basically the same in taste and quality. Olive oils differ from one another, not only in quality and price, but also with respect to their culinary uses.

Take, for instance, cold-pressed, extra-virgin olive oil, the most expensive type. Its high price doesn't mean it is the best olive oil to use for everything. Since extra-virgin olive oil is generally the most flavorful, it is ideal for salads, tomatoes, and maybe (but sparingly!) even on vegetables cooked Greek style. On the other hand, a less expensive and less flavorful olive oil will not compete with other flavors in a dish. (For cooking purposes, the oil doesn't have to be cold-pressed, since it's going to be exposed to heat anyway.) And don't be misled into thinking that the new, expensive "light" olive oil is lower in calories; it's just lighter in flavor. This means that other, much cheaper, and relatively bland olive oils will do as well. Most "light" olive oils have relatively more polyunsaturated fatty acids, which can oxidize easily and form dangerous peroxides.

The bottom line on olive oil is that it is acceptable in a health-promoting diet—if used in moderation! Do we use it? Yes, but much less frequently and in much smaller quantities than most people. For instance, we may use a teaspoon of extra-virgin olive oil to give an additional accent to a salad or a cooked vegetable. But we would never pour it onto anything—as many people unfortunately tend to do, having been lulled into a false sense of security by the overblown publicity its allegedly cholesterol-reducing effect has received in the media. Our motto, "The only good fats are the ones you don't eat," applies also to olive oil.

SUNFLOWER OIL

Regular sunflower oil is so high in linoleic and linolenic acids that it is particularly vulnerable to oxidative deterioration. Soviet scientists have developed a sunflower-oil hybrid containing high levels of *oleic acid*, a much more stable, oxidation-resistant fatty acid.

This modified, high-oleic sunflower oil (mod-SFO) is now available in the United States. Its oleic-acid content is 80 percent, and research is under way to create a genetically modified variety of sunflower that will provide 100 percent oleic acid.

Meanwhile, the available mod-SFO is already highly resistant to oxidative assault and heat-induced breakdown because of its high smoke point. It also has a high viscosity and a bland flavor that makes it ideal in order to avoid taste distortion in food. It is necessary to look for the term "mod-SFO" on the label, since conventional sunflower oil is still commonly sold.

REFINED RAPESEED OIL

In 1987 the American Health Foundation declared Procter and Gamble's Puritan Oil (identical to Canola), an improved form of rapeseed oil,* the health-promoting "product of the year." They did so because Canola or Puritan Oil is lower in saturated fat than any other vegetable oil. It contains 6 percent, compared with safflower oil's 10 percent, the next lowest among vegetable oils.

This does not mean that Canola or Puritan Oil is superior to olive oil, for although it contains about 56 percent oleic acid—the same acid that's in olive oil and in genetically modified sunflower oil—it also contains 32 percent polyunsaturated linoleic acid, compared with olive oil's 7 to 8 percent. In that respect, Canola or Puritan Oil resembles peanut oil. It is more liable to autoxidation, and probably contributes more to triglyceride blood levels than olive oil. On the other hand, of the 32 percent polyunsaturated fatty acids, about 10 percent is alpha-linolenic acid, an omega-3 fatty acid that some researchers think is almost as health-protective as omega-3 marine oils.[1]

Also, refined rapeseed oil has several other features to recommend it—bland flavor, a light color, and good flow properties, all of which have quickly made it a favorite with the food-processing industry. It does not cloud much under refrigeration, which makes it the oil of choice for commercial salad dressings. However, in making your own salad dressing, we suggest using cold-pressed, extra-virgin olive oil, or a mixture of rapeseed and olive oil.

---

* Refined rapeseed oil, marketed in North America as either Canola or Puritan Oil, contains only traces of the toxic and possibly carcinogenic erusic acid, contrasted with 45 percent in regular rapeseed, because the oil is extracted from a modified, specially bred variety of the rapeseed plant (*Brassia rapus*) that has very little of this undesirable substance.

More important for the restaurant chef or home cook is refined rapeseed oil's high smoke point. It is very stable at high temperatures, which makes it an excellent choice for quick sautéing. We recommend it for cooking wherever higher temperatures are involved.

FAT SUBSTITUTES

Fat substitutes are certainly nothing new. Modified starches have been used for some time to replace about half of the real fat in some diet salad dressings and mayonnaise. In other low-cal salad dressings, some of the oil is replaced by gums.

Unfortunately, these starches and gums can't be used for cooking, which is exactly where a fat substitute is needed most. Some products that are under development, and are currently awaiting FDA approval, have certain distinct drawbacks of safety or taste.

One of these products, Simplesse, has been developed by the NutraSweet Company, which gave us the deservedly popular sugar substitute Equal. NutraSweet's new fat substitute is made from milk proteins and egg white. Its biggest plus is that it has the creaminess of fat without the calories. Its big *technical* minus is the same as with the fat substitutes based on starches and gums—it can't be used for frying or baking because it gets tough when exposed to heat (it coagulates). It's okay, however, to use it to make ice cream, salad dressings, or spreads.

From a nutritional point of view, there is another problem: Many people are allergic to milk proteins (casein and other proteins). In addition, although milk proteins don't raise cholesterol levels, they do contribute to atherosclerosis in other ways (see pages 329–330).

Another fat substitute awaiting FDA approval is a gelatin-and-water mixture, developed by Unilever, that cuts fat calories in half. Its advantage is that it can be used for baking and what the company calls "light frying." But thus far not enough data have been published for us to form an opinion of it.

The most promising of the upcoming fat substitutes is probably Procter and Gamble's Olestra, made of synthetic calorie-free sucrose polyesters (combinations of sugar and fatty acids). Not only does Olestra have no cholesterol of its own, it may actually inhibit the absorption of cholesterol from other foods. Its biggest plus is that it can be used for frying, as well as for replacing fat in such products as margarine, chocolate, and ice cream. On the negative side, Olestra may cause diarrhea if it is used too generously—but only in home cooking, because Procter and Gamble has requested FDA approval for their product to replace only 35 to 75 percent of fat in commercial food products.

In fact, Olestra may not even be marketed for home use right away. However, in the future you may be eating it unwittingly in some prepared foods, a possibility that could become a point of contention with consumer groups. The Center for Science in the Public Interest already claims that Olestra has caused leukemia, tumors, and liver problems in laboratory animals. Procter and Gamble plays down these objections, stating that other studies show no evidence of such health risks.

We suggest that you stick with olive oil, Procter and Gamble's Puritan or Canola Oil, for your home cooking. At least your body is used to these fats, so they won't pose any real health risks if used sensibly.

FISH OILS

Fish oils are the only exception to our motto "The only good fats are the ones you don't eat." They are polyunsaturates (PUFAs) like the vegetable oils, about whose overuse we have warned you repeatedly because of high oxidizability and, hence, implied cancer risk. But, unlike PUFAs, fish oils contain a group of long-chain fatty acids, called *omega-3*, consisting of eicosapentanoic acid (EPA) and docosahexanoic acid (DHA), which are the beneficial fractions of these special types of fats.

The present popularity of fish oils goes back to a study in 1977 by two Danish scientists, Jorn Dyerberg and Hans Olaf Bang. Dyerberg and Bang compared the effects of the typical, high-saturated-fat, high-cholesterol diet of the Danes with the high marine oil diet of Greenland Eskimos.[2] The Eskimos, they found, have virtually no heart disease, even though they eat more (but differently) than the Danes. The Danes, in contrast, have a very high coronary heart disease rate. The following years saw a number of articles in medical journals, reporting on studies about fish oils. As in the earlier findings, these articles credited fish oil consumption with the prevention of atherosclerosis and heart disease, reduction of cholesterol levels, and even with a degree of cancer protection.

By the time the popular media got through with these early reports from the scientific community, fish oils had become the new "snake oil" of our era. As a result, people who had despised cod liver oil as children began to gulp it down by the quart. Some even managed to overdose on vitamin A and D, both of which are plentiful in fish oils.

It didn't take the pharmaceutical industry long to catch on to the commercial prospects of these new discoveries. Soon commercials appeared on television, featuring Eskimos darting across Arctic waters in their kayaks, with voice-over commentaries extolling the virtues of fish oil capsules. There was perhaps nothing wrong with all this—a certain degree of hucksterism may be the price we have to pay for living in a free society. However, the idea that the Eskimos' relative freedom from heart disease is due only to the fish oils in their diet is certainly exaggerated.

The truth is that the diet of the Eskimos is absolutely atrocious. Sure, they eat a lot of fish, but they also devour huge amounts of meat, fats, and cholesterol from warm-blooded animals—from seals and whales to polar bears. The only reason they get away with such a high-saturated-fat, high-cholesterol diet—just as do the Masai of Africa with their diet of fermented milk and blood—is because they have a vigorous, active, high-energy life-style that prevents them from developing atherosclerosis. In addition, the subzero climate in which the Eskimos live makes a high-fat intake a necessity rather than the liability it would be for anybody else.

Having said all this, there is one factor—and an important one—in the low incidence of coronary heart disease among Eskimos: the omega-3 fatty acids from the fish they eat. It is these fish oils that prevent blood platelet aggregation and hence the formation of atherosclerotic plaque that can lead to clogged-up coronary arteries.[3] This protective effect is further enhanced by the ability of fish oils to slow down the production of the blood-thickening, clot-forming thromboxane B_2, produced by free-radical autoxidation of arachidonic acid and similar polyunsaturated lipids in our bodies.[4]

Since fish oils will prolong bleeding time, some researchers, among them Dr. Charles Hennekens, associate professor of medicine at Brigham and Women's Hospital at Harvard Medical School, have voiced concern that some people might suffer "significant hemorrhages" by taking too much fish oil. Cerebral hemorrhages are a leading cause of death among Eskimos. That may be true for excessive intakes, especially by people who have a preexisting tendency to prolonged bleeding, such as hemophiliacs. For most of us, however, this should not present a problem; other researchers from Holland, Norway, and the United States do not seem to think that there is any danger from relatively high fish and fish oil consumption for the average, normal person—in fact, quite the contrary.[5,6]

Perhaps even more important than the blood-thinning effect of fish oils is their well-established ability to significantly lower serum triglyceride levels. To quote just one outstanding researcher, Dr. Paul J. Nestel of the Division of Human Nutrition, Adelaide, South Australia, on this point: "The triglyceride-lowering effect of this group of fatty acids is dramatic and probably exceeds the capacity of most current drugs."[7,8] A study from The Netherlands[9] found that people who were on a fat-fish (mackerel) diet for no more than three weeks experienced an average drop in triglycerides by an incredible 35 percent. On the other hand, cholesterol levels were reduced only 7.5 percent, a significant decrease but a clear indication that one should not take fish oils in the mistaken belief that they are the best way to lower cholesterol.

An English study not only confirmed that fish oils do indeed dramatically reduce plasma triglycerides, but at the same time also noted a significant increase in the "good" HDL (high-density lipoprotein) fraction of cholesterol. The researchers also noted that the mackerel diet used in the study resulted in a lower production of thromboxane B_2, which has a major role in normal blood coagulation, and in excess can produce dangerous blood clots.[10]

Another favorable shift in lipoprotein composition that fish oils have been shown to bring about is their ability to reduce the VLDLs (very low-density lipoproteins).[11] This is important because the VLDLs can be converted in the liver to "bad" LDLs (low-density lipoproteins), which are the main culprits in the whole cholesterol saga. This is probably the reason for the small reduction in cholesterol levels observed with fish diets and fish oils.

The ability of fish oil supplements—and apparently a fat-fish diet—to control triglyceride and VLDL levels is of special interest to all who are on low-fat, high-carbohydrate diets because such diets can seemingly produce a rise in these blood lipids. For example, Dr. Nestel observes that triglyceride levels tend to rise when fat intake has been restricted to less than 25 percent,[12] as on our Nutrition for Life diet (15 to 20 percent of calories from fat, with no restriction on fruits).

From our own experience and that of others—famous diet specialists Dr. William E. Connor and his wife, Sonja Connor, the late Nathan Pritikin, and Dr. John A. McDougall and his wife, Mary A. McDougall— such a rise in triglycerides seems to be only temporary (our own triglyceride and VLDL levels fall within the lowest quartile of the general population). Still, it is a comforting thought that omega-3 fish oils may exert an equalizing influence right at the outset of any low-fat, high-complex-carbohydrate diet so that even a temporary rise in triglycerides can probably be avoided.

In this connection, you may have heard or read somewhere that fish oils are contraindicated for diabetics. Such statements in the popular media are based on earlier studies that gave that impression. However, more recent studies, such as a very important one by Dr. Leonard H. Storlien and colleagues from two leading Australian medical research centers, show quite the opposite. Dr. Storlien's study points out that if laboratory rats on high-fat diets are fed fewer omega-6 polyunsaturated fats of plant origin and more omega-3 fatty acids from fish oils, they do not develop insulin resistance. These researchers therefore felt that their findings had implications for humans, and suggested that "therapy combining modest increases in omega-3 fatty acid intake with general reduction in total fat may be particularly effective in the dietary treatment of non-insulin-dependent diabetes mellitus."[13]

To return to the Eskimos: They not only have less coronary heart disease than Americans, Europeans, and even contemporary Japanese, they also suffer less from chronic inflammatory disorders such as rheumatoid arthritis, which is practically unknown among them. That, too, has been shown to be due to their higher intake of marine oils, the omega-3 fatty acids EPA (eicosapentanoic acid) and DHA (docosahexanoic acid) in an otherwise not-so-great diet. Dr. Joel M. Kramer and colleagues at the Division of Rheumatology, Albany Medical College, New York, have been able to duplicate this anti-inflammatory effect by supplementing the diets of rheumatoid arthritis patients for fourteen weeks with 1.8 grams of EPAs and DHAs, provided by nineteen MAX-EPA capsules a day. The result was that the fish oils produced, as the researchers put it, "subjective alleviation of active rheumatoid arthritis."[14]

The mechanism that triggers the anti-inflammatory effect of fish oils is somewhat complicated, but here's a simplified version. Another researcher in this field, Dr. Ranjit Kumar Chandra at the Health Sciences Center of Memorial University of Newfoundland in Saint John's, Canada, explains it as follows: The typical manifestations of inflammation—swelling, heat, redness, and pain—are caused by the oxidation products of the arachidonic acid that the body produces from the essential linoleic acid in our diet. Among these metabolites of arachidonic acid are certain "bad" prostaglandins and leukotrienes. Furthermore, since we are talking about an oxidation process, free radicals cannot be far away, as are certain oxidized enzymes, all of which are causing tissue damage. On the other hand, the EPAs of the fish oils produce "good" types of arachidonic acid products that compete with the synthesis of their bad cousins that are promoting the inflammation.[15]

Oxidation products of arachidonic acid seem to play a crucial role in the distressful and disfiguring skin disease called *psoriasis*. It is therefore not surprising that fish oils can at least help reduce the pain, itching, flaking, and caking of the skin that are characteristic of psoriasis. While fish oils in and of themselves are no real "cure" for psoriasis, Drs. Knud Kragballe and John J. Voorhees of the Department of Dermatology, University of Michigan Medical School, Ann Arbor,

ANTI-INFLAMMATORY EFFECTS
OF FISH OILS*

CHEMICALS INVOLVED IN THE INFLAMMATORY RESPONSE	PRIMARY SOURCE(S)	MAJOR EFFECT(S)	EFFECT OF FISH OIL SUPPLEMENTS
1. Leukotrienes	neutrophils and other white cells; mast cells	neutrophil activation; histamine release from mast cells	marked decreases in leukotriene biosynthesis
2. Prostaglandins & Thromboxanes	neutrophils and mast cells	enhancement of inflammatory response	beneficial changes in types produced and in the ratio of prostaglandins to thromboxanes
3. Oxygen Radicals	neutrophils and other white cells	tissue damage; production of class 1 and 2 chemicals	reduction in damage from oxygen radicals noted, but not yet proven
4. Histamine & Other Vasoactive Molecules	mast cells and certain white cells (basophils)	increased capillary permeability & vasodilation leading to further inflammation	reduced mast cell activation and histamine release

* From: *Nutrition Update,* compiled and edited by Brian E. Leibovitz, Ph.D., published by Advanced Research Press, Inc., a subsidiary of Twin Laboratories, Inc. Reprinted by permission, Steve Blechman, vice-president, Research and Development, Twin Laboratories, Inc.

experimenting with EPAs, have at least been able to confirm symptomatic relief from such treatment in about one third of patients.[16] Our guess is that much better results could be obtained if not only saturated but also polyunsaturated fats were restricted in the diet, and if fish oils were supported by an effective spectrum of anti-oxidants and vitamin cofactors.

Still another area currently under investigation is the potential application of fish oils in the control of allergies. The theoretical basis for such possibilities lies in the fact that fish oils tend to inactivate mast cells and, as pointed out earlier, inhibit the synthesis of leukotrienes, both key factors not only in inflammatory but also allergic reactions.

Fish oils have been shown to help relieve certain types of migraine headaches, probably by vasodilation of the small blood vessels in the brain.* Vasodilation appears to be the physiological reason why fish oils seem to relieve high systolic blood pressure in laboratory rats subjected to isolation stress.[17] We are happy to report that German scientists at the Academy of Sciences in Berlin (Eberhard's former hometown) have been able to duplicate this blood-pressure–lowering effect of fish oils in men who suffer from borderline or mild hypertension. They therefore recommend fish oil supplementation as an alternative treatment in such cases.[18,19]

Much less is known about the alleged beneficial effects of fish oils on the immune system and about their anticancer potential. At least one study by a widely recognized expert, Dr. Bandaru Reddy, seems to support such a possibility. Dr. Reddy and a co-worker, Dr. H. Maruyama, compared the effects of dietary fish oil and corn oil on colon cancer in male laboratory rats.[20] The rats fed corn oil had over five times more artificially induced colon tumors than rats given high levels of fish oils. The researchers were not certain whether the latter effect was due to the fish oils themselves, or to reduced food consumption in the high fish oil group.

On the other hand, there can be no doubt about the protective effect of fish oils on the immune system. This was confirmed by a recent study on the postburn metabolism and immunity of guinea pigs conducted by Dr. Orrawin Trocki and colleagues at the Shriners Burns Institute in Cincinnati, Ohio. Clearly, animal studies like these may, in the words of the researchers, "have application in the nutritional support of burn patients."[21]

---

* In cases of migraine headache, fish oils should be supplemented by 200 to 400 milligrams of magnesium to help prevent the spasms in the smooth-muscle walls of large and small arteries that seem to play a role in migraines. Also people who suffer from migraines should definitely abstain from foods that contain large amounts of the amino acid tyramine, such as avocados, sour cream, aged cheese, pickled herring, beer, and red wine, most of which are on the no-no list anyway.

EAT MORE FISH OR TAKE SUPPLEMENTS?

In light of the healthful benefits of fish oils, especially with regard to cardiovascular problems, the question arises as how best to incorporate them into a comprehensive health-maintenance and life-extension program like ours. Our first instincts favored an exclusively dietary approach rather than a supplementary one. If people just ate enough fish, we thought, they should get enough beneficial fish oils and wouldn't need supplements.

To a point, that's true. However, the most popular types of fish consumed in the United States (Europe and Japan are a little better in that respect) are of the low-fat type that don't contain many protective EPAs and DHAs. So, as we started looking more deeply into the matter, we began to lean toward the combination of dietary and supplemental sources in order to get the full benefit of the fish oils.

Another reason for changing our opinion is that, although some studies indicate that eating more fish produces the desirable effects of the fish oils,[22] other studies seem to indicate that even high fish consumption does not necessarily mean a high enough intake of EPAs and DHAs to make any difference. The classical study illustrating this point is that of Dr. Terje Simonsen and colleagues at the University of Tromsø, Norway.[23] Dr. Simonsen compared two Norwegian communities—a coastal one and an inland one—with regard to the development of coronary heart disease (CHD) in the two communities. The results confirmed those of two previous studies from Hawaii and Norway:[24,25] In some instances, there appeared to be no relation between fish intake and mortality from heart disease.

The Tromsø study found that the coastal community with a tradition of high fish consumption actually had a higher mortality from CHD than the inland community whose diet was different. The researchers are only saying that "the dietary intakes of saturated fatty acids were similar in the two communities." Which leads one to assume therefore that, thanks to modern food transportation, the people in the coastal communities of Norway must be eating as much red meat, butter, and other animal fats as the people of the highlands and in the *dals* (valleys) of the interior. No wonder that eating a lot of fish can't make up for so much saturated fat.

On the other hand, several studies show that following a general low-fat diet and eating high-fat fish like mackerel, bluefish, herring, or salmon several times a week will have a very beneficial effect. But eating so much high-fat fish is probably not very practical for most people. It's more than likely that you eat some kind of fish or seafood maybe a couple of times a week, and not necessarily always high-fat fish. But if you eat mostly the leaner fish—like red snapper or flounder—the total fat content will have no more than 8 to 12 percent EPA and 10 to 20 percent DHA, not enough to make much of a difference. So, it's only common sense to take some fish oil in the form of supplements.

Another good reason for not relying only on heavy fish consumption is that if you do, you also ingest a fair amount of cholesterol with the fish. For instance, a 347-gram serving of chum salmon is not only rich in the beneficial omega-3 fatty acids of the fish oil, but also includes 74 milligrams of cholesterol—roughly one fourth of the maximum amount you can safely have for the whole day. On the other hand, three capsules of MAX-EPA provides you with fully 1 gram of omega-3 fatty acids and, at most, only 18 milligrams of cholesterol (many recently developed fish oil supplements are even higher in EPA and DHA, while being practically cholesterol-free).

Still another factor is that fish—and especially fresh-water varieties like catfish or lake trout (high in EPA and DHA)—are often heavily contaminated with chlorinated hydrocarbons and other chemicals from the runoff of agricultural pesticides and herbicides, not to mention those from industrial pollution, like the notorious PCBs—all the more reason to eat fish in moderation and as only one albeit important part of a varied, health-promoting diet.

FISH OILS: OUR BOTTOM-LINE RECOMMENDATION

If your cholesterol level and especially your triglyceride level are already on the low side, there is no urgent need to take fish oil supplements. Just include more of the oil-rich type of fish and seafood in your diet. On the other hand, since fish oils have a decided anti-inflammatory effect as well as other medicinal properties, we still think it is a good idea to take some fish oil supplement.* Dr. Demopoulas feels that fish oil manufacturers should use nitrogen gas processing to decrease the possibility of EPA and DHA oxidizing. He has

---

* At a recent symposium on the health effects of fish and fish oils at the Health Sciences Center, Memorial University of Newfoundland, Saint John's, Canada, it transpired that emulsified fish oils are ten to twelve times better absorbed than nonemulsified ("straight") fish oils. Since we both have a tendency toward painful joints, mitigated only by our anti-oxidants and exercise routine, we take Twinlab's Emulsified Norwegian Cod Liver Oil, which has a very agreeable orange taste, and is well protected against peroxidation by a synergistic mixture of anti-oxidants. (There is also an encapsulated form of emulsified and anti-oxidant–protected cod liver oil available from Twinlab, as well as a "devitaminized" version, from which vitamins A and D have been removed. This is the type of fish oil to take if you are using Twinlab's MaxiLIFE formula, or a similar product that includes vitamin A rather than only beta-carotene (pro-vitamin A), as with the Demopoulos spectrum.

found considerable lipid peroxides in EPA and DHA capsules in several commercial preparations.*

The following table shows fish and other seafood items that have the highest marine oil content:

OIL CONTENT IN FLESH OF FRESH FISH*	
	Total oil (wt. %)
Eel	20–22
Herring (fresh)	11
Sardines (fresh)†	9–10
Channel catfish†	9–10
Tuna (fresh or water-packed)	7–7.5
Coho salmon	7+
Sturgeon	(high, but no figures available)
Mackerel†	7+
Bluefish	6–7
Mullet	5–6
Carp	4.5
Pompano	4+
Black bass	4+
Smelt†	4+
Pink salmon	4
Boston and ocean perch	3–4
Porgy	3

* All figures are rounded out and adapted from T. L. Hearn et al. "Polyunsaturated fatty acids and fat in fish flesh for selecting species for human health benefits," *J. Food Sci.*, 1987; 52:1209.
† These fish also contain the highest amounts (40% or more) of total marine oils in omega-3 fatty acids.

Dr. Thomas L. Hearn and colleagues from the Department of Pathology and Laboratory Medicine of Emory University in Atlanta, Georgia, point out that the fat of most common fish contains 8 to 12 percent of EPA and 10 to 20 percent of DHA. The fats of scallops, oysters, and red caviar contain more than 20 percent of either EPA or DHA. But red caviar is also high in cholesterol, with oysters and squid medium-high (acceptable), and scallops very low in cholesterol. Out-

* Twinlab's fish oil preparations are all processed under nitrogen.

side some of the above-mentioned fish, scallops are one of the most ideal sources of marine oils.

Remember also that smoked, pickled, and fermented foods are *not* "friendly" foods by our definition. Pickled herring and smoked fish or smoked shellfish are not recommended.

You also cannot use fast-food fish sandwiches or their English equivalent, fish-and-chips, to increase your omega-3 fatty acids intake. Aside from being fried, such fish foods contain much more problematic omega-6 acids than protective omega-3 fatty acids.

Similarly, while fresh sardines are excellent sources of omega-3 fish oils, canned sardines are not, because they are invariably packed in oil (only the ones packed in pure olive oil are marginally acceptable).

On the other hand, fresh foods are "friendlier" than canned ones. The high heat used in the canning process always generates some compounds that have been found mutagenic or carcinogenic in various studies. Canned salmon has actually been found to be the most mutagenic canned food in one recent study by scientists from the Institute for Food Science and Technology at the University of Washington and the National Marine Fisheries Service in Seattle, and the Department of Agriculture in Honolulu.[26] Water-packed tuna, on the other hand, as well as water-packed clams, contained either no mutagens at all or only very low levels. Next to fresh tuna, our nod therefore goes to water-packed canned tuna, while salmon is better eaten fresh only.*

The reasons for the wide differences in mutagenicity of canned foods are not fully understood. However, one reason for the low, and probably not very problematic mutagenicity of canned tuna could be that the fish is precooked under steam *before* being packed into cans and thermally processed. As these scientists point out, this pretreatment removes some of the fats and water-soluble components of the flesh. Salmon, on the other hand, is placed directly into the cans, sealed, and processed without any pretreatment.

It is known that the lipids in fish contain several highly unsaturated fatty acids that are very vulnerable to autoxidation. We suspect that it is the autoxidation of the lipids, which forms free radicals, that accounts for by far the major part of mutagenicity in any canned foods that contain lipids. This is all the more plausible since the researchers report that the addition of 1 percent of ascorbic acid (vitamin C) decreased mutagen formation "significantly" in the canned salmon. It is for precisely this reason that we and Dr. Demopoulos have been suggesting for some time that fish products (and undoubtedly many other foods) should have the

---

* There are many species of tuna, but mostly blue fin and albacore tuna are seen in America. However, occasionally you can also find Tungo and flake white tuna on grocery store shelves. Both are very tasty and offer some variety. Why buy the more expensive brand-name tuna if the store has "generic tuna," which is just as good and costs a lot less?

MICROWAVE OVEN COOKING
MAKES IT EASIER TO EAT RIGHT*

1. Place raw vegetables on a plate with seasonings and cook them for 1 minute in the microwave oven. They retain more of their vitamins and minerals, look fresher, and taste better. This works best for:

snow peas	cauliflower	carrots	cabbage
asparagus	broccoli	squash	potatoes

   It does not work well with green beans. Blanch the green beans first, then reheat them in the microwave.

2. Combine microwave cooking with more traditional cooking methods. Example: ratatouille (a dish of mixed vegetables like zucchini, eggplant, tomato, bell peppers).

   The traditional method of stewing the vegetables destroys too many nutrients and negatively affects taste. Instead try the following:

   a. Simmer garlic and onions in a small amount of olive oil in a nonstick pan, add tomatoes, and cool.

   b. To this cooked mixture add raw vegetables: small pieces of zucchini, eggplant, bell peppers, and spices—rosemary and thyme or others if you prefer.

   c. Cook this mixture in the microwave oven 1 or more minutes, depending on the desired consistency.

*Adapted from recipes of St. Andrew's Café, the nutritional restaurant at the Culinary Institute of America, Hyde Park, New York.

---

most appropriate and most effective anti-oxidants added to them before processing (rosemary extract would be perfect in most cases).*

As far as the beneficial EPA and DHA marine oils are concerned, canning does not seem to affect them, according to a recent study by the MIT Sea Grant Program and Foster-Miller, Inc., an independent research group. (Remember, this is something quite different from the autoxidation problem discussed above.) Furthermore, only 3 percent of the good omega-3 fatty acids is lost by draining a can of tuna, in contrast to a 25 percent loss with salmon. There is no need to lose even 3 percent by draining water-packed tuna, because you can use the water in preparing tuna salad or in tuna casserole. With canned salmon, on the other hand, you have to drain the oil because it's autoxidated and able to do free-radical damage to lipid-containing

* The best rosemary extract is produced by Kalsec, Inc., P.O. Box 511, Kalamazoo, Mich.

TIPS TO EXPERIMENT WITH IN THE KITCHEN

Preparing sauces:

1. Start with a good stock. Different stocks can be made by adding the following combinations to water:
   lean meat with bones
   lean chicken (no skin or fat) and bones
   fish
   vegetables
   Vegetables may be added to the first three to make different types of sauces.

   To remove all fat from the meat and chicken stock, freeze and remove the fat, which will rise solid to the top of your container.

   An unusual stock can be made from the shells of fresh crab, shrimp, or lobster by sautéing them first in a nonstick pan with a little olive oil and then simmering in water.
2. The more you reduce the stock, the stronger the flavor. You do *not* need to skim the stock to prevent it from becoming cloudy. If the stock simmers just below boiling, it will remain clear without skimming.
3. Complement the stock's flavor with garlic, thyme, shallots, red or white wine, or any other spices and flavors of your choice.

Cooking Soup in Advance:

Cook the soup, cool it, measure it out into individual servings, and refrigerate or freeze for later use. Just before serving, reheat in the microwave oven or on a traditional stove. This way, the soup retains its fresh flavor, color, texture, and nutrients.

Sautéing:

Use a nonstick pan and sauté foods either in a light amount, a haze, of oil or in a small amount of stock. (This method is technically more like poaching or steaming.)

A Substitute for Frying:

If you can't live without deep-frying: Combine bread crumbs, a small amount of olive oil, finely chopped shallots, garlic, and any other spices you prefer. Moisten this mixture with a dash of either water, stock, wine, low-salt soy sauce, tamari, horseradish, mustard, or lemon juice so that the bread-crumb mixture will pack around the fish, meat, or skinless chicken (preferably breast), and bake it in the oven. The bread-crumb coating should become a firm crust, similar to the breading of deep-fried food, but without all the fat (this may require some experimentation before you get the consistency of the mixture just right).

(continued)

Healthful Desserts and Baked Goods:

Use skim milk instead of whole milk (you can actually modify some recipes that call for whole milk by using three fourths skim milk and one fourth water). Try using more egg whites instead of whole eggs, with perhaps one or, at the most, two added yolks. Use only one half the sugar that is called for in the recipe (sometimes only one third or one fourth is enough). People who have reduced their daily intake of sugar, fat, and salt prefer these modified pastries and desserts because they find the ones that are made the traditional way too sickeningly sweet and rich (fat).

body tissue, so there's no way of avoiding the substantial loss of marine oils that are mixed up with the packing oil.

Finally, with regard to shellfish as sources of omega-3 fatty acids, we recommend mollusks like oysters, clams, and mussels over crustaceans like crab, shrimp, or lobster, although both have appreciable amounts of omega-3 fatty acids. This does not mean that we consider crustaceans are "unfriendly" foods; it is not even that they contain more cholesterol than most fish and mollusks. The point is, it has been shown that oysters and clams (and, by implication, other mollusks) actually inhibit cholesterol absorption by 25 percent, while lobster, shrimp, and crab do not.[27] Mollusks also make for a healthier HDL_2:LDL_3 ratio in the diet, in favor of beneficial high-density lipoproteins (HDL_2).

Prawns and fresh-water crayfish should not provide your main sources of marine oils because a high proportion of these crustaceans are raised in ponds on pelleted soya meal, which is much higher in omega-6 fatty acids than the foods these creatures would eat in their natural habitat. The same applies to pond-reared fish, like commercial catfish.[28]

Our recommendation therefore is occasionally to enjoy lobster, prawns, and crayfish for flavor and variety, but not for their marine oils (many people are allergic to them, too, often without knowing it, which is another reason for urging caution).

For dietary fish oils it is therefore advisable to rely on the listed ocean fish like tuna, fresh salmon, mackerel, bluefish, fresh herring, fresh sardines, and fresh squid. Lake and river trout as well as eels are all right too, but be sure they are not pond-grown. Mollusks like oysters and mussels are generally not reared artificially. Even if they are, they are farmed in the sea and feed on the same algae and other microorganisms as mussels and oysters harvested from their natural habitat. Their EPA and DHA content is therefore equivalent, so they are good sources of marine oils, as are scallops.

UPDATE   A recent study,[29] conducted at the Veterans Administration Medical Center in Dallas, found that fish oil reduces the chances of coronary arteries becoming clogged up again after angioplasty,* an alternative to an arterial bypass operation. This discovery is highly important because in about one third of the estimated 200,000 angioplasty cases that will be performed in America alone per year, the arteries normally soon get clogged up again, a condition called *restenosis.*

With fish oil supplementation, most restenosis can for all practical purposes be avoided, especially, we may add, if the patient follows a low-fat, high-complex-carbohydrate diet like ours. Within such a health-promoting diet, fish oils have now proven themselves immensely helpful in this serious complication of angioplasty. In fact, Dr. Gregory J. Dehmer, now at the University of North Carolina, who headed the study, said in a *New York Times* interview that fish oil "is the only agent so far that has even shown a hint of having an effect."[30]

True, by the same token that fish oil thins out the blood, it can also encourage bleeding, although this has not been found to be a realistic problem with the vast majority of people, including angioplasty patients. However, there can be a risk with certain patients. In angioplasty cases, fish oil supplements should therefore not be taken without a supervising physician's consent. However, the same *Times* report quotes Dr. Eric H. Eichhorn, a co-author of the above-mentioned study, saying that if he were to undergo angioplasty, "I would take it myself."

A FINAL WORD OF CAUTION

We consider it extremely unwise to take any fish oil supplement that does not have the protection of added anti-oxidants. If it does not specifically state so on the label, we would advise not using the product.† Even if the fish oil supplement does contain added anti-oxidants, we still consider it extremely ill-advised to take such a supplement by itself alone without the benefits of a broad-spectrum anti-oxidant program, as outlined in this book.

---

* Angioplasty is a procedure in which a tiny inflatable balloon is inserted into the clogged artery in order to destroy or push aside the obstructing atherosclerotic plaque.

† For the majority of people, the most practical way of providing for such a full spectrum would be by supplementing a health-promoting diet with either HMP's Performance Packs or Ascorbic-B capsules, or with Twinlab's new MaxiLIFE formula.

SOURCES

1. Simopoulos, A. P., and N. Salem. *N. Eng. J. Med.,* (Correspondence), 1987; 316:628.
2. Dyerberg, J., H. O. Bang, E. Stoffersen, et al. "Eicosapentaenoic acid and prevention of thrombosis and atherosclerosis." *Lancet,* 1978; 2:117–119.
3. Weiner, B. H., et al. "Inhibition of atherosclerosis by cod-liver oil in a hyperlipidemic swine model." *N. Eng. J. Med.,* 1986; 315:14.
4. Chandra, R. K. "There is more to fish and fish oils." *Nutr. Res.,* 1988; 8:1–2.
5. Brox, J. H., J. E. Killie, A. Nordøy, and S. Gunnes. "The effect of cod-liver oil and corn oil on platelets and vessel wall in man." *Thromb. Haemost.,* 1981; 46:604–611.
6. Simons, L. A., J. B. Hickie, and S. Balasubramaniam. "On the effects of dietary (n-3) fatty acids (Maxepa) on plasma lipids and lipoproteins in patients with hyperlipidemia." *Atherosclerosis,* 1985; 54:75–88.
7. Nestel, P. J., W. Connor, et al. "Suppression by diets rich in fish oil of very low density lipoprotein production in man." *J. Clin. Investig.,* 1984; 74:82–89.
8. Nestel, Paul J. "Polyunsaturated fatty acids (n-3, n-6)." *Am. J. Clin. Nutr.,* 1987; 45 (Supplement 5):1161–1167. Also: Miettinen, T. A., and Y. A. Kasäniemi. "Cholesterol Balance and Liproprotein Metabolism in Man." In: *Bile Acids and Atherosclerosis,* Vol. 15, S. M. Grundy, ed. New York: Raven Press, 1986, p. 120. See also: Nestel, P. J. "Fish oil fatty acids—the answer to heart disease." *Austr. Fam. Physician,* 1987; 16(5):624–627.
9. Von Lossonczy, T. O., A. Ruiter, H. C. Bronsgeest-Schoute, et al. "The effect of a fish diet on serum lipids in healthy human subjects." *Am. J. Clin. Nutr.,* 1987; 31:1340–1346.
10. Sanders, T.A.B., et al. "Influence of mackerel diet on plasma lipoproteins and platelet function." *Proc. Nutr. Soc.,* 1987; 46:1–12.
11. Nestel, P. J., W. Connor, et al. "Suppression by diets rich in fish oil of very low density liproprotein production in man." *J. Clin. Investig.,* 1984; 74:82–89.
12. Ibid.
13. Storlien, L. H., et al. "Fish oil prevents insulin resistance induced by high-fat feeding in rats." *Science,* 1987; 238:885–888.
14. Kremer, J. M., et al. "Fish oil fatty acid supplementation in active rheumatoid arthritis." *JAMA,* 1987; 258:962.
15. Chandra, op. cit.
16. Kragballe, K., and J. J. Voorhees. "Arachidonic acid in psoriasis. Pathogenic role and pharmacological regulation." *Acta Dermatonever* (Stockholm), 1987; Supplement 120.
17. Mills, D., and R. Ward. "Effects of eicosapentenoic acid on stress reactivity in rats." *Proc. Soc. Experim. Biol. and Med.,* 1986; 182:127–131.
18. Singer, P., et al. "Influence on serum lipids, lipoproteins and blood pressure of mackerel and herring diet in patients with type IV and V hyperlipoproteinemia." *Atherosclerosis,* 1985, 51:111.
19. Singer, P., et al. "Blood pressure—and lipid-lowering effect of mackerel and herring diet in patients with mild essential hypertension." *Atherosclerosis,* 1985; 56:223. See also: Singer, et al. "Slow desaturation and elongation of linoleic and α-linoleic acids as a rationale of eicosapentaenoic acid-rich diet to lower blood pressure and serum lipids in normal,

hypertensive and hyperlipemic subjects." *Prostaglandins, Leukotrienes & Medicine,* in press.
20. Reddy, B., and H. Maruyama. "Effect of dietary fish oil on azoxymethane-induced colon carcinogenesis in male F 344 rats." *Cancer Res.,* 1986; 46:3367–3370.
21. Trocki, O., et al. "Effects of fish oil on postburn metabolism and immunity." *J. Parent. and Enterol. Nutr.,* 1987; 11:521–528.
22. Kromhout, D., et al. "The inverse relation between fish consumption and 20-year mortality from coronary heart disease." *N. Eng. J. Med.,* 1985; 312:1205–1209. See also: Nishizawa, K. Y., et al. "Eicosapolyenoic acids of serum lipids of Japanese islanders with low incidence of cardiovascular disease." *J. Nutr. Sci. Vitaminol.* (Tokyo), 1982; 28:441–453. Also: Weiner, B. H., et al. "Inhibition of atherosclerosis by cod-liver oil in a hyperlipidemic swine model." *N. Eng. J. Med.,* 1986; 315:841–846, and Dyerberg, op. cit.
23. Simonsen, T., et al. "Coronary Heart Disease, Serum Lipids, Platelets and Diet: Fish in Two Communities in Northern Norway." *Acta Med. Scand.,* 1987; 222:237–245.
24. McGree, D. L., et al. "Ten year incidence of coronary heart disease in the Honolulu Heart Program: relationship to nutrient intake." *Am. J. Epidem.,* 1984; 119:667–676.
25. Bjelke, E. "Kostdata brukt i analyse av senere krefthyppighet og dødelighet—og i en case—control studie av kreft i magesekk og tarm" (in Norwegian). *Vår Föda,* 1982; 34 (Supplement 4):277–297.
26. Krone, C. R., S.M.J. Yeh, and W. T. Iwaoka. "Mutagen formation during commercial processing of foods." *Environmental Health Perspectives,* 1986; 67:75–88.
27. Child, M. T., et al. "Effect of shellfish consumption on cholesterol absorption in normolipidemic men." *Metabolism,* 1988; 36:31–36.
28. Chanmugam, P., et al. "Differences in the omega-3 fatty acid contents in pond-reared and wild fish and shellfish." *J. Food Sci.,* 1986; 51:1556–1557.
29. *The New York Times,* September 22, 1988.
30. Dehmer, G. J., et al. "Reduction in the rate of early restenosis after coronary angioplasty by a diet supplemented with n-3 fatty acids." *N. Eng. J. Med.,* 1988; 319:733–740.

CHAPTER 58

YOGURT

FRIENDLY BACTERIA

Genuine yogurt is made by fermenting milk with the help of certain added bacteria. Usually it's made with *Lactobacillus bulgaricus* and *Streptococcus thermophilus;* sometimes *Lactobacillus acidophilus* is used. We prefer yogurt made with active cultures of all three bacteria, because each of them seems to provide different health benefits; there also appears to be a synergistic effect by the interaction of these three types of cultured bacteria.*

Yogurt has long since been considered a "friendly," health-promoting food. Remember Gaylord Hauser, America's most popular nutrition guru during the 1940s and 1950s? He was best known for his advocacy of yogurt and molasses. Around the turn of the century, long before Hauser, there was a famous Russian-born scientist, Dr. Elias Metchnikoff, who worked at the Pasteur Institute in Paris and insisted to an incredulous medical establishment that yogurt could prevent diseases of the gut caused by microbial putrefaction. He felt that yogurt was a life-extending food, since the Bulgarians, who traditionally had always eaten large quantities of yogurt, were considered unusually long-lived. Be that as it may, the bacteria from which Dr. Metchnikoff made his first batch of yogurt had been imported from Bulgaria, hence the name *bulgaricus.*

* In the United States, some unscrupulous manufacturers produce a type of phony yogurt not made with active bacteria cultures at all. It simply consists of milk that has been soured with some kind of acid, then given the appearance of yogurt by adding a thickening agent like carrageenan or some other type of artificial thickener. Therefore, if the label on the yogurt container does not say that it contains "active cultures," the product must be considered suspect.

Besides, he might not have been so far off the mark with regard to his life-extension hunch about yogurt, as we shall presently see. Today, scientists know more about yogurt, and basically the news is all good.

IMPROVED LACTOSE TOLERANCE

First of all, yogurt is better tolerated than milk, even by those with a deficiency in the enzyme lactase, without which they cannot digest milk sugar lactose. As mentioned in the chapter on milk, a large percentage of the world population lacks this enzyme and therefore cannot digest milk. Even those who in their youth have sufficient lactase activity and have no problem digesting milk, experience a gradual decline in this enzyme with age. Newborn infants, on the other hand, have high lactase activity. But right after weaning, the gene that controls lactase activity starts putting it on "slow"—nature's broad hint that milk may be all right for little humans, but not for grownups.

What happens with yogurt is that it seems actually to stimulate lactase activity.[1] Even more surprisingly, studies show that bacterial fermentation products in yogurt can actually substitute for the missing endogenous (body-produced) enzyme lactase.[2] As a result, even lactase-deficient people can generally handle the lactose in yogurt much better than that in milk,[3] although some individuals cannot even digest it in that form.

ANTIBIOTIC ACTION

It was not until 1963 that research fully corroborated Dr. Metchnikoff's half-century earlier hunch that yogurt does indeed have a decided antibiotic effect in the gut. The study showed that for forty-five infants under one year of age who had to be hospitalized for severe diarrhea, giving them 100 milliliters (approximately 1 cup) of yogurt three times per day was more effective than the standard medical treatment of 1 teaspoon of Kaopectate, fortified with 50 milligrams of neomycin, three times per day. The children who got the yogurt recovered, on average, in less than three days, while those on kaolin and neomycin medication needed almost five days to recover.[4]

Ten years later (1973), Italian researchers demonstrated in a study on adults that giving patients yogurt "significantly reduced" the number of dangerous E. coli bacteria in the intestines.[5] Even earlier, it had become evident, though largely ignored, that yogurt was able to control the diarrhea that frequently results from antibiotics.[6]

The same antibiotic activity of yogurt against various pathologic gut bacteria was observed in several animal studies. In one study young pigs were deliberately infested with disease-producing *E. coli* bacteria; one group was given a broth with the benign *L. bulgaricus* bacteria that are present in yogurt, and the other group, likewise infested, did not receive the *L. bulgaricus* broth. The piglets who had had the benefit of the *L. bulgaricus* broth had a better survival rate and showed more growth than the control group.[7] Similarly, yogurt-fed rats survived inoculation with *Salmonella enteritidis,* bacteria notorious for causing severe dysentery, much better than those given milk only.[8]

These researchers noted in this and a subsequent study that rats who were kept continuously on a yogurt diet, before as well as after exposure to disease-producing microorganisms, survived best.[9] Interesting too, is that test-tube studies showed that yogurt does, in some instances, have a potent antimicrobial effect even against a variety of microorganisms resistant to a great number of antibiotics.[10]

The mechanism by which yogurt exerts this antibiotic effect is not fully understood. Experimental evidence suggests that it is the cultured lactobacteria themselves in yogurt, rather than any fermentation products, that are responsible. One of the country's foremost experts on yogurt, however, Dr. Khem Shahani, of the Department of Food Science at the University of Nebraska, claims to have isolated two antibiotic compounds in yogurt—one, produced by *L. acidophilus,* which he named "acidophilin," and another one from *L. bulgaricus,* which he calls "bulgarican."[11] There is no doubt that by whatever mechanism, yogurt is able to exert a powerful antibiotic effect on harmful microorganisms in the gut that may rival those of the best synthetic antibiotics.

YOGURT, IMMUNITY, AND CANCER

We've known since at least 1980 that yogurt positively strengthens the immune system of laboratory animals. That same year, a group of French researchers published the results of their mice studies showing that when yogurt was added to the diet, it greatly increased antibody production. Also, the spleens—which are reservoirs of large numbers of phagocytes and lymphocytes, capable of destroying bacteria and viruses—of the yogurt-fed mice were hyperactive compared with those of the mice whose diet had not been supplemented with yogurt.[12] In short, the immune systems of the yogurt-fed mice were working overtime.

In 1986 a group of Italian researchers demonstrated that yogurt was able to strengthen the immune system not only in animals, but also in humans. These medical scientists discovered that yogurt increases the production of a type of immune interferon (gamma IFN), which in turn is capable of stimulating antibody production. Moreover, there was increased NK (natural killer) cell activity, which is known to suppress certain tumor cells. The scientists credited *L. bulgaricus* and *S. thermophilus* for these protective effects, giving a slight edge to *S. thermophilus.*[13] (This is a good reason to make certain that your yogurt contains both of these cultures!) Furthermore, a comparison between yogurt and Levaelsole, a drug frequently used to strengthen the immune response, resulted in yogurt being at least equally effective— and minus the common side effects of the synthetic drug!

The *L. bulgaricus* bacteria in yogurt are, however, not to be deprecated. A Yugoslavian group of researchers found that a substance (blastolysin) from the cell wall of *L. bulgaricus* is effective against a malignant type of tumor, called *sarcoma S180.*[14] It is not known whether the blastolysin from *L. bulgaricus* also works against other sarcomas, as for example, Karposi's sarcoma, frequently associated with AIDS. Follow-up studies are certainly long overdue, especially in view of the AIDS crisis (we strongly advise anyone with immune deficiency disease to eat plenty of "friendly," immune-system– strengthening foods like yogurt, along with plenty of fresh fruits and vegetables and less animal fats and proteins).

There are also indications that yogurt is protective with regard to breast cancer[15] and, of course, cancer of the colon.[16] The way this anticancer effect may come about in the case of colon cancer seems to be that the *L. acidophilus* of the yogurt deprives potential carcinogens in the gut of its "energy of activation" to cause malignant cell growth. That energy is usually supplied when certain intestinal enzymes turn otherwise harmless substances into cancer initiators or promoters. *L. acidophilus* apparently is able to block the enzymatic transformation. In one study done in the United States, people who were given acidophilus milk to drink had 200 to 400 percent less of this potentially cancer-causing enzyme activity than those who drank plain milk.[17] Clearly, yogurt with all three *Lactobacillus* cultures—*acidophilus, bulgaricus,* and *thermophilus*—should be even more protective, as well as being better digested and posing less of a casein problem.

CHOLESTEROL-LOWERING EFFECT

A study with men of the Masai tribe in Africa during the early 1970s discovered, to the surprise of medical scientists, that the more lactobacillus-fermented milk these men drank (4 to 8 liters per day!) the larger the decrease in their serum cholesterol levels.[18] Since normally, high milk consumption results in high cholesterol levels, there was at the time no logical explanation for this strange reversal of established scientific fact.

Subsequently, however, Dr. George Mann, who had directed the Masai study, started thinking that Masai yogurt must contain some as yet unidentified factor, which would account for this difference. In 1976 Dr. Mann published a paper explaining that this mysterious anti-cholesterolemic factor could only be a substance that inhibits the synthesis of cholesterol in the liver. He identified that substance as HMG (hydroxymethyl glutarate), a compound produced by *L. acidophilus* in yogurt.[19]

Several later studies confirming these findings included the observation that a yogurt-supplemented diet resulted (in humans) in an increase in the protective HDL_2 (high-density lipoprotein) fraction of cholesterol.[20] Still another study with humans also showed a cholesterol-lowering effect of yogurt, which varied, depending on the type of yogurt culture used.[21]

THE BOTTOM LINE ON YOGURT

No doubt, yogurt is one of the "friendliest" foods around. It has antibiotic, immunity-strengthening, anticancer, and cholesterol-lowering effects. We ourselves eat low-fat yogurt frequently and would do so even if it did not have all these splendid protective properties, simply because we like its nicely balanced taste and its cooling effect with hot curries and other spicy foods.

But frankly there is still another reason why we eat yogurt: The different beneficial bacteria it contains make for a healthier microbial balance in the intestines. They prevent putrefaction and reduce the production of intestinal gas, a distinct bonus with a high-fiber diet such as ours.

SOURCES

1. Kilara, A., and K. M. Shahani. "Lactase activity of cultured and acidified dairy products." *J. Dairy Sci.*, 1976; 59:2031–2035.
2. Kolars, J. C., et al. "Yogurt—an autodigesting source of lactose." *N. Eng. J. Med.*, 1984; 310:1–3.
3. Cochet, B., et al. "Effects of lactose on intestinal calcium absorption in normal and lactase-deficient subjects." *Gastroenterology*, 1983; 84:935–940.

4. Niv. M., and N. M. Greenstein. "Yogurt in the treatment of infantile diarrhea." *Clin. Pediatr.*, 1963; 2:407–411.

5. Salvador, P., and B. Salvadori. "Studio sulle variazioni coprocolturali nell'uomo in rapporto alla somministrazione di yogurt." *Minerva Diet.*, 1973; 14:8–12.

6. Shapiro, S. "Control of antibiotic induced gastrointestinal symptoms with yogurt." *Clin. Med.*, 1960; 7:295.

7. Mitchell, I. de G., and R. Kenworthy. "Investigations on a metabolite from *Lactobacillus bulgaricus* which neutralizes the effect of enterotoxin from *Escherichia coli* pathogenic for pigs." *J. Appl. Bact.*, 1976; 41:163–174.

8. Hitchins, A. D., et al. "Amelioration of the adverse effect of a gastrointestinal challenge with *Salmonella enteritidis* on weanling rats by a yogurt diet." *Am. J. Clin. Nutr.*, 1985; 41:92–100.

9. Hitchins, A. D., et al. "A gastrointestinal and nonsystemic dietary effect of yogurt in the alleviation of rat salmonellosis." *Nutr. Rep. Int.*, 1985; 31:601–608.

10. Yazicioglu, A. von, and N. Yilmaz. "Untersuchungen über die Mikroflora von Joghurt und dessen antibakterielle Wirkung." *Milchwissenschaft*, 1966; 21:87–92.

11. Shahani, K. M., et al. "Properties of and prospects for cultured dairy foods." *Soc. Appld. Bacteriol. Symp. Ser.*, 1983; 11:257–269.

12. Conge, G., et al. "Effets comparés d'un régime enrichi en yoghourt vivant ou thermisé sur le système immunitaire de la souris." *Reprod. Nutr. Dev.*, 1980; 20:929–938.

13. De Simone, C., et al. "The adjuvant effect of yogurt on production of gamma-interferon by Con A-stimulated human peripheral blood lymphocytes." *Nutr. Rep. Int.*, 1986; 33:419–433.

14. Bogdanov, I. G., et al. "Antitumor action of glycopeptides from the cell wall of *Lactobacillus bulgaricus.*" Bull. Exp. Biol. Med., 1978; 84:1750–1753.

15. Le, M. G., et al. "Consumption of dairy produce and alcohol in a case-control study of breast cancer." *J. Natl. Cancer Inst.*, 1986; 77:633–636.

16. Reddy, G. V., et al. "Antitumor activity of yogurt components." *J. Food Prot.*, 1983; 46:8–11.

17. Goldin, B. R., et al. "The effect of milk and lactobacillus feeding on human intestinal bacterial enzyme activity." *Am. J. Clin. Nutr.*, 1984; 39:756–761.

18. Mann, G. V., et al. "Studies of a surfactant and cholesteremia in the Masai." *Am. J. Clin. Nutr.*, 1974.

19. Mann, G. V. "A factor in yogurt which lowers cholesteremia in man." *Atherosclerosis*, 1977; 26:335–340.

20. Bazarre, T. L., et al. "Total and HDL-cholesterol concentrations following yogurt and calcium supplementation." *Nutr. Rep. Int.*, 1983; 28:1225–1232.

21. Jaspers, D. A., et al. "Effect of consuming yogurts prepared with three culture strains on human serum lipoproteins." *J. Food Sci.*, 1984; 49:1178–1181.

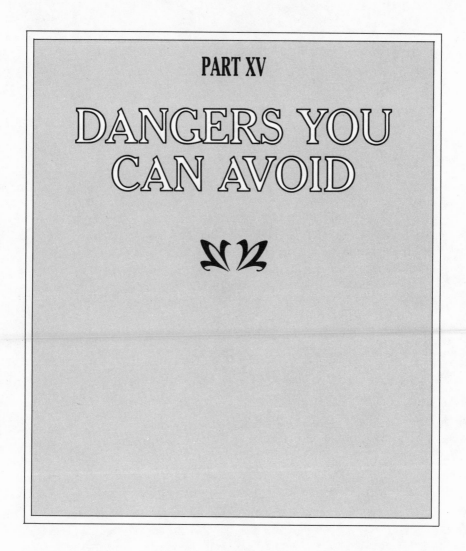

PART XV

DANGERS YOU CAN AVOID

CHAPTER 59

SMOKING

SUICIDE ON THE INSTALLMENT PLAN

A WORD TO THE NONSMOKER

If, like us, you are a nonsmoker, you might assume this chapter would be of little interest to you. You may be in for as much of a surprise in reading it as we were when doing research for it.

At the outset, we thought we already knew as much as there was worth knowing about the much publicized health risks of smoking. We soon discovered we hadn't known the half of it—the worst half, that is—such as recent research that leaves little doubt that smoking exposes both smokers *and* nonsmokers to ionizing radiation thousands of times more damaging than fallout from nuclear power-plant accidents, like the one at Chernobyl.

Nor did we realize that the mutagenic activity of cigarette smoke produces ten thousand times the mutagenic effect of its benzo(a)pyrene (BP) content.* Adding the effects of other factors that contribute to the degree of mutagenic activity of cigarette smoke, we find that it has not just ten thousand but twenty thousand times the mutagenicity one would expect from its BP content alone. The principle involved is the same as that which applies to any products of combustion or burning, as, in charred animal proteins produced by grilling or barbecuing, or by burning cooking oil.[1]

There are other surprises too. Everybody realizes, of course, that smokers must be getting something out of smoking or they wouldn't be doing it.[2] But we failed to fully appreciate the very real psychological "benefits" (yes, benefits!) that smokers derive from smoking. Our

---

* In scientific assessments of the mutagenicity of any substance, the mutagenic activity is commonly expressed in BP (benzo[a]pyrene) equivalents regardless of whether the substance contains any BP or not. Cigarette smoke condensate does of course contain BP, just as does any burned or charred protein of animal or vegetable origin.

473

research gave us a whole new outlook on how this strange habit of burning dried tobacco leaves and inhaling the smoke succeeded in conquering every tribe and nation on our planet.

We also gained a better understanding about the much underrated addictiveness of nicotine. With these insights came increased sympathy and tolerance for those who, once hooked on this seductive social drug, find it as difficult to give up as heroin or cocaine addicts do to face life without *their* fix. (Experiences with many clients whom we have helped quit smoking have given us the distinct impression that nicotine addiction is often tougher to kick than alcohol addiction.)*

The nonsmoker may also find of interest our discussion of the different (though by no means lesser) health risks of pipe and cigar smoking, as well as of the problems associated with snuff, chewing tobacco, and marijuana.

Last but not least, you may want to do a friend who smokes a great favor by letting him or her read this chapter. It could just mean the difference between health and sickness, life and death.

THE BIOCHEMISTRY OF SMOKING

Basically there are six factors involved in smoking that cause severe damage to the body.

(1) TARS: Tobacco smoke, like any other kind of smoke, contains certain "tars." These tars, in turn, contain chemical compounds called polynuclear aromatic hydrocarbons (PAH). Many free-radical pathologists, Dr. Demopoulos among them, feel that these PAH from various external sources are responsible for approximately 40 percent of all internal human cancers.

The reason is that the PAH can bind to nucleic acid (DNA) molecules in our cells. Since DNA carries our genetic blueprint, other cells then receive misinformation from "DNA headquarters," may mutate (undergo a permanent, transmissible change in genetic material) or start multiplying wildly, thus causing malignancy (cancer).

This, incidentally, can happen as easily from smoking marijuana or crack as from smoking tobacco. It may also occur from inhaling the hydrocarbons in gasoline or diesel fumes, some industrial emissions, from smoldering leaves, or even from the barbecue grill.

Many of the tar substances are present in tobacco smoke as free radicals and can be detected by electron paramagnetic resonance (EPR) spectrometry. Some are relatively long-lasting and stay around

---

* It is interesting to note that recovered alcoholics who, in sobriety, also stopped smoking often say at A.A. meetings that it is easier to stop drinking than to give up cigarettes.

long enough to get deeply into the lungs, then dissolve in the bloodstream. They are perhaps the most damaging aspect of the chemistry of tobacco tars.

(2) ACETALDEHYDE: The second most vicious chemical in tobacco smoke is a substance called *acetaldehyde,* closely related to the better-known chemical formaldehyde (a powerful disinfectant used mainly in solution to preserve body organs following autopsies).

Related to the hydrocarbons (but with a double oxygen bond, whereas hydrocarbons proper are composed of only hydrogen and carbon) acetaldehyde is also present in smog. Furthermore—as we will point out in our discussion on alcohol—it is the primary metabolite of alcohol (ethanol). What makes it so dangerous is that it spontaneously oxidizes with air, or with oxygen in the bloodstream or body tissues.

When it autoxidizes, it produces an organic peroxide called *peracetic acid,* as well as large quantities of free radicals. It is this combination of factors that makes acetaldehyde so carcinogenic and which sets into motion a process called *cross-linking* of connecting tissue that occurs with both alcohol and smoking.

In either case, the acetaldehyde and its metabolites bring about abnormal chemical bonds between certain molecules in the body—for example, between proteins and nucleic acid. Like so many other normal and abnormal physiological functions of our body, this one, too, is dependent on free-radical reactions. If these free-radical reactions remain under the control of other physiological mechanisms in the body, everything is fine. Without cross-linking, the tissues of our bodies would not be able to hang together. We'd literally be like jellyfish.

However, when cross-linking gets out of hand—as with free-radical chain reactions—it can produce the bonding of molecules exactly where we don't want it. For instance, cross-linked proteins in the skin are the cause of wrinkles in the face, on the neck, the hands, and elsewhere, wherever ultraviolet rays from the sun have penetrated our skin. Smoking only accelerates this process, which is why smokers get more wrinkles, and get them earlier, than nonsmokers. (With alcohol, the cross-linking is more internal, because other aspects of alcohol metabolism—notably the production of estrogens—inhibit, to some extent, the cross-linking of collagen and elastin in the skin.)

The cosmetic damage of smoking is the least of the trouble: Smoking produces much more serious types of cross-linking. First, it causes hardening of the arteries, making them less able to help the heart to get the blood through the body. This condition is a major contributing factor in strokes and heart attacks. Smokers tend to have more atherosclerotic plaque in their arteries from peroxidized fats—thanks mainly to the aldehydes in the smoke—which further impedes the blood flow. As a result, they frequently suffer from high blood pressure.

Smoking also makes blood platelets very sticky, so blood clotting is exaggerated in smokers.

The best-publicized result of cross-linking induced by acetaldehyde is emphysema, a frequently fatal disease in which the lungs gradually lose their elasticity until the victim is no longer able to breathe. Finally, acetaldehyde can produce cancers on its own and in concert with other carcinogens in cigarette and other tobacco smoke—hence the high incidence of lung cancer and a variety of other cancers in smokers. To make matters worse, acetaldehyde also destroys cysteine, a vital anti-oxidant and an important ingredient of glutathione.

(3) CARBON MONOXIDE AND NITROGEN OXIDE: These are the two dangerous gases in cigarette and other tobacco smoke. You know about carbon monoxide poisoning by inhaling automobile exhaust or from burning other materials without sufficient ventilation. Smoking tobacco produces the same kind of effect except that in this case the carbon monoxide gas is rendered even more toxic by the nitrogen oxide in the smoke, which damages the throat, lungs, and the DNA in cell nuclei. It is able to produce carcinogens in the body by abnormally oxidizing body fats as a result of free-radical chain reactions. Obviously, all these toxic effects are heightened if smoking takes place in poorly ventilated places like closed rooms, cars, or telephone booths. Just as obviously, the danger to nonsmokers because of "secondhand smoke" is greatly increased.

Smoking can become immediately life-threatening when (1) the carbon monoxide creates a state of hypoxia (decreased oxygen in the bloodstream), and (2) this coincides with a preexisting heart condition called *myocardial insufficiency.* (The myocardium is the thick middle layer of cardiac muscle tissue that is responsible for forcing the blood out of the heart chambers.) If the heart muscle is overstimulated by nicotine under those conditions, the result may be a myocardial infarct (a type of heart attack) and even sudden death. The role of nicotine in these cases is, unfortunately, often overlooked.

When smoking reduces oxygen in the bloodstream, the entire body suffers. For instance, bone marrow, which is the body's main factory of hemoglobin, overcompensates by producing too many red blood cells to replace the ones knocked out by the carbon monoxide. As a result, the blood becomes too thick and the heart has to pump all the harder to get the thickened blood through the arteries and to every part of the body. Moreover, nicotine constricts the blood vessels, thus putting still more strain on the heart. This means the blood it is delivering is already "polluted," not only by the carbon monoxide, but also by the nitrogen oxide and all the other toxins of tobacco smoke.

(4) HEAVY METALS: Smoking damages the body's enzyme systems

through the presence in tobacco of a number of highly toxic heavy metals, like radioactive polonium, lead, and arsenic. These poisonous substances are particularly hard on protective compounds in our body that contain sulfhydryl (SH) groups and are potent free-radical scavengers, such as cysteine. In other words, the heavy metals contribute to the suppression of the body's immune system, along with all the other immunosuppressive effects of smoking.

(5) IONIZING RADIATION: Most recently, tobacco smoking has come under serious scientific consideration for yet another record-breaking "distinction": namely, as possibly "the largest single worldwide source of effectively carcinogenic ionizing radiation."[3]

The Israeli scientist Dr. Jerome B. Westin, of Hebrew University in Jerusalem, has made some very interesting calculations, comparing the effect of radioactive fallout from the Chernobyl nuclear accident on Israel's population to that from smoking cigarettes. He arrived at the astonishing conclusion that ionizing radiation from cigarette smoking—calculated on a one-pack-per-day habit—would expose the average Israeli annually to 12,500 times the whole body dose received by persons exposed to the radiation from the Chernobyl disaster.

This translates, over the next thirty years, to four extra deaths from Chernobyl fallout among Israel's population of four million, as against eighty thousand excess cancer deaths due to smoking, "the majority of which may possibly be due to tobacco-related radiation," according to Dr. Westin. To this must be added all the untimely and unnecessary deaths from heart disease, lung disease, and other tobacco-caused illnesses.

This radiation would certainly amplify the free radicals in tobacco tar, since radiation causes its damage by producing still more free radicals right in the important parts of the cells, like the DNA, the proteins, and the cell membranes. It is no wonder that tobacco abusers have so little cysteine, vitamin C, and vitamin E in their bodies. The free radicals in tobacco smoke and the radiation actually "use up" these anti-oxidants.

(6) NICOTINE: We have deliberately put nicotine last on our list of noxious substances in tobacco smoke, even though it is a dangerous alkaloid. Fortunately, it is less hazardous than it could be because the smoker automatically adjusts his intake by inhaling it in longer or shorter puffs, the length of time he inhales, and his timing between puffs. Smokers, of course, do not engage in this intricate ritual because they are aware of the dangers that await them if they don't. Their purpose is to achieve just the right pharmacological level of nicotine to give the maximum physiological reward—that is, to tone down disturbing external or internal stimuli and, at the same time, provide a heightened sense of well-being.

THE PSYCHOLOGY OF SMOKING

The ease with which the smoker can regulate nicotine intake by subtly adjusting his smoking technique to obtain, maintain, or change the desired nicotine level in the brain may actually be the main factor why smoking established itself so early and universally in the history of human civilization. No other drug is nearly so flexible and adjustable in this respect, including alcohol.

The other big advantage nicotine has over other mind drugs is that it does not interfere with mental functioning, judgment, or motor coordination. Nor does it have the potential of upsetting interpersonal relations, as is the case with alcohol or the harder drugs.

With nicotine, it is not so much its toxicity or direct social consequences in terms of undesirable behavior, but its addictive effect that makes it more dangerous than any other ingredient of tobacco. Nicotine is, after all, the substance in tobacco that makes people smoke in the first place and makes it so hard to quit. It is what filters and buffers irritating or annoying stimuli—from crying babies, ringing phones, howling fire sirens, to the boss's criticism, the children's demands, a spouse's nagging—and gets the smoker through the day. The stimuli-softening effect is probably the result of the nicotine binding to the same receptors in the brain as do the morphine-like brain chemicals, the endorphins and enkephalins, an excess of which produce similar effects.

Unfortunately, while nicotine serves as a stimulus barrier to the smoker, there is a rebound effect when the nicotine is withdrawn: External irritants, together with any internal problems and conflicts, suddenly seem a hundred times more aggravating than ever before. All these external and internal stresses are back with a vengeance for the smoker who is trying to quit, because his brain is now overreacting to them, handling the stress in a worse way than if no attempt had ever been made to put a nicotine filter between him and the world. That's why people who have recently given up smoking have such a hard time concentrating.

Nicotine is not only responsible for cushioning disagreeable stimuli from without and within, it is also credited with those good feelings that make smoking doubly worthwhile to the smoker. The point has frequently been made that nicotine is a paradoxical drug. For people under stress, it can work as an anti-anxiety and mellowing agent; for those who need more get-up-and-go, it can act as a stimulant or energizer.

THE MEDICAL EFFECTS OF SMOKING

The medical effects of smoking are serious enough in and of themselves, as are those of drinking ethanol in the form of alcoholic beverages. Unfortunately, smoking and drinking frequently go hand in hand because people want to combine the psychological "benefits" of both. What they don't know is that the combined health effects of smoking and drinking are more than additive.

Ethanol and the combustion products of tobacco synergize, a combined effect that is responsible for many cancers, including those of the mouth, larynx, and esophagus. Together they also accelerate the production of atherosclerotic plaque, which accounts for much of the high incidence of heart disease and death due to heart attack among heavy smokers who are also heavy drinkers.

Smoking by itself, however, is quite enough to bring about, over time, a staggering deterioration of health—not just from lung cancer and emphysema, but all across the board. The general health-threatening effects of smoking arise from the interaction of the various toxic substances in tobacco smoke. Since few smokers have a very clear idea of what these specific effects are, we shall list the most prominent ones:

(1) STROKE: A carefully conducted six-year study, published in 1986, confirmed beyond any reasonable doubt that, compared with nonsmokers, male cigarette smokers are running a considerably increased risk of stroke *regardless of the number of cigarettes smoked;* and that among those who smoke heavily, the risk of stroke is three to four times that of nonsmokers.[4]

If anyone thinks that women smokers are better off in that respect, a more recent study (1988) ought quickly to dispel such misplaced optimism. Researchers from some of the most prestigious medical centers of America unequivocally state that their findings "support a strong causal relationship between cigarette smoking and stroke among young and middle-aged women."[5] Women who take birth control pills and smoke are at even greater risk.

Smokers who drink alcohol are subjected to a major increase in risk of a stroke from the alcohol.

If a stroke does develop in a smoker, it will be worse than in a nonsmoker because the tobacco smoke causes spasms of blood vessels that decrease the flow of blood from alternative vessels ("collaterals") that try to supply the tissues from the stroke zone.

A smoker and drinker who gets a stroke will fare worse because the alcohol, which precipitated the stroke in the first place, also makes the extent and severity of the stroke worse.

(2) RESPIRATORY PROBLEMS: Some of the toxins in tobacco smoke

damage microscopically small, hairlike projections in the lungs called *cilia.* The cilia's job is to sweep—by gentle and rhythmic movements—dust, chemical pollutants, and bacteria from our lungs. Smoking first slows them down and eventually makes them disappear altogether. That's one more reason why smokers have so many respiratory problems, from chronic "smoker's cough" to bronchitis and pneumonia. In addition, tobacco smoke causes an increased production of bronchial mucus, which then causes plugging of the bronchial tubes. This leads to more chronic bronchitis and "air-trapping" in emphysema.

(3) INFERTILITY AND GENETIC DAMAGE: It has been known for some time that the mutagens present in tobacco smoke can induce sperm abnormalities in animals. There is now little doubt that this also applies to humans. In fact, there is evidence that the degree of sperm abnormalities is directly proportional to the number of cigarettes smoked per day, as well as to their tar content, the greatest incidence being in men who smoke unfiltered high-tar cigarettes.[6]

It is therefore not surprising to learn that there seems to be an increased rate of perinatal (i.e., referring to the period before and shortly after birth) infant mortality and congenital abnormality not only among the offspring of cigarette-smoking women, but also among cigarette-smoking men. As one researcher put it, "Smoking may be a mutagenic pastime."[7]

It is also a deadly pastime, considering the annual figure of 350,000 deaths directly attributed to smoking. Research has shown that not only is it more deadly in proportion to the number of cigarettes smoked per day and their tar and nicotine content, but that mortality rates increase the longer one smokes.[8]

(4) MANY DIFFERENT TYPES OF CANCER: Tobacco smoke leads not only to cancers of the bronchial branches of the lungs, but also to cancers of the stomach, kidneys, urinary bladder, and pancreas. In conjunction with alcohol, it causes cancers of the mouth, tongue, pharynx, larynx, and esophagus. It now seems as though breast cancer in women can also be added to this unfortunate list.

SNUFF AND CHEWING TOBACCO

You may have heard or read that you can avoid the health risks of smoking by using snuff or chewing tobacco. Unfortunately, this is an illusion, as witness the case of Sean Marsee, a young American athlete who abstained from cigarettes and used only snuff or chewing tobacco to get his "nicotine fix." He developed cancer of the mouth and died a protracted, painful, smokeless death.

What he—like most people—didn't realize is that the chemical interaction of saliva and tobacco produces an overabundance of cancer-causing nitrosamines in the mouth. "Snorting" snuff can have the same effect on the mucous membranes of the nostrils. A single dip of snuff, containing roughly the same amount of nicotine as one cigarette, produces ten times the amount of nitrosamines that a cigarette contains.

In spite of much publicized cases like that of Sean Marsee, chewing tobacco and snuff remains popular among young athletes. In 1986 statistics showed that over the last twelve-month period in that year at least ten million Americans used snuff or chewing tobacco, with three million being under twenty-one. In keeping with this trend, the mortality rate from tongue cancer for white males in the ten-to-twenty age group more than doubled in the period 1950 through 1982, the last date for which there are any reliable figures.

CIGAR SMOKING

Although cigar smokers usually don't consciously inhale, the same nitrosamines are formed in the mouth as with chewing tobacco. In fact, some cigar smokers actually "chew" as much as smoke their cigars. In addition, the absence of a filter and the direct contact of the tobacco with the lips and tongue often produce cancer at these sites. In short, cigar smokers should consider themselves no "safer" than cigarette smokers. Cigar smokers in fact do inhale their own smoke since it surrounds them. They are at high risk, therefore, for the same disorders caused by cigarettes.

PIPE SMOKING

Pipe smoke, unless it passes through a special replaceable filter in the pipe stem, contains even more tar than cigarettes or cigars. Nor can any amount of filtering take care of all the toxins in the tars or get rid of all the carbon monoxide, nitrogen oxide, and, naturally, nicotine. Like cigars, pipe smoking leads to the same risks as cigarette smoking.

MARIJUANA SMOKING

Smokers of marijuana, much like users of chewing tobacco and snuff, usually consider themselves "safe" or "safer" than cigarette smokers. We will try to dispel this kind of self-deception, but first, and paradoxically, we must say a couple of good things about marijuana.

First of all, marijuana can be very helpful in overcoming the nausea that frequently accompanies chemotherapy for cancer patients. Many years ago the word had gotten around about this beneficial effect and thousands of chemotherapy patients have been helping themselves quietly to this unorthodox therapy with—and more often without— their physicians' knowledge.

More recently, however, the cat was let out of the bag when *The New York Times* of July 28, 1987, published an article with the headline CANCER PATIENTS SHOULD GET MARIJUANA, written by Dr. Lester Grinspoon, a psychiatrist and author of several books on marijuana and other drugs. In this report, Dr. Grinspoon confesses that he had to allow his own son, who was undergoing chemotherapy for acute lymphatic leukemia, to smoke marijuana before his chemotherapy sessions, because after a while he could no longer tolerate them any other way.*

Another possibly redeeming feature about marijuana is that it may be useful in relieving the dangerous buildup of pressure in the interior of the eye called *glaucoma,* which can lead to blindness. Even so, most ophthalmologists feel that there are safer and more effective drugs available.[9]

On the other hand, there is now mounting evidence that free radicals generated by light might be the culprits in destroying the trabecular meshwork cells, which are like membranes through which excess fluid in the interior of the eyeball must be able to drain. So, while drugs and maybe *Cannabis* (marijuana) are useful in alleviating the *symptoms* of glaucoma, only anti-oxidants will be able to scavenge and neutralize the free radicals that seem to be the *cause* of the problem.[10]

Marijuana's only socially redeeming features are as a symptomatic glaucoma treatment and as an antinausea remedy for chemotherapy. All the rest spells nothing but trouble, very serious trouble.

To begin with, the chemical compound tetrahydrocannabinol (THC) in marijuana is highly immunosuppressive. As it happens, THC is metabolized in the spleen, the largest of the lymphatic organs in the human body and a key element of our immune system. The spleen is

---

* For a discussion of how clinical hypnosis can have the same effect in overcoming cancer pains and anticipatory nausea in chemotherapy, see page 211–214.

AMONG THE KNOWN OR SUSPECTED CHRONIC EFFECTS OF MARIJUANA USE ARE:*

- impaired short-term memory and slowed learning;
- impaired lung function similar to that found in cigarette smokers (indications are that more serious effects may ensue following extended use);
- decreased sperm count and sperm motility;
- interference with ovulation and prenatal development;
- impaired immune response;
- possible adverse effects on heart function; and
- by-products of marijuana remaining in body fat for several weeks with unknown consequences. The storage of these by-products increases the possibilities for chronic effects as well as residual effects on performance even after the acute reaction to the drug has worn off.

* Statement by C. Everett Koop, Surgeon General of the U.S. Public Health Service, *Marijuana and Health,* 9th Report to the U.S. Congress from the Secretary of Health and Human Services, 1982.

the home of T4 lymphocytes and phagocytes,[11] the paramount importance of which to our immune system we have emphasized throughout this book. In fact, a rare immune-function disease called *systemic lupus erythematosus* (SLE) can be brought on or promoted by marijuana smoking.[12]

A study conducted at Columbia University's College of Physicians and Surgeons showed that the immunosuppressive effect of marijuana was longer-lasting than had been believed. As long as five weeks after people had stopped smoking marijuana, their antibody production was found to be still deficient, meaning that their immune systems had not yet returned to normal levels.[13]

An earlier report by the National Academy of Sciences had already indicated that marijuana smoking can cause anxiety attacks, confusion, impaired motor coordination (similar to that caused by alcohol), reduced learning ability, and, in cases of gross abuse, even delirium (as in alcoholic psychosis). More recently, the New York State Division of Substance Abuse Services confirmed that marijuana smoking disrupts short-term memory as well.

Marijuana produces a memory loss for recent events similar to that which accompanies aging. This memory loss has recently been confirmed by animal experiments showing that THC is capable of reducing the density of brain cells in the hippocampus by 20 percent.[14]

Did you know that—
about 5,000 extra perinatal deaths of babies are caused every year by maternal smoking?

Did you know that—
smoking during pregnancy can affect the child's physical growth, intellectual development, emotional maturity, and behavior pattern?

Source: Norman H. Edelman, M.D.,
Consultant for Scientific Affairs,
American Lung Association

As pointed out earlier, we lose a certain percentage of brain cells continuously merely through aging. If we now add to this normal brain-cell attrition, the 20 percent loss from smoking marijuana and another percentage from alcohol consumption, a pot smoker who drinks may be speeding up the aging process of the brain by 50 percent or more.

In 1986 it was also established that marijuana smoking can cause fungus infections like fungal sinusitis.[15] Nor is this particularly strange. Rather, it should have been expected all along, because marijuana plants are not exempt from fungal infestations in the field, just as is true for tobacco. However, while tobacco is commercially dried and stored under proper conditions, marijuana is allowed to absorb moisture during its clandestine harvesting and storage.

One final word of warning: The hybrid marijuana that is currently being grown in America and elsewhere contains much larger amounts of THC than the pot smoked in the sixties and seventies. We personally know of at least one case where a friend who had been a user for a number of years passed out after smoking only one joint of the new, "improved" marijuana. Since the trend is toward even higher levels of THC—and since the effects of THC in the body have been known for years to be cumulative—this makes marijuana a progressively dangerous social drug.

SMOKING MAY CAUSE IMPOTENCE

It has long been known that habitual drinking has an emasculating effect. But until now it was not suspected that cigarette smoking has a similar effect. A new study by researchers from the Department of

Did you know that—
about 33% of low birth weight in babies is due to maternal smoking?
(If you weren't aware of this, you're only one of 47% of American
smokers who don't realize this medically important fact.)

Source: A 1987 Gallup survey commissioned by the American Lung Association.

Urology, University of California School of Medicine, and the Clinical
Pharmacology Unit at San Francisco General Hospital suggests that
"cigarette smoking impairs erective function in patients with moderate
arterial insufficiency." In other words, cigarette smoking may contribute to the progressive impotence experienced by a large percentage of
middle-aged men, many of whom are known to have insufficient arterial
blood flow—including blood flow to the pelvic area—due to varying
degrees of atherosclerosis.

The exact mechanism by which this impotence-producing effect of
cigarette smoking is achieved is not yet fully understood. However, the
researchers suspect that "the erection-blocking effect of nicotine is
related to a catecholamine effect on the corporeal and vascular
smooth-muscle tone [of the penis]." The scientists are basing this
hypothesis on the observation that when the neurotransmitter norepinephrine ("the brain's adrenaline") was administered to male animals,
it "clearly caused detumescence." It is further known from recent
findings, as these researchers point out, that the "blood levels of
circulating catecholamines increase with smoking or nicotine administration." But, they admit, further studies are needed to come to more
definite conclusions.[16]

Meanwhile, it appears to be sheer folly for any middle-aged male to
continue smoking if he is at all interested in sexual activity. This is
especially so since a certain degree of impairment of arterial blood flow
is almost universal in American and European men past fifty.

SOURCES

1. Sugimura, T., and T. Matsushima, et al. (University of Tokyo). "Mutagen-
   carcinogens in food, with special reference to highly mutagenic pyrolytic
   products in broiled foods." *Origins of Human Cancer.* Cold Spring Harbor,
   N.Y.: Cold Spring Harbor Laboratory, 1977.
2. Dawley, H. H., Jr. "Attitudes toward smoking and smoking rate: implications
   for smoking discouragement." *Internat. J. Addictions,* 1985; 20(3):483–488.
3. Westin, Jerome B. "Ionizing radiation from tobacco." *JAMA,* 1987; 257:2169.
4. Abbot, R. D., M. A. Yin Yin, D. M. Reed, and K. Yano. "Risk of stroke in male

cigarette smokers." *N. Eng. J. Med.*, 1986; 315(12):717–720. Also: Benowitz, N. L., J. Peyton III, L. T. Kozlowski, and L. Yu. "Influence of smoking fewer cigarettes on exposure to tar, nicotine, and carbon monoxide." *N. Eng. J. Med.*, 1986; 315(21):1310–1313.

5. Colditz, G. A. "Cigarette smoking and risk of stroke in middle-aged women." *N. Eng. J. Med.*, 1988; 318(15):939–941.

6. Evans, H. J., and J. Fletcher. "Sperm abnormalities and cigarette smoking." *Lancet*, March 21, 1981; 627–629.

7. Ibid, p. 629.

8. Moody, P. M., and J. V. Haley. "Quantified human smoking behavior among various disease categories." *Publication of the Department of Behavioral Science*. Lexington: University of Kentucky, College of Medicine, 1985.

9. Liu, J. H. "Central nervous system and peripheral mechanisms in ocular hypotensive effect of cannabinoids." *Arch. Ophthalmol.*, February 1987; 105(2):245–248. Also: Nahas, Gabriel G. *Marijuana—Deceptive Weed*. New York: Raven Press, 1972.

10. Kolata, Gina. "Glaucoma and Cataract: Closing in on Causes." *The New York Times*, July 12, 1988.

11. Klein, T. W., et al. "Inhibition of natural killer cell function by marijuana components." *J. Toxicol. Environ. Health*, 1987; 20(4):321–332. Also: Specter, S. C., et al. "Marijuana effects on immunity: suppression of human natural killer cell activity of delta 9-tetrahydrocannabinol." *Intl. J. Immunopharmocol.*, 1986; 8(7):741–745.

12. M. Frajman, M.D., Director, Department of Immunology, INCIENCIA, Costa Rica, personal communication.

13. Kerr, Peter. "Increases in Potency of Marijuana Prompt New Warnings for Youths." *The New York Times*, September 25, 1986.

14. Essmen, E. J. "Marijuana intoxication in rats: interruption of recent memory and effect in brain concentration of delta 9-tetrahydro-cannabinol." *Psychol. Rep.*, October 1984; 55(2):563–567.

15. Brummund, W., V. P. Kurup, G. J. Harris, et al. "Allergic sino-orbital mycosis." *JAMA*, 1986; 256:3249–3253. Also: Kagen, S. L. "Aspergillus: An inhalable contaminant of marijuana," *N. Eng. J. Med.*, 1981; 304:483–484; Kagen, L. L., V. P. Kurup, P. G. Sohnle, et al. "Marijuana smoking and fungal sensitization." *J. All. and Clin. Immunol.*, 1983; 71:389–393; Kurup, V. P., A. Resnick, S. L. Kagen, et al. "Allergenic fungi and actinomycetes in smoking materials and their health implications." *Mycopathologia*, 1983, 82:61–64; Schwartz, I. S. "Marijuana and fungal infection." *Am. J. Clin. Pathol.*, 1985; 84:256; "Fungal Sinusitis and Marijuana" (Letters). Schwartz, I. S., W. Brummund, and J. G. Harris. *JAMA*, 257(21):2914–2915.

16. Juenemann, K. P., T. F. Lue, et al. "The effect of cigarette smoking on penile erection." *J. Urol.*, 1987; 138:438–441.

CHAPTER 60

SIDESTREAM SMOKE

NOT ALTOGETHER AVOIDABLE

*In cities, our homes and places of work are where we spend 90 percent of our time. The quality of the air in these indoor environments is obviously more crucial to our health than the air we may be exposed to during the other 10 percent of the day.

There are many sources of indoor pollution: air conditioning and heating systems, unvented gas ranges, radon gas from the ground, certain formaldehyde-containing building materials like plywood, flake board, or particle board, not to mention asbestos with its own well-known, but, in this case, grossly exaggerated health risks. But no matter how serious any of these pollutants are, the *single most important source of indoor air pollution is tobacco smoke.*

Let us submit, for a start, the following facts:

(1) Over a decade ago, the Environmental Protection Agency established the increased rates of many forms of cancer in coke-oven workers. What most people don't realize is that the tobacco smoke that escapes into the air is chemically very similar to coke-oven emissions and hence just as dangerous.[1]

(2) A decade ago animal studies demonstrated that the combustion products in tobacco smoke contain numerous potent carcinogens known to be tumor initiators, promoters, and accelerators.[2] All these carcinogens get into the air breathed by smokers and the nonsmokers with whom they live and work. The risk to the nonsmoker has been revised upward with every new study.

(3) It is a well-established fact that cigarette smoke contains over

two thousand compounds—many of which are known to be carcinogens, irritants, and asphyxiants that have a suffocating effect because
they take oxygen out of the air while raising the level of carbon
monoxide, nitrogen oxide, and other toxic gases.[3]

(4) Some highly toxic chemicals are present in much higher concentrations in sidestream smoke than in the mainstream smoke that the
smoker himself is inhaling. When you breathe in sidestream smoke, you
are getting 52 times as much dimethylnitrosamine, 16 times as much
naphthalene, 3.4 times as much benzo(a)pyrene, and 5.6 times as much
toluene as the smoker.[4] As a result, approximately 4,666 nonsmokers
die each year in the United States from lung cancer as a result of
involuntarily inhaling the tobacco smoke of others. In other words, 5
percent of all annual lung cancer deaths and 30 percent of nonsmoker
annual lung cancer deaths—2,400 casualties—are due to sidestream
smoke.[5]

If you happen to wear contact lenses, you will have noticed that
being in a smoke-filled room is especially hard on the eyes. Others
suffer from headaches, rhinitis, chest colds, and coughing when
exposed to smoke—which will come as no surprise to those readers
who are nonsmokers. And sidestream smoke very often causes throat
irritations.

Those of you who are particularly sensitive or allergic to tobacco
smoke may even start wheezing, sneezing, and becoming nauseated as
well. Most affected, of course, are persons with cardiovascular or
respiratory disease[6,7]—although ironically the mainstream smoker
may often belong to one of these high-risk groups himself!

Since considerably more nonsmoking women live with men who are
smokers than the other way around, studies that try to assess the
damage of sidestream smoke are usually done on populations of
women or children. Such research has shown that *women who are
nonsmokers themselves but are married to smokers run a two- to
threefold risk of developing lung cancer* compared with nonsmoking
women not living with smokers.[8,9] These women's chances of developing and possibly dying from emphysema are also much greater than if
they are not exposed to their husbands' secondhand smoke.[10] By the
same token, it was found that nonsmoking men who are married to
cigarette smokers are more likely to suffer from heart disease than the
husbands of nonsmoking women.[11]

An interesting study from Japan included a fourteen-year follow-up
on the effects of the husbands' smoking on their wives' chances of
developing lung cancer. First of all, if a Japanese woman gets lung
cancer at all, it is almost certainly either the result of sidestream smoke
or air pollution, because only 15 percent of Japanese women smoke. In
contrast, fully *73 percent of Japanese men smoke cigarettes!*

The study showed that "continued exposure to their husbands' smoking increased mortality from lung cancer in non-smokers up to twofold." But the most fascinating finding was that in younger agricultural couples, whose general life-style is healthier than that of city people, the lung cancer risk for nonsmoking wives was twice as high as that for their nonsmoking urban counterparts.

At first glance, there seems to be no logical explanation. But if we look more deeply into patterns of Japanese family life, we soon discover that in large cities like Tokyo, Kyoto, and Osaka, many couples meet for only a very short time in any twenty-four-hour period. Wives are therefore often spared most of the ill effects from their husbands' smoking—though they are at risk nevertheless. Young couples in the Japanese countryside, however, spend much more time together—a togetherness that ironically increases the prospects of the women contracting lung cancer.[12]

Incidentally, laws to protect nonsmokers from sidestream smoke in public places are very difficult to pass in Japan. One of the key factors in this resistance is a traditional reverence for *okami,* or higher authority. The Japanese feel—not without some justification—that if the government makes cigarettes and sells them (which it does in Japan), smoking cannot possibly be harmful.

It is now known beyond any reasonable doubt that women who are exposed to secondhand smoke not only have a significantly higher chance of developing lung cancer but also have a considerably higher *overall* risk for cancers that are not usually thought of as smoking-related. Researchers have, for instance, found a *twofold cervical cancer risk,* as well as an *increased risk of breast cancer among women exposed to sidestream smoke.*[13,14]

All this unexpected information seems less surprising when you consider the fact that tobacco smoke mutagens—substances that can induce genetic changes in cells and thus produce cancer—have been measured in the urine and other body fluids of people exposed to sidestream smoke. Passive exposure to tobacco smoke has also been found to activate certain enzymes that metabolize toxic substances like benzo(a)pyrene, a known carcinogen.[15]

A number of studies link not only active maternal smoking but also passive smoking to increased prenatal and postnatal infant mortality, lower birth weight, and other genetic abnormalities.

There is no doubt that intrauterine exposure to smoking-related toxins closely parallels the well-known "fetal alcohol syndrome" especially if the mother herself is an active smoker during pregnancy. The mother's smoking is experienced very directly (transplacentally) by the fetus, leading to increased perinatal mortality of up to 35 percent.[16] A child whose parents smoke during his or her early years is also more prone to develop various types of cancer in adulthood. This predisposition comes particularly into play if the person who has been exposed to sidestream smoke during childhood is exposed to it again as an adult.

For instance, it has been established that maternal smoking includes effects on fetal lung development.[17,18] Studies show that the fetus of smoking parents is definitely exposed to components of cigarette smoke and that these toxins are capable of affecting the embryo's living tissue in a way that can lead to anatomical abnormalities and/or later disease.[19] Cancer-causing metabolites of nicotine such as cotinine,[20] benzo(a)pyrene, and thiocyanate have been discovered and measured in the urine and placentas of women who smoke, and even in those women who are exposed only to sidestream smoke. Even more disturbing, high levels of toxic substances from tobacco smoke have been found in the tissues of the fetuses as well as in exposed infants.[21,22]

A recent study from Southampton, England, shows devastating effects of smoking during pregnancy. Thirty-two percent of pregnant women in Southampton were smokers; about half of the remainder were exposed to the sidestream smoke from their husbands. Not surprisingly, even the nonsmoking women had relatively high cotinine levels in their urine (9 nanograms per milliliter). Worse, the husband of the woman who had the highest cotinine level turned out to be smoking more than seventy cigarettes a day! The researchers' dismal conclusion: "One-third to two-thirds of all fetuses in this area are either secondary or tertiary smokers."[23]

Findings such as these have been implicated in long-term health hazards. Maternal smoking was found to be related, for instance, to an

A COUNTERBLAST TO TOBACCO

Have you no reason then to bee ashamed and to forebeare this filthie noveltie, so basely grounded, so foolishly received, and so grossely mistaken in the right use thereof? In your abuse thereof sinning against God, harming your selves in persons and goods, and raking also thereby the markes and notes of vanitie upon you: by the custome thereof making your selves to be wondered at by all forraine civil Nations, and by all strangers that come among you, to be scorned and contemned. A custome lothsome to the eye, hatefull to the Nose, harmefulle to the braine, daungerous to the Lungs, and in the blacke stinking fume thereof, neerest resembling the horrible Stigian smoke of the pit that is bottome lesse.

—Written by King James, 1604, and published anonymously. *The New York Times,* August 24, 1987 impressively increased risk of blood cancers such as leukemia, lym-phomas, and Hodgkin's disease. The offspring of women who smoked had nearly twice the leukemia rate of children whose mothers did not smoke.[24]

Another group of researchers found a *fivefold increase* in the tendency to develop brain tumors among children whose mothers continued to smoke during pregnancy.[25]

Even more surprising is the finding that the general cancer risk of children whose fathers smoked increased by 50 percent![26] Involved in this finding were cancers not usually associated with smoking, such as colorectal, breast, and even cervical cancers. All risks were highest, as one might expect, when both parents smoked during the mother's pregnancy or during their offspring's early childhood. Double exposure to secondhand smoke from both parents, either before or after birth, not only dramatically affects later cancer risk, but also greatly increases the chances of the child's developing bronchitis, asthma, and emphy-sema later on in life. For example, the odds of a male child developing asthma before reaching the age of nineteen are 2.16 times as great if he has been passively exposed to sidestream smoke from both parents than if he has not been exposed at all. The increase in risk of developing cancer is somewhat less for girls, though it is not clear why. Neverthe-less, their risk of respiratory disease is also higher.[27]

Approximately 54 to 70 percent of children in the *United States live in homes where one or more people smoke.* A woman who smokes during pregnancy generally continues to do so after the baby is born, thus placing the child in double jeopardy during the most formative years of its life. If we add to that the possibility of exposure to secondhand smoke from the father, the jeopardy is tripled.

Parental smoking clearly is a case where, to quote the Old Testament, the sins of the fathers (and mothers!) shall be visited unto the third and fourth generation. Studies also show that the smoking habits of the parents strongly influence the smoking habits of their offspring. Heavy smokers, in particular, were likely to have had smoking parents.[28]

The closer one looks at the way sidestream smoke can affect children, the worse the picture gets. For example, nicotine has been detected in the breast fluid of nonlactating women who smoke.[29] That being so, you may be sure that it is also present in the milk of lactating mothers who smoke as well as in the milk of nonsmoking women exposed to heavy sidestream smoke from their husbands or others around them. In that case the fetus is first exposed to nicotine (and other toxic substances) through the placenta, then to nicotine (and possibly other toxins) from mother's milk, and finally to secondhand smoke from the mother and maybe the father as well.

Unfortunately, there is a not too far-fetched possibility in many cases that that child has also been exposed, even before birth, to alcohol and alcohol metabolites (even if the mother has only been drinking "moderately" during pregnancy). Thus, a situation has developed that can result in milder and probably never-recognized degrees of *"fetal smoking-related syndrome"* and *"fetal alcohol syndrome"* (FAS) *at the same time.* Talk about being born to lose!

UPDATE It was found that among fifty-one countries, those having high mortality rates for male lung cancer generally also have high rates for female breast cancer (the rate is highest in England, Scotland, and The Netherlands). The researchers' interpretation: "Because women in many of these countries account for only a small fraction of the tobacco consumption, the conclusion is that the risk of the female disease is closely related to the extent of male smoking. Thus, breast cancer [in these cases] is apparently initiated by the involuntary inhalation of indoor tobacco smoke for more than two decades on the average before diagnosis."[30]

A new study adds further weight to earlier findings that maternal smoking during pregnancy is not only related to lower birth weight, but also that "respiratory deaths and sudden infant death syndrome deaths may be related to the effect of passive exposure of the infant to smoke after birth."[31]

SOURCES

1. Repace, J. L., and A. H. Lowrey. "Indoor air pollution, tobacco smoke, and public health." *Science;* 1980, 208:471.
2. Elliott, L. P., and D. R. Rowe. *J. Air Pollut. Control Assoc.,* 1975; 25:635.
3. Spengler, J. D., and K. Sexton. "Indoor air pollution: a public health perspective." *Science,* 1983; 221:11.
4. Sandler, D. P., R. B. Everson, and A. J. Wilcox. "Passive smoking in adulthood and cancer risk." *Am. J. Epidem.,* 1985; 121:38.
5. Repace, J. L., and A. H. Lowrey. "A quantitative estimate of nonsmokers' lung cancer risk from passive smoking." *Environmental International,* 1985; 1:3–22.
6. *Smoking and Health: A Report of the Surgeon General Publication 79-50066.* Washington, D.C.: Dept. of Health, Education, and Welfare, 1979.
7. Speer, F. *Arch. Environ. Health,* 1968; 16:443. Also: Savel, H., ibid, 1970; 21:146; Greene, G. *JAMA,* 1978; 239:2125; Barad, C. B. *Occup. Health Saf.,* 1979, 48(1):21.
8. Spengler and Sexton, op. cit., p. 12.
9. Sandler et al., op. cit., p. 37.
10. Ibid.
11. Result from the Multiple Risk Factor Intervention Trial as reported at the annual meeting of the American Heart Association, Washington, D.C., 1985.
12. Hirayama, T. "Non-smoking wives of heavy smokers have a higher risk of lung cancer: a study from Japan." *Brit. Med. J.,* 1981; 282:183–185.

13. Buckley, J. D., R.W.C. Harris, R. Doll, et al. "Case control study of the husbands of women with dysplasia or carcinoma of the cervix uteri." *Lancet,* 1981; 2:1010–1015.
14. Brown, D. C., L. Pereira, and J. B. Garner. "Cancer of the cervix and the smoking husband." *Can. Fam. Physician,* 1982; 28:499–502.
15. Sandler, D. P., R. B. Everson, A. J. Wilcox, and J. D. Browder. "Cancer risk in adulthood from early life exposure to parents' smoking." *Am. J. Pub. Health,* May 1985; 75(5):487–491.
16. Whidden, P. "Effects of passive smoking." *Lancet,* January 18, 1986; p. 150.
17. Tager, I. B., et al. "Longitudinal study of the effects of maternal smoking on pulmonary function in children." *N. Eng. J. Med.,* 1983; 309:699–703.
18. Tager, I. B. (Editorial). " 'Passive smoking' and respiratory health in children—sophistry or cause for concern?" *Am. Rev. Respir. Dis.,* 1986; 133:959.
19. Abel, E. "Smoking during pregnancy: a review of effects in growth and development of offspring." *Hum. Biol.,* 1980; 52:593–625.
20. Matsukura, S., T. Taminato, N. Kitano, et al. "Effects of environmental tobacco smoke on urinary cotinine excretion in nonsmokers." *N. Eng. J. Med.,* 1984; 311:828–832.
21. Smith, N., J. Austen, and Chr. J. Rolles. "Tertiary smoking by the fetus." *Lancet,* May 29, 1982; 1252.
22. Sandler, D. P., R. B. Everson, A. J. Wilcox, and J. P. Browder. "Cancer risk in adulthood from early life exposure to parent's smoking." *Am. J. Pub. Health,* May 1985; 75(5):487–491.
23. Smith et al. op. cit.
24. Sandler et al., op cit., pp. 487–488, see footnote 26.
25. Gold, E., L. Gordis, J. Tonascia, and M. Szklo. "Risk factors for brain tumors in children." *Am. J. Epidem.,* 1979; 109:309–319.
26. Sandler et al., op. cit.
27. Burchfiel, C. M., et al. "Passive smoking in childhood." *Am. Rev. Respir. Dis.,* 1986, 133:966–973.
28. Correa, P., et al. "Passive smoking and lung cancer." *Lancet,* September 10, 1983; 595–597.
29. Petrakis, N. L. "Nicotine in breast fluid of nonlactating women." *Science,* 1978; 199:303–305.
30. *Cancer,* 1988; 62:6–14.
31. Malloy, M. H., J. C. Kleinman, G. H. Land, and W. F. Schramm. "The association of maternal smoking with age and cause of infant death." *Am. J. Epidem.,* 1988; 128:46–55.

CHAPTER 61

ALCOHOL

THE "NICE, WARM GLOW"

THE POLITICS OF ALCOHOL

If you think the United States has a big alcoholism problem, you're right. But if it's of any comfort, we can tell you that the Soviet Union—which prides itself on being a relatively drug-free society, in contrast to our own—has a much bigger alcohol monkey on its back than the United States does.

Example: In 1984 (the last year for which there are reliable statistics) the Soviet Union consumed the equivalent of 15.6 liters of *pure* alcohol per person over the age of fifteen, a figure that includes a generous margin for home-brewed alcoholic beverages, which are much more of a factor there than in the United States. The comparable figure for the U.S., according to a 1987 report published in the *Journal of the American Medical Association (JAMA)*[1] was 10.9 liters, or roughly 30 percent less than the per-capita consumption of alcohol in the Soviet Union.*

Consider these facts:

• Sixty-seven percent of the total alcohol consumed in 1984 in the Soviet Union was in the form of hard liquor (mostly vodka). This compares with about half that figure in the United States, since much more beer and wine is drunk here than in the Soviet Union.

• Alcoholism is the third most prevalent disease in the Soviet Union

* Home-brewed spirits are not a statistically significant factor in the United States.

next to cancer and heart disease, according to the same report. It also substantially affects the crime rate there, as it does in the United States, if not more so.

- The majority of birth defects in the Soviet Union are attributed to fetal alcohol syndrome.

- In 1979 there were about fifty-six thousand cases of acute, fatal alcohol poisoning in the Soviet Union, according to Dr. Vladimir Treml, a professor of economics at Duke University, Durham, North Carolina, a foremost expert on such matters. That figure, as he states in the 1987 *JAMA* report, "is totally out of range of international experience." In the United States that year, for instance, there were four hundred to five hundred such cases, a mere fraction of the Soviet fatalities.

Not surprisingly, in the light of such grim statistics, General Secretary Gorbachev has, since May 1985, launched a vigorous attack on alcoholism. He has sponsored the creation of the All-Union Voluntary Temperance Society (TPS). As its name implies, its immediate purpose is to promote "temperance," that is, the prevention of alcohol abuse, but not (yet) to turn a nation of vodka-guzzling Russians into teetotalers overnight. "We are forced temporarily to compromise in this regard," said Nikolai S. Chernykh, first vice-chairman of TPS. However, the quasi-governmental objective is ultimately total abstinence and total prohibition.

Making the Russians quit celebrating birthdays, weddings, and even governmental events without the traditional downing of vodka won't be easy. Foreign journalists are already reporting there is widespread grumbling about even the relatively mild curbs on liquor consumption enacted thus far, such as alcoholic beverages not being sold before two o'clock in the afternoon and limits on how many bottles can be sold per person.

Moscow taxi drivers have been quoted using colorful vernacular to describe their disgust with such measures. Home distilling of moonshine (*samogon*) is said to have become a specialty of housewives, who thereby double and triple their husbands' official salaries. It has also caused a run on already limited sugar supplies, much of which is imported from Cuba, and has brought about sugar rationing.

But not even the 390,000 arrests for home brewing of spirits since the new laws were enacted have been able to stop the spontaneous and totally unanticipated expression of economic self-initiative that Gorbachev has been encouraging in other areas. Another sign of how deeply ingrained alcohol dependency is in the Russian psyche can be guessed from the officially acknowledged fact that even government drivers have been known to give themselves straight alcohol enemas to avoid detection from any smell on their breath!

Looking back into recent Russian history, there was a previous attempt at prohibition, enacted in 1914 by the czarist regime. Needless to say, it failed dismally, as have several national anti-alcoholism campaigns since then. A curious historical item: In 1917 the Bolshevik revolution was, for a curious moment in history, almost aborted when the Red troops who stormed the Winter Palace got drunk for days in the czarist wine cellars!

When the Bolsheviks subsequently assumed total power, they publicly denounced the disgraceful incident in the Winter Palace as a serious infraction of Communist morality and revolutionary discipline. Social drinking, the new Soviet morality declared, was nothing but "a pre-revolutionary myth" and alcoholism was branded as a "disease of social decadence," destined to disappear in the new, postrevolutionary society. Contemporary events have proven such revolutionary ambitions to be yet another myth. The reality is that alcohol consumption in Russia has not decreased one iota since then, but rather has risen to new historical heights.

Nor is such fantastic alcohol consumption in the Soviet Union anything but what one might have expected. Lewis Hyde, an American poet and writer, remarked in an essay on alcoholism in literature that "alcoholism spreads when a culture is dying as rickets appears when there is no vitamin D. It is a sign that the culture has lost its health-granting cohesion."[2]

Hyde, a recovered alcoholic himself, was able to see such psychosocial connections with much greater clarity than others. He did, of course, have the United States in mind when making this statement. However, it is at least equally applicable, we think, to social conditions in the Soviet Union.*

Hyde's unintentionally apropos referral to the Soviet Union becomes even stronger when he says further on that when a society deprives its members of "authentic expressions of creative energy," the individual is left with only "a vague longing to feel creative energy." Such a person, he says, becomes "a sitting duck for alcoholism." All the more reason for the urgency of Mr. Gorbachev's initiatives to allow for the expression of more individual creativity.

We now know that alcoholism, or the tendency toward alcoholism, may be passed on from one generation to the next by a certain gene that some scientists believe they have identified. In the Soviet Union, that gene may be present in large numbers of people, making any attempts to encourage temperance—not to speak of total prohibition and abstinence—perhaps the biggest challenge to contemporary Soviet society.

According to the Soviet press,[3] alcohol abuse plays a part in 60

---

* Hyde's words seem to apply more to cocaine and other illicit drug use in the United States than to alcoholism.

percent of all larcenies, 75 percent of murders and rapes, 80 percent of robberies, and more than 90 percent of misdemeanors.* Also, while Soviet divorce statistics are about the same as in the United States (one in three marriages fail), the reasons for divorce are quite different. In our country a number of social and economic factors conspire against the success of marriages. In the Soviet Union, where, according to *Literaturnaya Gazeta,* women initiate seven out of every ten divorces, the most common reason cited is their husbands' excessive drinking.[4]

In the light of all the damage wreaked by alcohol abuse, Soviet authorities would obviously like to rid the country of this social disease. The trouble is that such measures as restricting the hours during which alcoholic beverages can be sold, limiting the quantity that can be purchased, and inflicting heavier penalties on public drunkenness don't work. As we saw during Prohibition in the U.S. and at present in the Soviet Union, people will simply make their own booze or drink after-shave lotion if they cannot buy liquor legitimately. And no alcoholic has ever been permanently weaned of his or her alcohol dependency in jail.

The only thing that is likely to work in the Soviet Union, as it is essentially the only thing that works here, is an approach to the problem like that taken by Alcoholics Anonymous (A.A.). But much as the Soviet government would like to curb alcoholism, it is reluctant to allow an organization like A.A. to operate freely there, because of A.A.'s spiritual or quasi-religious approach to alcoholism. A.A. insists that members admit their own powerlessness to conquer their alcohol dependency and turn over their lives "to the care of God." However, in an attempt to overcome this ideological obstacle and not offend the atheist sensibilities of the Soviet leadership, A.A. literature, at one point distributed experimentally in the Soviet Union, was translated from a version developed by a New York A.A. chapter for atheists and agnostics in which all references to God have been replaced by the words "a higher Power."

Even so, there are still other problems, as far as establishing A.A. in the Soviet Union is concerned: There are misgivings by Soviet officials because A.A. is an organization that works outside government control. On the other hand, A.A. cannot put itself under bureaucratic control, if for no other reason than nobody would believe that all private communications, records, and public confessions in A.A. meetings would be kept strictly confidential.

Still other obstacles to establishing A.A. in the U.S.S.R. are certain basic differences in social psychology, that is, between prevailing

* Only in alcohol-related traffic accidents, do we, not surprisingly, surpass the Soviet Union.

mental attitudes among the Soviet and American publics. Principles at the very core of A.A., such as self-help, noninvasion of privacy, and absolute honesty about what's happening in one's life, including confession about the most shameful behavior, are totally alien concepts to the Soviets, as many expert observers have pointed out.[5] Paradoxically, there is more social stigma attached to alcoholism in the Soviet Union than in the United States despite its being more widespread there: No former First Ladies like Betty Ford or celebrities like Elizabeth Taylor have publicly admitted their alcoholism in the U.S.S.R.

Notwithstanding all the psychosocial handicaps that complicate the fight against alcoholism in the Soviet Union, there would still be hope for success if—but *only* if—the Soviet leaders would take a calculated risk and give a Russian A.A. the social space and freedom to operate along the lines that have proved themselves so successful here. On the other hand, we cannot help but feel that the leadership of A.A. also might have to show some flexibility to adapt its system even more to the realities of Soviet society. Reliance on "a higher Power" could, for instance, be an understood but unspoken premise in order to remove this last ideological stumbling block. We think this could be done without reducing the effectiveness of the program. For A.A.'s success is more than anything due to its thorough, experiential understanding of the dynamics of alcoholism, the quasi-therapeutic group support it is able to provide, its totally nonjudgmental attitude, and above all to the palpable evidence of genuine *caring* for every member—and of the members for each other—on the most intimate, personal level.

It is conceivable that the program would actually work without some of its ideological trappings, no matter how important they may appear in theory. Giving an ex-alcoholic a sense that he or she—in having taken that first step toward full recovery by renouncing dependency on a substance—has, in effect, signed the death warrant to his/her old self, and all its destructive, self-defeating ways, and been reborn into a new, saner, more affirmative kind of life, ought to be sufficient.

WHY ALCOHOLICS ARE "DIFFERENT"

Some people are especially vulnerable to the psychological "benefits" (the "nice, warm glow") of alcohol. This may in many cases be due as much to hereditary factors as to emotional and environmental ones.

For a long time, the well-known fact that the children of heavy alcohol consumers are likely to become heavy drinkers too has been attributed to imitation of parental drinking habits. Now, however, we know that for at least half of all alcoholics, a hereditary predisposition toward alcoholism is the deciding factor. Researchers have actually identified the gene that makes for that inherited "weakness," and known too are the biochemical mechanisms that determine the differences among individuals as to how they metabolize alcohol. It is clear now that alcohol has different hormonal and behavioral effects on predisposed people, and that they can quickly build up a tolerance toward alcohol that makes them consume more and more of it.

Even if you are not the child of a heavy-drinking parent, but only the grandchild or a blood relative of one, you may still be at considerable risk. The trouble is that the vast majority of people in these high-risk groups are not at all aware of their hereditary inclination and vulnerability. They therefore "innocently" follow the general drinking behavior of their social environment, not realizing that, while others might be able to get away with it, they will get hooked on alcohol.

It is therefore important for you to know whether you must take special care in not exposing yourself to the lures of alcohol, because of a familial predisposition to become overly dependent on this social drug. Forewarned is forearmed. Studies have shown that children of heavy drinkers who are not aware of their special hereditary inclination toward alcohol abuse are drinking several times as much and more often than those who are aware of their predisposition. It is also known that those who recognize a familial tendency do not let themselves get drunk nearly as much as those who do not make these mental connections.*

People who are heavy drinkers generally show other physiological abnormalities: They have, for example, lower levels of the enzyme monoamine oxidase in the tiny organelles called *mitochondria* in the cells of the central nervous system. This may be the reason, some specialists think, why heavy drinkers process environmental information so differently—a factor that makes them so hard to reason with.[6]

Many heavy drinkers also have low cerebrospinal fluid levels of the inhibitory neurotransmitter serotonin, which is important for sound sleep, and which seems to be the reason why heavy drinkers generally have sleeping problems. They are usually also short of the neurotransmitter dopamine, which affects body movement, motivation, sex drive, and plays a role in the functioning of the immune system.[7] These are all well-known physiological differences among those who regularly consume significant† amounts of alcohol and those who do not.

---

* In some American cities—for example, in the St. Paul-Minneapolis area, and in Dallas and San Francisco—there are chapters of an organization, Children Are People (CAP), which is geared to children of alcoholics between the ages of five and thirteen. Your local A.A. chapter would know whether such a support group for children exists in your area.
† More than two to three drinks per day would be considered "significant."

TWO DIFFERENT TYPES OF ALCOHOLICS

According to Dr. C. Robert Cloninger of Washington University, St. Louis, Missouri, a psychiatrist and geneticist and America's foremost authority on the genetic aspects of alcoholism, there are marked differences in the brain-wave patterns of heavy drinkers, compared with nondrinkers,[8] as well as a number of other characteristics that must be considered as genetically determined rather than "learned" or "conditioned" by the social environment.

Dr. Cloninger distinguishes between what he and other scientists who have looked extensively into these matters think of as two different types of alcoholics—type 1 and type 2. The type 2 alcoholic usually starts having problems in controlling his drinking only in late adulthood. At first, drinking may have been socially encouraged— for instance, in the working class by socializing after work with companions in bars; or in managerial and executive circles during business lunches (the notorious three martinis during the discussion before the meal is served, followed by wine or beer during the meal).

Generally, the type 1 drinker is characterized by a basically passive-dependent or "anxious" personality, even though this may be overlaid by a show of spurious "aggressivity" and bravado. Such people are usually warm and sympathetic, eager to help, sentimental, and sensitive toward the feelings and moods of others. What distinguishes them from the type 2 drinker—aside from their starting to drink more heavily only later in life—is that, having basically an anxious personality, they are rather shy and prefer avoiding circumstances that might expose them to obvious harm. In other words, they tend to be cautious, often to the point of being apprehensive, inhibited, easily fatigued, and pessimistic in outlook.

In contrast, the typical type 2 drinker is impulsive and likes to take all kinds of physical, social, and economic risks. He's the kind of guy who literally "asks for trouble." If type 2 drinkers are men, they're the ones who get into barroom fights, or have recurrent auto accidents and get booked for drunken driving. If they're women, they may go on irresponsible buying sprees, abuse their credit cards, pass uncovered checks, and enter into reckless relationships with men. Most important, type 2 drinkers of either sex distinguish themselves from type 1 by starting to drink in adolescence or early adulthood without much need for social encouragement.

Of course, these are not rigid categories, and a heavy drinker may show personality traits from both types. Most women drinkers, however, are of the type 1 variety. They start drinking later in life, but typically suffer more from guilt feelings, depression, and medical complications, such as cirrhosis and other liver abnormalities. Men drinkers, on the other hand—although they can be of either type—are more likely than women to be type 2.

The important thing is that recent research has shown both types of heavy alcohol consumers to have very distinct neurological and physiological characteristics, including, as noted, quite different brain-wave patterns. These characteristics are being passed on genetically; only, with a type 1 background (characterized by the later onset of heavy drinking, absence of criminality, etc.) the genetic predisposition alone is not enough to produce alcoholism, unless there is also a social factor (like heavy drinking in the social or occupational group) that favors alcohol abuse. Specialists therefore speak of "milieu-limited" alcoholism with the type 1 drinker.

In the case of the type 2 personality, however, the inherited neurophysiological traits suffice to lead to heavy drinking, regardless of whether the social environment favors drinking or not. In these families the research referred to earlier has shown that "the risk of alcohol abuse in the adopted-away sons of type 2 alcoholic fathers was nine times that in the sons of all other fathers."[9] Since this kind of type 2 alcoholism (characterized by "sensation-seeking," recklessness, and impulsiveness) is much more common in men, it has also been called "male-limited."

It is against genetic backgrounds such as these that we must view the social, psychological, and biochemical factors, all of which enter into the final causation of alcoholism. A person may have all the genetic markings for the disease, but never become an alcoholic unless one or another of these additional factors push him or her over the brink.

This is not the place to go into the social and psychological dimensions of alcoholism—whole libraries have been written on the subject. Less, however, is known about certain biochemical factors in our physical environment that also seem to determine whether or not predisposed persons will become alcoholic.

Researchers at Texas A & M University, under the direction of Dr. Jack Nation, found that laboratory rats fed a diet containing cadmium developed a taste for alcohol in preference to plain water. (Contrary to many humans, rats are not very fond of alcohol and reject it in even small amounts.) Why would cadmium—one of the metallic poisons from pollutants that scientists today increasingly detect in our foods—turn these teetotaling rodents into lushes?

Dr. Nation thinks that cadmium, which is known to cause anxiety states in humans, does so also in animals, and that they learn to overcome their dislike for alcohol in order to reduce the anxiety. Whatever the causes of anxiety in humans—whether possibly genetic in origin, as in the type 1 alcoholic described by Dr. Cloninger, or purely psychologically determined—many try to cope with the anxiety by using alcohol as a kind of tranquilizer. If Dr. Nation is right, as he just might be, we now also have to take into account a new type of anxiety, caused by toxic cadmium levels in the environment.

This theory has interesting ramifications. Cadmium is a component of tobacco smoke. If at least part of the motive for smoking is the unconscious desire to reduce anxiety through taking in nicotine, it would mean the existence of a heretofore unrecognized vicious circle: The smoker tries to reduce anxiety by smoking, the tobacco smoke produces cadmium ions that increase anxiety, which leads to more smoking to cope with that anxiety, and so on.

It is also tempting to think of the cadmium factor in terms of the type 1 alcoholic, who has a tendency toward anxiety. If such a person lives in an environment where he or she is exposed to high levels of cadmium pollution, either through smoking or inhaling the sidestream smoke of others, or lives in an area where vegetables and fruits have high levels of cadmium because fertilizers made from sewage sludge are being widely used, the anxiety would be increased, reinforcing any preexisting tendency toward alcoholism.

These are just our own speculations, which the Texas A & M researchers might want to explore in future studies. At any rate, we agree with Dr. Nation when he says that there may indeed "be some relation between the pollution problem in the country and the No. 1 drug problem, which is alcohol abuse."

FINDING YOUR WAY OUT OF THE BOTTLE

As mentioned earlier in this discussion, a special vulnerability toward alcohol is very often due to a genetic defect that can be passed on from generation to generation. Here we must add that this genetic peculiarity enables a person to build up alcohol tolerance more quickly than others. As a result, such individuals tend to drink much larger amounts of alcohol than the rest of us who are not predisposed to alcohol dependency. It appears that the different alcohol metabolism of these people results in their deriving more pleasure or psychological "benefits" from alcohol than people without this "alcoholism gene."

But let us hasten to add that none of this should be interpreted to mean that nothing can be done about it, and that such a person is condemned to spend the rest of his or her life in dependence on alcohol. For alcoholism is not only an inheritable disease of the body, it is also a malaise of the mind and a sickness of the spirit. It was this broader concept of alcoholism, first crystallized in the 1930s in the

United States, that led to the almost simultaneous founding of Alcoholics Anonymous and the first recovered alcoholics.

Up till then, all attempts at helping people overcome their craving for and dependence on alcohol by using conventional psychotherapy had failed dismally. It transpired that neither psychoanalysis nor uncovering the psychological aspects of a person's dependence on alcohol, nor any amount of psychological "insight"—much less good intentions and heroic efforts of willpower—were a match for this strange affliction.

The first psychotherapist to realize this limitation of his craft was none other than Freud's perhaps most famous but dissident pupil, Carl Jung. The story of how Jung arrived at this conclusion, as told in an essay on alcoholism in American literature by Lewis Hyde, is most revealing. In 1931 an American alcoholic came to Jung for treatment. They made nice psychoanalytic progress, and the patient gained all kinds of interesting insights into many aspects of his drinking behavior, but none of it prevented the man from continuing to drink.

As Jung pondered the case, he gradually arrived at the conclusion that, as he put it thirty years later in a letter, the "craving for alcohol was the equivalent, on a low level, of the spiritual thirst of our being for wholeness . . . [for] the union with God." To illustrate the point, he included a line from the Forty-second Psalm: "As the heart panteth after the water brooks, so panteth my soul after thee, O God." And he concluded his letter: "You see, 'alcohol' in Latin is *spiritus,* and one uses the same word for the highest religious experience as well as for the most depraving poison. The helpful formula therefore is: *spiritus contra spiritum* (freely translated, "holy spirit to conquer base spirit" [alcohol])." He therefore bluntly informed his patient that his only hope to liberate himself from his otherwise unshakable dependence on alcohol lay in undergoing a profound spiritual, conversion-like experience.

Alcoholics Anonymous bases its whole rehabilitation program on this deeper understanding of alcoholism as not only a "physical compulsion" (which we now know to be based on various neurophysiological and inheritable factors) and a mental obsession with alcohol, but also as a symptom of the soul's alienation from its spiritual source, that is, what we call "God." It is for this reason that A.A. insists that its members freely admit their powerlessness over the physical predisposition and mental compulsions involved in alcohol dependence.

The only problem is that such "surrender to a higher Power" can be misinterpreted to mean that this is all there is to it, and that one has to make no effort of one's own whatsoever. Quite the contrary is the case. All of us—alcoholic or not—have to face the sick part of ourselves and reject it ("die to it") on a daily, hourly, even moment-to-moment basis.

It is interesting and revealing to note in this connection that Lewis

Hyde cites *anger, resentment, self-pity,* and *willfulness* as the primary emotions that "booze will latch on to and keep a person drinking." He singles out self-pity as a particularly pernicious form of self-indulgence on which alcoholism can feed. He calls it "the poor me's," which turn into *"Poor me, poor me, pour me a drink!"*

Lewis Hyde says that, for these reasons, "an alcoholic must deal daily with his own anger, self-pity, willfulness, and so on." On closer look, this means dying daily to the old self and its self-centered mechanisms, of which early Christian mystics like Meister Eckhart and Saint John of the Cross, as well as the late religious philosopher Krishnamurti, have spoken with such emphasis and urgency.

But "dying to the self" is not only part of every genuine religious experience, it is eminently practical. It means paying close attention to the "content of our consciousness" (to use Krishnamurti's terminology) and catch ourselves at the silly and self-defeating "games we play" (as psychiatrist Eric Berne has described them in a best-selling psychological self-help book).*

The religious teachings of the mystics and the admonitions of Krishnamurti to "die to the self" and "reincarnate *now*" coincide with the words of Lewis Hyde about alcoholism. One could therefore say that the way to overcome alcoholism (the way out of the bottle) is also the way out of the bondage of the ego and the point at which the secular and the sacred roads to physical and mental health converge.

HOW ALCOHOL DOES ITS DIRTY WORK

Not only is alcohol abuse a symptom of a sick society, as well as a perpetual reinforcer of that sickness, it also has the most serious health consequences for the individual in that society. Alcohol—in much smaller quantities than you might think—damages mental health, the immune system, the central nervous system and brain, the liver, the spleen, the pancreas, the kidneys, the digestive system, the bone marrow, the cardiovascular system, female orgasmic response, and male sexual functioning. It causes malnutrition, wrinkles the skin, greatly increases women's risk of breast cancer, shortens life span, and tragically affects the lives of thousands of children born each year to women who consume even relatively small amounts of alcohol during pregnancy.

Let us take a quick look at some of the health hazards of even moderate alcohol consumption that are less well known and appreci-

* Eric Berne, *Games People Play* (New York: Grove Press, 1964).

ated by many people, including not a few physicians. Even negligible amounts of alcohol (ethanol) can produce permanent paralysis (paraplegia or quadriplegia) under certain conditions. Experiments with cats given alcohol have shown that it takes no more than the equivalent of a single drop (yes, one drop!) of alcohol in the spinal fluid of a cat to produce total and permanent paralysis of the limbs, if the slightest spinal cord injury is induced.[10] The same accentuation of trauma by alcohol is seen with injuries to the brain or heart.

This translates into taking no more than one drink of whiskey or one bottle of beer and subsequently having a car accident involving a minor spinal cord, head, or chest injury that would otherwise have been inconsequential. However, in the presence of *any* amount of alcohol in the bloodstream (and hence also in the spinal cord), that person is likely to wind up in a wheelchair for the rest of his or her life. Many young lives have been ruined just that way, and without anybody having made the connection.*

Alcohol is also a very definite threat to a man's sexuality. It is a well-known medical fact that with excessive alcohol consumption, testicular weight decreases and the testicles shrink, sometimes to half their normal size. Two factors are involved in this demasculinization process. First, alcohol depresses testosterone levels. Second, heavy drinkers develop increased levels of estrogen (the female sex hormone) because alcohol impairs the liver's ability to destroy excess estrogen. (This, incidentally, is why so many heavy drinkers have deceptively healthy-looking, ruddy faces.)

These hormonal changes, along with direct free-radical damage from alcohol's principal metabolite acetaldehyde, may account for the fact that the sperm of men who consume larger amounts of alcohol are known to be less vigorous and often seriously defective. This factor has only come to light in recent years, but the ancient Greeks knew enough to prohibit bride *and groom* from drinking on the wedding night, lest any future offspring be damaged.[11]

Originally, only the results of *heavy* maternal drinking during pregnancy were medically recognized. The real shocker came when subsequent research revealed that even minor consumption of alcohol during pregnancy can have drastic effects on fetal development,

* Dr. Demopoulos has found that only if massive doses (30 milligrams per kilogram) of the powerful anti-oxidant methylprednisolone (MP) are injected intramuscularly or intravenously within one to two hours after spinal cord injury, can free-radical chain reactions be stopped and the resulting paralysis prevented in a high percentage of cases. After three to five days, Dr. Demopoulos suggests, this dosage should be cut in half (15 milligrams per kilogram). The patient should also be monitored for (1) bleeding from gastric or duodenal ulcers, and (2) for predisposition to infections as a result of steroid suppression of the immune system. Usually, victims of central nervous system (CNS) trauma are given no specific treatment for the first three to twenty-four hours. After that, Dr. Demopoulos remarks, if MP is administered at all, it is usually given much later and in too small doses—a typical case of too little, too late.

especially with regard to the brain. "As little as two drinks a week by a pregnant woman throughout her pregnancy puts her child at risk for significant brain damage," explains Dr. Demopoulos.

His statement is echoed by psychiatrist Ann Streissgut of the University of Washington in Seattle, who has studied the problem in depth and is alarmed at its social implications. "The fact that a variety of adverse outcomes [for the unborn child] are being reported at levels of alcohol use that are well within the rubric of 'social drinking,' " Dr. Streissgut says, "raises concern about the extent of the effects within normal populations of nonalcoholic pregnant women.[12]

The full significance of such statements can only be appreciated in light of the finding that the proportion of women who drink during pregnancy is much higher in some American populations than is the proportion of women who smoke.[13,14] Also surprising is the fact that more middle-class American women (80 percent)[15] drink some alcohol during pregnancy than lower-class women (70 percent).[16]

A study by the Harvard School of Medicine, published in *The New England Journal of Medicine*,[17] reveals that as few as three alcohol drinks a week put a woman at a higher risk of developing breast cancer. If the woman has one drink or more a day, researchers at the National Cancer Institute found, she faces a 50 percent greater chance of developing breast cancer. On the average, a woman has a 10 percent chance of breast cancer. If she has three or more drinks a week, the risk increases to 15 percent. This confirms earlier studies by British, French, and Japanese researchers that alcohol consumption increases the risk of breast cancer in women.[18]

More than men, women tend to become secret, or closet, drinkers, probably because women drinkers are still less accepted socially than male drinkers. Recent research reveals women are more susceptible to alcohol addiction and more vulnerable to the effects of alcohol itself than men. Women need much less alcohol to become intoxicated—not, as you may think, because the average woman has less body weight and thus reacts quicker to smaller quantities of any drug than the average, heavier man. Rather it's because women have a greater proportion of body fat and less body water than men, so the alcohol reaching the central nervous system is less diluted and consequently has a greater impact on it.[19]

Women, as a group, frequently have lower levels of an enzyme that also makes whole ethnic groups (for example, Jews, Japanese, and Native Americans) more prone to feel the effects of alcohol than most Caucasian men. This enzyme is cytochrome P-450, which breaks down the toxic substance acetaldehyde that is metabolized in the body from alcohol.

In the case of the Japanese, low levels of cytochrome P-450 may not only make them feel the effects of alcohol much more strongly, but some as yet not fully understood mechanism may also make them more attracted to it. Be that as it may, there are surely sufficient sociopsy-chological reasons in the contemporary Japanese life-style to turn a majority of stressed-out businessmen there into confirmed alcoholics. Now also, more Japanese women are becoming secret "kitchen drink-ers," as they are derisively called. Along with this we might expect a rising incidence of breast cancer among Japanese women, a cancer rate that has traditionally been one of the lowest in the world.

There are still other factors to consider: Animal experiments show alcohol to be linked with the opiate system in the brain. Certain enzymes in the brain are able to metabolize alcohol into opiate-like compounds that fit into the same nerve receptors as the body's own opiates, our old friends the "endorphins" and other endogenous opioids like the enkephalins.

If we produce an excess of endorphins under physical and emotional stress, we can become lethargic and depressed, sometimes to the point of suicide. On the other hand, life without a certain level of these natural tranquilizers and pacifiers would be unbearable. We need the endorphins to cope, but if our bodies make too many of them we enter a black, hopeless cloud. And endorphins play a problematical, para-doxical role in alcohol addiction.

The overproduction of endorphin-like compounds due to ingestion of alcohol blackens the drinker's outlook. However, many researchers, like Dr. Kenneth Blum of the University of Texas Health Science Center, believe that people particularly susceptible to alcohol abuse lack a natural ability to make enough of their own endorphins. Experiments with successive generations of the offspring of alcoholic animals show low levels of endorphins in generations that have never been given any alcohol.[20]

Regardless of whether your brain produces plentiful endorphins or relatively few, the consistent heavy use of alcohol signals it to shut down its own endorphin factory. Once your body has gotten used to this shutdown, it cannot easily pick up endorphin production again, and you have a continuing need for alcohol. It is extraordinarily difficult to escape from this biochemical trap.

We know for certain that alcohol interferes with the normal trans-mission of nerve impulses in the brain. There is no doubt that the acetaldehyde metabolized in the body from alcohol leads to uncon-trolled free-radical activity, which is extremely damaging to the delicate fibers called *neurites* that are the connective links between the brain's nerve cells. Without neurites there is no communication between nerve cells. Intoxicated people cannot "think straight" because their brains can no longer process incoming information the way normal, nonintoxicated brains do.

Why are the brain and the liver so sensitive to alcohol? And why is the brain particularly vulnerable to its effects?

Alcohol (ethanol) is converted in the liver to acetaldehyde through the action of an enzyme called *alcohol-dehydrogenase* (ADH). At this point, a second enzyme system, acetaldehydrogenase, goes into action and converts acetaldehyde to peracetic acid. The metabolism of alcohol is not over yet, but continues along complicated biochemical pathways that involve further direct or indirect damage to the brain, liver, pancreas, and other organs.

On a practical level, if you drink just one glass of wine or beer, the alcohol-dehydrogenase system handles it. This is not to say that a glass of wine is harmless; *some* harm is always done when you drink any amount of alcohol. But the point is that with so little alcohol you won't get any warm glow or the happy feelings until all of the ADH in both the liver and the brain has been saturated. From that point on, we're talking about alcohol intoxication—and with it, still another enzyme system comes into play, the catalase.

The specific problem is that the brain has only one tenth the catalase activity of the liver. So, if you drink more than the alcohol-dehydrogenase can handle, you end up with a lot of highly toxic hydroxyl radicals in your brain. This is probably the reason why the brain is so much more vulnerable to alcohol intoxication than the liver. The sad reality is that with every drink you take you kill a thousand brain cells that can never be replaced. If you look at a dedicated drinker at age fifty, you know that person has already lost one third of his or her brain weight. The brain will have shrunk from three pounds to two pounds, just as it does in the normal aging process—and for the same reason: free-radical damage—unless stopped in time by anti-oxidants.

Worst of all, alcohol seems to have a predilection for the processing neurons. You have probably heard that we never use all of our brain, but only a small part of it. The extra neurons, however, are mostly utilized for memory storage; they can't make up for the loss of information-processing neurons.

We know today that alcohol causes a significant reduction in the number of receptor sites for the brain chemical gamma aminobutyric acid (GABA), a crucial inhibitory neurotransmitter in the central nervous system. GABA decreases the activity of GABA-specific neurons and is essential for the regulation of hormones—in particular, prolactin, a hormone of the anterior pituitary.

Prolactin stimulates and sustains milk production in nursing mammals, including the human female. Prolactin production must be controlled by GABA to prevent lactation in nonnursing women, as well as to prevent female-like breast development in men and its accompanying drop in male sex drive. Alcohol-induced prolactin production is a frequent cause of impotence in middle age, when the male body produces more prolactin anyway.

In men *heavy* drinking, which leads to shrinking of the testicles (hypogonadism) and, consequently, abnormally low testosterone levels, has now also been shown to be associated with increased risk for myocardial infarct, "analogous to smoking and hypertension."[21]

Although cancers directly induced by alcohol constitute only one tenth of the figure for smoking-induced cancers, it is obvious that an immune system weakened by alcohol will put a person not only at greater risk for developing infectious diseases, but nonalcohol-related cancers too. Lowered immune system functioning also undoubtedly plays a role in those cancers that have been more directly linked to alcohol consumption, such as those of the colon, rectum, stomach, liver, and pancreas, as well as of the upper gastrointestinal tract, the larynx, pharynx, and esophagus. Alcohol can even play a role in cancers of the breast and in the very dangerous form of skin cancer called *malignant melanoma.*[22,23]

A combination of alcohol and tobacco use, of course, greatly increases such vulnerability. One study, for instance, found that alcohol consumption and heavy smoking increased the risk of oral cancer fifteenfold, compared with that of people who neither drink nor smoke.[24]

Most important among these alcohol-related cancers are those of the large intestine and rectum. Animal experiments suggest that alcohol encourages the production of certain toxic, mutagenic, and possibly cancer-causing chemicals (nitrosamines) in the gut.[25]

The link between alcohol consumption and pancreatic cancer has been suspected for some time.[26] In fact, it has been discovered that the risk of pancreatic cancer is twice as great in men who regularly consume alcohol as in nondrinkers.[27] (Alcohol seems to cause even more liver damage in women than in men: Given the intimate connection between liver function and the pancreas, we would assume that women who are heavy drinkers are at least as vulnerable to pancreatic cancer as their male counterparts.)

As to the role of alcohol in cancer of the stomach, drinking increases stomach acidity, which, in turn, irritates and injures the mucous membranes. It is these premalignant alcohol-produced lesions—often aggravated by aspirin,[28] commonly used by heavy drinkers for hangover symptoms—that, together with disordered nutrition and smoking, may lead to malignancy.

In the early stages of alcohol-related heart disease, injury to heart muscle cells can only be seen with the electron microscope. As the patient's drinking continues, the ability of the heart muscle to produce sufficiently strong contractions for adequate circulation becomes more and more impaired. In the end, it takes as little as two ounces of whiskey (about the amount in a single generous highball) to severely suppress the heart's pumping contractions, once the heart muscle has been weakened by some years of significant alcohol consumption.[29] In fact, at this stage, just having the proverbial "one drink too many" can result in the heart stopping altogether. Even if the victim of such a heart attack survives, the heart is usually too weak to function unaided by itself, and the patient requires a permanent pacemaker.[30]

The most interesting thing, from the point of view of free-radical pathology, is that heart muscle cells cannot process alcohol and metabolize it into acetaldehyde, as can liver and brain cells. Heart cells can and do, however, destructively metabolize acetaldehyde,[31] in a process that is known to throw off highly injurious free-radical species. No wonder researchers have found leakage of cellular contents in animal hearts subjected to alcohol stress[32,33] and thus, by implication, to free-radical assault.

Indirect proof that free-radical activity can damage myocardial (heart muscle) cells can also be deduced from the established fact that heart-muscle cell damage is one of the outstanding and most troublesome side effects of a much used anticancer drug, Adriamycin, known as a powerful free-radical generator. (Another, though fortunately not life-threatening, side effect of Adriamycin is cataracts, highlighting at last the long-suspected connection between that common degenerative symptom of aging and free-radical activity.)[34]

Finally, alcohol consumption (even social drinking) can produce serious nutritional deficiencies. Not only does alcohol destroy essential vitamins and important trace minerals, it can inhibit their proper absorption from the colon—all the more reason for those who drink to stick religiously with the full Demopoulos spectrum of anti-oxidants and vitamin co-factors. Selective mineral supplementation (as discussed in Chapters 18–22, pages 145–173) may also be a good idea, if you consume significant amounts of alcohol.

SOURCES

1. Kirn, T. F. "In time of change, USSR seeks to end tradition of extensive alcohol use by majority of citizens." *JAMA,* August 21, 1987; 258(7):883–885.
2. Hyde, L. "Alcohol and poetry: John Berryman and the booze talking." *The American Poetry Review,* 1975, 1986; 811(54):1–18.
3. Kirn, op. cit., p. 883.
4. *Time,* June 6, 1988.
5. Keller, Bill. "American alcoholics lend Russians a hand." *The New York Times,* August 17, 1987.
6. Pace, N. A. "Why doctors treat alcoholism as a disease" (Letter). *The New York Times,* November 27, 1987.
7. Cloninger, R. C. "A unified biosocial theory of personality and its role in the development of anxiety states." *Psychiatr. Dev.,* Autumn 1986; 4(3):167–226.
8. Cloninger, R. C. "Neurogenetic adaptive mechanisms in alcohol." *Science,* 1987; 236:410–416.

9. Ibid.
10. Seligman, M. L., E. S. Flamm, B. D. Goldstin, R. G. Poser, H. B. Demopoulos, and J. Ransohoff. "Spectrofluorescent Detection of Malonaldehyde as a Measure of Lipid Free Radical Damage in Response to Ethanol Potentiation of Spinal Cord Trauma." In: *The 1984 Olympic Scientific Congress Proceedings, Sport, Health, and Nutrition,* Vol. 2, F. I. Katch, ed. Champaign, Ill.: Human Kinetics Publishers, Inc., 1984.
11. Van Thiel, D. H., et al. "Alcohol-induced testicular atrophy: an experimental model for hypogonadism occurring in chronic alcoholic men." *Gastroenterology,* 1975; 69:326. Also: Haggard, H. W., and E. M. Jellinek. *Alcohol Explored.* New York: Doubleday, 1942; "Notes and News: Alcohol and Health." *Lancet,* April 11, 1987; 876. Additional reading: *A Great and Growing Evil: The Medical Consequences of Alcohol Abuse.* London: Royal College of Physicians, 1987; Available from Tavistock Publications, 11 New Fetter Lane, London, EC414EE; *Alcohol: Our Favourite Drug.* London: Royal College of Psychiatrists, 1986; *Alcohol—A Balanced View.* London: Royal College of General Practitioners, 1986.
12. Streissgut, A. P. "Fetal alcohol syndrome: an epidemiologic perspective." *Am. J. Epidem.,* 107:476.
13. Little, R. "Alcohol consumption during pregnancy and decreased birth-weight." *Am. J. Pub. Health,* 1977; 67:1154–1156.
14. Streissgut, A. P., et al. "Alcohol, nicotine and caffeine ingestion in pregnant women." Presented at the Western Psychological Association meetings, Seattle, Washington, April 1977.
15. Ibid.
16. Rosett, H. L., et al. "A pilot prospective study of the fetal alcohol syndrome at the Boston City Hospital. Part I: Maternal drinking." In: *Work in Progress on Alcoholism.* F. A. Seixas and S. Eggleston, eds. *Ann. N.Y. Acad. Sci.,* 1976; 273:118–122.
17. Schatzkin, A., et al. "Alcohol consumption and breast cancer in the epidemiologic follow-up study of the first national health and nutrition examination survey." *N. Eng. J. Med.,* 316(19):1170–1173; Willett, W. C., et al. "Moderate alcohol consumption and the risk of breast cancer." *N. Eng. J. Med.,* 316(19):1174–1179.
18. Enstrom, J. E. "Colorectal cancer and beer drinking." *Brit. J. Cancer,* 1977; 35:674–683. Also: Kono, S., and M. Ikeda. "Correlation between cancer mortality and alcoholic beverage in Japan." *Brit. J. Cancer,* 1979; 40:449–455; Lê, M. G., C. Hill, A. Dramer, and R. Flamant. "Alcoholic beverage consumption and breast cancer in a French case-control study." *Am. J. Epidem.,* 1984; 120(3):350–357.
19. "Women Alcoholics' Treatment Needs Studies." *The New York Times,* September 21, 1986, quoting Sheila Blume, State University of New York at Stony Brook.
20. Franks, L. "A New Attack on Alcoholism." *The New York Times Sunday Magazine,* October 20, 1985.
21. Swartz, D. M., et al. "Low serum testosterone and myocardial infarction in geriatric male inpatients." *J. Am. Geriatr. Soc.,* 1987; 35:39–44.
22. Williams, R. R., and J. W. Horn. "Association of cancer sites with tobacco and alcohol consumption and socioeconomic status of patients: Interview study from the Third National Cancer Survey." *J. Natl. Cancer Inst.,* 1977; 58:525–547.
23. *Fifth Special Report to the U.S. Congress on Alcohol and Health.* Rockville, Md., December 1983, p. 59.

24. Lemon, F. R., et al. "Cancer of the lung and mouth in Seventh-Day Adventists." *Cancer,* 1964; 17:486–497.
25. Wynder, E. L. "The Environment and Cancer Prevention." In: Demopoulos, H. B., and M. A. Mehlman. *Cancer and the Environment.* American Cancer Society, Inc., 1980, pp. 179–181.
26. Lieber, C. S. "Pathogenesis of alcoholic liver disease: An overview." In: *Alcohol and the Liver,* M. M. Fisher and J. G. Rankin, eds. *Hepatology: Research and Clinical Issues,* Vol. 3, N.U. New York: Plenum Press, 1977, pp. 197–255.
27. Burch, G. E., and A. Ansari. "Chronic alcoholism and carcinoma of the pancreas: A corrective hypothesis." *Arch. Int. Med.,* 1986; 122:273–275.
28. Robert, A., et al. "Aspirin combined with alcohol is ulcerogenic" (Abstract). *Gastroenterology,* 1980; 78 (5, part 2): 1245.
29. Newman, W. H., and J. F. Valicenti. "Ventricular function following acute alcohol administration: A strain-gauge analysis of depressed ventricular dynamics." *Am. Heart J.,* 1971; 81:61–68.
30. Leier, C. V., et al. "Heart block in alcoholic myocardiopathy." *Arch. Int. Med.,* 1974; 134:766–768.
31. Forsyth, G. W., et al. "Acetaldehyde metabolism by the rat heart." *Proc. Soc. Exp. Biol. and Med.,* 1973; 144:498–500.
32. Garcia-Buñuel, L. "Oxygen radicals and cell damage" (Correspondence). *Lancet,* September 8, 1984; 577.
33. Del Maestro, R. F., et al. "Free radicals as mediators of tissue injury." *Acta Physiol. Scand.* (Supplement), 1980; 492:43–57.
34. Dormandy, T. L. "An approach to free radicals." *Lancet,* October 29, 1983; 1030.

CHAPTER 62

"A LITTLE ALCOHOL IS GOOD FOR YOU"— OR IS IT?

A few studies have suggested that drinking *some* alcohol may be better for us than drinking none.[1–4] One study, for example, reported a "negative association" between "small to moderate" alcohol consumption and heart attack. You may have read about these studies in the newspapers and rejoiced in the knowledge that we now have it on good medical authority that it is actually better to have a bottle of beer, a glass of wine, or a shot of whiskey than not to have any.

What can we say about this, having just told you how hard alcohol is on the heart and the whole human system?

We don't question the reported findings that light-to-moderate drinkers seem to have fewer heart attacks. The question is how to interpret these findings and what conclusions to draw from them. What could be the real reason or reasons why people who drink some alcohol seem to be better protected from heart attacks than those who don't?

It could be that alcohol, being an organic solvent, might be able to dissolve atherosclerotic plaque. Perhaps it works in our arteries like Drano in a clogged pipe. That's one medical theory. Next, there is alcohol's relaxing effect. Merely by reducing tensions, alcohol can reasonably be expected to reduce one's chances of suffering a heart attack.

Third, alcohol initially has a dilating effect on blood vessels, which causes a temporary drop in blood pressure, and may therefore play a role in preventing a certain percentage of heart attacks. A couple of hours later, the alcohol constricts the blood vessels and thereby raises the blood pressure again. But the initial dilating effect combined with the relaxation of tensions may well account for some of the protective effect—especially in tense, high-strung individuals. For these people, having a glass or two of wine or a single shot of whiskey may be preferable to swallowing tranquilizers—certainly it is more pleasurable. It is, however, not without its own risks, as we shall explain in some detail, especially if no anti-oxidants are taken.

ALCOHOL AND SEX

Men who drink may have fewer sexual encounters. As we have said, even relatively small amounts of alcohol can have a pronounced negative effect on male sexual capacity and performance.

Incidents of middle-aged men suffering fatal heart attacks during sexual intercourse are far more frequent than is generally realized, and for a very simple reason—they usually remain unreported. Families tend to keep quiet about such incidents (witness the death of Nelson Rockefeller, a case whose sex-related nature came to light only accidentally). Men often die of heart attack during sex because they are atherosclerotic and, as Dr. Demopoulos has delicately put it, "their imagined sexual capacity is greater than their aerobic capacity."

Perhaps the best way for a man to avoid even the possibility of expiring under such pleasant circumstances would be simply to drink a small amount of alcohol. That will automatically decrease his sexual potency, and therefore his risk of heart attack. For this reason, heart attack statistics might indeed show a decrease for men who consume small-to-moderate amounts of alcohol (thereby bringing down the overall statistics on heart attack for both men and women).

ALCOHOL, VASOSPASMS, AND STROKES

But make no mistake—alcohol, in *any* quantity, is definitely detrimental to your health, as we hope to have shown in the preceding discussion. Let us give you one more example, which applies to circulatory problems in general and strokes in particular:

An enzyme in our cells, called *xanthine dehydrogenase,* helps digest nutrients on the cellular level, turning them into energy and discharging the rest into the bloodstream to be eliminated by the kidneys and liver. So long as this elegant system is working properly, everything is fine. But if the heart, the brain, the liver, the kidneys, or even the sex organs aren't getting quite enough blood and oxygen (a condition called *ischemia*) because the arteries are narrowed by small clumps of platelets and plaque, a big problem arises if any amount of alcohol is taken in.

Before telling you what happens then, we must remind you that—the typical American diet being what it is—most of us suffer from at least a mild degree of atherosclerosis, and, hence, an inadequate blood supply in one or another of our internal organs. Chances are, too, that we are not aware of this state of affairs, because in the early stages of ischemia there are no gross clinical symptoms. But the evidence of thousands of autopsies is clear: There is some ischemia on the *molecular,* or *subclinical,* level in some of our tissues, often even long before we reach middle age (see our discussion of atherosclerosis in young people, page 224).

When such a state of developing ischemia exists anywhere in our body tissues—which it very likely does in men over forty or women over fifty—decreased oxygen availability will produce a concomitant drop in the cells' pH in those tissues, in other words, the tissues will become more acid. That ischemic tissue environment in turn changes the molecular configuration of the benevolent enzyme xanthine dehydrogenase into xanthine oxidase.

If you now take a drink, you know that your body will convert the alcohol (ethanol) into its metabolite, acetaldehyde, which will spread throughout your system. It will certainly go to your brain, which is particularly vulnerable to acetaldehyde.

The trouble is that xanthine oxidase seems to have a special affinity for acetaldehyde. It will interact with xanthine oxidase wherever it can and in so doing produce myriads of superoxide free radicals, causing tremendous amounts of damage to cell membranes and other tissues. "It's like getting the equivalent of whole body radiation damage," Dr. Demopoulos says. Any ischemic tissue that gets involved in this destructive process simply doesn't have the slightest chance of surviving. In medical terms, this is called *necrocytosis,* meaning the death and decay of the affected cells.

Aside from all this, it is well known from clinical experience that alcohol—in the presence of ischemia—can cause stroke in the brain. Here's how that happens: When you have partially obstructed blood vessels, due to atherosclerosis, and you get a vasospasm—a sudden, convulsive narrowing of a blood vessel—the blood flow is cut off some more or even altogether. If that happens in the brain (as explained earlier in a different context), the result is a stroke; if it occurs in a coronary artery, the result is a heart attack.

The risk to the heart is not necessarily as great as that to the brain because the arteries of the heart are generally of larger diameter. A spasm has to be powerful to shut off a coronary artery completely. The blood vessels of the brain, on the other hand, have a narrow diameter, and if they have been partly occluded by atherosclerotic plaque, it doesn't take much of a spasm to shut some of them off totally. In that case, you get what in medical parlance is called a *cerebrovascular accident*—a stroke. The equivalent phenomenon can also occur in the heart, that is, a spasm of a partially atherosclerotic vessel, which by itself would not cause symptoms.

Any number of things can trigger a vasospasm, the above-mentioned conflagration of free radicals in oxygen-depleted tissue being only one of them. Physical or emotional stress alone can set the whole process in motion and cause the coronary arteries to go into spasm, causing what is called *ventricular arrhythmias*—wild, uncontrolled heart contractions that may lead to instant death. That's why a person may have a stress test to check his heart function in the morning, and suffer a heart attack that afternoon.

DRINKING TO RELAX?

Might not our hypothetical patient have been helped by taking a couple of drinks to relax? Would the two drinks be clearly beneficial?

First, the "therapeutic" maximum is so frequently and easily exceeded that the consequences of doing so bear a closer look. The same studies that suggest drinking small amounts of alcohol to prevent heart attacks warn that a third drink already turns the odds against the drinker; from that point on, blood pressure and pulse rise—greatly *increasing* the chances for heart attack. What's worse, the risk of stroke for those who exceed the two-drinks-a-day limit goes up to four times that of nondrinkers.[5] Second, even the drinker who does *not* exceed the limit is likely to be paying for a possibly protective heart attack factor with an increased risk of stroke.

The reality is that many doctors advise a patient who doesn't seem to be able to relax any other way to have a glass of wine or a highball at the end of the working day. Of course, the patient could relax just as well or better by doing some simple breathing exercises or a little meditating, or just by taking a walk, none of which would have side effects. But chances are, most people will opt for relaxing with the help of alcohol. And if they're on our anti-oxidant program, and can stay within the two-drinks-a-day limit, they're probably fairly safe.

On the other hand, a person not taking anti-oxidants should not use alcohol for relaxation or for possible protection against heart attack— or for any other reason. In fact, we fully agree with Dr. Robert G. Niven of the National Institute on Alcohol Abuse and Alcoholism: "Physicians should avoid prescribing alcohol or sanctioning its use for medical purposes." He adds: "I know of no medical condition in which the consumption of beverage alcohol is the preferred treatment."[6]

ALCOHOL FOR THE ELDERLY—BOON OR BUST?

Apparently some doctors find the condition of old age suitable for the prescription of alcohol—some even installing a "happy hour" in nursing homes for the elderly. Every so often one comes across yet another "study" proclaiming the virtues of alcohol for the institution-alized elderly, who are already too handicapped by "old age" (read: degenerative diseases) to fend for themselves. Such reports tend to be given much more publicity than are studies dealing with the dangers of alcohol consumption. That those dangers are considerably more acute for the elderly than for any other group, except children, is a matter of common sense—or ought to be.

If we can be sure of anything with elderly people, it is that most are suffering from more or less advanced stages of atherosclerosis with at least partial occlusion of large, medium-sized, and small blood vessels, including these of the heart and brain. We can also safely assume that an older patient has areas of ischemia in one or more of the internal organs—again probably including the heart and brain. To administer alcohol under these conditions is clearly to place the patient in jeopardy.

One report, for example, proclaimed that "two months after the staff of a Boston-area hospital for the aged started serving cheese and beer in the afternoon, the number of patients who could walk on their own had risen from 21 to 74 percent."[7] The unspecified type of cheese was probably high enough in fat content to raise the patients' cholesterol still higher, but they and the staff weren't aware of it—nor of the free radicals generated from the peroxidized rancid fats. What mattered to the staff was that their elderly patients suddenly were able to move about a lot better with the beer and cheese regimen than before when they had been doped up with the powerful tranquilizer Thorazine.

*   *   *

We cannot leave this discussion without a few words about the effects of wine and beer—the choice of the more moderate drinker—compared with those of whiskey and other stronger drinks.

First of all, the actual amount of alcohol (ethanol) in a shotglass of whiskey or vodka is approximately the same as the amount in a normal-sized glass of wine or a bottle of beer. So, as far as net alcohol consumption is concerned, it really doesn't matter what type of beverage you drink.

Here is how it actually works:

AMOUNT OF ETHANOL IN A DRINK

BEVERAGE		UNIT OF MEASURE		
TYPE	ETHANOL CONTENT (%)		OZ	(ML)
Whiskey (80 proof)	40	1-oz shot (30 ml)	0.40	(11.83)
Table wine	12*	3½-oz glass (104 ml)	0.42	(12.42)
U.S. beer	3.5†	12-oz bottle (355 ml)	0.42	(12.42)

* Most table wines contain 11 to 13% ethanol. Fortified wines, such as sherry and port, contain approximately 20% ethanol.
† Most U.S. brands contain 3.2 to 4.0% ethanol.

So, while it doesn't really make much difference in terms of total alcohol intake whether you drink beer, wine, whiskey, or anything else, some of the other compounds in alcoholic beverages can definitely make a difference, as we shall presently see.

WINE: RED OR WHITE?

Of all alcoholic beverages, wine is the one health-conscious people are most likely to drink or consider drinking. In our opinion, it's also the most pleasant and "civilized" of all alcoholic drinks. We still on occasion sip a glass of a particularly nice wine, if offered. Needless to say, we do it to enjoy the taste rather than for the effect of the alcohol.

Also, our one-glass limit is not because we fear that two glasses might do us any serious harm (our anti-oxidant program would prevent that), but because we no longer have the acquired alcohol tolerance we used to have, and our bodies seem to be telling us that they don't want any more.

However, we feel duty-bound to tell you that even with good wines and staying within limits—enjoyment of the fermented fruit of the vine is not without health risks. For one thing, some wines already naturally contain sulfites, and current wine-making techniques rely on adding sulfites to control fermentation. Unfortunately, both kinds of sulfites are highly toxic, and can cause serious allergic reactions in predisposed individuals (500,000 to one million people in this country).

It was found that there are varying amounts of a cancer-causing compound called *urethane* (ethyl carbamate) in many wines. Since urethane is not an additive but a common by-product of fermentation, it is present in other drinks and fermented foods, too.

The Center for Science in the Public Interest, a health-advocacy organization, has issued a seventy-page report and guidebook, *Tainted Booze,* in which urethane-containing alcoholic beverages are identified by brand names along with the amounts of urethane that are in them.* More than one hundred wines and liquors sold in the United States contain urethane at levels that are illegal in Canada, which is generally more lenient (and reasonable) in these respects than the FDA. In this instance, however, the Canadian health authorities acted more prudently than the FDA, having learned that even if you drink only moderate amounts of urethane-contaminated liquor—say, the equivalent of two shots of bourbon a day—you may contract cancer.†

The most heavily and frequently contaminated liquors are bourbons, sherries, and fruit brandies, but many other whiskeys, dessert wines, brandies, and liqueurs are listed by the center as containing potentially hazardous amounts of this common carcinogen. (Only a few types of beer seem to contain urethane, although beers in general are well known to have numerous potentially health-endangering chemicals in them.)

Some wines also contain impressive amounts of iron, which can cause a problem because iron accumulates in the liver[8] and can catalyze dangerous free-radical reactions. In addition, alcohol consumption enhances iron absorption from the gastrointestinal tract, thereby increasing the likelihood of undesirable iron accumulations.[9] If

* For a copy of the report you may write to: Center for Science in the Public Interest, 1501 16th St., N.W., Washington, D.C. 20036. Tel. (202) 332-9110.
† The United States government agreed to accept voluntary industry guidelines to reduce urethane levels in alcoholic beverages marketed here to below 125 parts per billion as of January 1989. The Center for Science in the Public Interest considers these guidelines inadequate and unsafe.

larger amounts of wine are drunk on a daily basis, as in France, Italy, Spain, and Portugal, iron toxicities are not uncommon. Regular wine drinkers should definitely not take iron supplements (nor should anyone else, unless a deficiency has been established by blood test).

Having said all these bad things about wine, we are glad to be able to say a few good things about it. Claims have been made that red wines (especially the dry Bordeaux) may have some antibiotic properties. Dry red wines are rumored to be especially effective for gastrointestinal infections. There is, however, little more than purely ancedotal "proof" for such claims—from Saint Paul giving his young disciple Timothy, leader of the early Christian church at Corinth, special dispensation to "use a little wine for your stomach's sake," to wine drinkers who supposedly survived the cholera epidemic of Paris in 1892 better than teetotalers. (How much one can trust such claims in the absence of reliable health statistics in that early time is another matter. Also, the protective effect of drinking wine rather than contaminated water during a cholera epidemic does not prove the wine itself had any antibiotic action.)

Nevertheless, there is some contemporary evidence that dry red wine may indeed have medicinal properties—if one can be satisfied with two early studies, which, to our knowledge, have not been confirmed by more recent investigations. The first of these studies concerns the work of Jacques Masquelier, a professor of pharmacology at the University of Bordeaux during the 1950s. Masquelier claimed to have discovered that the alleged antibacterial and antiviral activity of red Bordeaux wine was due not to its alcoholic content, but to certain compounds called *polyphenols*—especially one called *malvoside*—in the pigment of grape skins. Just eating grapes or drinking grape juice doesn't have the same medicinal effect as drinking red wine, he claimed, because the antibiotic properties of the polyphenols have to be fully activated by fermentation during the wine making.[10]

It certainly is a nice theory for wine lovers, and there might be something to it. But additional evidence is scanty at best. The only serious corroboration, to our knowledge, comes from work done by Dr. Jack Konowalchuk in Canada during the 1970s.[11] Konowalchuk's theory was that the tannins in wine (which are also phenols) will coat viruses and somehow inactivate and eventually kill them. He also claimed that the tannin concentrate from red wine could cure cold sores, caused by the herpes virus.

We know that while plant phenols can work as anti-oxidants, they can also become toxic and even turn into carcinogens, depending on the dosages and circumstances. The same is true specifically for tannins. In some areas of England, for instance, significant losses of farm animals occur every year from their overconsumption of tannin-rich acorns.[12] Hence, the relatively small amount of tannin in even the driest of Bordeaux wines may have a beneficial, antibiotic effect, whereas larger amounts could easily become toxic.

BEER

Beer, like wine, contains greater or lesser amounts of sulfites and other toxic substances, depending on the type of beer and in what country it was brewed. Germany has strict century-old laws regulating what may and especially what may *not* be used in the preparation of beer. Still, even the best German beer contains many harmful chemicals. But there are thresholds below which toxicities are not really that serious. Ultimately, the alcohol in either beer or wine is a great deal more worrisome than the hundred-some other natural or added chemical compounds it may contain.

We should mention that there are also those who attribute medicinal properties to beer. One researcher, Dr. Hans Stich, credits the phenolics in both wine and beer with an antimutagenic (anticancer) effect similar to that which he also claims for coffee and tea.[13] Needless to say, Dr. Demopoulos and we remain highly skeptical.

There are also certain scientists who feel that small-to-moderate amounts of beer produce a more favorable profile of blood lipids in favor of the "good" high-density lipoproteins (HDLs). In fact, alcohol increases only the wrong kind of HDLs (a subfraction known as HDL_3), another study insists that beer drinking increased the right HDL_2 subfraction.[14]

So, every one of us has to decide what and whom to believe. Perhaps there are some health-protective benefits connected with beer, wine, or any other type of alcoholic beverage. However, the overwhelming weight of evidence seems to be very much on the opposite side.

Not just drinking beer but drinking alcoholic beverages in general has been definitely linked to a long list of human ills, ranging from encouraging gout and raising blood pressure, to promoting and possibly even initiating cancers of the urinary system, to being implicated in colorectal, breast, and even lung cancers and, as we pointed out earlier, greatly increasing the risk for stroke due to vasospasm. Therefore, if both of us drink a glass of wine on special occasions, we are not kidding ourselves that it is doing us some good because it contains phenolics or anything else. Neither do we think that, given the protection of our anti-oxidant spectrum, we are doing ourselves any serious harm.

SOURCES

1. Klatsky, A. L., et al. "Alcohol consumption before myocardial infarction." *Ann. Int. Med.,* 1974; 81:294–301.
2. Leger, A. S. St., A. L. Cochrane, and F. Moore. "Factors associated with cardiac mortality in developed countries with particular reference to the consumption of wine." *Lancet,* 1979; 1:1017–1020.
3. Hennekens, C. H., B. Rosner, and D. S. Cole. "Daily alcohol consumption and fetal coronary heart disease." *Am. J. Epidem.,* 1978; 107:196–200.
4. Yano, K., et al., "Coffee, alcohol and risk of coronary heart disease among Japanese men living in Hawaii." *N. Eng. J. Med.,* 1977; 297:407–409.
5. Gill, J. S., et al. "Stroke and alcohol consumption." *N. Eng. J. Med.,* 1986; 315:1041–1046.
6. Niven, R. G. "Alcoholism—a problem in perspective" (Editorial). *JAMA,* 1984; 252:1912–1914.
7. Hales, Diane, and R. E. Hales. "Thinking About Drinking." *Eastern Airlines' Review,* February 1987; pp. 19–25; reprinted from *American Health,* n.d.
8. Aron, E., et al. *Arch. Mal. Appar. Dis.,* 1961; 50:745.
9. Charlton, R. W., et al. "Effect of alcohol on iron absorption." *Brit. Med. J.,* 1964; 2:1427.
10. Masquelier, J. "The Bacterial Action of Certain Phenolics of Grapes and Wine." *The Pharmacology of Plant Phenolics.* New York: Academic Press, 1959.
11. Konowalchuk, J., et al. "Virus inactivation by grapes and wines." *Appld. Env. Microbiol.,* 1976; 32:757–763.
12. *Toxicants Occurring Naturally in Foods.* Washington, D.C.: National Academy of Sciences, 1973; p. 329.
13. Stich, H. F., et al. "Inhibition of mutagenicity of a model nitrosation reaction by naturally occurring phenolics, coffee and tea." *Mutat. Res.,* 1982; 95:119–128.
14. Burr, M. L., et al. "Alcohol and high-density-lipoprotein cholesterol: a randomized controlled trial." *Brit. J. Nutr.,* 1986; 56:81–86.

IMPORTANT ADDITIONAL READING

Sixth Special Report to the U.S. Congress on Alcohol and Health from the Secretary of Health and Human Services. Peter L. Petrakis, ed. Rockville, Md.: National Institute on Alcohol Abuse and Alcoholism, 1987.

CHAPTER 63

SUN EXPOSURE

"DEADLY PLEASURE #4"

12 The excessive sun exposure so many of us experience unknowingly while sunbathing is indeed a "deadly pleasure," as Dr. Thomas B. Fitzpatrick of the Harvard School of Medicine describes it.[1] In fact, as a health hazard, getting too much sun ranks right after smoking tobacco, drinking alcohol, and eating the wrong kinds of food. Specialists, for once, are in agreement on this point. And they are not talking only about skin cancer, as we will show.

WANTED: SUN-LIGHT, NOT SUN-BURN

Before discussing what sun exposure can do *to* us, we'd like to talk about what it does *for* us. We all know that without sunlight there would be no photosynthesis, the conversion of carbon dioxide and water in the air into carbohydrates that makes plant life possible. And without plant life, there would be no animal or human life.

According to Dr. F. Hollwich,[2] an international authority on the mental and emotional effects of sunlight, creative life flourishes mainly in sunshine and languishes in its absence. He quotes Richard Wagner: "If only the sun would come out, I would have the score finished in no time!" and the composer Humperdinck: "The sun is indispensable for my work; that is why it is important for me to have my study face east or south." Similarly, Bernard Shaw preferred working in a bungalow especially built for him on a movable platform so that it could be turned in order to always receive maximum sunlight.

No artificial light can duplicate the benefits of natural sunlight. In fact, Hollwich proved that people exposed to bright white artificial illumination for a couple of weeks experienced considerable stress, whereas daylight of the same intensity had a beneficial, vitalizing effect. And recent experiments with people hospitalized for depression have demonstrated that the patients experienced a dramatic lift in spirits when they were exposed to several hours a day of full-spectrum light, the artificial illumination that most closely resembles sunlight.

The energizing benefits of sunlight come to us by a totally different pathway from that of vision. The stimulus of light that is not defined on the visual receptors of the retina (the back part of the eye) is carried to the pituitary and pineal glands through which it exerts its activating effects. In contrast, vision itself "proceeds independently via the 'optic portion' of the optic pathway."[3]

The practical implications of recent medical discoveries about sunlight are far-reaching. They leave no doubt about the importance of natural sunlight—including the ultraviolet portion of its spectrum—for mental and physical health. They also explain why being deprived of natural sunlight is so harmful to our well-being.

When light is cut off completely, as in the case of blindness, much more is involved than just the loss of vision. The blind person is also deprived of the stimulatory and regulatory effects of light—specifically, those sunlight provides. That's why the rhythmic fluctuations that normally regulate our daily waking-sleeping cycle are barely discernible to the blind person.

The importance of the diurnal rhythms that depend on natural sunlight is dramatically illustrated by the plight of people living near the Arctic Circle. In these latitudes, sunlight is scarce, if not totally absent, during the long winter months—and insomnia and chronic depression are widespread. Researchers at the University of Trondheim, the Norwegian city closest to the Arctic Circle, found that these serious symptoms are promptly relieved by providing the sufferers with short periods of full-spectrum artificial sunlight.

It is a well-known medical fact that our metabolism and crucial hormone systems are disturbed when we are deprived of sunlight. For example, children who are born blind or have gone blind before reaching puberty commonly have underdeveloped sex glands. Their growth is often stunted, bone development can be poor, and there may be other physiological deficiencies. Frequently, mental retardation and serious psychological problems are associated with congenital or early acquired blindness. All these problems are of course determined by many factors, but the absence of sunlight entering our bodies through the channel of the eyes is generally considered the determining factor underlying many other psychological and social factors.

Blindness is, of course, not the only way in which drastic sunlight deprivation can come about. Prolonged imprisonment in semidarkness can produce many of the same effects. And our urban life-style has created an environment in which millions of people are almost as deprived of sunlight as any prisoner in a windowless cell. Because architects no longer are concerned about allowing as much natural daylight as possible into apartment buildings, classrooms, offices, and factories, huge buildings proliferate in which the "inmates" live and work for many hours of the day without the activating and life-sustaining benefits of natural sunlight. The PanAm Building in New York City is a typical example of how one can go directly from a subway or commuter train to an "imprisoned" work environment, without the benefit of a single moment of natural daylight.

As a result, countless people have had to become "adjusted" to living under lighting conditions that are definitely harmful to good health. The shadowless lighting from fluorescent ceiling fixtures commonly used in schools interferes in many subtle ways with a child's natural development. Fluorescent fixtures used in factories and offices put workers under inordinate stress. The bright light shining down on workers has an overstimulating effect on their eyes, tiring them inordinately, creating early fatigue, and interfering with their accurate perception of spatial relationships—something workers engaged in manfuacturing processes that require precision frequently complain about.

If only for the sake of increasing efficiency and productivity, industrial management should insist on a building design that allows as much natural daylight to enter offices and factories as possible. Another step would be to provide full-spectrum, daylight-simulating lighting, which should probably include a small amount of non-erythema (burn) producing UV light, as Dr. John Ott suggests.[4] Finally, the light source should come not just from above, but also from other angles so as to simulate normal daylight conditions more fully.

THE GREAT TANNING MANIA

When you consider the enormous importance of sunlight to human well-being, it's not surprising that people are instinctively drawn to it, since it promotes health and strengthens vital processes. Unfortunately, overexposure to the sun can also endanger our health and weaken our resistance against infectious diseases and cancer.

In simple terms, if sun exposure is not of the erythematous (burning)

THE TRUTH ABOUT SUNGLASSES

Only those OTC lenses that are marked Z-80.3 Standard provide the needed eye protection against UV radiation.

type, it is health-promoting. That's why most of us feel so invigorated after having been outdoors for a while on a sunny day. We ourselves enjoy these good feelings without risking sunburn. On the farm in Costa Rica, we do a few bends and stretches on our balcony first thing in the morning, before the tropical sun turns too fierce. We also spend time on the beach, taking walks and swims at sunrise or sunset. However, lying around sunbathing poses risks that neither of us is willing to take.

Sun worshipers sometimes say yes, they know sunlight can cause skin cancer, but skin that tans easily is less susceptible. To a certain extent, they're right. People who tan easily have enough melanin pigment in their skin to provide a certain amount of protection—but not immunity, by any means! They can still get skin cancer, including melanoma, which metastasizes and can travel anywhere in your body, like other kinds of cancer.

The only people who are virtually resistant to the damaging effects of UV radiation are the black- and brown-skinned races. But even they are at serious risk if there are high enough concentrations of certain photosensitizing chemicals in their skin. There are a number of commonly used bactericidals (halogenated salicylanides) in some deodorants and medicated soaps, some broad-spectrum antibiotics, oral contraceptives, hypoglycemic or antidiabetic drugs (for instance, Diabinese), some major and minor tranquilizers (for instance, Librium and Thorazine), some antihistamines (phenothiazines), coal tar and coal tar derivatives used in a number of shampoos, and even otherwise harmless essential oils used in many cosmetics and beauty aids.[5]

Needless to say, the risk with these constituents in many cosmetics is much greater with white-skinned people. But both blacks and whites had better watch out, especially if they use any skin creams for acne because they frequently contain retinoids, which can promote cancer when skin is exposed either to natural sun irradiation or to simulated sunlight, as in tanning salons.[6] (Ask your pharmacist or doctor whether the acne medication you are using contains any of these retinoids. If the answer is yes, just stay out of the sun and give tanning salons a wide berth.) This applies also to Retin-A cream, which is used to eliminate wrinkles (sometimes it works, sometimes it doesn't). Although Retin-A is a prescription drug in this country, doctors sometimes fail to mention the greatly increased cancer risk with sun exposure associated with this kind of cream.

Despite all the public health warnings about UV radiation and skin cancer, there are still more than 400,000 cases of skin cancer per year in the U.S. Fortunately, most of them are of the highly curable basal or squamous-cell types. "Only" 22,000 people a year develop the most serious type of skin cancer, malignant melanoma, and of these "only" 7,400 die from it. That's relatively few fatalities as health statistics go—unless you happen to be one of those statistics. With increasing travel and social movements to more sunny areas, the incidence of melanoma has risen dramatically. It is now approximately double what it was just fifteen years ago, and it continues to climb!

HOW TO DETECT MELANOMA

If you ever notice an irregularly shaped area of dark brown or black pigmentation on your skin, be sure to have it checked by a dermatologist. Usually, melanomas start as small, flat, molelike growths that increase in size, produce a black lump, change color, and sometimes become ulcerated. Another tell-tale sign: They tend to bleed easily from the slightest injury.

Malignant melanomas (in contrast to the other, more common skin cancers) are dangerous because they can spread to other parts of your body very quickly. Fortunately, with early detection and treatment, a complete cure is almost assured. Why, then, are there 7,400 deaths from malignant melanomas each year? Because many people don't know how to recognize these cancers and assume they are just harmless moles. By the time they do seek medical advice, the cancer may already have spread and taken its deadly course. Also, these early melanomas may be in parts of the body that cannot be easily detected by self-examination.

WHO'S AT GREATEST RISK?

The most likely candidates for melanomas are those who have suffered painful sunburn during childhood or adolescence, particularly if more than once or twice. A study by scientists at the University of California in San Francisco and at the Northern California Cancer

Center suggests that the number of moles* on a person's body is linked to melanoma risk.[7] They found that if you have twenty-six to fifty moles you are three times more likely to develop malignant melanoma than if you have fewer than ten. A person with fifty to one hundred moles may be more than four times at risk. Since the average person has between fifteen and forty moles, most of us are definitely at some risk.

Contrary to what one might think, those who, because of occupation or for other reasons, spend a great deal of time in the sun during the *entire year* are not particularly prone to develop melanomas. Much more susceptible are people who normally live in temperate climates and spend most of their time indoors, but who expose themselves to intense sunlight by spending occasional weekends on the beach or by taking winter vacations under the tropical sun.[8]

UNFRIENDLY FOODS AND MELANOMAS

For people who have or have had melanomas—including those who suspect that they might be genetically predisposed toward this skin cancer—certain foods are definitely unfriendly to them and should be avoided or eaten only occasionally and in very small amounts.

The first thing to keep in mind is that not only animal fats but also vegetable oils are "unfriendly" in the sense that they contribute to cancer in general, and to melanoma in particular.[9] These fats and oils should be used only in the smallest quantities possible and with due respect for their cancer-promoting potential (as before said, mono-unsaturated olive oil is more benign than polyunsaturated vegetable oils, but should be used sparingly too).

Other unfriendly foods for the melanoma patient or melanoma-prone person are all shellfish—lobster, shrimp, mussels, clams, oysters, etc.—because of their high copper content (scallops being an exception). For the same reason, chocolate and broccoli stems are unfriendly to melanoma (broccoli florets, however, are just fine). High copper levels help the melanoma produce more energy and multiply faster.

Unfortunately, red meat and dairy products—including yogurt, cottage cheese, and, of course, milk itself—must be considered unfriendly in this case because they contain high levels of tyrosine. The amino acid is well known to promote the growth of melanoma. It is best to avoid excessive amounts of tyrosine and its immediate precursor, phenylalanine. Certainly these two amino acids should *not* be taken as

---

* Moles are harmless, pigmented, sometimes warty growths that can vary considerably in size, shape, and color. Sometimes melanomas are thought to be moles and are therefore neglected. If you have any suspicions, let a dermatologist decide what kind it is.

supplements. They can promote the development and progression of melanomas, in addition to aggravating cardiac arrhythmias and disturbing the brain's chemistry.

Our bottom-line recommendation, therefore, is that melanoma patients ought to beware of all the foods that are especially unfriendly to them, and not precisely friendly to anyone else. Should you shun them altogether? Well, we would certainly do just that. But since not everybody feels as strongly on these points as we do, our recommendation is: Only *taste* these foods, don't actually eat them, so you won't feel frustrated and yet will not do yourself any serious harm.

SUNBURN AND THE IMMUNE SYSTEM

The sun-cancer connection has been known for a long time, but only recently have the profoundly damaging effects of ultraviolet (UV) radiation on the immune system been studied. These effects include a predisposition to infectious diseases that feeds directly into skin cancers, regardless of whether the affected site on the skin was directly exposed to UV radiation.

Exposure to excessive UV radiation has two direct effects on the immune system: It leads to impaired proliferation of the protective T cells[10] and the disappearance of suppressor T lymphocytes in the spleen and lymph nodes. The combined effect is a critically reduced immunity against UV-induced skin cancers.[11] By the same token, it is also true that exposure to excessive UV radiation, as in sunbathing, would have a particularly devastating effect on persons with already suppressed immune systems, like diabetics or others who are especially prone to infectious diseases. As one noted dermatologist, Dr. Richard D. Granstein, put it: "Immunosuppressed patients have increased rates of skin cancer . . ."[12] And, most unfortunately, people suffering from recurrent infections—especially respiratory infections—frequently sunbathe deliberately in attempts to "cure" themselves (the ultimate, and possibly fatal, error would be for an AIDS carrier to expose himself unwittingly to such a risk).

When UV radiation hits the melanin pigment in our skin, it generates free radicals. If we don't stay out in the sun too long, the melanin itself paradoxically is able to quench the singlet-oxygen radicals produced by the action of the UV rays upon it.[13] However, exposing ourselves beyond a certain point (certainly beyond the point at which actual sunburn occurs) means exceeding the melanin's free-radical–quenching capacity. Once that happens, another chain of events is set

THE "ABCD" OF MELANOMA*

Asymmetry—Most common moles are symmetrical but early melanomas tend to be asymmetrical.

Border—Most moles have very clear–cut borders, but early melanomas tend to have very irregular borders, resembling the coast of Maine or Greenland.

Color—While most moles are uniform in color, early melanomas are often variegated.

Diameter—Most common moles are less than the size of a pencil eraser, about 6 millimeters, but early melanomas are usually larger.

* D. S. Rigel, "ABCD," *Emergency Medicine*, 1987; 19, 51.

in motion that suppresses our immune system in a number of different ways.

For one thing, when the skin is exposed to full sunlight for an extended period of time, it receives not only UV rays but infrared rays as well. This heat-producing radiation renders the skin highly overperfused; that is, all the superficial blood vessels are opened up wide so that blood flow to the skin is twenty to forty times greater than normal. To put it differently, during the time that it takes to develop a mild sunburn, an equivalent of the entire blood volume of the body may pass through the skin two or more times.[14] This, in turn, means that enormous numbers of circulating lymphocytes—the core of the immune system—will be exposed to a high dose of ultraviolet radiation in the superficial blood vessels. Such prolonged UV radiation damages the lymphocytes in peripheral blood and can even destroy them entirely. According to Dr. Warwick L. Morison of the Harvard Medical School, a leading authority on photoimmunology, this damage "could ultimately result in defects of immune function of clinical importance."[15]

The harm done by no means stops there. Sunburn destroys the membranes of important small organelles called *lysosomes* inside the cells of our skin. This results in a literal outpouring of lysosomal enzymes that cause serum and neutrophils (a special type of leukocyte) to leave the blood vessels and enter the tissues, thereby causing painful swelling. It is not clear whether this damage to lysosomes is due to being directly hit by ultraviolet photons or caused indirectly by the generation of free radicals. We are, however, inclined to suspect free radicals—if only on the grounds that they are known to damage lipid-

(fat-) containing membranes that form lysosomes and other cell structures and cause cell death.[16]

Considering all the dangers of sun exposure, many of them well publicized, we are often asked why so many people go right on baking themselves. Dr. W. Mitchell Sams, Jr., a noted dermatologist with the University of Colorado Medical Center, puts it this way: "Sunburning is such a common and accepted event that it seems more a part of man's normal and expected exposure to his environment"[17] than a disease process or a situation that involves risk of injury.

Another factor is that it may take decades before there are many visible signs of photoaging of the skin. If a dedicated sun worshiper finally comes to realize at age fifty that his or her skin is dry, leathery, inelastic, and full of wrinkles—to say nothing of the probability that he or she has a number of benign, premalignant, or even malignant skin cancers—the damage has already been done and is irreversible. At that point, the sun worshiper can only envy the smooth, elastic, cancer-free skin of the dyed-in-the-wool photophobes among his acquaintances who have avoided the sun—while dedicated photophobes have to reconcile themselves to the idea that they may have missed out on some of the very real benefits of moderate exposure to natural sunlight.

However, there is a safe and happy middle ground between the photophobes on the one side and the sun worshipers on the other. So, we say: Let's worship the sun, but let's do it wisely and with all due respect for both its healing and destructive properties.* As we tried to show earlier in our discussion of oxygen and the free radicals, the forces of nature are usually both life-supporting and life-threatening. Keeping that in mind, we need not phobically avoid the sun, thereby depriving ourselves of its potential benefits. But neither should we risk sunburn with all its cancer-causing and immune-system–suppressing consequences.

SOURCES

1. Fitzpatrick, T. B. "The Trends and Future of Photobiology: Medical Aspects." In: *Trends in Photobiology,* C. Hélène, ed. New York: Plenum Press, 1982.
2. Hollwich, F. *The Influence of Ocular Light Perception on Metabolism in Man and in Animal.* New York: Springer-Verlag, 1979, p. 1.

* Whenever you must be exposed to the sun, we urge that you use a good sunscreen with a minimum sun-protection factor (SPF) of 25 or more. The sunscreen should be applied about half an hour *before* exposure, and applied again if you have been in the water.

We noticed that the beta-carotene on our personal anti-oxidant program (we take more of it for cancer protection than most people: 150 milligrams, or 250,000 I.U.) also gives us a little sun protection. But beta-carotene must never be considered an alternative to an effective sunscreen.

3. Ibid., p. 2.
4. Ott, J. N. *Light, Radiation and You.* New York: Devin-Adair, 1983. Also: *How to Stay Healthy.* New York: Devin-Adair, 1985.
5. Fitzpatrick, T. B., et al. "An Introduction to the Problem of Normal and Abnormal Responses of Man's Skin to Solar Radiation." In: *Sunlight and Man, Proceedings of the International Conference on Photosensitization and Photoprotection,*" T. B. Fitzpatrick, ed. Tokyo: University of Tokyo Press, 1974.
6. Kennedy, A. "Prevention of radiation transformation in vitro." In: *Vitamins, Nutrition, and Cancer,* S. Prasad, eds. Basel, Switzerland: S. Karger, 1984.
7. Rampen, F. H., et al. "Frequency of moles as a key to melanoma incidence?" *J. Am. Acad. Dermat.,* December 15, 1986; 6:1200–1203.
8. Fitzpatrick, T. B., and A. J. Sober. "Sunlight and skin cancer." *N. Eng. J. Med.,* 1985; 313:818.
9. Mackie, B. S., L. E. Mackie, et al. "Melanoma and dietary lipids." *Nutr. Cancer,* 1987; 9:219–226.
10. Stingl, L. A., et al. "Mechanism of UV-B-induced impairment of the antigen-presenting capacity of murine epidermal cells." *J. Immunol.,* 1983; 130:1586–1591.
11. Kripke, M. L. "Immunological Aspects of UV Carcinogenesis." In: *Trends in Photobiology,* C. Hélène, ed. New York: Plenum Press, 1982, p. 235.
12. Granstein, R. D. "Photoimmunology." In: *Dermatology in General Medicine,* 3rd ed., T. B. Fitzpatrick et al., eds. New York: McGraw-Hill, 1987.
13. Fitzpatrick, T. B. "Ultraviolet-induced pigmentary changes: benefits and hazards." *Curr. Probl. Derm.,* 1986; 15:28.
14. Parrish, J. A. "Ultraviolet radiation affects the immune system." *Pediatrics,* 1983; 71:130.
15. Morison, W. L. "Photoimmunology." *J. Investig. Dermatol.,* 1981; 77:73.
16. Sams, W. M. "Inflammatory Mediators in Ultraviolet Erythema." In: *Sunlight and Man, Proceedings of the International Conference on Photosensitization and Photoprotection,* Tokyo, Japan, 1972, T. B. Fitzpatrick et al., eds. Tokyo: University of Tokyo Press, 1974.
17. Ibid.

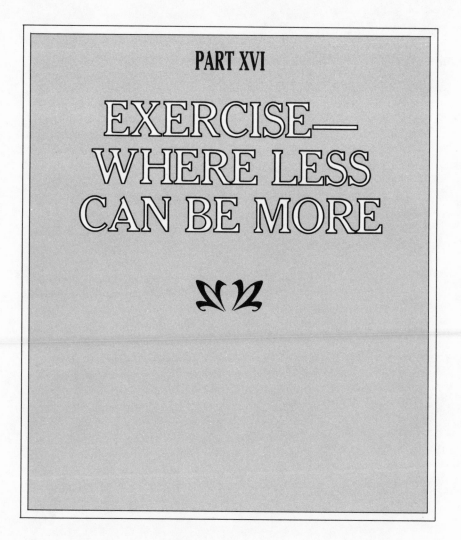

PART XVI

EXERCISE—WHERE LESS CAN BE MORE

12 There are those who religiously run several miles every day, play tennis, swim, or go to the health club and work out—but pay no attention to proper nutrition. They think that by paying their dues to some kind of "fitness" program, they've bought insurance against the effects of the wrong diet. We are sure you know some people like that (we do). But they are only deluding themselves. As Dr. Richard Remington, dean of the University of Michigan School of Public Health, says: "Someone who thinks he's protecting his heart by running around the track but continues to eat a high-fat diet is just kidding himself."[1]

Fortunately, these individuals are in the minority among those who believe in regular exercise. For most of them, the words of Drs. Edward W. D. Colt and Sami Hashim, two noted experts in sports medicine at St. Luke's-Roosevelt Hospital Center in New York City, happily apply: "There can be little doubt that people who exercise regularly are particularly health-conscious and more likely to make health promoting changes in all aspects of their lives."[2]

Most people who exercise regularly also want to take care of themselves in other ways, including their diet. The problem is they often lack the necessary information to implement their good intentions: "Most athletes have little or no idea what it means to eat a good, nutritionally sound diet," as another outstanding specialist in sports medicine flatly puts it.[3]

Then, there are those who take pretty good care of themselves as far as not smoking, not drinking too much alcohol, and eating a sensible diet are concerned. They may even be taking supplemental anti-oxidants, vitamins, and minerals. However, many of them do not seem to appreciate the importance of regular exercise. That's too bad because they are cheating themselves of a large part of the benefits from all the other things they are doing right.

We've even run into some people who figured they had laid up enough credit from their earlier sporting days so they could now afford just to sit in front of the TV and watch others do the running, catching, and pitching. They, too, are kidding themselves. Studies of middle-aged men have shown that the ones who were very active in sports in their younger years had no fewer heart attacks later on in life than those who had not engaged in sports—unless they continued keeping in shape.[4]

On the other extreme, there are middle-aged people who exercise all right but are overdoing a good thing. You know who they are—they're the ones you keep reading about in the newspapers who suddenly collapse with heart attacks on their daily jogging run. For the most part, they are men past forty—women seem to be smarter about such things, or is it because they don't have that monkey called macho on their backs, spurring them on beyond their limits?

Remember the case of the runner-writer Jim Fixx, written up many times in magazines and newspapers? He had been running seventy miles a week for years. Then, in July 1984, he noticed some chest pain. In analyzing his case, Drs. Colt and Hashim comment that instead of seeing a physician and having a stress test, Fixx figured that if he kept running he could overcome whatever was hurting him. Runners don't have heart attacks, right? But Jim Fixx, the seasoned marathon runner, suddenly collapsed and died of myocardial infarction while jogging.

WHAT MAKES ENDORPHIN JUNKIES?

Aside from the machismo problem, what can also lure the unwary runner—or any dedicated practitioner of endurance sports—to his or her doom are our old friends the endorphins.* They are responsible for the notorious "runner's high"—that euphoric feeling of well-being that keeps the endorphin junkie running. In fact, the endorphins are what cause the runner not to feel the pain in the chest, or to disregard what's left of it, and to want to keep going even after he or she collapses.

This excess endorphin production has been clinically demonstrated not only in connection with prolonged jogging and other endurance sports, but with such diverse things as childbirth, surgery, extended fasting, examination anxiety, and so on.[5] But, you might ask, why is that so bad?

Well, the trouble is that the excess endorphins are awfully hard on our NK (natural killer) lymphocytes, which are, by all odds, the most intelligent of our defender cells. Nobody knows exactly how they work. But without any previous information or prior exposure to invading bacteria, viruses, or cancer cells, the NK lymphocytes know exactly what to do when they encounter any of them—they zero in and kill them. It is exactly because of this wonderful and still somewhat

---

* Endorphins, as used here, include the enkephalins and other opium-like molecules that our bodies can produce.

mysterious ability of theirs that the NK lymphocytes are considered the centerpiece of our immune system.

There's a catch though: The NK cells also have receptors on them for endorphins. Therefore, an overproduction of these opiate-like substances—which have a tranquilizing, pain-killing, or anesthetizing effect—can, by the same token, put the protective lymphocytes temporarily out of commission. This is why after surgery, accidental injuries, childbirth, and competitions, people are notoriously prone to infectious diseases they would normally be able to shake off without so much as developing the first symptoms.

The only good news is that if all goes well—say, after overexerting yourself in sports or at work, or having delivered the baby, or when that big emotional crisis is finally over—the NK lymphocytes bounce right back. Normally it doesn't take them more than a day or so to be right up to par again. That's one of the reasons Marc Bloom, former editor of *The Runner* magazine, counsels that for the average person "daily running is self-destructive."[6] You must, Bloom and other experts say, give your system some time to recover from the stress of exercise. Unfortunately, not everybody is listening.

HOW MUCH IS ENOUGH?

Let's stay with running as an example to make a point that applies to exercise in general: Less can sometimes be more. First of all, no exercise should be experienced as stressful or a chore. All too often on our walks, we encounter pale-faced, sweat-dripping runners who by their huffing and puffing clearly indicate that they are overexercising and harming themselves. (Incidentally, these runners look pale because, under all the stress, the blood has gone out of the head, brain, heart, and other internal organs in order to supply the leg muscles.) "Recreational runners, growing into athletic maturity," says Marc Bloom, "are finding that the conspicuous consumption of high mileage is a foolish excess, bound to result in injury, emotional scars and infringement on other aspects of life." Amen.

We feel sorry for those runners whose only time out in nature is when they are running in the park but can't possibly appreciate the beauty of their surroundings because of the stress they are under. That's one reason we ourselves prefer brisk walking, which does allow for contemplation of nature's beauty. Such contemplation not only has its own esthetic rewards, but it also brings city dwellers into closer contact with the outdoors, and has been shown to have medical and psychological benefits by reducing anxiety and lowering blood pressure.

Since running is such a popular pastime, just how much should anyone run? According to Ted Corbitt, a New York physical therapist and long-distance pioneer who ran in the Olympic marathon some thirty years ago, you don't need to run very much once you have reached a certain fitness level. He thinks twenty miles of "low-impact" running a week is quite enough to keep in shape, if you do it consistently.

The consensus of opinion among sophisticated, health-conscious experts seems to be that running three to five miles no more than five days a week should be optimal for most people, and that daily running is counterproductive. They also think that middle-aged people are better off leaving competitive running to the younger crowd because underlying heart problems are not as common among them as in those over fifty. Furthermore, people in the know, whose judgment we can trust, favor having a short fast run one day, and a long, slow one the next day. Doing this involves some speed training instead of constantly trying to stretch the distance run; plus it alleviates the boredom and monotony of running the same way every day.

DON'T NEGLECT THE REST OF THE BODY

One mistake many devoted runners make is to neglect all other forms of exercise. It is true that you can get your heart rate up by nothing more than just running or brisk walking. But it is advisable not to totally neglect all the other muscles that are not involved in running, but which build upper-body strength, or help out areas like the lower back and the abdomen.

To overcome this problem, former Pittsburgh psychiatrist Leonard Schwartz developed special, rubber-cushioned, easy-to-grasp hand weights (marketed under the trade name Heavyhands). The idea is that by swinging these weights as you run, you use more muscle groups and achieve maximum oxygen consumption by muscle cells. The idea is as simple as it is logical—by running you are getting your heart rate and lung capacity up while using your leg muscles, plus—courtesy of Dr. Schwartz's clever weights—you are building up your arms, shoulders, and neck muscles at the same time.

Another way of avoiding muscle imbalances by single sports like running or, to some extent, even tennis is to vary your physical exercise. However, if you are a middle-aged runner, the two days you're "off," perhaps you should relax and give your body a total rest. That's why Dr. Schwartz's hand weights are especially practical. You can use them even with brisk walking, and if you do a few yoga stretches in addition, that's all you really need to do to keep in perfect shape.

WHAT ABOUT AEROBICS?

The Jane Fonda-type high-impact aerobics are definitely for the younger set only, or for that minority of middle-aged people who have kept up daily exercise throughout life and are in perfect condition. Many have found out the hard way that high-impact aerobics is not for them: chondromalacia (softening of the cartilage in the knees), strained or ruptured tendons and ligaments, stress fractures, and worse. The constant pounding and jumping has a way of taking its toll.

Even Jane Fonda now advocates low-impact aerobics for most people. Aerobic dancing is one way of enjoying the physical and emotional benefits of low-impact aerobics without the drawbacks of its more strenuous forms. The idea is always to keep one foot on the floor, so there can be no jumping and hence no jumping-related injuries. Still, aerobic dancing can burn up six hundred calories an hour, making it a very time-effective form of low-impact exercise.

The only trouble is that most aerobic dance classes are considered a group activity; there is less concern on the part of the instructors to individualize the intensity of the workout for individual participants. Furthermore, as Drs. Patricia A. Gillet and Patricia A. Eisenman, leading health and fitness experts at the University of Utah, Salt Lake City, point out, there often is "no progression in the exercise intensity, but rather each class is of a similar intensity."[7]

These experts advocate an "intensity-controlled format" for aerobic dancing, with exercise intensity and duration based upon the individual's level of fitness. They also urge safety features, such as a long warm-up and cool-down, as well as periodic pulse monitoring for middle-aged participants. For beginners, they suggest twelve- to fifteen-minute sessions, gradually increasing them to twenty-five-minute sessions over an eight-week period.

There is also the "brave new world" type of computerized video exercise equipment that makes individualizing and gradating exercise easier for gyms and health clubs owning these newfangled machines. For example, there is the Powercise system, which works exactly like a personal-fitness trainer. Its computer, which assesses the exerciser's fitness level and ideal workout, is programmed to keep motivating you to go on and succeed, and it chirps sweet words of encouragement and a face on the monitor flashes broad smiles of satisfaction at your accomplishments. Maybe such computerized programs motivate some people who might otherwise stop exercising, and they do at least prevent you from overdoing it. But we personally feel there is no substitute for real contact with real people—and especially with nature—when it comes to exercise.

HOW LITTLE EXERCISE IS ENOUGH?

For those of us in the older age brackets who have allowed ourselves to get all out of shape, even less initial exercise is indicated. It is good news that even minimal exercise can be of tremendous medical benefit. It has, for instance, been scientifically established that "as little as climbing five flights of stairs a day reduced the incidence of heart attacks by 25%."[8]

Today, not many peole have the dubious privilege of living in a five-story walk-up (this happens to be our current situation, so we consider walking up the stairs part of our daily exercise). However, it is easy to translate this activity into five minutes of brisk walking, swimming, a few minutes of aerobic dancing, hatha yoga, or other physical exercise.

Recent findings confirm earlier ones that very moderate physical activities such as walking, gardening, yardwork, doing home repairs, and so forth, may be at least as protective against heart disease as more strenuous exercising, jogging, or tennis for those who are not in very good physical condition. One study found that fifteen to forty-five minutes of these daily activities, normally not even considered legitimate physical exercise, had proved helpful beyond the researchers' own expectations.[9]

Three retired women from Brooklyn have made a video exercise tape for seniors called "Fit After 50."* We have not had a chance to view it, but William Stockton, health columnist for *The New York Times,* says the tape is "quite good."[10] It's aimed at older people with basically sedentary life-styles and little or no previous exercise experience. According to Mr. Stockton, the routines are "built around a straight-backed chair, two Frisbees and a piece of elastic that a seamstress would sew into the waistband of a dress."[11] Much of the forty-five-minute routine is spent doing a series of leg and arm movements while sitting on the chair or skipping around it. Admittedly, the purpose is not to get the heart rate up, but just to

* The videotape is available for $39.95 from Three J Productions, 2 Pineridge Road, White Plains, New York 10603.

improve circulation and flexibility. That's not bad for starters, if you've been completely out of it exercise-wise for some time. But we hope that most older people would graduate from that to something more active that would get their heart rate up and improve their lung capacity.

THE FUN OF ROPE JUMPING

Middle-aged and older people can get themselves into better shape by rope jumping. One reason we encourage you to pick up what must, for many, be an old, happily remembered childhood game is that it's so easy to self-regulate your degree of exertion by either speeding up the jumping or slowing it down, just as you do with walking. And yet once you go beyond getting tangled up in the rope every other jump, you're able to raise your heart rate as quickly with rope jumping as with running—and it doesn't matter whether it's raining or snowing outside. On the other hand, there's no reason why you can't jump rope outside too, weather permitting. In fact, it's more fun to take your rope along when you walk in the park. You can stop at a nice place and do some jumping, just for a change.

Sports writer and health columnist William Stockton advises you to buy a rope that has handles attached by bearings rather than swivel hooks, and to use a pair of cushioned basketball shoes instead of running shoes. Good advice. But even more important, you should land from the low jumps on the *balls* of your feet, rather than on the whole foot, otherwise the impact is too hard, no matter how cushioned your shoes are.

Mr. Stockton also advises to select the right rope length. "A rope is the correct length," he says, "if, when you place one foot on its middle, the tops of the handles extend to the middle of your chest."[12] Fair enough, but as kids we never worried about the right length of the rope. If there were any handles at all (most of the time, there weren't), they were just held in place at the far end by a simple knot. We only wish we could jump as well today, in our cushioned shoes and the deluxe commercial rope with its roller-bearing handles, as we did as children, barefoot or in sneakers with an ordinary length of rope.

The advantage of working with the right kind of rope and shoes at our age is of course that we can gradually polish our skills and increase our aerobic workout, depending on our state of health. If you keep practicing and watching more experienced rope jumpers, you can actually build up your rope jumping to where it is no longer a minimal to moderate exercise just to keep you in reasonable shape, but becomes one of the best aerobic exercises for your cardiovascular system. Rope jumping burns up fat and calories almost as efficiently as high-impact aerobics—but with a greatly reduced possibility for self-injury. If you wear cushioned shoes and jump on a yielding surface (not concrete), it won't jolt your joints the way jogging can.

Also, rope jumping is great for improving hand-eye coordination and making you faster on your feet. That, of course, is exactly why boxers routinely include rope jumping in their daily practice (it's a must for people who practice the martial arts too, and even improves competence in recreational dancing).

But start in easy—no more than, say, three rounds of thirty seconds each, with thirty-second rest periods in between, boxing trainer Al Gavin recommends. You can build up from there, he says, until you can jump for three minutes at a time, and that's about all most of us should ever aspire to anyway.

THE MEDICAL REWARDS OF REGULAR EXERCISE

Exercising admittedly requires sacrificing a certain amount of time in one's busy day. But it surely has its own rewards, the first one being immediate—you simply feel better right away. Not only does exercise make you feel better; it makes you *look* better.

EXERCISE AND CARDIOVASCULAR DISORDERS

We know from numerous studies that people who do *not* exercise are at much greater risk of heart attack and stroke. On the other hand, it is equally well known that regular exercise increases the percentage of the HDL fraction of lipoproteins in our bloodstream that carry cholesterol from the tissues back to the liver, where it is processed into bile acids and eliminated via the gut (especially with the help of a high-fiber diet). By the same token, exercise reduces the "bad" LDL fraction, the main building block of cholesterol, and also reduces the VLDL triglyceride content, also a contributor to total blood cholesterol. Furthermore, regular exercise causes a reduction in total triglycerides, another important factor in preventive health care, especially with regard to diabetes.

Exercise also helps lower blood pressure, a fact that is frequently overlooked by those on blood-pressure–lowering medication. Generally, this reflects that those who suffer from hypertension are simply unaware that exercise can provide this benefit. We have noticed that many patients who are on medication for chronic conditions have a strange kind of emotional passivity. It is as if they had signed over all responsibility for their well-being to the pills prescribed for them.

EXERCISE AND DIABETES

Regular exercise is especially important for both insulin-dependent and non-insulin–dependent diabetics. As early as 600 B.C., the Indian physician Sushutra urged patients with diabetes mellitus not to neglect physical exercise.[13] Likewise, the Roman physician and scientist Celsus, at the beginning of our era, prescribed exercise for patients with sugar (glucose) in their urine.[14] But it was not until the eighteenth century that the importance of exercise for diabetics gradually became more fully recognized by Western medicine, although it had been of much greater importance in pre-insulin times.

Just how important exercise is for diabetics is best appreciated from the fact that, as Drs. Stephen H. Schneider and Hassan Kanj of Rutgers University Medical School at New Brunswick, New Jersey, remind their colleagues, "physical inactivity, even a few days of bed rest, can result in glucose intolerance and insulin resistance" in normal people.[15] How much more is this true for diabetics!

On the other hand, diabetes specialists point to studies showing that exercise results in reduced fasting blood sugar and plasma insulin levels in these patients.[16] Still other studies have shown that "a single bout of exercise can increase insulin receptor sensitivity," and there is evidence that regular exercise training increases the number of insulin receptors and improves glucose tolerance.[17]

Specialists have even figured out the best way for insulin-dependent diabetics to exercise: First, upon arising have a small snack, then do your exercise, after that give yourself your regular insulin injection, and only then sit down for your low-fat, high-carbohydrate breakfast. In fact, having a light snack—maybe half an apple or a piece of whole wheat or rye bread—before doing your morning exercise, and only after that eating something more, is a good routine for anybody to follow, especially for those with non-insulin–dependent diabetes mellitus.

EXERCISE AND OSTEOPOROSIS

In addition to all the other benefits from a regular exercise program, it protects against the softening of the bones called *osteoporosis,* a condition that can, as noted bone specialist Dr. Morris Notelovitz of the University of Florida at Gainesville points out, "cause premature death."[18] The statistics are grim: Every year over 200,000 women in the United States will fracture their hips as a result of osteoporosis, and 10 to 15 percent of them will die within six months of complications arising from this serious condition. Only one third of these women will ever return to normal, active life. And yet, Dr. Notelovitz notes, "osteoporosis can, in all probability, be prevented by the simple expedients of appropriate exercise and good nutrition." Included in such "good nutrition" should be the taking of an efficient calcium supplement with a proven capacity of being well absorbed.*

Exercise, correct nutrition, and calcium supplementation, in that order, are the three cornerstones of prevention of osteoporosis. Once the bone loss has started, the damage has occurred and precious little can be done about it. What it boils down to is that the more bone mass a woman has, the more she can afford to lose—and exercise is the one thing that will give her that extra reserve.

A regimen of preventive exercise, diet, and calcium supplements should be started long before hormonal changes during menopause hasten bone loss. As many specialists have emphasized, "changes in diet and physical activity at older ages occur too late to have much effect."[19] Once a woman is into menopause, she is probably well advised not only to use a good calcium supplement, but to have estrogen-replacement therapy that includes progesterone too. In that way, she can at least prevent further serious bone loss.

The question remaining is how much exercise is optimal for a woman to conserve and build bone mass while she is still in her prime? We know for certain that overexercising is counterproductive: Women marathon runners who had brought on exercise-induced amenorrhea (abnormal cessation of menses) were found to have more rather than less bone loss, caused mainly by an estrogen deficiency that was brought on by overexercise.[20, 21]

In other words, moderate exercise is important for women of pre- and postmenopausal age to prevent bone loss—but overly strenuous exercise can result in excessive loss of body fat and in estrogen deficiency. This, in turn, produces the "masculinization" many women

---

* For more specifics on the role of calcium in a broad-spectrum micronutrient program, see our discussion on pages 145–151 and Appendix C, List of Suppliers, for recommended calcium preparations.

athletes experience, including stopping menstruation and an increased bone loss. The watchword again is: "Everything in moderation."

Should women with established osteoporosis engage in any physical exercise at all? The answer is, yes, but one should take into consideration that there probably already exist microfractures and other abnormalities in some bones that could be aggravated by too much stress, as occurs in aerobic jumping or lifting weights. However, the medical experts say, "light to moderate exercise in older women has resulted in an improvement of the cortical bone mass."[22]

A group of sports physicians and bone specialists even designed an exercise program for elderly women suffering from osteoporosis (average age, eighty-one), with activities built around a chair, similar to the previously mentioned minimum-exercise video (see page 540). Over a three-year period, a group of older women following these minimal exercises actually had a 2.29 percent increase in mineral bone content, while a matched control group that did not exercise lost 3.29 percent of bone mineral content.[23] But, Dr. Morris Notelovitz adds, barring such a specialized program, "walking is the safest and most effective form of exercise for women with osteoporosis."

THE PSYCHOLOGICAL BENEFITS

Last but not least, exercise has been shown to reduce anxiety[24] and depression,[25] both of which have, Drs. Colt and Hashim point out, been associated with coronary heart disease.[26] One study of the effects of exercise and diet states, "a regimen of diet and exercise, besides producing a decided change in blood chemistry, and an improvement in circulatory efficiency, vitality, and stamina (measured by the treadmill stress tests), also results in improved psychological and personality factors as well as increased mental acuity."[27]

SUMMING UP

We found that it is easy for people to forget the basic purpose of physical exercise and to let it become an end in itself. Let us therefore remind you that exercise is to maintain aerobic capacity—that is, to prevent your heart muscle from deteriorating and to keep your body supple—as well as helping to control your weight!

The only thing to add is that a complete exercise program should, as physical education specialist Dr. Bernard Gutin of Teachers College, Columbia University, New York City, indicates, "attend to strength and flexibility of the trunk and hip areas to help prevent back problems."[28] Our own exercise routine therefore includes some sit-ups and toe-touching, arms-over-head back bends, and side bends (the half-moon position of hatha-yoga).

Dr. Gutin makes two other important points: First, the routine should be "pleasurably tiring." If it's just pleasurable, chances are you're not pushing yourself enough. If it's too tiring, you may be pushing yourself too much. In our experience, fifteen to thirty minutes is not only sufficient for most people, but few of us have more time than that to exercise during the weekdays. If you can add another 15 to 30 minutes more on weekends (preferably outdoors), so much the better. But remember—if running is part of your exercise routine—do not run more than five days a week.

The other important point Dr. Gutin makes: After any exercise routine, you should spend a few minutes in total relaxation. It's best to lie down on a comfortably soft surface, like an exercise mat or a foam-rubber mattress. You can combine this relaxation period with your personal meditation technique; for instance, Dr. Benson's relaxation response, or whatever is most compatible with your personality and philosophy of life. You'll find that the short period of complete relaxation and meditation will recharge your batteries and add a whole other dimension to your exercise routine.

In our "Formula for Life," that kind of attention to your mental and spiritual well-being is the necessary element without which even the best anti-oxidant program, the most health-promoting diet, and the most perfect exercise program will always remain partial and ultimately disappointing.

SOURCES

1. Anon. *A Complete Guide to Sports Nutrition,* Part I, Food. Mt. View, Calif.: Vitamin Research Products, 1987.
2. Colt, E.W.D., and Sami Hashim. "Effect of exercise and diet on lipids and cardiovascular disease." Chapter 8, in *Nutrition and Exercise,* M. Winick, ed. New York: John Wiley & Sons, 1986, p. 127.
3. *Nutrition and Exercise,* p. 92.
4. Paffenbarger, R. S., Jr., et al. "Energy expenditure, cigarette smoking, and blood pressure are related to death from specific diseases." *Am. J. Epidem.,* 1978; 108(1):12–8.
5. Kalin, Ned H., and B. L. Loevinger. "The Central and Peripheral Opioid Peptides." In: *Psychiatric Clinics of North America, Symposium on Endorphins,* September 1983; 6(3):421.
6. Bloom, M. "Finding Out That Less Can Sometimes Be More." *The New York Times,* November 23, 1987.

7. Gillet, P. A., and P. A. Eisenman. "The effect of intensity controlled aerobic dance exercise on aerobic capacity of middleaged, overweight women." *Research in Nursing and Health,* 1987; 10:383–390.
8. Paffenbarger et al. op. cit.
9. Leon, A. S. "Age and other predictors of coronary heart disease." *Med. Sci. Sports Exerc.,* April 19, 1987; 2:159–167.
10. Stockton, W. "Retirees Make Exercise Video for People Over 50." *The New York Times,* July 25, 1988.
11. Ibid.
12. Stockton, W. "If He's in the Swing of It, Rope-Jumper Can Have Serious Sort of Workout." *The New York Times,* November 30, 1987.
13. Sushruta, S.C.S. *Vaidya Jadavi Trikamji Acharia,* 11/11, 12, 13, rev. 3rd ed. Bombay: Nirnyar Sagar Press, 1938. The original text dates from about 500 B.C.
14. Grasset, H. *La Médecine Naturiste.* Paris, 1911.
15. Schneider, St. H., and H. Kanj. "Clinical aspects of exercise and diabetes mellitus." In: *Nutrition and Exercise,* p. 149.
16. Bjorntorp, P. *Clin. Endocr. Metab.,* 1976; 5:431.
17. Barnard, R. J., et al. "Response of non-insulin-dependent diabetic patients to an intensive program of diet and exercise." *Diabetics Care,* 1982; 5:370–373.
18. Notelovitz, M. "Interrelations of exercise and diet on bone metabolism and osteoporosis." In: *Nutrition and Exercise,* p. 203.
19. Kelsey, J. I., and S. Hoffman. "Risk factors for hip fractures" (Editorial). *N. Eng. J. Med.,* 1987; 316:404–406.
20. Drinkwater, B. L., et al. *N. Eng. J. Med.,* 1984; 311:277.
21. Cann, C. E., et al. *JAMA* 1984; 251:626.
22. Notelovitz, op. cit., p. 213.
23. Smith, E. L., et al. *Med. Sci. Sports Exerc.,* 1981; 13:60.
24. Morgan, W. P. "Influence of acute physical activity on state anxiety." *Proc. Nat. College Phys. Ed. Assoc. for Men,* 1973; pp. 113–121.
25. Greist, J. H., et al. *Comp. Psychiatr.* 1979; 20:41.
26. Jenkins, C. D. *N. Eng. J. Med.,* 1976; 294:987, 1033.
27. Merzbacher, C. F. "A diet and exercise regimen: its effect upon mental acuity and personality, a pilot study." *Perceptual and Motor Skills,* 1979; 48:367–371.
28. Gutin, B. "Prescribing an exercise program." In: *Nutrition and Exercise,* p. 34.

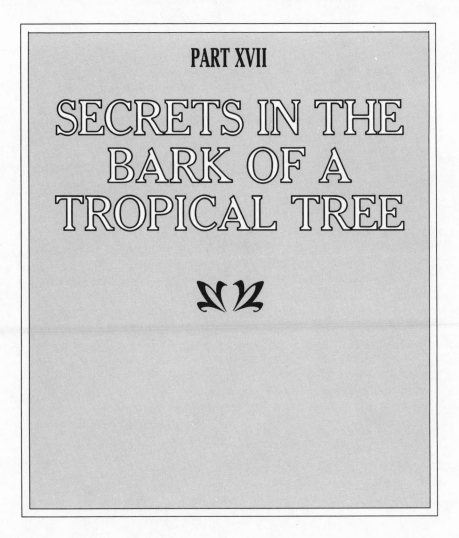

PART XVII

SECRETS IN THE BARK OF A TROPICAL TREE

CHAPTER 64

SCIENCE REDISCOVERS A NATURAL APHRODISIAC

12 Twenty-some years ago, a Danish specialist in artificial insemination of livestock demonstrated—to our amazement—the almost instant aphrodisiac effects of a substance called *yohimbine* when given to sexually sluggish bulls and stallions. It worked in a similar fashion for male dogs, inducing strong erections within less than half an hour. Perhaps if yohimbine were administered to the adorable but listless Chinese panda couple Ling Ling and Yong Yong, and the whole tribe of undersexed pandas, this adorable species of animals wouldn't become extinct!

Since at that time it was impossible to know whether the mysterious aphrodisiac (sexual stimulant) was safe for human use, we did not dare experiment with it ourselves. To be perfectly truthful, we totally forgot about yohimbine until, many years later, we came across two research reports, describing the effect of yohimbine on the sexual behavior of male laboratory rats.[1] This research confirmed scientifically exactly what we had witnessed earlier in Denmark, namely that this remarkable substance acts as a powerful sexual stimulant, as proved by the increased copulatory behavior of these animals.

Our curiosity rekindled by these studies, we did some research of our own on yohimbine, and soon discovered some very interesting facts. For one thing, we found out that natural yohimbine from the bark of a group of tropical trees,* known by different names in many parts of the world,

---

* A group of trees or shrubs of the family *Rubiaceae,* principally *Corynanthe yohimbe* and *Pausinystalia yohimbe,* growing wild in West Africa and elsewhere. In Central and South America, another variety (*Aspidosperma quebracho*) of the same botanical family is popularly known as *quebracho blanco.*

had been used for centuries in herbal medicine to cure impotence.

A check into the history of western medical practices revealed, to our surprise, that yohimbine's lore had evidently reached Victorian England, perhaps from the colonies, where it was said, not without a certain cynicism, to be "the refuge of aging Don Juans."[2] In England, natural yohimbine was used in the form of a "tea" made from the bark of the African yohimbehe tree. However, during the Industrial Revolution the emphasis in western medicine shifted ever more radically toward man-made, chemical drugs and away from the natural remedies of what is referred to disparagingly as "folk medicine." Therefore, the use of yohimbine fell victim to this bias against anything that did not come out of a pharmaceutical laboratory test tube. Thus, yohimbine became for over a century a "forgotten" treatment for one of the human male's most vexing problems—the inability to produce a satisfactory erection.

It was not till the late 1960s and mid-1970s that medical researchers started experimenting with some drugs—including compounds containing yohimbine[3]—to treat impotence. These early trials involved only a very few patients, but they were successful beyond all expectations. For instance, in a group of four cardiac transplant patients treated with a combination of male hormone and yohimbine, only one did not tolerate the treatment, while, the doctors reported, "within a month . . . the other three patients were having satisfactory sexual relations."[4]

The real breakthrough, however, did not come until 1982, when a group of physicians at Queens University in Kingston, Ontario, Canada, embarked on a well-designed and controlled study of organic impotence, using *only* yohimbine as the therapeutic agent.[5] This study included twenty-three patients between thirty-two and seventy-two years of age, almost half of whom were diabetics, the rest suffering from high blood pressure and other circulatory problems for which they were taking antihypertensive drugs, which often produce impotence.

In this treatment, the patients were given 6 milligrams of synthetic yohimbine hydrochloride* three times a day for a minimum of ten weeks. That amount of yohimbine does represent pretty much a maximum dose, and at the outset a few of the patients did experience some side effects like "nervousness," unspecified gastric effects, and mild tremors. These patients were therefore told to reduce the dose to 2 milligrams three times daily, then to increase it progressively until they were back up to 18 milligrams a day. This strategy worked, and

---

* The most common form in which yohimbine is taken in this country is as the prescription drug Yohimex, each pink tablet containing 5 milligrams of chemically pure yohimbine hydrochloride. If it is taken as a natural tea brewed from the bark of the West African yohimbehe tree, or from the quebracho blanco tree of Central and South America, it is difficult to judge the dosage per cup. The bark also contains another alkaloid (aspidospermine), about which little is currently known. We therefore much prefer to use the prescription drug whenever possible.

eventually all of the men were able to tolerate this relatively high dosage without any further problems.

The results of this clinical study were most encouraging: Six of the twenty-three men were able to experience again sustained erections and resume satisfactory sexual relations—not bad, we'd say, following a lengthy period of total impotence. Another four patients reported partial but not fully satisfactory erections.

The six patients in this study who regained complete potency represent statistically a success rate of 26 percent, an impressive figure in itself. But you may be sure that, as far as these men themselves were concerned, the experiment was not 26 percent but 100 percent successful! Equally important, the yohimbine was, in the words of the researchers, "well tolerated" after the slight initial side effects a few of the patients experienced (such psychological problems as "nervousness" and "anxiety" could have been avoided if vitamin C had been administered simultaneously, as we will explain further on).

These results are all the more remarkable, since they were achieved by simply giving these men, who were in poor general health, nothing more than yohimbine. Even though they might not have been allowed to drink alcohol during the actual treatment period (the published results do not specify this prohibition), one could safely assume that at least some (and more likely most) of the men were doing so during the follow-up period. Since alcohol is a well-known sex depressant, any consumption of alcohol would of course have reduced the effectiveness of the yohimbine therapy.

Another factor that might have artificially depressed the treatment results, excellent as they are, is that the patients had apparently been allowed to smoke cigarettes, probably even during the treatment period; there is no indication to the contrary in the published study. This is likely, since not very many people realize that cigarette smoking can seriously affect potency as well.

There is also the distinct probability that some of the men were, like most middle-aged people, suffering from at least "moderate arterial insufficiency."[6] This condition can also affect blood flow to the pelvic area. If there is severe atherosclerotic obstruction in the iliac arteries leading to that area, no natural or synthetic aphrodisiac, or even the best sex therapy, can be of any help. The only solution would be either a bypass operation, as is done when coronary arteries are blocked, or a penile implant.*

* In some cases, the penile valves through which the blood flows out through the veins become leaky, making it impossible to maintain necessary engorgement for an erection. Here, too, surgery is sometimes possible; otherwise the only other remedy is a penile implant.

There are also some rare cases of impotence due to temporal lobe epilepsy. These cases must be treated with anticonvulsant drugs and sex hormones (chorionic gonadotropin and/or testosterone). Only the most sophisticated diagnostic techniques are adequate for making such differential diagnoses.

One thing that puzzled the doctors in this yohimbine study was that it took the patients two to three weeks before any aphrodisiac effects were noticeable. Frankly, that is puzzling us too. Our own experience, corroborated by physician friends of ours who use yohimbine in the treatment of potency problems, is that the substance almost consistently has the desired result if 10 milligrams (two 5-milligram Yohimex tablets) are taken on an empty stomach. We can therefore only assume that the poor general health of that particular patient group accounted for the strangely delayed reaction.

On the other hand, there was one happy surprise benefit in the same impotence study: Three of the diabetic patients who had been suffering from the typical paresthesias of the legs and feet (a prickly sensation as if the limb were going to sleep) that frequently accompany diabetes were suddenly relieved of this disagreeable symptom. The researchers offered some informed guesses, but had no definitive explanation for this welcome side effect.[7] Another researcher suggested that, since yohimbine selectively blocks certain nerve cell receptors, the increased norepinephrine release might be the mechanism involved.[8] Be that as it may, for any patients suffering from paresthesias and impotency, yohimbine represents a double blessing.

There are several theories on how yohimbine might work as a direct-acting sex stimulant, whether to cure impotence or just to promote libido and improve sexual performance. However, the theories are so complicated and technical that even most physicians, let alone the average layman, cannot possibly follow them.

Trying to simplify these often contradictory theories, focusing on only the most promising "explanations," and to summarize what is known thus far about the way yohimbine works, we would say the following:

Considering that yohimbine blocks certain nerve receptors in the penis, called *alpha-2 adrenergic receptors,* and considering too that the cavernous spongy tissue of the penis is full of them, one might think that this would normally cause a loss of erection rather than produce one. What suggests itself therefore is that there must exist a more powerful central nervous system mechanism that overrides the negative effects of these nerve receptors. In other words, yohimbine produces erections, not because but *despite* the fact that it blocks the peripheral, alpha-2 adrenergic receptors in the penis.

How yohimbine accomplishes this paradoxical feat, nobody seems to know. All we can say at this point is that from a strictly clinical point of view, the parasympathetic nervous system is clearly enhanced after taking yohimbine.

Scientists feel that yohimbine's enhancement of the parasympathetic system is indirect and relative, and is achieved by the substance suppressing the sympathetic system to some extent. This, in turn, would put the parasympathetic system more in control, and that, by itself, often results in erections. But *how* yohimbine affects blood flow not just *to* but, more important, *within* the erectile tissue of the penis, is still a matter of scientific speculation. A urologist we consulted made the following interesting observations:

> My own guess is that yohimbine probably affects in a positive way the many little valves, called arterial sphincters, that regulate blood flow within the penis. The neurological control of those sphincters is critical. That's the bottom line on whether there will be an erection or not.
>
> You may be getting plenty of blood flow in the large arteries and into the smaller arterioles branching out from them—and yet you may not be getting any blood into the network of tiny capillaries [in the penis], simply because the precapillary sphincters have never opened up.
>
> Actually, the precapillary sphincters, which control blood flow into the capillaries of the penis, are still a mystery. And these capillaries—spongy areas where blood sort of pours in and out—are extremely complicated. There are still many unknown areas in the microcirculation of the penis. But one thing seems certain to my mind—if yohimbine is producing erections, as we know it does, it must be by affecting all these little valves or sphincters that have to open up to let the blood into the penis, and others that have to close down to keep it inside, if there's to be an erection. Only that I don't think there's anybody today who knows exactly by what mechanism yohimbine is able to accomplish this.

The fact that yohimbine is able to restore erectile ability in many cases of organic impotence was further corroborated by a double-blind follow-up study,* conducted by the same group of Canadian researchers who had done the previous breakthrough study. Again, the results were excellent, showing a combined total and partial success rate of better than 40 percent.[9]

With this second study, scientific research had finally caught up with the ancient practical knowledge that yohimbine can indeed cure impotence. At least, at the conclusion there was proof positive that yohimbine could cure impotence due to *organic* causes.

But what of those countless cases of impotence for which there seems to be no underlying *physical* cause? This type of impotence is technically referred to as "psychogenic" or "situational impotence."

Until now there was only one way of treating psychogenic impotence, and that was through a gradual reeducation and reconditioning of a

---

* A double-blind study refers to one in which scientific research conducted in such a way that neither the human subjects, nor the researchers know which group is receiving the substance to be tested (in this case, the yohimbine), and which group is being given an innocuous look-alike placebo, a substance that has no effect whatever. Only at the end of the study is the code broken and the results evaluated.

person's attitudes toward his own body, his principal sex partner, the opposite sex in general, and what he knows or how he feels overall about human sexuality. In short, psychogenic impotence could be treated only with the kind of psychological explorations and educational techniques (including touching, massage, or even a surrogate sex partner) that falls under the general heading of sex therapy.

Fortunately, it has now been scientifically established that yohimbine also works in a high percentage of people suffering from psychogenic impotence. The researchers at Kingston General Hospital, Queens University, in Ontario, Canada, along with a psychologist, Dr. K. Reid, recently conducted a study on forty-eight men suffering from psychogenic impotence that equals or betters the good results of the previous studies of organic impotence: Thirty-eight percent experienced complete restoration of potency and satisfactory sexual relations (compared with 26 percent for organic impotence), and an overall success rate of 46 percent, if one includes all those cases in which there was at least a partial restoration of sexual functioning.[9]

These success rates are very similar to those obtained by sex therapy alone,[10] without any pharmacological support. In other words, in terms of results, the two techniques are about equal. In our opinion, however, being equal in effectiveness does not mean that since yohimbine can do as good a job as sex therapy, we might as well forget about sex therapy altogether. True, sex therapy is by its very nature time-consuming and costly. So is psychotherapy. But does that mean we ought to use only tranquilizers and antidepressants to treat neurotic and psychotic disturbances? Certainly not.

We believe the same pertains to psychogenic impotence. In fact, we think that "curing" psychogenic impotence with yohimbine, or any other pharmacological therapy alone, would be on very shaky grounds as far as lasting results are concerned. All too often, the problem is a result of faulty sex attitudes, or sexual ignorance, or an inability to "pleasure" one's partner or to enjoy being "pleasured." Ideally, therefore, some kind of psychological counseling and/or sex therapy ought to accompany the administration of yohimbine whenever available or economically feasible.

Admittedly, the initial success rate might not be greatly increased by the two-pronged approach we are proposing. However, it is reasonable to expect that the results would ultimately be more solid and longer-lasting. A well-designed study along these lines would be an important counterpart to the one done by the Kingston researchers.

Another study that ought to be undertaken as soon as possible is to ascertain whether yohimbine therapy might not also be effective with women who are unable to achieve satisfactory orgasm. Contrary, however, to what is true for male sexual dysfunction, we believe that most of these women, once having "learned" to achieve orgasm with the help of yohimbine, might not have to continue taking yohimbine afterward.

What is the most important fact about yohimbine therapy for either organic or psychogenic impotence is that in their new study, the Canadian researchers again found that yohimbine therapy is "a *safe treatment* for psychogenic impotence,"[11] just as had been the case in their earlier experiment (emphasis ours). We can only confirm this from our own observations of many cases in which both men and women took yohimbine under medical supervision for its aphrodisiac effects and experienced no mental or physical problems whatsoever.

We hasten to add, however, that in all these cases, the yohimbine was taken with no less than 6,000 milligrams (6 grams) of ascorbic acid (vitamin C) per day (in three divided doses). This counteracts, as we shall explain in the chapter that follows, the anxiety and nervousness that are sometimes reported to accompany yohimbine therapy without the addition of vitamin C.

In the next part of our discussion of yohimbine, we shall be focusing on its considerable mood-enhancing and mental-energizing properties, which are often overlooked. We will discuss the probable reasons for this oversight, as well as the additional therapeutic benefits of yohimbine as a fast-acting antidepressant, if it is used with proper medical controls and supervision.

SOURCES

1. Clark, John T., Erla R. Smith, and Julian M. Davidson. "Enhancement of sexual motivation in male rats by yohimbine." Reprint supplied by the Department of Physiology, Stanford University, Stanford, CA 94305. Original source not given.
2. Arena, J. M. *Poisoning: Toxicology, Symptoms, Treatments.* Springfield, Ill.: Chas. C. Thomas, 1979, p. 94.
3. Margolis, R., and C. H. Leslie. "Review of studies on a mixture of nux vomica, yohimbine and methyl testosterone in the treatment of impotence." *Curr. Ther. Res.,* 1966; 8:280.
4. Walpowitz, A., and C. N. Barnard. "Impotence after heart transplantation" (Letters to the Editor). *S. Afr. Med. J.,* 1978; 53:693.
5. Morales A., et al. "Nonhormonal pharmacological treatment of organic impotence." *J. Urol.,* 1982; 128:45–47.
6. Juenemann, Klaus-Peter, et al. "The effect of cigarette smoking on penile erection." *J. Urol.,* 1987; 138:438–441.
7. Morales, A., et al. "Yohimbine for treatment of impotence in diabetes" (Letters to the Editor). *N. Eng. J. Med.,* 1981; 305:1221.
8. Steinmetz, Laura L., in a response to "Is yohimbine an effective treatment for impotence?" *Drug Intelligence and Clin. Pharm.,* 1986; 20:950–951.

9. Reid, K., et al. "Double-blind trial of Yohimbine in treatment of psychogenic impotence." *Lancet,* August 22, 1987; II(8556):421–423.
10. Reynolds, B. "Psychological treatment models and outcome results for erectile dysfunction: A critical review." *Psych. Bull.,* 1977; 14:545.
11. Morales, A., et al. "The effectiveness of yohimbine in the treatment of organic impotence: a controlled trial." *J. Urol.,* 1988.

CHAPTER 65

A NEW ANTIDEPRESSANT AND MENTAL ENERGIZER

12 It took a hundred years for us to catch up with what the witch doctors of Africa and the *curanderos* of Central and South America had known for ages: Yohimbine can indeed cure many types of impotence.

Yohimbine can be produced synthetically in its pure chemical form, yohimbine hydrochloride. It is now possible for doctors to prescribe the right dosage (normally between 15 to 20 milligrams per day), if they want to use it to treat impotence. That this is by no means widely known and done in actual medical practice is another matter.

Much less known and appreciated is the fact that not only is yohimbine about the only medical treatment for many forms of impotence, but it is a first-class antidepressant and general mental stimulant. It is also apparently relatively safe, if used correctly and under medical supervision.

The trouble is that its potential to relieve depression and make the mind work better is not widely known. Nor is this surprising, if we consider that it works that way only if taken with plenty of vitamin C. The researchers who studied yohimbine as a treatment for impotence did not and could not use anything but yohimbine in their tests because they wouldn't have known what effect was due to what.

On the other hand, when we experimented with yohimbine, we had plenty of vitamin C on board as part of our regular anti-oxidant program, and therefore noticed its extraordinary mental effects right away. There was an astounding clarity of thought and a greatly heightened state of mental alertness. For the time that the yohimbine was active (something like two to three hours), our brains were firing even more happily and efficiently on all cylinders than usual—but without the unpleasant sensation of "speeding" one can get with too much caffeine or other stimulants.

Another thing we noticed immediately was a greatly enhanced verbal facility. During writing or lecturing, it was much easier to find the right turn of phrase or way of saying something. Also, we were "wittier" than usual, readily able to see the funny side of things, and more inclined to laughter than usual. Our basic mood was very good anyway, thanks to our regular anti-oxidant program, only with yohimbine, it became even better, especially at times when the going was rough, and we would have been a little down without it.

Best of all, we found that yohimbine was highly effective even if taken only in mini-doses. To treat impotence, three or four 5-milligram tablets of Yohimex are generally taken in the course of a day. However, we discovered that we could break a 5-milligram tablet in half or into quarters, taking as little as 1¼ milligrams to 2.5 milligrams at a time, and still enjoy all the mental and emotional benefits. Of course, we made sure to take the yohimbine with at least 6,000 milligrams of vitamin C per day as part of our broad-spectrum anti-oxidant program.

Because of yohimbine's almost instant mood-elevating capacity (effects are noted in thirty to sixty minutes on an empty stomach), we feel that it ought to be seriously considered as an alternative treatment for depression. The dosage would have to depend on the severity of the condition. If the depression is relatively mild, 5 milligrams to 10 milligrams per day should be perfectly adequate. It might, however, take the maximum dosage of 15 milligrams to 20 milligrams of yohimbine and 10,000 milligrams to 12,000 milligrams of vitamin C per day to relieve a more serious depression.

We have actually seen this happen more than once, and as clinical psychologists, we would like to point out that in these cases, yohimbine has the edge over other antidepressants unless there are counterindications (for instance, underlying psychosis with potential for violent or manic acting out). Our reason for feeling so strongly on this point is that most antidepressants require one to several weeks of buildup in the brain before they become fully effective. With yohimbine plus vitamin C, the effect is immediate.

On a lighter note: We noticed right away that yohimbine made all our senses more acute. This can actually become too much of a good thing, especially with regard to the sense of smell. Yohimbine slightly magnifies not only the pleasant aromas, but unfortunately also the less agreeable ones. It reminded us of the supposedly true story of a man whose sense of smell became, by some neurological accident, as acute as that of a dog's—and the problems it posed for him!

Even more pronounced is yohimbine's effect on the auditory sense. That, too, can be pleasant or otherwise, depending on the situation. To enjoy to the fullest all the overtones and undertones of a fine symphony orchestra is one thing—but it's quite another to have the noise of a jackhammer or the cacophony of city traffic amplified so that it becomes even more intolerable.

As far as the effect of yohimbine on the sense of sight is concerned, it is definitely not hallucinogenic. You don't see flowers "breathing" or have "visions" of things that aren't actually there, as with hallucinogens like LSD or mescaline. All that yohimbine does is to make one see objects somewhat more distinctly or sharply and colors slightly more pronounced. But there is no distortion of perception whatsoever.

Important, too, is yohimbine's effect on the sense of touch. One area, for instance, in which it would be of obvious advantage to use yohimbine/vitamin therapy is in certain cases of sexual dysfunction. As is well known, the sense of touch is very important in human sexuality, but many people have an underdeveloped sensory apparatus, which is often an important part of the problem. The use of yohimbine/vitamin therapy in medically supervised sex therapy should therefore be a promising area of future research.

A heightening of the sense of touch is, however, by no means the only or most important way in which vitamin C supplementation can render yohimbine more effective as an aphrodisiac. One hardly need point out that a depressed person feels less sexy than a happy one. Yohimbine's mood-enhancing capacity in the presence of vitamin C could therefore be another helpful tool in sex therapy, if depressive trends are part of the problem.

How are these various mental and psychological effects of yohimbine achieved if it is used together with vitamin C, and why do they come into play *only* in the presence of vitamin C?

From the sparse scientific literature, the only thing that seems really clear is that yohimbine affects a brain area called the *locus ceruleus,* which to a large extent controls mental alertness. Now, when you stimulate the firing of the neurons in the locus ceruleus, it sends noradrenaline (the brain's version of adrenaline) to the hippocampus, an important part of the limbic system that has a lot do with our emotions, including fear. If you stimulate this area with yohimbine, you will not only produce a state of high alertness, but also the kind of anxiety and nervousness that some of the patients in the Canadian impotence studies, mentioned in the previous chapter, seem to have initially experienced.

Why doesn't this happen when yohimbine is administered together with vitamin C? Actually, one might expect an increase rather than a decrease in anxiety and nervousness with vitamin C. The reason is that vitamin C is known to prevent the endorphins from attaching to nerve receptors in the locus ceruleus,[1] and keeps them from exerting their normal calming, antianxiety effect.[2] It should therefore theoretically make you more nervous and anxious, perhaps even panicky, when you take yohimbine with vitamin C. And yet we know from experience that quite the opposite is true.

Feeling that the medical intricacies to explain this puzzling and apparent contradiction were well beyond our own expertise, we turned to a neurologist friend of ours, who we knew had studied yohimbine in some depth, to give us (and you) the benefit of his special knowledge on this difficult subject.

"Well, the effect of vitamin C in connection with yohimbine is, as you say, paradoxical," he began.

> By blocking the endorphin receptors in the locus ceruleus, it actually enhances the activity of the yohimbine. In so doing, it removes a natural brake on the yohimbine which would otherwise be exerted by the suppressing effect of the opioid endorphins. At the same time, yohimbine comes in and acts as an accelerator. It's pushing on the gas and stimulating the locus ceruleus directly. Now you've got a marked acceleration and a true synergism between the yohimbine and the vitamin C, both acting on the locus ceruleus.
>
> That, in fact, could be a potentially dangerous situation, not a beneficial one, because it could produce exaggerated yohimbine effects. It could, as you suggest, cause outright panic. Yet it doesn't do anything of the kind because vitamin C works not only on the locus ceruleus, but also on other parts of the brain.
>
> Panic is a cerebral cortex event; it is not a locus ceruleus event. To explain the rest, I'll have to digress for a moment: As you will recall from your work as clinical psychologists, it has become almost common practice in psychiatry to administer the antipsychotic drug haloperidol [Haldol], together with about two thousand milligrams of vitamin C. The reason for that—though it is not generally recognized—is that vitamin C makes the receptors on the brain cells a lot more receptive to the haloperidol.
>
> Now obviously the body didn't make nerve receptors for a man-made substance like haloperidol. It made it for a natural, antipsychotic compound we are producing ourselves, but which hasn't as yet been isolated.

What our neurologist friend was referring to goes back to certain animal studies with haloperidol,[3,4] which showed that the drug was more effective if it was administered along with vitamin C. Looking for an explanation of this phenomenon, the researchers recalled that the popular tranquilizers Valium and Librium owe their effectiveness to the fact that they fit, like a key in a lock, into certain brain cell receptors that are made for some natural tranquilizing substance that as yet has not been isolated either. The researchers therefore suspected that such was the case with haloperidol and vitamin C, an assumption that was borne out by subsequent investigations. Thus far, we know only that the respective mystery substances X and Y for the tranquilizers and the haloperidol are not the brain-manufactured endorphins, which also have tranquilizing properties. Some day, undoubtedly, we shall know exactly what these natural substances actually are and be able to synthesize and use them instead of the toxic chemical analogs with which we have presently to content ourselves.

Continuing his explanation about the strange synergism between yohimbine and vitamin C, this nutrition-oriented neurologist said:

> Keeping in mind that vitamin C binds to the same nerve receptors in the cerebral cortex that the antipsychotic drug haloperidol binds to, we must conclude that vitamin C has very positive, cerebral-cortical properties. It has a *normalizing* effect, but at the same time it has an *awakening* effect.
>
> You want to be very alert, but cool and able to think clearly—not panicky, but sharp. Vitamin C does that for you. That's why the brain has so much vitamin C in it. It has as much vitamin C as an orange.
>
> In the presence of yohimbine, the vitamin C allows the locus ceruleus to keep going, because it is blunting the tranquilizing effects of the endorphins. That produces a sense of alertness. At the same time, it acts on the cerebral cortex to produce a frame of mind that is calm. So, with enough vitamin C, you get the ideal person: calm, cool, and collected—but very sharp!

The neurologist felt that the mood-enhancing effect of yohimbine, if taken together with vitamin C, is due to still another, related mechanism. Here's how he explained it:

> One must remember that when you increase the firing of the locus ceruleus [with yohimbine], that, in turn, feeds into the hippocampus. There are actually nerve cell bodies [axons] in the locus ceruleus that go directly to nerve cells in what is called the cortex of the hippocampus gyrus. It's a direct, nerve-to-nerve transmission, and that's how it elevates the mood.

In this connection, he pointed out the difference between the action of a substance like cocaine, which produces a similar mood elevation, and yohimbine:

> Cocaine has effects all over the body, centrally [meaning within the brain itself], and peripherally. It does not distinguish—everyplace you've got a synapse of a sympathetic nerve, where dopamine is the neurotransmitter that fills the synaptic gap—cocaine prevents the reabsorption [of the neurotransmitter].
>
> Normally, any dopamine that's secreted gets reabsorbed right away, so that the stimulation stops. If anything like cocaine prevents that prompt reabsorption [of the neurotransmitter], that can be very dangerous. Keep in mind that all these neurotransmitters don't only work on the cerebral cortex, but also on the brainstem that regulates the heart rate, respiratory rate, and other fundamental life processes. So, if these transmissions are not promptly

extinguished, because the cocaine blocks the reabsorption of the neurotransmitters, you not only get a high, you also get a high myocardial output—and
that would be very serious.

Emphasizing the importance of the nervous system being able to stop
nerve transmissions in a timely fashion, our neurological consultant
said, "The most dangerous thing you can do to the nervous system is
to make the neurotransmitters persist in the synaptic gap [as happens
with cocaine]." In that case, he pointed out, "it's like high voltage going
through the circuits persistently." We would like to add that if there is
any heart problem, like the very frequent arrhythmias many people
experience but are not even aware of, the result from using cocaine
may be tragic indeed—as we all know too well from periodic news
reports of sudden death following the use of cocaine.

The difference between what occurs with cocaine and with yohimbine is that with yohimbine the norepinephrine (a) never gets outside
the brain, and (b) its reabsorption is not blocked, so it gets reabsorbed
in the normal fashion.

Our consultant added:

> If the locus ceruleus is activated by yohimbine, the norepinephrine that's
> released actually travels inside the axon as a droplet and is deposited right
> on the nerve cells of the hippocampus. It's like water flowing through a
> pipeline; it's not like a stream flowing outside that you can see. It never gets
> outside the brain itself—it's an "inside job."
>
> That's why you'll never find it [the norepinephrine, released by the action
> of yohimbine] in increased circulating blood levels. You don't even find an
> increase of norepinephrine in spinal fluid, if you take a sample of it after
> yohimbine use. That's why it's a relatively safe drug in medical hands. Still,
> it's got to be used with certain precautions, and some medical conditions
> preclude its use altogether. That's why it's got to be a prescription drug.

Some medical conditions—aside from any kind of heart disease—in
which the use of yohimbine is definitely counterindicated, are renal
(kidney) or hepatic (liver) problems. Also, people with Parkinsonism
should probably not be treated with yohimbine, since it might interfere
with dopamine function.[5,6] In short, wherever there is some doubt
about safety, it would seem best to err on the side of prudence.

On the other hand, yohimbine is, in some respects, much safer than
many other, commonly prescribed drugs. To keep relative risks in
some perspective, let us just remind ourselves that Americans consume
a staggering 3.7 billion (yes, 3.7 *billion!*) dollars' worth of Valium and
similar drugs of the benzodiazepine family a year to calm their nerves.
And if these drugs are taken with alcohol, as they often are, the effects
can be devastating, even lethal.

In contrast, with yohimbine—if used in concert with vitamin C and, better still, with other anti-oxidants—the worst that can happen if it is taken irresponsibly along with alcohol is that the alcohol will nullify the benefits of the yohimbine. While alcohol synergizes with tranquilizers like Valium, yohimbine is antagonistic to it, and anti-oxidants tend to ameliorate alcohol's negative effects.

Yohimbine does, however, synergize with some far-too-frequently-taken single amino acids, like tyrosine or phenylalanine, thereby potentiating each other's effects. We do not think it is a good idea to take these single amino acids, because they all increase the circulating levels of powerful neurotransmitters. If you add to that another potent neurotransmitter, norepinephrine, which is released by the yohimbine, who can tell what the mixture of these neurotransmitters will do? It would be especially risky in view of the fact that yohimbine, as we know, blocks the alpha-2 adrenergic receptors, about which we still know little.

All tranquilizers and sleeping pills—and "uppers" like amphetamines—gradually lose their effectiveness with prolonged use, so that the dosage has to be increased more and more over time. By the same token, all these types of drugs are by definition habit-forming. Before a person realizes it—perhaps some readers will be able to confirm this from their own sad experience—he or she has already become thoroughly hooked and can no longer get along without the drugs.

On the other hand, we have noticed nothing of this sort in our medically controlled experimentation with yohimbine—provided the substance is taken together with vitamin C and other anti-oxidants. Nonetheless, we do not advise taking yohimbine as a steady diet. It is totally different from all the health-promoting, anti-aging substances on our regular program. It should therefore never be used for anything but very specific purposes, as an aphrodisiac or for its mood-elevating and activating properties—and then only on a temporary, short-term basis, as a prescription pharmaceutical, by a physician.

SOURCES

1. Dr. Harry B. Demopoulos, verbal communication.
2. Gold, M. S., and W. S. Rea. "The role of endorphins in opiate addiction, opiate withdrawal, and recovery." *Psychiatric Clinics of North America,* September 1983; 6(3):497.
3. Rebec, G. V., et al. "Ascorbic acid and the behavioral response to haloperidol: Implications for the action of antipsychotic drugs." *Science,* 1985; 227:438–440.

4. Dorris, R. L., and R. E. Dill. "Potentiation of haloperidol-induced catalepsy by ascorbic acid in rats and nonhuman primates." *Pharmacol. Biochem. Behav.,* 1986; 24:781–783.
5. Scatton, B., et al. "Antidopaminergic properties of yohimbine." *J. Pharmacol. and Exper. Therapeutics,* 1980; 215:494–498.
6. Goldberg, M., et al. "Influence of yohimbine on release of anterior pituitary hormones." *Life Sciences,* 1986; 39:395–398.

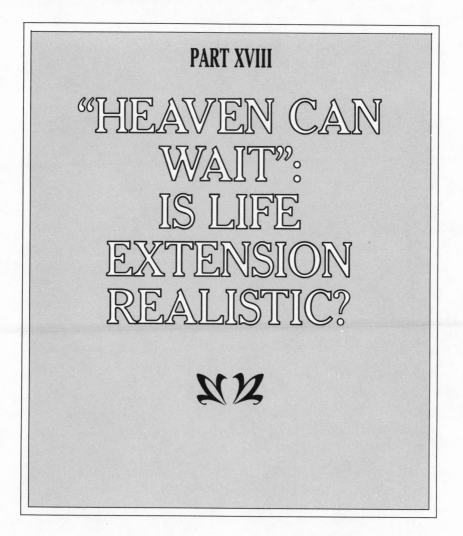

PART XVIII

"HEAVEN CAN WAIT": IS LIFE EXTENSION REALISTIC?

12 A reporter asks an old man what he's done to live to such a great age. The old man says his secret is a quart of whiskey, two packs of cigarettes, and three square meals a day. So the reporter asks him how old *is* he, and he says, "Thirty-two."

Longevity jokes have been around for centuries, as have news stories about men and women who live to be 120 or even 139 years old. Usually the stories concern tribal people like the Hunzas of Kashmir or the Vilcabamba Indians of Ecuador—and unfortunately do not stand up to closer investigation. The longest life span on reliable record thus far seems to be 113 years, and the maximum span for our species is thought to be somewhere around 115 years.

What interests us even more than the question of whether human life span is relatively fixed or potentially expandable is the question of *individual* life span. That, after all, is the more immediate—and practical—reality for each one of us.

It's fair to assume that if people are known to be able to live close to 113 years without special diet, aerobic exercise, or anti-oxidants, they could live even longer under more ideal conditions. In other words, 113 years are definitely not the best humans can do in terms of longevity. Speaking for ourselves, we'd settle for 113, provided we stayed in reasonably good shape.

Why are we so interested in longevity? Because even though we are already pushing the life-expectancy statistics, we feel that we've only now come into the fullness of life. Our entire previous existence—everything that's ever happened to us, good and bad—seems to have only been so much preparation for where we are today.

Of all the factors affecting individual life span, the dominant one is genetic. If your forebears were generally long-lived, the chances are that you too will reach a ripe old age. The opposite, of course, is equally true.

Genetic predisposition plays a major role in the rate at which each of us becomes old *and* the age to which any of us is likely to live. However, environmental and life-style factors also have a profound influence on life expectancy. Over some of these factors we may not

569

have much control—or may *think* we don't—like where we live and what we do for a living. Other matters are more definitely self-determined: Nobody's forcing us to smoke or to drink more alcohol than we should; nobody's telling us what we should have for lunch or dinner.

Whatever genetic patterns are factored into any individual life expectancy equation, we ourselves supply—to a much greater extent than we imagine or care to admit—the *determining* factor. It's perfectly clear that, as one doctor put it recently, "the great majority of our major illnesses are largely self-inflicted by self-destructive lifestyle and dietary habits. They are therefore largely preventable."[1]

Even so conservative a body as the National Cancer Institute has acknowledged that not a single new breakthrough in cancer diagnosis or treatment is needed. In fact, the much publicized war on coronary heart disease and on cancer, the two major killers, has *theoretically* already been won. At least 85 percent of heart disease and cancer—like most other degenerative diseases—don't have to happen.

Dr. Demopoulos agrees, but sees possibilities far beyond simply preventing or avoiding heart disease and cancer:

"We can already stop the extensive, rapidly spreading free-radical chain reactions in experiments that simulate free-radical damage in the central nervous system. It should therefore be much easier to halt the much slower, less energetic, ongoing free-radical reactions that seem to underlie the pathology of strokes and cancer, and very possibly of cell-aging itself. Put differently, in principle, I see no reason why we should not be able to inhibit the insidious atrophy and shrinkage of our internal organs that is one of the main characteristics of aging."

Seen in this light, a very high percentage of deaths attributed to "old age" are actually premature. For that matter, we don't really know what the term "aging" means. As one specialist in aging and nutrition put it: "In man, aging is so modified by disease that its truly uncomplicated course is unknown. When an elderly man dies, he dies from disease or accident, although his demise may euphemistically be attributed to 'old age.' "[2]

In practical terms, let's assume that your genetic makeup gives you a life expectancy of around one hundred years. Whether you'll actually reach anything like that age will, barring accidents, depend largely on how well or how poorly you take care of yourself between now and then. Since most of us don't give much thought to such matters until late middle age, it's comforting to know that this one factor can make a tremendous difference at any stage of life. As Samuel Goldwyn is said to have quipped on his ninety-fifth birthday, "If I'd known I'd ever get this old, I'd have taken better care of myself!"

Taking better care of ourselves—a subject we have discussed earlier in the book—obviously involves changes in our life-style. Some of these changes are easy enough to make: walking instead of driving short distances, or choosing to have cereal and fruit instead of bacon and eggs for breakfast. Or, as life-extension specialist Dr. Roy Walford emphasizes, restricting our total calorie intake—in short, eating less.

Other changes might be considerably more difficult to make, especially where smoking, alcohol, and other drug dependencies are concerned. Life extension interests might even force occupational and residential changes.

The degree of change required to maximize any individual's life span depends on many different factors for each person. Some people may only need to increase their amount of exercise and to start taking anti-oxidants. Others may need to take up exercise and anti-oxidants and abandon cigarettes and alcohol. Still others may need to do all of the above, and move to Vermont.

There are, of course, people who won't make the choices that would enable them to live longer—either because they don't care enough or because the prospect of longevity itself serves to frighten them rather than to act as an incentive. Many who equate advanced age with disability would far rather die prematurely than stay around to become feeble and feeble-minded.

This fear, however understandable, is unfounded—because the common disabilities of old age, like premature death itself, *are* so often avoidable. The term "golden years" needn't refer to the cruel irony of having to be dressed, bathed, fed, and toileted, to be a burden to oneself and others. How to grow old in years while staying young in mind and body is exactly what our program is all about.

Still others may wonder whether it is really worth surviving too far into the twenty-first century. They are concerned about overpopulation, or depletion of natural resources, or the progressive pollution of the environment.

But here again, we are not merely helpless victims of outside forces beyond our control. None of these possibly catastrophic developments is inevitable. Problems are still solvable—provided we put our wills and minds to solving them. If we don't, they will be "solved" for us.

There is no reason why each of us should not seek, first of all, to fulfill our own personal life-span potential, whatever that may be, and to fulfill it in good health and with a clear mind. Next, we may want to extend that life span beyond the point set by genetic predisposition and whatever damage has already been done to our system. Finally, having glimpsed the theoretical possibilities for extending not only our individual life span but also that of the whole human race, we may stop considering that maximum life span as if etched in stone and unalterable. In fact, as biotechnology enters the twenty-first century, it is only reasonable to assume that maximum life span for the human race will become expandable.

On what are we basing these grand hopes and expectations? First, on the fact that anti-oxidants have already been shown in animal experiments to increase maximum life span in rats, mice, fruit flies, and other species. Second, the aging rate in humans during the last 100,000 to 200,000 years has been slowing down, scientists have determined, by about 12.5 percent. During that same period, maximum human life span has been increasing by about ten years.[3–5] There is no way to determine for sure whether this trend will continue. But we should soon be able to *make* it continue, and even at at a faster pace than it has been doing on its own.

The third reason for our belief in the expandability of human life span lies in recent advances in genetic engineering. It appears that the longer-lived species—the tortoise (150 years), man (113 years), the Asian elephant (60 years), other primates like the orangutan, gorilla, and chimpanzee, along with the whale and the golden eagle (50 to 60 years)—all have more effective DNA repair mechanisms than do shorter-lived creatures. All we have to do to reset the genetic clocks that make for these differences in longevity is first to find out exactly which genes control these cell repair mechanisms.

Making some genetic improvements shouldn't be all that difficult. The most up-to-date studies of the aging process place the rate of physiological decline at an average of only 1 percent per year.[6] This means that even a very small improvement in the ratio of cell repair to cell damage will have a tremendous effect on human life span. All we have to do is help our bodies to repair cell damage at a rate a little closer to that which occurs "naturally" as we age—a repair that would involve only fractions of 1 percent—in order to double and triple maximum life span.

If such speculations about life extension sound more like science fiction than science, consider that for a queen bee nothing more than a different kind of nutrition—royal jelly—is able to extend that bee's life span by a factor of seventy to ninety times. In human terms, this translates to a life span of seven thousand to nine thousand years— virtual immortality!

Consider these biological facts:

- The trees on the Mount of Olives in Jerusalem are estimated to have been alive for more than a millennium.
- The bristlecone pine of the American Northwest is known to live as long as four thousand to five thousand years.
- The chaparral bush, scientists now know, has a life span of ten thousand years or more, as measured by radiocarbon techniques.

Who knows how long the olive tree, the bristlecone pine, the chaparral bush, and other extraordinarily long-lived organisms might last if they were fully protected and nurtured? When they finally do die, it's not from old age but from accidental death: struck by lightning, parched by drought, starved for nutrients, attacked by insects or fungi. It's a wonder they survive to such extraordinary lengths at all. If it weren't for all these environmental hazards, what could their life spans be?

To those of us working with the concept of free-radical pathology (the theory that free-radical activity is the root cause of disease and aging), their longevity comes as no surprise. Analysis of the chemical compounds making up the dry mass of long-lived plants has revealed an extraordinarily high level of anti-oxidants in all of them. The chaparral bush, for example, has a level of 60 percent. No wonder it can live to be ten thousand years old!

To our knowledge, no one has attempted to determine the percentage level of anti-oxidants in human beings; but it's reasonable to assume that it is extremely low. However, unlike other living organisms, humans can do something about our anti-oxidant household. Unfortunately, most of us move in the opposite direction. Instead of eating the foods that contain the most anti-oxidants, we seem to prefer those that use them up. When you add to an anti-oxidant–poor diet such factors as smoking, pollution, stress, drinking alcohol, using "recreational" drugs, overworking, overeating, and overplaying, you're placing a tremendous strain on your body's anti-oxidant defenses.

The good news is that we can compensate for this ongoing anti-oxidant drain. Not one of the factors listed above is entirely beyond our control, and most are subject to dramatic changes through adjustments in life-style—including, if need be, reevaluating our values, goals, and philosophy of life.

If we do our part in taking good care of ourselves and our environment, there is no good reason why nature should put any insurmountable obstacles in the way of a longer life span. True, nature does not seem interested in keeping us going for much longer than it takes to reach reproductive age. Add to that maybe another twenty years or so until our offspring, if any, also reach reproductive age. That takes no more than forty years or so. Yet nature seems to have no interest in killing us off at that stage.

In the animal kingdom, shorter life spans force prolific reproduction to ensure the survival of the species. They also help to prevent exhaustion of limited food supplies or living space in the ecological niches or habitats peculiar to such species.

This survival factor, fortunately, does not have to apply to humans. Unlike animals, human beings are not restricted to any ecological niches—we have, in fact, the widest ecological adaptability of all creatures on the planet. Eskimos can eventually adjust to the tropics; a tribe from equatorial Africa can adapt with ease, if not grace, to life in

Siberia. We have even demonstrated our ability to survive underwater (as in SeaLab) and in outer space. There is, therefore, nothing in the nature of things that would present an insurmountable barrier to the eventual extension of maximum life span for the human race.

On the practical level, there is certainly nothing to prevent us from fulfilling and even extending our own personal life span potential. All we need do for that to become a reality is apply the message of this book to ourselves: Say no to disordered nutrition and life-styles that clearly undermine our health; disavow negative, hostile, and other destructive mental attitudes and cultivate positive, life-enhancing ones; avoid, to the extent that we have control over these matters, exposure to environmental hazards and refrain from unnecessary risk taking; last but not least, commit ourselves—if for nothing more than good health insurance!—to an effective anti-oxidant program, as we have taken pains to outline in several different ways so as to accommodate differing circumstances and economic realities.

Granted, true immortality is not of the flesh but of the spirit and, as Krishnamurti has said, "that is the beauty thereof." But a happy, productive, energetic old age, the completion of a life enjoyably and productively lived, is a fountain of youth available right now. To us, that's a very real and tangible symbol of ultimate immortality.

SOURCES

1. Bailie, Ira E. "Educating the public about lifestyle and national practices" (Correspondence). *Western J. Medicine,* April 1987.
2. Watkin, D. M. "Nutrition for the Aging and the Aged." In: *Modern Nutrition in Health and Disease: Dietotherapy,* fifth ed. R. S. Goodhart and M. E. Shils, eds. Philadelphia: Lea & Febiger, 1973, p. 681.
3. Cutler, R. "Evolution of Human Longevity." In: *Advances in Pathobiology: Aging, Cancer, and Cell Membranes,* Borek, Fenoglio, and King, eds. New York: Georg Thieme Verlag, 1980.
4. Cutler, R. "Evolution of human longevity and the genetic complexity governing aging rate." *Proc. Natl. Acad. Sci. USA,* 1975; 72(11):4664–4668.
5. Sacher. "Longevity and aging in vertebrate evolution." *Bioscience,* August 1978; 28 (8): 497–501.
6. Winfree. "Resetting biological clocks." *Physics Today,* March 1975; pp. 34–39.

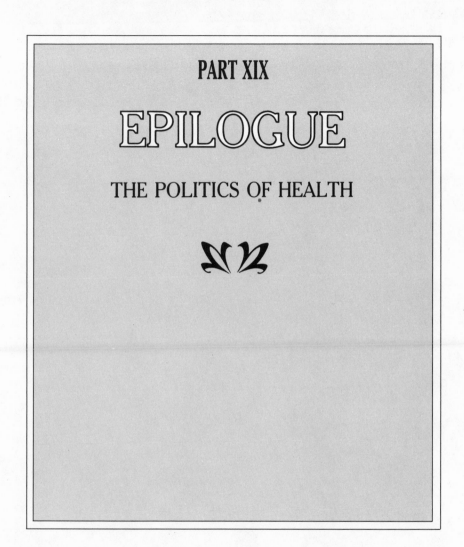

PART XIX

EPILOGUE

THE POLITICS OF HEALTH

12 We have been focusing throughout this book on the health of the individual and how to realize one's life span in a functioning body and with a sound mind. But nobody—even the most reclusive among us—lives in isolation. We live within a society. Therefore, the nature of that society has a great deal to do with our being well or sick, fulfilling our life-span potential, or the thread of our life being cut short before its time.

Obviously, the most affluent are the least affected by the social climate around them, just as they are the least affected by the physical climate in which they live. If it gets too cold in the winter, they can fly to a tropical resort, and if it gets too hot in the summer, they can just turn up the air conditioning or go to the mountains. That way, they may not get as many colds and escape the flu in winter, or avoid the effect of oppressive heat in summer.

Nor are the most affluent members of society greatly affected by the unemployment rate in the country, lack of affordable housing, skyrocketing medical costs, and inadequate or absent health insurance. But all these things do matter a great deal and affect the health of thirty million to forty million Americans who live right on or below the poverty line.

The physical and mental health of most of us is very much affected by social and economic factors. Take, for instance, unemployment. Sure, sickness and disability can ultimately result in unemployment. But, more often, the reverse is true: Unemployment or worry about unemployment produces illness, even death.

Any outpatient clinic at any major hospital can attest to the well-known medical fact that the unemployed frequently come in with typical "psychosomatic" problems like headaches, backaches, eczema, and with gastrointestinal complaints, such as peptic ulcers, gastritis, diarrhea, spastic colon, and so forth. With unemployment and financial worries, asthma attacks become more frequent and severe, stomach ulcers may start bleeding, and those who in the past had overcome recurrent disabilities suddenly suffer unexplainable relapses on losing their jobs, or under the threat of losing them. Even the spouses and children of the unemployed are known to develop more illness.

577

There is a great deal of psychological fallout from unemployment or the threat of unemployment. There may be acute anxiety attacks with heart palpitations and difficulty in breathing, sleeplessness (insomnia), chronic fatigue, lack of appetite, and, of course, depression, self-blaming, and a sense of worthlessness.

Thousands of underprivileged in the inner cities (not to mention the homeless) are sick in body and mind, and there seems to be no way out. What folly it would be to tell them that the cigarettes or the booze they are wasting their begged change on are killing them. Or to talk to them about correct nutrition, or the necessity for regular exercise. Doing so would border on obscenity—*real* obscenity.

Perhaps we can all agree that what matters is not only the health of the individual in society, but the health of society as a whole. It does matter very much because it affects us all—yes, even the most affluent. Ultimately, what good is it to be rich or superrich, never have to worry about paying the rent or meeting the mortgage payment, or how to buy food for yourself and the kids, and at the same time constantly live in fear that some half-crazed have-not will rob your home at night or stick you up in the street to get money for the next fix? It wouldn't have to happen, would it? if that person were employed rather than chronically unemployed, or if—though temporarily unemployed, as can happen in any society—he still has a decent home and hope for a better future.

We suggest that it is the priorities of our society that we have to reexamine, if the health and productive longevity of all the citizenry is the agreed-upon objective. Only if we can agree on this basic assumption will this discussion make any kind of sense and not be a total waste of time.

With these priorities in mind, we would like to start with the special nutritional and other needs of children. First, let's look at some animal studies, discussed by Dr. M. Winnick of Columbia Presbyterian Hospital in New York City. These studies show that food deprivation among animals during certain crucial periods of growth results in "aberrant behavior which persists throughout the animal's life."[1] Dr. Winnick goes on to say that these studies show further that such deprived animals engage in "less exploratory activity," overreact to adverse stimuli, and "exhibit increased emotionality." These malnourished animals do not learn as well as others, for instance, how to find their way out of a maze. And, worst of all, "this behavior pattern persists even after rehabilitation."

Let's go on to the human case: At a recent conference about the special educational problems of underprivileged children, organized by the City University of New York, D. Ernest L. Boyer, president of the Carnegie Foundation for the Advancement of Teaching, had this to say: "I am convinced that there is an absolute connection between poor nutrition among pregnant teen-agers and their children's performance in school later on."[2] And while the nutrition of underprivileged teenagers is notoriously poor, that of underprivileged mothers is not much better.

The poor educational performance record, the high rate of emotional disturbance, and the appalling school drop-out rate among these youngsters, and their equally known propensity to drift into drugs and crime, are too distressingly familiar. We would like to tell you, however, that there are societies—admittedly with more manageable social problems than ours because their populations are smaller—where this vicious process is prevented from developing right at the start.

One of these societies is in Scandinavia, where we have spent a great deal of time, and which is about the only place on earth where enlightened social policies are even thinkable. In Denmark, Norway, and Sweden, prenatal care is writ large (it is for everyone!), and the preschool child's physical and mental health, as well as its nutrition, are considered the first priorities of organized society. In West Germany and The Netherlands, similar policies prevail.

From two months before the birth of a baby, a specialized public health nurse starts making regular visits to poorer mothers, not only to give advice, but also to provide for material help, if needed. In Denmark, even when the baby is only two months old (eight months in Sweden), if the mother is working or cannot properly take care of it, the child is promptly admitted into a child-care center. And at that center, it is not the families who can pay the most, or who are better connected, but, as Fred M. Hechinger pointed out in an article in *The New York Times* (August 31, 1988), those who are the neediest, single parents, immigrants and political refugees, are given preference.

Fred M. Hechinger stresses that such social policies in Scandinavia are considered anything but "applied communism" there; as Mr. Hechinger says, "Scandinavians despise Soviet-style regimentation and any infringement of freedom." And well they might, for the Soviet system of health care in general, and maternity care in particular, is nothing short of scandalous, as Mr. Gorbachev himself admits.

Life expectancy in the Soviet Union has declined, and mortality rates both for infants and for the total population are climbing. Murray Feshbach, an expert on the Soviet Union at the Georgetown University Center for Population Research in Washington, D.C., points out, "No other industrialized country in the postwar period has experienced a sustained falloff in even one of these indicators."[3,4]

According to the same reliable source, the infant-mortality rate, kept secret since 1974, was recently revealed to have risen from a low of 22.9 in 1971 to 26.0 in 1985. Professor Feshbach says, "That is 2.5 times higher than the United States rate and ranks the U.S.S.R. 50th in the world, just behind Barbados."

There are more reasons than one for this sorry state of affairs in

Soviet medicine. Health care workers, including physicians, are poorly paid and, as might be expected under these conditions, hopelessly corrupt. As anyone who knows the Soviet Union well will tell you, there is a bribe price to be paid for any special service in the hospital, even to get the sheets on the bed changed, or to have any bed at all. If you have to have an operation, you'd better make some amicable financial arrangements with the surgeon, or you may find yourself long enough on the waiting list that you'll need a coffin more than an operation.

Clearly, these conditions are a hundred times worse than what can, in all fairness, be said to exist in our own badly flawed health care system. This is not to say that it, too, does not desperately need long-overdue reform. Every day of the year, people are dying from curable diseases because they cannot afford the expensive treatments. Others lose their homes and their last savings to pay for treatments they cannot afford.

Tens of millions of Americans are, at this moment, not covered by any kind of health insurance. A recently published book, *Medical Care, Medical Costs,* * by Dr. Rashi Fein, a professor of medical economics at Harvard Medical School, analyzes the American medical dilemma. Interestingly enough, Dr. Fein, a highly regarded expert and critic of the present system, does not advocate national health insurance—at least not in its classical form—much less some kind of "socialized medicine."

What Dr. Fein favors instead—and his approach appears to us the most reasonable proposal to date—is federally mandated universal health insurance coverage for everyone, but with some built-in budget control and sufficient flexibility to allow for variations in its application, depending on the differing situations among the states. Dr. Fein believes such health insurance would preserve our competitive medical system while curbing its excesses.

The philosophy underlying Dr. Fein's proposal is remarkably close to our own, which, as the reader will recall, is based on a recognition that if the physical or mental health of one segment of society is put in jeopardy by social injustices or neglect, we are all ultimately bound to suffer the consequences. Dr. Fein states: "The health of others affects our psychological well-being," and, as we pointed out earlier, it often also affects our physical well-being and very existence. All ethical considerations aside, it is no more than in our own enlightened self-interest that we voluntarily make ourselves our brother's keepers.

There is also the purely humane side to the problem. Let Dr. Fein speak to this point: "Decent people—and we are decent people—are offended by unnecessary pain and suffering." He arrives at the inevita-

* R. Fein, *Medical Care, Medical Costs: The Search for a Health Insurance Policy* (Boston, Mass.: Harvard University Press, 1988).

ble conclusion at which any decent person will ultimately arrive: It is unacceptable that relief from pain and suffering—to which we would add the enjoyment of good health and longevity—should be "available only to those who can pay for it out of their own means."

It is also imperative that such a new approach to universal health insurance definitely not be modeled on our present insurance system (where it exists at all). As pointed out by Dr. Bernie S. Siegel—surgeon and author of *Love, Medicine, and Miracles,* to which we referred in our discussion of the mind-body connection in diseases like cancer—our present health and life insurance systems "reward illness by penalizing those who take care of themselves." If insurance premiums were based on a person's commitment to health, Dr. Siegel suggests, there would be considerably more incentive for people to take better care of themselves (see our chapter on this subject, pages 29–40). "We should establish certain basic requirements," Dr. Siegel says, "controlling weight, not smoking, and so on. When these are met for a minimum fee, all medical expenses would be covered."

Under a truly equitable health insurance system, those who refuse to take better care of themselves would pay more for their coverage. Such an insurance system makes eminently good sense. What is strange is that it should not have been put into practice long ago.

A great deal more revision of current thinking on health care matters seems called for: This country is well ahead of others in developing sophisticated life-support systems for the terminally ill. Many thoughtful people, including not a few physicians, feel that some dying patients are kept "alive" far too long by artificial feeding and other life-support systems—especially if their families can pay for this care. Sometimes, for legal or other reasons, even the indigent are kept on costly and, more often than not, utterly futile life supports. Is it not legitimate to ask whether the time and the material resources for such extravagant health care should be lavished rather on those, rich or poor, for whom there is still reasonable hope for recovery?

This brings us to the whole problem of preventive health care. As an editorial in *The Lancet,* the official journal of the medical profession in England, puts it: ". . . we are in danger of devoting so much time and so many resources to rescuing the lives of people who have become ill that we fail to pay proper attention to removing the reasons why they fall ill in the first place."[5]

Very true. But can we, in all fairness, lay this societal problem solely at the feet of the medical profession? Frankly, we do not think so. Physicians in private practice are generally overworked, trying to deal with the acute diseases of their patients; or, in hospital settings, they are mainly concerned with emergency situations. In addition, these days many hospital physicians are literally driven beyond their physical and emotional limits by the ever-increasing number of AIDS patients they must care for. There is precious little room, under these conditions, to worry about preventive health care.

Also, our present insurance system, with its stipulated fees for strictly therapeutic services, does not provide reimbursement for preventive health counseling or preventive health care. Even if the system were changed—as it should and, we hope, will be—it may not be practical or desirable that physicians' time and skills should be squandered on services that other health professionals might render as well or better. Perhaps a new class of specially trained preventive health care professionals, knowledgeable in the basics of medicine, nutrition, and exercise physiology, ought to be created. Such health professionals might work in private practice, some might team up with individual physicians or groups of physicians, while others might work within the framework of private industry. Here might be a practical solution to a problem that until now has been considered only in philosophical and critical terms, but without the slightest prospect for actual change.

Needless to say, there ought to be more emphasis on preventive health education from as early as kindergarten throughout later education on all levels. And such education, to be most effective, must be supported by appropriate action and example in school and university cafeterias and by the constant encouragement of health-promoting life-styles. It is intolerable that 26 percent of eighth graders and 38 percent of tenth graders in our schools were found, by a national survey conducted in 1987, to have had "five or more [alcoholic] drinks on one occasion in the two weeks preceding the survey."[6] Nor is it comforting to know that "at least 100,000 elementary school children report getting drunk on a weekly basis," according to the American Council for Drug Education. Needless to say, there is far too much cigarette smoking among teenagers, nor has the message that marijuana is a very dangerous and addictive drug really gotten through to this age group.

While findings such as these are a clear indication that health consciousness in the home is largely absent and that health education in the school has failed, the blame is not with the individual family, nor even with the school. If we want to be perfectly candid, it is rather the result of a split in public consciousness and the consequent failure of public policy. In short, it is no more than the expression of our ambivalence, as a society—of all societies—about our two favorite social drugs, alcohol and nicotine.

Take, for instance, the U.S. government's attitude about smoking tobacco. On the one hand, the current surgeon general, Dr. C. Everett Koop, a public servant of rare courage and candor, tells our nation in unmistakably clear terms that smoking kills. On the other hand, another branch of the government is subsidizing American tobacco growers instead of advising and helping them *not* to grow tobacco. It's as if the Colombian or Peruvian governments were subsidizing farmers in the Andes to grow coca leaves rather than encouraging them to plant alternative crops, as our government is urging them to do. In either case the trouble is that virtually no other crop would give these North American or South American farmers, on the small acreage available, the kind of high and secure income that is possible only with tobacco or coca leaves. The plain fact that governments will therefore have to face sooner or later is that there are simply no "alternative crops" for tobacco or coca leaves, unless heavy subsidies are paid for *not* growing them.

In addition, there is, for the United States, the issue of being against smoking cigarettes here while promoting the export of American cigarettes to other countries, notably Japan and China, to improve our negative foreign trade balance. Some are comparing this situation to the nineteenth-century dispute between the British and the Chinese governments over the importation of opium into Canton and Macao, and they called it the "new Opium War." Without wanting to go so far ourselves, we can only agree again with Dr. Koop's lone voice of conscience in Washington's bureaucratic wilderness on this issue. "I don't think," he says, "that we as citizens can continue to tolerate exporting disease, disability, and death." If our government had what we like to call a "politics of health," it would undoubtedly have to adopt Dr. Koop's position, and policy decisions would have to be made on that basis.

If countries had a genuine "politics of health," there could be little dispute over the necessity to stop production of acid rain that is already killing the forests and lakes of Europe, and is about to do the same in the United States and Canada—and enact the necessary legislating to do so *now*.

The same applies to the threat posed by the greenhouse effect and the destruction of the protective ozone layer in the stratosphere through certain volatile industrial chemicals, automobile emissions, smoke—as from the large-scale burning of trees in the Amazon basin—and so forth. True, there is still some scientific controversy or uncertainty at this moment whether these are really the actual causes of the problem, or whether the thinning of the ozone layer is due to atmospheric conditions in the stratosphere over which we have no control. Be that as it may—and in view of the most serious, realistic threat that the greenhouse effect would have on all life on this planet—should a "politics of health" not err, if need be, on the side of caution and shouldn't we begin *right now* to take the necessary measures to prevent such a global disaster, assuming we can do anything about it at all?

We could go on and on—about the need for more protective clean water and clean air acts; about checking more seriously into indoor air pollution and workplace illness caused by radon gas from the ground, carbon monoxide from underground garages, and infectious diseases that spread through air-conditioning and ventilation systems in hermetically sealed office buildings, factories, schools, and even hospitals, and about many other such threats to public health. However, we want to make one more point, the threat to our planet and our lives by overpopulation—still the most taboo subject of our time.

If we really wanted to face the facts, we would soon discover that overpopulation is at the root of many of the other problems we have just touched upon. Briefly, here are just a few representative examples from recent news items: General Jaruzelski of Poland was recently asked why the Polish economy was in so much worse shape than that of East Germany, and why were living standards in Poland so much lower than those there. The general thought for a moment and then reminded his questioner that East Germany's population had remained stable since 1951 at about seventeen million, while Poland's had swelled in that period from twenty-three million to thirty-eight million.[7]

We see the same situation reflected in the youth riots in Algeria. People are protesting high food prices and widespread unemployment there, and they are no doubt justified in their discontent. But few will realize the grim statistics at the root of Algeria's economic problems: More than 50 percent of Algerians are younger than twenty, and the population has soared from 9.4 million in 1954 to 22.7 million.[8] A "politics of health" would certainly have to address the problem of that country's exploding birth rate, if any basic improvements in the economy are to be realized. The same could, and must of course, be said about many other countries.

In sub-Saharan Africa, matters are very much worse than any of the examples thus far given. Millions die every year of malnutrition, lack of medical care, and—civil wars. And what is the most basic root cause of all this? Again, overpopulation. As *The New York Times* of May 19, 1987, reported, the annual growth rate of the population in Africa south of the Sahara is 3.2 percent, which makes it the world's highest. And predictions are that this galloping population growth rate will not only continue, but actually rise well into the next century. This will mean Africa's population will double approximately to one billion by the year 2000. Wouldn't a "politics of health" practiced on an international scale, as implemented by the United Nations, be forced to face this serious problem, rather than ignore the whole matter of population control simply because it is "not politic," or "politically unfeasible"?

The same points can of course be made—and with the same urgency—for the Indian subcontinent and large parts of Southeast Asia, as well as for Central and South America. It therefore ought to be fairly obvious that if governments do not soon stop putting Band-Aids on economic problems that can only be solved by determined efforts at population control, we won't have to worry about acid rain and the greenhouse effect anymore. We'll have bred ourselves unthinkingly out of existence even before these calamities can do us in.

If there was ever a time for a global "politics of health," it would be now. Such an approach also has to recognize that in a technological age, and with dwindling unrenewable global resources, international conflicts will have to be settled by other means than warfare. If we may be allowed to close a discussion of as serious a matter as this with a quip, we would like to say that for a "politics of health," war is the ultimate health hazard.

SOURCES

1. Winnick, M. *Malnutrition and Brain Development.* New York: Oxford University Press, Inc., 1976, p. 114.
2. *The New York Times,* December 1, 1987.
3. *The Wall Street Journal,* August 18, 1987.
4. Ryan, M. "Life expectancy and mortality data from the Soviet Union." *Brit. Med. J.,* 1988; 296:1513–1515.
5. Anon. "An Apple a Day." *Lancet,* 1988; 2:408.
6. *The New York Times,* August 10, 1988.
7. Tagliabue, J. "Jaruzelski Encounters His Complaining People." *The New York Times,* October 8, 1988.
8. Delaney, P. "Algiers Riot Toll Put at Dozens Dead and 900 Hurt." *The New York Times,* October 8, 1988.

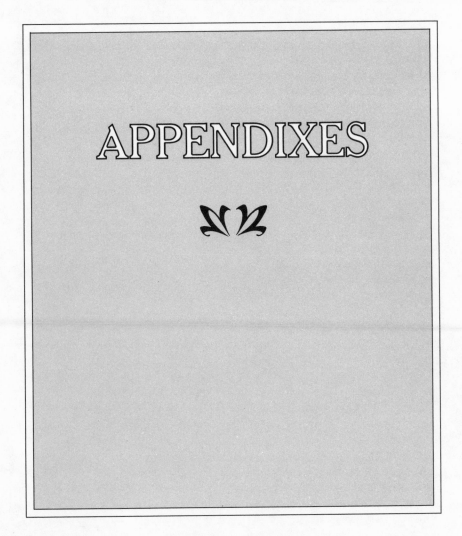

APPENDIXES

APPENDIX A
HOW TO IMPLEMENT OPTION 2

You can put together the Full Menu, Short Order, or Short-Short Order of our anti-oxidant program by using carefully chosen individual micronutrients from any one of several recommended suppliers. We suggest that you take these micronutrients in capsule form, since tablets or pills have too many binding agents to hold them together, and often have lacquers in their coatings as well. On the other hand, if you do not use the Health Maintenance Programs (HMP) Performance Packs or Ascorbic-B capsules (identical to our Short-Short Order) taking the required additional capsules can be hard on your stomach, which has to cope with all those extra gelatin capsules.

VITAMIN C

To reduce the number of capsules you take with this option, we recommend to take the most basic and also the most voluminous anti-oxidant, ascorbic acid (vitamin C) in loose powder form rather than in capsules.

While vitamin C is quite acidic, somewhat like lemon juice, it does not taste unpleasant at all. Eberhard takes a level teaspoon of it first thing every morning before breakfast and washes it down with a few sips of water. You can also dissolve it first in water and drink it that way.

You can take vitamin C either as a straight crystalline powder, or as a mixture of 75 percent ascorbic acid and 25 percent calcium ascorbate, a buffered form of C, to reduce the acidity.

One level teaspoon of crystalline ascorbic acid equals approximately 6,000 milligrams (6 grams) of C, and one level teaspoon of calcium ascorbate equals about 4,250 milligrams (4½ grams) of C, plus about 1,500 milligrams (1½ grams) of calcium. If you prefer the straight crystalline vitamin C, be sure to get your calcium in some other form.

Most health-food stores carry several varieties of powdered vitamin C, but you can also get it in more economical bulk form from Vitamin Research Products. Twinlab offers a well-buffered form in their Ascorbate-C powder, which also includes the entire bioflavonoid complex (see our discussion of "Bioflavonoids: The Other Half of the Vitamin C Equation?" pages 105–107). Each teaspoon of Twinlab's Ascorbate-C powder gives you 2,000 milligrams of pure ascorbic acid (vitamin C), which corresponds exactly to the individual dosage of vitamin C on the Demopoulos spectrum (our Menu); so 3 to 5 teaspoons would give you 6,000 to 10,000 milligrams, respectively, for the day. That is equal to the minimum and maximum recommended dosages, respectively, for that key anti-oxidant on our program.

VITAMIN E

We prefer that you take this fat-soluble vitamin and anti-oxidant as pure *liquid* dl-alpha tocopheryl acetate (see our detailed discussion earlier in the book). Health Maintenance Programs and the Solgar Company offer it as such, and HMP also makes it in a soft-gel capsule combined with beta-carotene, for which it fulfills the simultaneous function of preservative, since it provides a lipoidal medium.

You can, however, take your vitamin E under this option as straight powder, using Vitamin Research Products (VRP) or Twinlab as suppliers, or you may use Twinlab's Hypo-E Caps.

Still another alternative is using the VRP combination capsule of 200 I.U. vitamin E with 2 milligrams of octacosanol (a substance reputed to be an "energizer," but we cannot be sure of its efficacy at this writing). The 200 I.U. in the capsule is twice the amount of each serving on our Menu (100 I.U.) so take these capsules so that they equal the total amount for the day.

In general, we prefer liquid dl-alpha tocopheryl acetate because the dry-base form oxidizes more quickly.

GLUTATHIONE

If you can possibly afford it, we urge you to take this triple amino acid and powerful anti-oxidant. It is available from various suppliers, but we favor the 100-milligram capsules from HMP or VRP because the easily degradable glutathione is put up in these preparations with four times its amount of ascorbic acid, which keeps it in its reduced, fresh state.

BETA-CAROTENE

If you're taking the vitamin E/beta-carotene capsules from HMP, you're all set. Otherwise, there are several alternatives. Twinlab offers Carotene Caps, each of which contains 15 milligrams of beta-carotene, the dose recommended on our Menu. We also like Twinlab's Marine Carotene, derived from certain single-cell algae. One "pearl" of this product is equivalent to the dose on our Menu (but it is more expensive than the Carotene Caps).

VITAMIN B CO-FACTORS

Twinlab makes 250-milligram B_5, 100-milligram B_1, 100-milligram niacin (B_3), and 100-milligram B_2 capsules. Their sublingual 400-microgram B_{12} tablet is exactly the right dosage prescribed on our Menu.

Since the amount of B_2 (riboflavin) in the Twinlab capsule is a bit too generous, we suggest taking only one capsule per day, or skip it altogether, unless you are a vegetarian.

CALCIUM

As for a good calcium supplement, aside from HMP's Calcium-D capsules (250-milligram calcium carbonate plus 125 I.U. vitamin D), there is now a very interesting liquid calcium plus vitamin D_3 product from Twinlab called Cal-Quick (½ tsp. equals 250-milligrams of calcium and 150 I.U. of vitamin D_3).

Still another way of getting calcium is to take three Tums per day. The best way to take Tums (or any calcium product) is right after the anti-oxidants and vitamin co-factors, some of which are rather acidic, so the calcium carbonate can work as a buffering agent.

VITAMIN D₃ (ERGOCALCIFEROL)

If you don't use HMP's Performance Packs, which include a calcium-D_3 supplement, or HMP's calcium-D_3 capsules, or Twinlab's Cal-Quick, or another calcium preparation with built-in vitamin D feature, don't take vitamin D_3 separately. It only serves to make the calcium more available, and is not absolutely essential (you can just take straight calcium, as in Tums).

We have offered the above suggestions for implementing option 2 merely as examples of several convenient and safe ways to do it. This does not mean that the products we suggest you use are the only ones worth taking.

On the other hand, we have taken great pains to check out all products recommended here. We know they are pure and safe, and that they offer approximately the right dosages for our anti-oxidant program. Even though there are undoubtedly other products of equal excellence, we suggest that you stick as closely as possible to the ones listed here—if for no other reason than playing it the safest and most convenient way possible.

APPENDIX B

HOW TO IMPLEMENT OPTION 3

12 If you choose option 3, making your own micronutrient powder mix, we suggest that you do not incorporate vitamin B_{12} or beta-carotene into the mix; for the average person, the procedures are just a bit too cumbersome. Using ready-made B_{12} and beta-carotene will of course bring up your costs, but savings will still be substantial.

To prevent the various ingredients from oxidizing and degrading chemically, prepare only enough powder mix for a week at a time. And since some micronutrients—glutathione, for instance—are also highly light-sensitive, your week's supply of powder mix should be placed in an opaque glass jar that isn't much larger than the quantity of powder. The less air space on top, the less oxidation.

We must warn you that the powder mix doesn't qualify as gourmet fare—in fact, it tastes terrible. However, we know quite a few dedicated life-extenders with limited budgets who take the mix either by the teaspoon, or mixed into applesauce or a nonacidic fruit juice.

To get around the nasty taste problem, it's best to encapsulate the powder mix yourself, something that's easily done at home with inexpensive devices offered by some suppliers (for example, Vitamin Research Products). Because the powder oxidizes less when it's in capsules, you can prepare a whole month's supply at a time. You can even put little pouches of Sorbit, a drying agent, into the bottles, just as commercial manufacturers do. (These bottles are available from a number of micronutrient suppliers, including Vitamin Research Products, as well as photographic supply houses.) Why put up with a bad-tasting mix when it takes only a small effort to put it into capsules and keep it fresh much longer?

You will find that vitamin C powder (either pure, crystalline ascorbic acid or calcium ascorbate) is much more palatable than the rest of the micronutrients on the Menu. There is therefore no advantage to encapsulating vitamin C and you gain an advantage by not having to take so many capsules.

Most health-food stores carry several forms of powdered vitamin C, but it is available in more economical bulk form from Vitamin Research Products (VRP). Twinlab offers a well-buffered vitamin C in its Ascorbate-C powder, which also includes the entire bioflavonoid complex. Each teaspoon of this product gives you 2,000 milligrams of pure ascorbic acid (vitamin C), which corresponds exactly to the individual dosage of the Demopoulos spectrum (our Menu); so 3 to 5 teaspoons would give you 6,000 to 10,000 milligrams, respectively, for the day. That is exactly equal to the minimum and maximum recommended dosages, respectively.

Here are some other helpful hints: You will recall from our discussion of option 2 that VRP supplies detailed information on how to make your own powder mix. The only additional information you might find useful is this: To make just enough mix for the week, multiply the amount of each nutrient per serving (as listed on the Menu) by the number of times per day you intend to take the whole combination. You will definitely want to take your micronutrients at least three times a day with your regular meals; so, if you want to make a week's supply, you first have to multiply the amount of the nutrient by 3 then multiply that figure by 7.

Let's take an example: You want to get the right amount of calcium pantothenate (vitamin B_5) for the week. The Menu calls for 240 milligrams per serving. Multiplying 240 by 3 gives you 720 milligrams per day. Multiplying 720 by 7 equals 5,040 milligrams, the total amount you need weekly.

Follow this same procedure for the other B vitamins (with the exception of those discussed earlier), and you have your own economical vitamin/anti-oxidant mix.

The last step, which is optional, is to put the mix into No. 0-size capsules. Then divide the total number of filled capsules by 7 to get your daily quota. Dividing the daily quota by 3 will give you the number of capsules you need to take per meal. (The one or two odd capsules can be taken between meals.)

With these suggestions and Vitamin Research Products' detailed instructions, you're on the road to putting yourself and your family onto our anti-oxidant program in the most economical manner possible. It all sounds a bit complicated, but don't let that discourage you. We personally know many life-extenders who have been happily using this money-saving method for several years. As for us, if we had the choice between making our own mix or being without any anti-oxidants, we'd know exactly what to do!

APPENDIX C
LIST OF SUPPLIERS

HEALTH MAINTENANCE PROGRAMS, INC.
7 Westchester Plaza
Elmsford, NY 10523
Phone: inside New York State: (914) 592-3155
(toll-free) outside New York State: 1-800-362-8673

The top of the list are the Performance Packs, which in three regular-sized and one tiny soft-gel capsule, contain the whole spectrum of anti-oxidants and vitamin co-factors as shown on our full micronutrient Menu (page 59). Recommended dosage: 3 to 5 packs per day.

HMP's economical Ascorbic-B capsules contain the same micronutrients (800 milligrams of vitamin C and all the B vitamins) as the Performance Packs, except for the vitamin E, beta-carotene, and expensive glutathione. Recommended dosage: 6 to 8 capsules per day.

Calcium Health Packets: same formula as the Performance Packs, but have only one Ascorbic-B capsule instead of two (contain also the full 50 milligrams of glutathione). In addition to 125 I.U. of cholecalciferol-D_3, as in the Performance Packs, the Calcium Health Packets contain 400 milligrams of calcium carbonate instead of 250 milligrams of calcium carbonate. Particularly suited for postmenopausal women. Recommended dosage: 3 to 5 packets per day.

Calcium Endurance Packs: same as the Calcium Health Packets, but *without* glutathione, hence more economical. Extra high in calcium (500 milligrams of calcium carbonate plus 250 I.U. of cholecalciferol-D$_3$. For "moderately paced adults" with special needs for calcium.

Endurance Packs: exactly the same as the Performance Packs, but *without* glutathione, hence more economical. Recommended dosage: 3 to 5 packets per day.

Our recommendation: Take 3 to 5 Performance Packs per day if you can possibly afford it. It's the Rolls-Royce formula of anti-oxidants and vitamin co-factors.

An economical alternative that still gives you some glutathione, pure liquid vitamin E, and beta-carotene: take at least 1 or 2 Performance Packs per day and fill in the full quota with 4 to 6 Ascorbic-B capsules during the rest of the day.

Health Maintenance Programs (HMP) also offers the following products:

Superkids: an excellent formulation with all the water-soluble anti-oxidants, vitamins, and minerals in medically correct dosages for children two to twelve years of age. Dosage: for children from two to four years: 1 tablet per day; for children over four: 2 tablets per day.

Seniors: especially formulated spectrum of anti-oxidants, vitamins, calcium, and magnesium in chewable tablets or powder form for older people who find it difficult to swallow capsules, or prefer not to be as highly energized as with the other preparations. Dosage: 1 tablet or 1 packet of powder at breakfast and 1 in midafternoon.

For Two: "Scientifically calculated, for pregnant and lactating women, to help provide the extra amounts of nutrients around the clock for mother and child." Dosage: 1 with breakfast and 1 at bedtime.

HMP also offers the following: Glutathione-C capsules, containing 50 milligrams of pure glutathione, protected from degradation by 200 milligrams of crystalline vitamin C. Now also available as energy boosters in capsules containing 250 milligrams of glutathione (expensive, but worth it!) plus 750 milligrams of vitamin C.

Calcium-D: bone-promoting formulation; each capsule contains 250 milligrams of calcium carbonate, plus 125 I.U. of cholecalciferol-D$_3$.

Carotene-E: pure beta-carotene in pure vitamin E. We highly recommend this product as a supplement to the Ascorbic-B capsules (1 to 3 soft-gel capsules per day).

Pure-E: pure liquid vitamin E (which we consider the best), as capsules or liquid. We feel taking ½ to 1 teaspoon of vitamin E in this form at bedtime greatly improves the quality of sleep (also improves the appearance of skin and hair).

TWIN LABORATORIES, INC.
2120 Smithtown Avenue
Ronkonkoma, NY 11779
Phone: (516) 467-3140

Twin Laboratories sells its products mainly through health-food stores. In Appendix A we explained how you can put together the Demopoulos spectrum of anti-oxidants and vitamin co-factors, using individual Twinlab or Vitamin Research Products products. Therefore, we will add only some additional Twinlab products (for Vitamin Research Products, see opposite page).

Twinlab has recently come out with a new formulation of anti-oxidants, vitamin co-factors, minerals, and trace elements* called MaxiLIFE. It contains a high percentage of ascorbic acid, the "regular," water-soluble form of vitamin C, plus a little (76 milligrams) of ascorbyl palmitate, the fat-soluble form of vitamin C—a good idea, we feel, since it might help to quench free radicals in lipid (fat) containing body tissues. It also contains some citrus bioflavonoids in order to supplement the vitamin C.

It also provides a good level of mixed tocopherols (vitamin E, and a fair amount of glutathione), bolstered by a nice dash (157 milligrams) of cysteine, which should enhance the free-radical scavenging capacity of the glutathione.

In its present form it is especially suitable for those with relatively high cholesterol levels, since this MaxiLIFE mixture is very high in niacin (B_3). By the same token, it presents somewhat of a problem to people who are sensitive to the "niacin flush." (We are told that in the spring of 1989, Twinlab is going to offer an alternative MaxiLIFE version with less niacin.)

Twinlab also offers an excellent 500-milligram time-release niacin capsule which makes the niacin gradually available over a seven-hour period. By taking the niacin in the time-release form, there is less chance for the "niacin flush" and you also avoid getting sleepy, a nice side effect at bedtime but not so good when you need to be firing on all cylinders during the day.

We also personally take Twinlab's liquid sugar and sodium-free potassium-magnesium supplement Liqui-K Plus, as well as either its Emulsified Norwegian Cod Liver Oil or its Emulsified Omega-3 fish oil concentrate, in which all vitamin A and D has been removed to prevent any possibility of overdosing on these fat-soluble vitamins.

Other Twinlab products we recommend include its Chromium-

---

* Dr. Demopoulos does not believe that there is any need for extra minerals or trace elements, aside from calcium, except for children and older people. His formulation for children, Superkids, by Health Maintenance Programs, therefore includes a medically dosaged mineral mix of iron, copper, zinc, and manganese. Likewise, his formulation for the elderly (Seniors) includes some magnesium as well as calcium.

GFT (Glucose Tolerance Factor) capsules, especially in case of diabetes, and its yeast-free sodium selenite capsules. (But do *not* take any additional selenium if you are using MaxiLIFE or any other formulation that already contains this trace element.)

For those who need a little help in staying regular—something that should never be a problem on our kind of diet—or who wish to control their appetite, we can recommend Twinlab's Fibersol, a soluble fiber mixture of psyllium seed husks (which, incidentally, have recently been found to lower cholesterol), guar gum, and apple pectin.

VITAMIN RESEARCH PRODUCTS
2044 Old Middlefield Way
Mountain View, CA 94043
Phone: (toll-free) outside California: 1-800-541-1623
                  inside California: 1-800-541-8536

In option 3 (see pages 63–64) we have been telling you how to put together the Demopoulos spectrum of anti-oxidants and vitamin cofactors in the most economical way by making your own micronutrient mix using bulk powders from Vitamin Research Products (VRP).

In addition, we can recommend some of this supplier's individual anti-oxidants and vitamins in capsule form as alternatives to Twinlab's, if you want to put the Demopoulos spectrum together that way (see option 2, pages 62–63). You can use VRP's crystalline ascorbic acid (vitamin C) powder, or a mixture of water-soluble ascorbic acid and lipid (fat)-soluble ascorbyl palmitate powder for option 2 or 3.

Also recommended is VRP's economical water-soluble (hydrate) L-Cysteine HCL powder (Code No. 413.1), a reasonable substitute for the costly glutathione. As an alternative to Twinlab's liquid potassium-magnesium supplement, VRP offers EM3 capsules, containing magnesium and potassium orotate together with the enzyme bromelain (Code No. 701.1).

VRP's alternative to Twinlab's Fibersol is Fiber-Rite capsules or powder. This is an excellent mixture of apple pectin, cholesterol-lowering oat bran, and guar gum, plus some zinc, calcium carbonate, magnesium, and potassium. Once again, we would like to emphasize that if you follow our nutritional guidelines, you will hardly ever need fiber supplements. On the other hand, well-formulated supplements like Fiber-Rite can be of great help to bedridden or very sedentary people, and to some elderly.

You can buy pure fructose in bulk from VRP (Code No. 670.2), which is more economical than buying it packaged from supermarkets and health-food stores. One kilogram (about 2 pounds) will cost about the same as ½ pound of store-bought packaged fructose.

Other food items from VRP that we like are a powder of freeze-dried cruciferous vegetables (cabbage, broccoli, Brussels sprouts, and cauliflower) (Code No. E110.0). Of course, it is better to eat fresh vegetables, but if you are one of those many busy people who don't always have time to go vegetable shopping and then clean and cook them, these vegetables come in handy as second-best for putting into soups, salads, casseroles, and so forth.

We can also recommend VRP's CV seasoning (Code No. E111.1), prepared from freeze-dried vegetables, but more concentrated than the above-mentioned products. This is another way to cut down on salt and provide more flavor to many dishes.

In discussing option 3 (pages 63–64), we mentioned that VRP offers empty capsules, encapsulating machines, a handy and economical measuring scale, measuring spoons, and other items you will find useful if you want to make your own mix from bulk raw materials. VRP provides detailed instructions on how to prepare your own anti-oxidant–vitamin mix.

VRP distributes excellent portable, table-top water purifiers, one made by the Brita Company, and the other one by Waterboy, as well as replacement filters for both. We actually take our portable water filter with us wherever we go. We wouldn't be without it, since so much of our municipal drinking water is contaminated, not to mention the unpleasant chlorine taste of unfiltered water.

OTHER RECOMMENDED ITEMS Since we are talking about water purifiers, if you want to go all out and are willing to spend a few hundred dollars to install a truly ideal, permanent water purifier, you should get in touch with the top experts in this field: Aqua-Kleen, Inc., 5715 Pacific Highway East, Tacoma, WA 98424. Phone: (toll free) 1-800-426-7777 or (209) 922-2442.

Another very helpful item to keep your neck from being sore in the morning, is a sculpted, comfortable therapeutic pillow that helps your neck and shoulder muscles relax during sleep. We understand there are several manufacturers making such pillows, but we have been buying ours from: The Pillow Company, 1307 Fifth Avenue South, Hopkins, MN 55343. Phone: (toll-free) 1-800-328-4827.

We also referred earlier to former Pittsburgh psychiatrist Dr. Leonard Schwartz's specially sculpted and rubber-cushioned hand weights called Heavyhands, for running (or brisk walking). The reason we like them is that our leg and thigh muscles get more of a workout than our arm muscles and upper torso. So, if you use these handweights when you run or walk, you will get a double benefit from the exercise. Many sporting-goods stores carry Heavyhands; they can also be ordered direct from: Sport Club, 615 W. Johnson Avenue, Building 3, Cheshire, CT 06410. Phone: 1-800-345-3610. Also available is a book:

L. Schwartz, *The Heavyhands Walking Books,* Panaerobics Press, 1988, 5526 Northumberland Street, Pittsburgh, PA 15217.

We also like a portable gadget called the Bicep Machine, which is cleverly designed to do just what its name says, strengthen your biceps, upper arm, and shoulder muscles by a combination of external rotation and extension of the wrists during exercise. It has three different spring settings so you can start building up your strength gradually, depending on what shape your arm muscles are in. The only trouble with this exercise machine is its price (about $60.00), but we think it's worth it. It is distributed by: The Bicep Machine, P.O. Box 187, Brookville, OH 45309. Phone (toll-free): 1-800-342-6451; from Ohio: 1-800-223-3103.

RECOMMENDED ADDITIONAL READING

Micronutrients

Hendler, Sheldon S., M.D., Ph.D. *The Complete Guide to Anti-aging Nutrients.* New York: Simon & Schuster (A Fireside Book), 1986.

Pearson, D., and Shaw, S. *Life Extension.* New York: Warner Books, 1982.

Both these books are excellent, quick-reference works that we urge any serious life-extender to purchase. With regard to *Life Extension,* we must call attention to the fact that while these authors recommend certain substances—for example, single amino acids like tryptophan, phenylalanine, argine, ornithine, and L-Dopa—Dr. Demopoulos and we consider them hazardous. We therefore urge you to use only the basic Demopoulos spectrum, possibly supplement it with certain minerals and trace elements (as are contained in Twinlab's new MaxiLIFE, or as are suggested by Dr. Hendler). Aside from these provisos, you will find *Life Extension* a constantly valuable source of information on life extension.

Pauling, Linus, *How to Live Longer and Feel Better.* New York: W. H. Freeman & Company, 1986.

The emphasis in this book is, as you may expect from Dr. Pauling, on vitamin C. However, he also discusses the role of other micronutrients in promoting human health and longevity. Dr. Pauling's advice on diet differs from ours in that he seems more concerned about there being too much sugar in the diet than fat, that he does not consider milk and cheeses as hazardous as Dr. Demopoulos and we do, and that he seems to be too fond of juicy steaks to appreciate the delights of our vegetarian-and-seafood oriented nutrition. Aside from these quibbles, we think you will find this book by a Nobel Prize-winning scientist fascinating and informative.

Medical Matters

McDougall, John A., M.D. *A Challenging Second Opinion.* Piscataway, NJ: New Century Publishers, Inc., 1985.

As we said previously in the main text, we can only urge you to purchase this inexpensive paperback, which is full of easily comprehended medical information on alternative treatments for many serious ailments, including cancer, diabetes, and kidney disease. The author is a strict vegetarian, and therefore differs from our beliefs in that he does not accept fish and other seafood, while we do. Although this is a small point of difference between us, we regret the fact that he does not include micronutrient supplements in his otherwise excellent medical advice. Nonetheless, we believe this unpretentious book belongs in the library of anyone who wants to stay or get well.

Diet and Nutrition

Pritikin, N., with P. M. McGrady, Jr., *The Pritikin Program for Diet and Exercise.* New York: Grossett & Dunlap, 1979.

Pritikin, N. *The Pritikin Permanent Weight-Loss Manual.* New York: Grosset & Dunlap, Inc., 1981.

Pritikin, N. *The Pritikin Promise: 28 Days to a Longer, Healthier Life.* New York: Pocket Books (Simon & Schuster), 1985.

Grenoble, P. B. *Pritikin People.* New York: Berkley Brooks, 1986.

We consider the books by the late Nathan Pritikin absolutely essential for anyone seriously interested in maintaining good health and following a more sensible diet. We must, however, advise our readers of two important differences between Mr. Pritikin's and our approach to diet in general and to supplemental micronutrients in particular:

(1) Pritikin felt that a good diet and regular exercise were enough to maintain good health without any need for supplemental anti-oxidants or vitamins. We have already discussed our contrary view on this point in the chapters contained in Part VI, "Stress: Another Good Reason for Anti-oxidants," and elsewhere. (2) While the Pritikin diet allows for only 5 to 10 percent of calories from fat, our Nutrition for Life diet provides 15 to 20 percent. We feel that going below this percentage of total fat in the diet is counterproductive, both medically and in terms of acceptability (compliance), nor is such a severely restricted diet necessary with the Demopoulos spectrum. Keeping these differences in mind, the reader will find all the Pritikin books a great source of inspiration and practical information, including many well-thought-out recipes.

Nutritive Value of Foods. Department 115-R, Consumer Information Center, Pueblo, CO 81009. $2.75.

The Mind-Body Connection

Benson, H. *The Mind-Body Effect.* New York: Simon & Schuster, 1979.

Benson, H., and M. Z. Klipper. *The Relaxation Response.* New York: Avon Books, 1976.

Benson, H., and W. Proctor. *Beyond the Relaxation Response.* New York: Berkley, 1985.

Borysenko, J. *Minding the Body, Mending the Mind.* New York: Bantam Books, 1988.

Chopra, D. *Creating Health.* Boston: Houghton Mifflin, 1987.

Cousins, N. *Anatomy of an Illness.* New York: W. W. Norton, 1979.

Gillespie, P, and L. Bechtel. *Less Stress in 30 Days.* New York: Plume Books, 1986.

Jampolsky, G. *Love Is Letting Go of Fear.* Berkeley, CA: Celestial Arts, 1979.

Jampolsky, G. *Teach Only Love: The Seven Principles of Attitudinal Healing.* New York: Bantam Books, 1983.

Locke, St., and D. Colligan. *The Healer Within: The New Medicine of Mind and Body.* New York: E. P. Dutton, 1986.

Matthews-Simonton, S., O. C. Simonton, and J. L. Creighton. *Getting Well Again.* New York: Bantam Books, 1978.

Pelletier, K. *Mind As Healer, Mind As Slayer.* New York: Dell Books, 1982.

Sagan, L. A. *The Health of Nations.* New York: Basic Books, 1988.

Siegel, B. *Love, Medicine and Miracles.* New York: Harper & Row, 1986.

Weil, A. *Health and Healing: Understanding Conventional and Alternative Medicine.* Boston: Houghton Mifflin, 1983.

Psychology and Philosophy

Aranya, S. H. *Yoga Philosophy of Patanjali.* Albany: State University of New York Press, 1963.

Bohm, D. *Wholeness and the Implicate Order.* Boston: Ark Paperbacks, 1980.

Krishnamurti, J. *Commentaries on Living Series I, II,* and *III. The Flight of the Eagle, You Are the World, The Ending of Time, Freedom from the Known, The First and Last Freedom, Krishnamurti's Journal,* and also *Notebook, The Future of Humanity* (dialogues between J. Krishnamurti and Professor David Bohm). An audiocassette—Krishnamurti and Dr. Jonas Salk, "Dialogue 1982."

The above-listed books by J. Krishnamurti are only a random selection from this great religious philosopher's published works. They are a fairly representative cross-section of his teachings. We recommend that all who are looking for a deeper meaning to life and a fuller understanding of human nature study *all* of Krishnamurti's works.

We have found that constantly rereading Krishnamurti's books over the years gives a different and more total view of what we thought we understood perfectly well the first time around.

J. Krishnamurti's books, audiocassettes and videocassettes are available from some major bookstores, or from The Krishnamurti Foundation, Box 216, Ojai, CA 93023. Phone: (805) 646-2726 or 646-5347.

Yogananda, P. *Autobiography of a Yogi.* Los Angeles: Self-Realization Fellowship, 1974.

Exercise and Yoga

There are so many good books on exercise and fitness that it would take several pages to list them. However, we found a small paperback very helpful to us:

Moorehouse, L. A., and L. Gross. *Total Fitness in 30 Minutes a Week.* New York: Pocket Books, 1975.

The title of this book is misleading; thirty minutes of total exercise a week is definitely not enough, but it does teach you how to gradually increase your heart rate. This book describes a number of basic and easily implemented exercises you can even do in cramped quarters (they were originally designed for use in submarines!).

There are also many excellent books on physical (hatha) yoga. It will be easy to find one that appeals to you and fits your particular circumstances. What you cannot find so easily are modified yoga instructions for children or older people. We would therefore like to call your attention to the following books:

Carr, R. *Be a Frog, a Bird or a Tree: Rachel Carr's Creative Yoga Exercises for Children.* New York: Doubleday, 1973.

Carr, R. *Yoga for All Ages.* New York: Simon & Schuster, 1972.

Fiction

Hesse, H. *Siddhartha.* New York: Bantam Books, 1983.

INDEX

Academic stress, 187–188
Acetaldehyde, 136, 515
    alcohol and, 506, 508
    in tobacco smoke, 475–476
Acetaldehydrogenase, 508
Acid rain, 583
Acid stomach, 289
Acne, 163
ACTH (adrenocorticotropic hormone), 185
Adrenaline, 52, 97, 184, 185
Adriamycin, 510
Adult-onset diabetes, *see* Diabetes mellitus
Aerobic dancing, 539, 540
Aerobics, 539–540
Age spots, 138, 139
Aging
    atherosclerosis and, 223–224
    beneficial micronutrients for, 23, 43, 71–
        72, 88, 116–117, 119, 120
    diverticulosis and, 279, 280
    free-radical effect on, 73–79, 570
    genetic improvements in, 572
    oxidized fats and, 314–315
AIDS, 53, 189–192
    high-colonic irrigation for, 278
    vitamin C for, 191
Air pollution, *see* Environmental pollution
Alcohol, 21, 34, 35, 44, 72, 494–522
    beer, 518, 521
    beneficial micronutrients for, 119, 120,
        124, 136
    cancer and, 51, 54, 195, 509
    cross-linking and, 475
    for the elderly, 517–518
    ethnic groups prone to effects of, 506–
        507

free-radical damage due to, 78
immune system and, 189, 190
peptic ulcer disease and, 269
politics of, 494–498
relaxation and, 516–517
selenium and, 156
sex and, 514
strokes and, 514–516
teenagers' use of, 582
U.S. cancer deaths/day due to, 51, 54
wine, 518–521
Alcohol-dehydrogenase (ADH), 508
Alcoholics, 87, 498–499
    Type 1, 500–502
    Type 2, 500, 501
Alcoholics Anonymous (A.A.), 497–498,
    503–504
Alfalfa sprouts, 344–345
Alginic acid in sea vegetables, 404
Allergies
    beneficial micronutrients for, 97, 102–103,
        132
    fish oil and, 454
    milk and, 330–331
All-Union Voluntary Temperance Society
    (TPS), 495
Almonds, 348
Alpha-2 adrenergic receptors, 554
American Cancer Society, 43
American Diabetes Association, 260
American Heart Association (AHA)
    dietary fat recommended by, 229, 317
    "prudent diet" of, 49
Ames, Dr. Bruce, 337, 338, 341*n*, 343,
    344, 345, 346, 354, 418, 428, 430,
    443*n*